Child and Adolescent Neurology for Psychiatrists

Editors
Audrey M. Walker, M.D.
Departments of Psychiatry and Pediatrics
Montefiore Medical Center
Bronx Children's Psychiatric Center
Associate Clinical Professor of Psychiatry
Assistant Clinical Professor of Pediatrics
Albert Einstein College of Medicine
Bronx, New York

David Myland Kaufman, M.D.
Departments of Neurology and Psychiatry
Montefiore Medical Center
Professor of Neurology and Psychiatry
Albert Einstein College of Medicine
Bronx, New York

Cynthia R. Pfeffer, M.D.
Department of Psychiatry
New York Presbyterian Hospital
Professor of Psychiatry
Weill Cornell Medical College
New York, New York

Gail Ellen Solomon, M.D.
Attending Pediatric Neurologist
Director of Electroencephalography Laboratory
New York Presbyterian Hospital/Weill Cornell Medical Center
Professor of Clinical Neurology and Professor of Clinical Neurology in Pediatrics and Psychiatry
Weill Cornell Medical College
New York, New York

Wolters Kluwer Health | Lippincott Williams & Wilkins
Philadelphia • Baltimore • New York • London
Buenos Aires • Hong Kong • Sydney • Tokyo

Acquisitions Editor: Charles W. Mitchell
Managing Editor: Sirkka E. Howes
Project Manager: Cindy Oberle
Manufacturing Manager: Benjamin Rivera
Marketing Manager: Kimberly Schonberger
Design Coordinator: Steve Druding
Production Services: Nesbitt Graphics, Inc.

© 2008 by LIPPINCOTT WILLIAMS & WILKINS, a Wolters Kluwer business

530 Walnut Street
Philadelphia, PA 19106 USA
LWW.com

All rights reserved. This book is protected by copyright. No part of this book may be reproduced in any form by any means, including photocopying, or utilized by any information storage and retrieval system without written permission from the copyright owner, except for brief quotations embodied in critical articles and reviews. Materials appearing in this book prepared by individuals as part of their official duties as U.S. government employees are not covered by the above-mentioned copyright.

Printed in the USA

Library of Congress Cataloging-in-Publication Data

Child and adolescent neurology for psychiatrists / [edited by] Audrey M. Walker ... [et al.].
   p. ; cm.
Includes bibliographical references and index.
ISBN-13: 978-0-7817-7191-7
ISBN-10: 0-7817-7191-9
   1. Child psychiatry. 2. Pediatric neurology. 3. Developmental neurobiology. 4. Nervous system--Diseases. I. Walker, Audrey M.
   [DNLM: 1. Nervous System Diseases--diagnosis. 2. Adolescent. 3. Child. 4. Diagnosis, Differential. 5. Diagnostic Techniques, Neurological. 6. Nervous System Diseases--psychology. 7. Neurologic Examination--methods. 8. Psychiatry--methods. WS 340 C5355 2008]
RJ499.C48225 2008
618.92'89--dc22
                     2008020769

   Care has been taken to confirm the accuracy of the information presented and to describe generally accepted practices. However, the authors, editors, and publisher are not responsible for errors or omissions or for any consequences from application of the information in this book and make no warranty, expressed or implied, with respect to the currency, completeness, or accuracy of the contents of the publication. Application of the information in a particular situation remains the professional responsibility of the practitioner.
   The authors, editors, and publisher have exerted every effort to ensure that drug selection and dosage set forth in this text are in accordance with current recommendations and practice at the time of publication. However, in view of ongoing research, changes in government regulations, and the constant flow of information relating to drug therapy and drug reactions, the reader is urged to check the package insert for each drug for any change in indications and dosage and for added warnings and precautions. This is particularly important when the recommended agent is a new or infrequently employed drug.
   Some drugs and medical devices presented in the publication have Food and Drug Administration (FDA) clearance for limited use in restricted research settings. It is the responsibility of the health care provider to ascertain the FDA status of each drug or device planned for use in their clinical practice.

To purchase additional copies of this book, call our customer service department at (800) 638-3030 or fax orders to (301) 223-2320. International customers should call (301) 223-2300.

Visit Lippincott Williams & Wilkins on the Internet: at LWW.com. Lippincott Williams & Wilkins customer service representatives are available from 8:30 am to 6 pm, EST.

This project would not have been possible without the inspiration, support, patience, and understanding of our families and mentors. Thank you to Robert Catenaccio, Caroline, Charlie, and Peter Walker Kaplan; Rita Kaufman and our children: Rachel, Bob, and Lila; Jennifer and William; and Sarah and Josh; Harvey Hecht, MD-husband; Samuel Solomon, MD-father; Sidney Carter, MD-mentor; and Ann C. Pfeffer, a loving mother whose nine-plus decades of wisdom, empathy, and intellect have enhanced her family.

Acknowledgments

We thank our LWW editors, Charles Mitchell and Sirkka Bertling, and Bonnie Boehme of Nesbitt Graphics, Inc., for their expertise and devotion to this project. We also thank the chapter authors for their tireless efforts to produce this ambitious and unique text.

We thank our chairmen, Drs. T. Byram Karasu and Mark Mahler, of Montefiore Medical Center/Albert Einstein College of Medicine; and Dr. Jack Barchas, of Weill Cornell Medical College/New York Presbyterian Hospital, for their visionary leadership and devotion to the interdisciplinary pursuit of knowledge in the fields of neurology and psychiatry. We also thank the Presidents and CEOs of Montefiore Medical Center and New York Presbyterian Hospital/Weil Cornell Medical Center—Drs. Spike Foreman, Steven Safyer, and Herb Pardes. They provided our professional homes, where we began, grew, and remain happy and successful.

Preface

The relationship between psychiatry and neurology remains complex, with twists and turns, approach and avoidance, interconnection, and divergence. At a time when neurology and psychiatry were not yet recognized as distinct medical specialties, Sigmund Freud's early work focused on neurological subjects, including aphasia and neuropathology. A psychiatrist, Hans Berger, was the principal inventor of the electroencephalogram (EEG) and coined the term "elektenkephalogram." Despite the fields' common ground, neurology and psychiatry split during the twentieth century: Neurologists claimed neuroanatomy as their province, and psychiatrists focused on pathological behavior and thinking. With the development of sophisticated diagnostic techniques and systematic empirical research to understand etiology, pathophysiology, and symptoms of brain functioning, greater overlap between neurology and psychiatry has diminished their distinctions. Psychiatrists realize the blurring of mind-brain dichotomies and neurologists appreciate the impact of emotional and environmental factors on disease manifestations.

This edition of *Child and Adolescent Neurology for Psychiatrists*, coming 16 years after the original, attempts to reconcile these sister disciplines. At the same time, this book elucidates the differences between diseases that affect adults and those that affect children. For neurologists and psychiatrists, children and adolescents are not diminutive adults. The afflictions of children and adolescents are often unique, with different manifestations than those encountered in adults, and requiring special treatment. The neurological disorders of childhood and adolescence deserve the combined, collaborative perspectives of these two distinct disciplines.

Child and Adolescent Neurology for Psychiatrists speaks to psychiatrists who treat children and adolescents. It reviews developments in the diagnosis and treatment of neurological illnesses that psychiatrists are likely to encounter in their clinical practice. Most chapters have been written collaboratively by teams of neurologists and psychiatrists who discuss the psychiatric comorbidity of neurological illnesses and the psychiatric ramifications of medications often prescribed by neurologists. As an extension of the customary topics in a neurology textbook, *Child and Adolescent Neurology for Psychiatrists* has included discussions of psychiatric aspects of congenital and acquired childhood visual and hearing impairments. Currently available imaging techniques and their appropriate applications are discussed and, acknowledging Berger's seminal invention, the role of EEG in the diagnosis of epilepsy is reviewed.

The book's chapters, written by multiple authors who are experts in their fields, are presented in an accessible format for the practicing psychiatrist. Most chapter text is supplemented with case discussions that illustrate the complexities of diagnosis and treatment. Chapters conclude with multiple-choice questions that allow for interactive learning.

In Remembrance of Paulina F. Kernberg, MD

Prior to her death, we discussed our concepts for this book with Dr. Paulina Kernberg, child and adolescent psychiatrist and psychoanalyst and Professor of Psychiatry and Director of Training of Child and Adolescent Psychiatry at the Westchester Division of New York Presbyterian Hospital-Weill Cornell Medical College. She enthusiastically remarked that "the collaboration and interspecialty communication between psychiatrists and neurologists is a must!" She emphasized that awareness of neurological problems is important in assessing what might appear to be psychiatric symptomatology. She remarked, "I remember my first paper, the problem of organicity; in those times, many years ago, language processing disturbances were erroneously diagnosed as schizophrenic disorder. As a child psychiatry resident, I felt like a magician when I noticed that a school-age child had responded correctly after a significant delay to the question of how long it took her parents and her to get from her home to the hospital. Approximately ten minutes later, she answered. So, I decided to slow down the speed of my language. Her speech and mood improved significantly in the two remaining diagnostic sessions—to the extent that all ideas of a formal thought disorder were ruled out."

Paulina noted, "The child psychiatrist can contribute uniquely to the child's awareness of his body and cognitive functions so that the child can accommodate, adapt, accept, and hopefully compensate for these deficits in an effective manner. The meaning of the illness for the patient and its impact on the siblings and parents are an additional input on the psychological dimension."

"My personal wish for the commendable work of the authors and editors is a successful, effective new book!"

We lament that Dr. Kernberg will not see the completed product of our work, a clearly written, informative, and concise reference on neurological problems often impacting children's psychosocial development.

Foreword

A textbook of clinical neurology for psychiatrists? The twenty-first century is indeed a brave new world for American psychiatry! Neuroscience at the dawn of the twenty-first century has revolutionized the field. Freud, who started his career as a clinician studying the neuropathology of infantile hemiplegia, would be pleased with this transformation, as he clearly believed that behavior belongs in the brain. Though a great divide still exists between our nascent understanding of the complexities of human behaviors and their neuroanatomic foundations, the coming decades hold great promise for breakthroughs in this important area of medicine.

The publication of *Child and Adolescent Neurology for Psychiatrists* signals the narrowing of the breach between psychiatry and neurology, which developed nearly a century ago. The book focuses on common neurological conditions that affect the immature brain and explores the psychiatric comorbidities that accompany them. It is enriched by cases that illustrate the fruitful collaboration that results from a joint neuropsychiatric approach to children whose presentations are at the border between psychiatry and neurology. It is hoped that this book will find a niche on the shelves of both psychiatrists and child neurologists, and bring greater sophistication to practitioners in both disciplines, ultimately for the benefit of the many children who enter our consulting rooms with vexing problems requiring mutual understanding and collaboration.

Isabelle Rapin, M.D.
Saul R. Korey Department of Neurology
Department of Pediatrics
Rose F. Kennedy Center for Research in Mental Retardation and Human Development
Albert Einstein College of Medicine
Bronx, New York

Contributors

Kenneth S. Allison, M.D.
Resident, Department of Radiology, Albert Einstein College of Medicine of Yeshiva University; Montefiore Medical Center, Bronx, New York

Karen R. Ballaban-Gil, M.D.
Professor of Clinical Neurology and Clinical Pediatrics, Albert Einstein College of Medicine; Director, Child Neurology Residency Program, Montefiore Medical Center, Bronx, New York

Jacqueline A. Bello, M.D., FACR
Professor of Clinical Radiology, Albert Einstein College of Medicine of Yeshiva University; Director, Division of Neuroradiology, Montefiore Medical Center, Bronx, New York

Lucy Ann Civitello, M.D.
Assistant Professor of Neurology, George Washington University; Attending Neurologist, Children's National Medical Center, Washington, District of Columbia

Lee Cohen, M.D.
Assistant Clinical Professor of Psychiatry, Columbia University College of Physicians and Surgeons; Attending Psychiatrist, New York Presbyterian Hospital/Columbia, St. Lukes–Roosevelt Hospital Center, Roosevelt Division, New York, New York

Michael E. Cohen, M.D.
Professor of Neurology and Pediatrics, State University of NY at Buffalo; Neurologist, Women and Children's Hospital of Buffalo, Buffalo, New York

Kelly A. Condefer, M.D.
Fellow, Department of Neurology, Beth Israel Medical Center, New York, New York

Martha Bridge Denckla, M.D.
Professor of Neurology, Pediatrics and Psychiatry, Johns Hopkins University School of Medicine; Director, Developmental Cognitive Neurology, Kennedy Krieger Institute, Baltimore, Maryland

Aleksandra Djukic, M.D., Ph.D.
Assistant Professor of Neurology and Pediatrics, Albert Einstein College of Medicine; Attending Physician, Neurology, Montefiore Medical Center, Bronx, New York

Patricia K. Duffner, M.D.
Professor of Neurology and Pediatrics, University at Buffalo School of Medicine; Attending in Child Neurology, Women and Children's Hospital of Buffalo, Buffalo, New York

David W. Dunn, M.D.
Professor of Psychiatry and Neurology, Indiana University School of Medicine; Director, Child and Adolescent Psychiatry Clinics, Riley Hospital for Children, Indianapolis, Indiana

Josephine Elia, M.D.
Assistant Professor of Psychiatry, University of Pennsylvania; Medical Co-director, ADHD Center, Child and Adolescent Psychiatry, The Children's Hospital of Philadelphia, Philadelphia, Pennsylvania

Howard L. Geyer, M.D., Ph.D.
Assistant Professor of Neurology, Albert Einstein College of Medicine; Attending Neurologist, Montefiore Medical Center, Bronx, New York

Rick O. Gilmore, Ph.D.
Associate Professor of Psychology, Pennsylvania State University, University Park, Pennsylvania

Elisabeth Guthrie, M.D.
Associate Clinical Professor of Psychiatry and Pediatrics, Columbia University; Director, Residency Training, Child and Adolescent Psychiatry, New York Presbyterian Hospital, New York, New York

Rana S. Jehle, PA-C.
Pediatric Physician Assistant, Department of Neurology, Montefiore Medical Center, Bronx, New York

David L. Kaye, M.D.
Professor of Clinical Psychiatry, University at Buffalo School of Medicine and Biomedical Sciences; Chief, Clinical Services, Division of Child/Adolescent Psychiatry, Women and Children's Hospital of Buffalo, Buffalo, New York

Robert A. King, M.D.
Professor of Child Psychiatry, Medical Director, Tourette's Syndrome/OCD Clinic, Yale Child Study Center, Yale University School of Medicine; Attending Physician, Yale–New Haven Hospital, New Haven, Connecticut

Lauren B. Krupp, M.D.
Professor of Neurology, SUNY Stony Brook; Director, National Pediatric MS Center; Co-Director, MS Comprehensive Care Center, Stony Brook University Hospital and Medical Center, Stony Brook, New York

Thornton B.A. Mason II, M.D., Ph.D.
Assistant Professor of Neurology and Pediatrics, University of Pennsylvania; Attending Neurologist, The Children's Hospital of Philadelphia, Philadelphia, Pennsylvania

Patricia Engel McGoldrick, N.P.
Adjunct Faculty in Nursing, New York University and Columbia University; Associate Director, DDC; Nurse Practitioner in Neurology, Beth Israel Pediatrics and St. Luke's Roosevelt, New York, New York

Todd S. Miller, M.D.
Assistant Professor of Clinical Radiology, Albert Einstein College of Medicine of Yeshiva University; Department of Radiology, Montefiore Medical Center, Bronx, New York

Stewart H. Mostofsky, M.D.
Associate Professor of Neurology and Psychiatry, Johns Hopkins University School of Medicine; Medical Director, Center for Autism and Related Disorders, Kennedy Krieger Institute, Baltimore, Maryland

Ngoc Nguyen, M.D.
Fellow, Child and Adolescent Psychiatry, Albert Einstein College of Medicine; Pediatric Psychosomatic Fellow, Child and Adolescent Psychiatry, Montefiore Medical Center, Bronx, New York

Wendy Osterling, M.D.
Pediatric Neurology Fellow, Department of Pediatrics, University of Utah, Salt Lake City, Utah

Maryland Pao, M.D.
Deputy Clinical Director, Office of the Clinical Director NIMH, National Institutes of Health, Bethesda, Maryland

John M. Pellock, M.D.
Professor and Chair, Division of Child Neurology, Vice Chair, Department of Neurology, Virginia Commonwealth University; Chief, Child Neurology, Medical College of Virginia Hospital, VCU Health System, Richmond, Virginia

Maris D. Rosenberg, M.D.
Associate Professor of Clinical Pediatrics, Albert Einstein College of Medicine; Developmental-Behavioral Pediatrician, Children's Evaluation and Rehabilitation Center, Rose F. Kennedy UCEDD, Bronx, New York

A. David Rothner, M.D.
Director Emeritus, Section of Child Neurology; Director, Children's Headache, Child Neurology Program; Staff, Section of Child Neurology, The Cleveland Clinic Foundation, Cleveland, Ohio

Rachel Saunders-Pullman, M.D., M.P.H.
Assistant Professor of Neurology, Albert Einstein College of Medicine, Bronx, New York; Attending Neurologist, Beth Israel Medical Center, New York, New York

Naalla D. Schreiber, M.D.
Assistant Professor of Psychiatry and Behavioral Sciences, Albert Einstein College of Medicine; Attending Psychiatrist, Montefiore Medical Center, Bronx, New York

Daniel J. Simmonds
Graduate Student, MD/PhD program, University of Pittsburgh, Pittsburgh, Pennsylvania

Tamar Steinberg, M.D.
Tutor, Department of Pediatrics, Tel-Aviv University, Tel Aviv, Israel; Senior Pediatric Neurologist, Schneider Children's Medical Center of Israel, Petah-Tikva, Israel

Susan Vig, Ph.D.
Professor of Clinical Pediatrics, Albert Einstein College of Medicine; Psychologist, Children's Evaluation and Rehabilitation Center, Rose F. Kennedy UCEDD, Bronx, New York

Rebecca J. Von Der Heide, M.A.
Department of Psychology, Pennsylvania State University, University Park, Pennsylvania

Joel M. Weinstein, M.D.
Associate Professor of Ophthalmology and Pediatrics, Pennsylvania State University, Hershey Medical Center, Hershey, Pennsylvania

Steven M. Wolf, M.D.
Associate Professor of Neurology and Pediatrics, Albert Einstein College of Medicine, Bronx, New York; Director, Pediatric Epilepsy, Beth Israel, Neurology; Director, Pediatric Neurology, St. Luke's-Roosevelt-Neurology, New York, New York

Kaleb H. Yohay, M.D.
Assistant Professor of Pediatrics, Division of Child Neurology, Weill Medical College, Cornell University; Assistant Attending, Pediatrics, Division of Child Neurology, New York Presbyterian Hospital, New York, New York

Contents

Acknowledgments iv
Preface v
Foreword vii
Contributors ix

1 Pediatric Neurological Examination for the Psychiatrist 1
STEVEN M. WOLF, PATRICIA ENGEL MCGOLDRICK, AND LEE COHEN

2 Neuroradiological Imaging in Children 13
KEN ALLISON, TODD MILLER, AND JACQUELINE BELLO

3 Movement Disorders in Children and Adolescents 47
KELLY CONDEFER AND RACHEL SAUNDERS-PULLMAN

4 Tourette Syndrome and Tic Disorders in Children and Adolescents 77
ROBERT A. KING AND TAMAR STEINBERG

5 Epilepsy 103
JOHN M. PELLOCK

6 Developmental Characteristics of Sleep and Sleep Disorders in Children . . 123
JOSEPHINE ELIA AND THORNTON B.A. MASON II

7 Headaches in Children and Adolescents 151
A. DAVID ROTHNER AND DAVID W. DUNN

8 Pediatric Brain Tumors 171
DAVID L. KAYE, PATRICIA K. DUFFNER, AND MICHAEL E. COHEN

9 Functional Neuroimaging in Pediatric Populations 189
DANIEL J. SIMMONDS AND STEWART H. MOSTOFSKY

10 Neurofibromatosis Type 1 and Tuberous Sclerosis Complex 205
KALEB H. YOHAY AND MARTHA B. DENCKLA

11 Static Encephalopathies and Common CNS Anomalies 225
ELISABETH GUTHRIE

12 Intellectual Disability/Mental Retardation 243
MARIS D. ROSENBERG AND SUSAN VIG

13 Neurobehavioral Aspects of Traumatic Brain Injury in Children 265
ALEKSANDRA DJUKIC

14 Neuropsychiatric Aspects of Pediatric HIV Infection 281
MARYLAND PAO AND LUCY ANN CIVITELLO

15 Pediatric Multiple Sclerosis 309
LAUREN B. KRUPP

16 The Development and Neuropsychology of Visual Impairment 323
RICK O. GILMORE, JOEL M. WEINSTEIN, AND REBECCA VON DER HEIDE

17 Challenges of Congenital Hearing Loss 349
WENDY OSTERLING

18 Neuromuscular Disorders 367
HOWARD L. GEYER AND NAALLA D. SCHREIBER

19 The Diagnostic Approach to
Neuropsychiatric Presentations 393
AUDREY M. WALKER, KAREN BALLABAN-GIL, NGOC NGUYEN, AND RANA JEHLE

Glossary 411

Index 423

CHAPTER 1

Pediatric Neurological Examination for the Psychiatrist

STEVEN M. WOLF, PATRICIA ENGEL MCGOLDRICK, AND LEE COHEN

This chapter should assist psychiatrists in detecting medical or neurological disorders that may masquerade as psychiatric ones. Among the children who present for psychiatric evaluation, some inevitably have symptoms or signs that may indicate an underlying neurological problem. Psychiatrists should be familiar enough with the neurological evaluation—whether they or a consultant neurologist performs it—to identify abnormal findings and to order appropriate testing.

The Neurological Examination

The neurological examination traditionally begins with assessment of the chief complaint, including changes in cognition, emotions, or behavior; slowing of development in a previously normal child; and loss of previously acquired milestones in growth and development. Physicians usually elicit the patient's medical history, including hospitalizations (medical and psychiatric), age at onset of the presenting symptoms, surgeries, illnesses, past and current medications, learning disabilities, and social history. In evaluating children, especially those who are developmentally delayed, the physician's pertinent questions include a full birth history with specific questions regarding whether (a) the child was full term (and if not, how premature); (b) the pregnancy was complicated by drug or alcohol abuse, illnesses, or trauma; (c) the infant experienced neonatal seizures, respiratory arrest, or hypoxic ischemic events; (d) any diagnosis was made of a neonatal stroke or intraventricular hemorrhage; or (e) the postnatal period was complicated by infections, seizures, trauma, or other potential insult. The physician should gather the results of prior neurological tests, such as ultrasound of the head, magnetic resonance imaging (MRI) of the brain and spine, and determinations of blood levels of amino acids and organic acids. The physician usually also inquires about a family history of epilepsy, psychiatric diagnoses, regression, mental retardation, consanguinity, and neurodegenerative disorders. The physician should also be particularly concerned about siblings with similar or other illnesses.

Pediatric neurologists usually begin the physical portion of the examination by noting the child's physical development (height, weight, and head size), appearance, and exposed skin surface. Then the physician assesses the child's behavior, thought processes, and thought content. As part of the mental status examination, physicians assess the child's affect, ability to respond to commands, and response to questions. Depending on the problem at hand, the physician may inquire about mood, visual or auditory hallucinations, illusions, delusions, and suicidality. The physician generally tests the child's higher functions, such as attention; short- and long-term memory; calculations; abstract thought; spatial, visual, and body perception; and praxis (ability to perform complex movements).

The physical portion of the examination begins with observation of the shape and size of the child's head, with attention to symmetry. For children younger than 2 years, examiners should measure and graph the circumference of the child's head on a normative graph. The head should be palpated for areas of tenderness and skeletal defect, and in young children, sutures and fontanelles should be assessed by palpation. The anterior fontanel closes usually at 12 to 18 months of age, whereas the posterior fontanel closes earlier, before 6 months of age. The ridges of the sutures (coronal, lambdoidal, metopic, and sagittal) should not be palpable. The examiner should also note asymmetry of the head. Flattening of the back of the head (found in infants and young children who spend much time lying on their backs) indicates *plagiocephaly*. If the head shape is more indicative of a parallelogram, the examiner should be concerned about craniosynostosis (premature closure of one or more of the sutures). Although plagiocephaly is usually managed by keeping the child off his or her back, the suspicion of craniosynostosis requires assessment with a three-dimensional computed tomography (CT) scan and immediate referral to a neurologist and neurosurgeon.

The examination then progresses to testing the cranial nerves (CNs) (Table 1.1), which are evaluated in the following manner: Inquire about a loss of the sense of smell, which usually suffices to evaluate CN I without formal testing. Looking at the level of the eyes, search for asymmetry of the eyelids, ptosis, and note whether the eyes are sunken (enophthalmic) or protruding (exophthalmic). Assess the pupils' symmetry, alignment, and response to light and accommodation. Observe the child's face for symmetry, lesions, and abnormal movements. Always test hearing by determining responses to spoken and whispered speech. Check lower CN function by asking the child to protrude and move the tongue, and observe palate movement.

Musculoskeletal Examination

Examination of the musculoskeletal system often gives important clues to neurological system abnormalities. Strength is tested in the upper extremities by having the child squeeze the examiner's hands. The child should then be asked to flex the arms and provide resistance as the examiner tries to pull the arms down and forward. To test the complementary muscles, the examiner asks the child to flex his or her arm muscles and push the examiner away.

In addition, the examiner, taking the child's hand as if to shake it, should pronate and supinate the forearm, and then roll the hand at the wrist. The examiner should check the arms for wasting and fasciculations and ask the child to extend his or her arms to check for involuntary movements (pronator test).

To test the lower extremities, the child should be seated with legs dangling and asked to raise the legs, with knees bent at a 90-degree angle, against resistance from the examiner's hand. Strength in both legs should be equal. The child should then be asked to kick against the examiner's hand. In this test, the examiner should separately test each leg. Again, strength should be equal. With the child relaxed, the examiner should check for hypertonicity or hypotonicity and for spasticity. In addition, the child should lie with legs

TABLE 1.1 EXAMINATION OF CRANIAL NERVES

Cranial Nerve	Function	Testing
I Olfactory	Sense of smell	Identify fruit, peppermint, ammonia (test each nostril separately).
II Optic	Vision, afferent arc of light reflex	Perform funduscopy (observe the disc's color, disc margins, optic cup, blood vessels). Evaluate visual fields. Determine visual acuity (use Snellen chart or available reading material).
III Oculomotor	Eye movements, pupillary response, efferent arc of pupillary reflex	Check vertical and horizontal movements, and then accommodation.
IV Trochlear	Inward-torsion eye movement	Test with CN III.
V Trigeminal	Sensory: ophthalmic (V_1), maxillary (V_2), and mandibular (V_3) sensation Motor: muscles of mastication	Determine jaw-muscle strength. Check facial sensation and corneal reflex. Look for wasting of temporalis muscles.
VI Abducens	Lateral eye movement	Test with CN III.
VII Facial	Muscles of facial expression; stapedius; taste; tearing	Observe nasolabial folds, and determine strength of opening and closing eyelids.
VIII Acoustic	Hearing	Using tuning fork, perform Rinné and Weber tests.
IX Glossopharyngeal	Taste, salivary response	Check taste, salivation.
X Vagus	Sensory: tympanic membrane, external auditory canal and external ear Motor: muscles of palate, pharynx, larynx Autonomic: carotid innervation	Check gag reflex and palate elevation.
XI Accessory	Sternocleidomastoid and trapezius muscles	Observe neck-muscle strength by turning head side to side and shrugging shoulders against force.
XII Hypoglossal	Tongue muscles	Determine tongue movements, bulk, and deviation.

CN, cranial nerve.

straight, and the examiner should roll the knee from side to side, and then rapidly flex and extend the lower leg at the knee. Similarly, holding the foot and lower leg, the examiner should flex and extend (plantar flex and dorsiflex) the child's foot. Normal tone is defined by slight resistance occurring through the whole range of movements; increased tone, by marked resistance; and decreased tone, by no resistance.

Examination of Reflexes

Deep tendon reflexes (DTRs) commonly tested in the office include those listed in Table 1.2

Examination of Gait

Of all the clinical assessments of the physical portion of the nervous system, none is more valuable than observing the child's gait. As the child walks into the examination room, the physician has the first opportunity to look for any indication of a neurological disorder.

TABLE 1.2 COMMONLY TESTED DEEP TENDON REFLEXES

Reflex	Innervation	How to test
Biceps	C5	The examiner should flex the child's arm at the elbow, swing the reflex hammer onto the child's biceps tendon, and watch the biceps muscle contract.
Triceps	C7	The examiner should draw the child's arm across the chest and, with the elbow at 90 degrees, strike the triceps tendon with reflex hammer, and watch the triceps muscle contract.
Brachioradialis	C6	The examiner should flex the child's arm onto the abdomen. Placing the finger on the radial tuberosity, the examiner should hit the finger with the reflex hammer and watch the brachioradialis muscle contract.
Patellar	L3L4	With the child's legs dangling, the examiner should strike the knee below the patella and watch the quadriceps muscle contract.
Achilles	S1	The examiner should hold the child's foot at 90 degrees, strike the Achilles tendon, and watch the calf muscle contract.
Babinski		Draw a sharp edge from the heel up and below the toes on the sole of the foot. The abnormal response, the Babinski sign, consists of extension of the big toe with fanning of the other toes. However, this is a normal response in infants, usually disappearing by age 2 years.

C, cervical; L, lumbar; S, sacral.

Because a normal gait depends on intact and delicately balanced motor, sensory, and coordination systems, a normally walking child probably has little or no impairment in the physical portions of the nervous system. Physicians should observe the child's gait for symmetry, size of paces, posture, arm swing, and smoothness of movements. *Tandem gait* should be assessed by having the child walk heel-to-toe, as if walking a tightrope. The examiner should also ask the child to walk on his or her heels and then toes. Having the child stand upright with arms outstretched, eyes closed (Romberg testing), will assess joint-position sense. The examiner can then gently push the child to see if he or she can maintain balance. If the child does not, a Romberg sign is said to occur. Table 1.3 lists common gait abnormalities.

TABLE 1.3 COMMON ABNORMALITIES OF GAIT

Description of Gait	Possible Diagnosis
Small paces, stooped posture, and reduced arm swing, with difficulty starting and stopping	Basal ganglia dysfunction, as seen in childhood Parkinson, Wilson, and juvenile Huntington diseases
Scissoring gait: adducted, straight legs	Spastic paraparesis, as in cerebral palsy, MS, spinal cord compression
Waddling gait	Weak proximal hip-girdle muscles, as in muscular dystrophy and other myopathies, and congenital hip dislocation
Bizarre, elaborate, inconsistent (including astasia–abasia)	Psychogenic disturbances
Ataxia: broad-based, lurching	Cerebellar dysfunction, as in drug or alcohol intoxication, MS, hereditary ataxias, posterior fossa tumor
Sensory ataxia with positive Romberg sign	Loss of joint-position sense, as in peripheral neuropathy or posterior column impairment; cerebellar disease
Hemiplegic gait: one leg swings out straight to side (circumduction)	Unilateral upper motor neuron disease, as in cerebral palsy, stroke, MS, or traumatic brain injury
Foot drop	Weakness on ankle dorsiflexor muscles, as in common peroneal palsy, L5 radiculopathy, peripheral neuropathy

MS, multiple sclerosis.

Abnormalities of Skin

Examiners look at children's skin for diagnostic clues. For example, petechiae may be indicative of a blood dyscrasia; striae may suggest Cushing disease or use of steroids; and "birthmarks" may indicate the presence of a neurocutaneous disorder. Because embryological ectoderm gives rise to both the central nervous system and the skin, many conditions—*neurocutaneous disorders*—consist of a cutaneous abnormality with an underlying neurological component. The examiner should undress the child and observe the skin for lesions that may indicate a neurocutaneous disorder. Physicians should note the distribution, size, and color of any lesion, and determine whether a change in its appearance has occurred (Table 1.4). They should always be on alert for signs of the above.

Helpful Clues on Examination

Although the examiner may use these physical findings to formulate a differential diagnosis and to order tests, the potential severity of an illness and the likelihood of its presence will determine whether further evaluation should be performed on an emergency basis.

Symptoms and examination findings that require immediate evaluation are the following:

- Severe headaches—worst of the patient's life, awakening from sleep, accompanied by vomiting, occurring in the early morning
- Inability to walk
- Unresponsiveness
- CN findings (abnormalities on examination)
- Apathy, depression of new onset, especially coupled with decline in performance

Symptoms that require neurological evaluation, but not as an emergency, include these:

- Abnormal gait (speak to a pediatric neurologist regarding whether to order radiographs of the spine or an MRI scan of the lumbosacral spine if a sacral dimple or hair tuft is found)
- Precocious puberty (order an MRI scan of the brain to rule out pituitary abnormalities)
- New onset of incontinence (discuss symptoms with a neurologist, especially regarding whether an imaging study and other referrals are needed)
- Back pain (MRI of the painful area usually can be performed while awaiting referral)

TABLE 1.4 LESIONS

Diagnosis	Type of Lesion	Color	Appearance	Distribution
Neurofibromatosis	Café-au-lait spots Lisch nodules Neurofibromas	Light-pigmentation masses	Flat	Axillary and groin freckling, Lisch nodules in iris, neurofibromas, and café-au-lait spots anywhere on the body
Tuberous sclerosis	Shagreen patch	Hypopigmented	Rough, irregular	Usually back, but can be anywhere
	Adenoma sebaceum	Brown	Raised	Malar region
Sturge–Weber syndrome	Vascular facial birth marks	Port-wine stain and facial capillary angiomas	Flat	Trigeminal distribution

- Weakness of one or more extremities [new onset requires referral; longstanding weakness without any previous testing may require MRI of the brain or spinal cord or electromyography (EMG)]
- Regression, including worsening of a previously diagnosed learning disability or attention deficit disorder [order an MRI scan of the brain; electroencephalogram (EEG); and metabolic workup, including urine for organic acids and toxicology, as well as blood for lactate, pyruvate, ammonia, and organic acids]
- Sudden change in vision (including loss of central or peripheral vision, onset of nystagmus, development of CN abnormalities) (order an MRI scan of the brain and orbits, and solicit an ophthalmology consultation)
- Change in gait (possibly consult with orthopedist)
- Change in level of consciousness (usually refer to the emergency room)
- Episodic events (for repeated, transient changes in the level of consciousness, delusion, hallucinations, or illusions, because they represent seizure activity, order an MRI scan of the brain and EEG)
- Headaches [if headaches occur more frequently than three times per week, without an obvious cause, such as lack of sleep or inadequate oral intake, consider an MRI scan of the brain and blood tests.

Psychiatric Comorbidities of Selected Neurological Disorders

Many neurological diseases, particularly epilepsy and migraine, have a high incidence of psychiatric comorbidities. Children with certain neurological disorders, such as autism, mental retardation, and cerebral palsy, carry a high incidence of behavioral problems usually treated by psychiatrists.

EPILEPSY

Persons with epilepsy have been found to have a higher incidence of psychiatric comorbidities than are found with any other chronic disease. Approximately 20% to 50% of epilepsy patients display clinical symptoms of depression. They also have high rates of attentional impairments, learning disabilities, sleep disorders, and oppositional defiant disorder. Children with epilepsy have higher rates of other diseases that also reflect unequivocal cerebral pathology, such as mental retardation, cerebral palsy, and autism. These problems lead to poor social outcomes.

Adults with epilepsy have increased incidences of the following:

- Unplanned pregnancies
- Heavy drinking
- Social isolation
- Psychiatric symptoms
- Economic dependency
- Lower educational levels
- Unemployment
- Lower marriage rate
- Higher rates of suicide, especially soon after a new diagnosis of epilepsy

MIGRAINES

Migraine patients have an increased incidence of depression, anxiety disorders, mania, and panic attacks. One long-term study found that, in children whose headaches were severe enough to cause functional impairment, 24% also met the criteria for depression within 7 years. A correlation also exists between problems in family relationships and incidence of headaches.

CEREBRAL PALSY

Cerebral palsy is a nonspecific term applied to central nervous system dysfunction resulting in abnormal motor function with changes in muscle tone. No clear predominance of psychiatric diagnoses is found in this population. The cognitively normal child with cerebral palsy has the same risk of a DSM-IV diagnosis as the average child. However, a higher incidence of learning disabilities is found, and about two thirds (40%) of patients will have some degree of mental retardation. Patients with cerebral palsy also have a high incidence of epilepsy, which adds to their risk of comorbid psychiatric issues.

Conclusion

Psychiatrists should readily consider the possibility of neurological comorbidity in their patients. Similarly, they should consider psychiatric comorbidity in patients with common neurological disorders, such as epilepsy, migraine, and cerebral palsy. They should also keep in mind that, in a young child, many psychiatric symptoms may actually represent underlying neurological illnesses that have not yet emerged. Consultations between pediatric neurologists and child psychiatrists may shed new light on the evaluation or treatment of each patient.

Case One

A 16-year-old boy presented with a gradual onset of behavioral problems, beginning with avoidance of engagement in social activities and progressing over several months to the point of frank paranoia, resulting in a psychiatric hospitalization. On initial examination after his hospital discharge, the adolescent boy was also noted to have dysarthric speech. The parents stated that this had begun in elementary school and had become slightly worse over the years, despite speech therapy. During the same time, they had also noted worsening gait (small steps, stooped posture) but had attributed it to his avoidance of exercise and his mild hypotonia. The examining psychiatrist noted rigidity, tremor, and slight drooling. The parents had attributed the drooling and the tremor to the antipsychotic medications that had been started recently.

Tests ordered included blood for copper and ceruloplasmin, 24-hour urine for copper, and an MRI scan of the brain. An ophthalmology consultation was requested.

Test results led to a diagnosis of Wilson disease (hepatolenticular degeneration). Wilson disease is transmitted by autosomal recessive inheritance. The defective gene is chromosome 13q14–q21. The abnormal gene product is the main copper transporter moving copper from the hepatocyte into the bile. Copper accumulates in the brain, liver, and cornea, causing tissue damage.

The disease is initially seen with hepatic, neurological, or psychiatric disturbances. Age at onset ranges from 3 to 50 years old. When onset occurs before 10 years of age, the most prominent feature is the hepatic manifestation. Neurological manifestations with minimal symptoms of liver disease are more common when onset is in the second decade of life, and psychiatric symptoms precede neurological abnormalities in 20% of cases. Symptoms include disturbance of speech and gait (often the initial feature, and it may remain unchanged for years), dystonia of bulbar muscles (dysarthria, pseudosmile, and a high-pitched whining noise on inspiration), and the presence of a Kayser–Fleischer ring (a yellow–brown granular deposit on the cornea. Diagnosis is made by liver biopsy or by the presence of the Kayser–Fleischer ring on slit-lamp examination. Of patients, 96% have a serum ceruloplasmin concentration of less than 20 mg per deciliter. Treatment is with copper-chelating agents that increase urinary excretion of copper. Siblings of patients with Wilson disease should be screened and treated early.

Case Two

A 5-year-old boy presented to a psychiatrist with parental concerns regarding his worsening academic problems and attentional issues. They were interested in trying medication to address the inattention. However, the psychiatrist immediately noted the boy's abnormal gait. On questioning, the parents stated that the child had always had "soft neuro signs," including low muscle tone, toe walking, and a speech delay. He was reluctant to engage in sports, and they thought that his gait had subtly worsened over the years because of his lack of exercise. The examiner noted a waddling gait and inability of the child to rise from a seated position on the floor without pulling himself up on a chair (positive Gower sign). He also had enlarged calf muscles, shortened ankle tendons, and 1+ (reduced) DTRs at the ankle and knee. Parents also noted that the child fell frequently.

The boy's blood was evaluated for creatinine kinase (CK), which was found to be elevated to 10 times the normal value. A genetics referral also was made, and chromosomal analysis resulted in a diagnosis of Duchenne muscular dystrophy (DMD).

Duchenne muscular dystrophy and Becker muscular dystrophy (BMD) are variable phenotypic expressions of a gene defect at the Xp21 site. The abnormal gene product is a reduced muscle content of the structural protein dystrophin. In DMD, the dystrophin content is less than 3% of normal, whereas in BMD, it is 3% to 20% of normal. The incidence of DMD is 1 per 3,500 males. BMD has a later onset. DMD presents initially with gait disturbance, always before the age of 5 and often before age 3 years. Toe walking and frequent falling, large calf muscles, short ankle tendons, and diminished tendon reflexes are often the first signs observed. Motor strength declines throughout childhood, and functional ability deteriorates rapidly. Most children require use of a wheelchair by age 12. Death occurs because of respiratory insufficiency and cardiomyopathy, as well as respiratory infections. DMD is treated with prednisone to increase strength and function.

Questions

1. A 3-year-old girl has a head circumference of 40 cm. Since birth, she has severely lagged in reaching developmental milestones. Of the following, which is the most likely diagnosis?
   A. aqueductal stenosis
   B. storage disease
   C. familial trait
   D. congenital rubella

2. A 2-year-old boy has a clumsy gait but appropriate cognitive and language development. He reaches for objects exclusively with his left hand and kicks a ball only with his left foot. He has right-sided hyperactive DTRs and a Babinski sign. Which of the following statements gives the most likely prognosis?
   A. Because his left hemisphere is damaged, aphasia will develop.
   B. Mental retardation will develop.
   C. As he matures, his right arm and leg will become foreshortened, and he will require tendon lengthening or other surgical procedures.
   D. He is at risk for primary seizures.

3. An 18-month-old girl is able to walk, manipulate objects, scribble, and interact normally with her parents and older siblings. Although she has garbled speech, she seems to understand her family members' wishes and requests. Which evaluation should be performed?
   A. hearing tests
   B. intelligence tests
   C. MRI
   D. autism evaluation

4. Which of the following conditions cannot be diagnosed by the physical examination?
   A. neurofibromatosis type 1
   B. Rett syndrome
   C. trisomy 21
   D. tuberous sclerosis
   E. Sturge–Weber syndrome
   F. Epilepsy

5. Match the gait (A–D) with the underlying cause (1–5):
   A. small-paced with stooped posture and reduced arm swing
   B. adducted, straight legs with scissoring
   C. waddling
   D. broad-based, lurching

   1. cerebellar dysfunction, as in spinocerebellar ataxia
   2. basal ganglia dysfunction, as in Parkinson, Wilson, and Huntington diseases
   3. muscular dystrophies, such as Duchenne muscular dystrophy
   4. spasticity, as in cerebral palsy, spinal cord damage, and multiple sclerosis
   5. psychogenic disturbance

6. Match the cutaneous disorder (A–D) with the associated neuropathological abnormality (1–5):
   A. café-au-lait spots
   B. adenoma sebaceum
   C. shagreen patches
   D. hemifacial hemangioma

   1. cortical tubers
   2. neurofibromas
   3. cortical hemangiomas
   4. cerebellar hemangiomas

7. Which set of physical findings is most closely aligned with cognitive impairment in a young child?
   A. from birth, right elbow and wrist flexion with muscle weakness and absent biceps, triceps, and brachioradialis DTRs
   B. since an infectious illness at age 12 months, flaccid, areflexic paresis of the right arm and left leg
   C. stable athetosis of all limbs since infancy
   D. since birth, seizures refractory to two antiepileptic drugs and spastic quadriparesis

8. Which of the following terms pertains to premature closure of one of a neonate's sutures—coronal, lambdoidal, metopic, or sagittal?
   A. craniosynostosis
   B. plagiocephaly
   C. microcephaly
   D. macrocephaly

9. A mother brings her 4-year-old boy for a psychiatric consultation because of a change in his personality and behavior. Previously he had been inattentive and hyperactive, for which he had required stimulant treatment. During the 3 to 6 weeks before the visit, he has become morose, inattentive, and noncommunicative. He denied physical symptoms to his mother. When entering the psychiatrist's office, the boy limps and, when sitting, he holds his head. On a neurological examination, he has normal head circumference, cranial nerves, motor strength, DTRs, and coordination. Movement around the left hip and right shoulder is limited by pain, and those joints are tender. He has ecchymosis over his left mastoid bone. Routine blood tests, a head CT scan, and an EEG show no abnormalities. Of the following, which is the most likely diagnosis?
   A. a systemic, inflammatory illness
   B. conversion disorder
   C. nonaccidental head injury
   D. withdrawal of stimulant medication

10. The school social worker refers a 6-year-old boy who, on most afternoons, has begun to act strangely. The social worker reported that over the previous month, the boy has started to mimic different physical disabilities, particularly the inability to walk, which caused him to miss his afternoon classes. Although the boy has never been a diligent or well-behaved pupil, he has shown normal intelligence, language, and learning skills, and he has had no physical impairments. More striking, he has had no problems in the morning classes. On neurological examination the next morning after the referral, he is found to have normal strength, reflexes, and gait. However, that afternoon, he has rigidity in his legs and abnormal posturing in all of his limbs, causing an abnormal gait and clumsy movements. His foster parents report that during the past 3 weeks, he has hobbled home from school and gone straight to bed. In the morning, he dresses, bathes, and runs to the school bus. Of the following, which is the most likely diagnosis?
    A. conversion disorder
    B. oppositional behavior
    C. cerebral palsy
    D. dopamine-responsive dystonia

11. While in psychotherapy, a 17-year-old girl describes recently developing afternoon and early evening weakness and intermittent diplopia. She reports that she even has difficulty speaking and chewing food at family dinners but not breakfasts. She has taken a variety of medications, including selective serotonin reuptake inhibitors, serotonin–norepinephrine reuptake inhibitors, stimulants, and antiepileptic drugs; however, she denies that she is currently taking any one of them or drugs of abuse. A neurological examination in the afternoon showed left ptosis, right lateral rectus muscle paresis, dysarthria, and a wan, expressionless face. Of the following, which is the most likely explanation?
    A. drug abuse
    B. anorexia
    C. a neuromuscular junction disorder
    D. dopamine-responsive dystonia

Answers

1. **D.** The head circumference of a 3-month-old infant is 40 cm, and that of a 3-year-old infant is 50 cm. This child has microcephaly

as well as retardation. "Primary causes" of microcephaly include genetic disorders, neural tube defects, migration defects, agenesis of the corpus callosum and other developmental anomalies. Any in utero or postnatal cerebral insult, a "secondary cause," can result in microcephaly. Secondary causes include in utero infections, such as congenital rubella; cerebral hypoxia; cerebrovascular accidents including stroke and hemorrhage; and systemic illness.

Although some families have many members with either large or small heads, these individuals typically have enjoyed normal growth and development. Physicians should examine the parents of children with an unusual-size head. In general, physicians should retrieve the growth and development charts of children to determine whether abnormalities have been present since birth or have appeared during infancy or later.

2. C. Most likely, he has cerebral palsy. During his childhood and adolescent growth spurts, his right-sided limbs will be less affected. They will remain shorter, and probably spasticity will develop. Orthopedic procedures can reduce the disability. Because his insult occurred in early infancy—long before age 5 years—the unaffected hemisphere will assume dominance for language. Moreover, if the lesion is restricted to a small area of the cerebrum, his cognitive abilities should be largely preserved. He is not at risk for primary generalized seizures, such as absences, but given the cerebral injury, he is at risk for partial seizures that may undergo secondary generalization.

3. A. In light of her overall development and communication, most likely her problem is hearing loss. She is able to understand her family members' wishes because they communicate with nonverbal cues, such as facial expression and gesturing. Also, she is probably able to hear some of their volume and tone. Detecting hearing impairment in infants is critical. They must be fitted with hearing aids, taught sign language, or prepared for cochlear implants.

4. F. The physical examination can allow the physician to diagnose innumerable conditions "by inspection." Some disorders, however, which usually occur in episodes, have no interval stigmata, such as migraine, metabolic aberrations, and epilepsy. Nevertheless, some stigmata, such as the neurocutaneous disorders and signs of cerebral palsy, indicate the likelihood of comorbid epilepsy.

5. A-2, B-4, C-3, D-1.

6. A-2 (neurofibromatosis type 1), **B-1** (tuberous sclerosis), **C-1** (tuberous sclerosis), **D-3** (Sturge–Weber disease).

7. D. This infant has sustained an extensive in utero cerebral lesion—for example, congenital infection, hypoxic ischemia insult, or congenital brain anomaly—that caused cerebral palsy and epilepsy. These injuries also cause mental retardation. The infant (A) with right arm areflexic weakness has a birth injury of the right brachial plexus. The one (B) with areflexic weakness in the right arm and left leg probably contracted poliomyelitis at 12 months and was left with residual motor neuron impairment. Cognitive impairment is not associated with either of these or most other neuromuscular conditions. Finally, as with the infant with athetosis of all limbs since infancy (C), cognitive impairment occurs in a minority of individuals with the athetotic form of cerebral palsy.

8. A. The posterior fontanel closes before 6 months, and the anterior fontanel, not until 12 to 18 months of age. Plagiocephaly is flattening of the back of the head, usually caused by the infant lying on it for excessive periods. Craniosynostosis, potentially a more serious condition, pertains to premature closure of one or more of the sutures. It can cause a misshapen or small head (microcephaly).

9. C. Nonaccidental head injury, which is a similar but less pejorative term than "child abuse," would explain not only this child's change in personality and behavior but also his mastoid area ecchymosis. This subcutaneous hematoma, often called a "battle sign," suggests a basilar skull fracture, which may not be seen on a head CT scan. The gait impairment and pain-limited joint mobility result from soft tissue injuries. Hyperactive children, compared with normally active children, are more prone both to trigger abuse and to injury from dangerous activities.

10. D. This diurnal dystonia probably indicates basal ganglia dysfunction. Most likely, he has dopamine-responsive dystonia, which is a genetic disorder in which the synthesis of dopamine is impaired. Small doses of L-dopa will completely and dramatically restore neurological function. Dopamine-responsive dystonia may mimic cerebral palsy or a psychogenic disorder. However, signs of cerebral palsy appear within the first 1 to 2 years after birth and thereafter persist with little change. Psychogenic movement disorders in children are rare and have not been reported to fluctuate in a diurnal pattern. Moreover, most psychogenic neurological problems in children are "seizures" and "deficits," such as weakness, inability to walk, or loss of vision.

11. C. She has the quintessential neuromuscular junction disorder, myasthenia gravis. This illness tends to affect young women and to present with paresis of CNs. As in this case, the examination typically shows weakness of the left levator palpebrae and right lateral rectus muscles. Her history also indicates weakness of jaw, laryngeal, and facial-expression muscles. Myasthenia gravis, which causes greater problems as the day wears on, is unrelated to medications or drugs of abuse. Its symptoms result from impaired acetylcholine transmission and not, like dopamine-responsive dystonia, from impaired dopamine synthesis, although symptoms of both illnesses are worse as the day progresses.

CHAPTER 2

Neuroradiological Imaging in Children

KEN ALLISON, TODD MILLER, AND JACQUELINE BELLO

Neuroradiological imaging plays a fundamental role in the diagnosis and management of neurological disease in children and adolescents. This chapter addresses the commonly available neuroimaging modalities and provides recommendations on how best to employ them in the evaluation of children, with particular attention to clinical conditions that the child and adolescent psychiatrist might encounter. In addition, it presents the neuroimaging characteristics of these conditions.

Neuroimaging Techniques

COMPUTED TOMOGRAPHY

Head computed tomography

The most readily available test for brain imaging is often computed tomography (CT). This modality is a quick and efficient screening tool for demonstrating intracranial structures and mass effect. Noncontrast head CT without sedation is usually tolerated by children as well as adolescents. It provides sufficient tissue contrast to demonstrate hydrocephalus, most tumors, infarcts, hemorrhage, and many infections. Compared to magnetic resonance imaging (MRI), CT provides better bony detail and spatial resolution. These attributes, most useful in an emergent situation, come at a cost. CT scan images are generated by passing x-ray beams through the patient. Although recent data suggest the radiation dose associated with head CT is not insignificant, this radiation exposure may be more significant in children than in adults. In addition, modern scanner designs, for the same test, deliver higher doses to a smaller patient than to a larger one (1).

Computed tomography angiography

Computed tomography angiography (CTA) is a head CT acquired rapidly (2 seconds) during an intravenous bolus injection of iodinated contrast timed to optimize arterial opacification. In order to maximize evaluation of the vascular structures, which are measured in millimeters, these scans are acquired with the thinnest slice width provided by scanner technology (as little as 0.625 mm). These factors combine to create one of the highest dose CT scans performed. While the radiation exposure is of some concern, CTA provides an unparalleled noninvasive three-dimensional demonstration of the intracranial vascular tree and

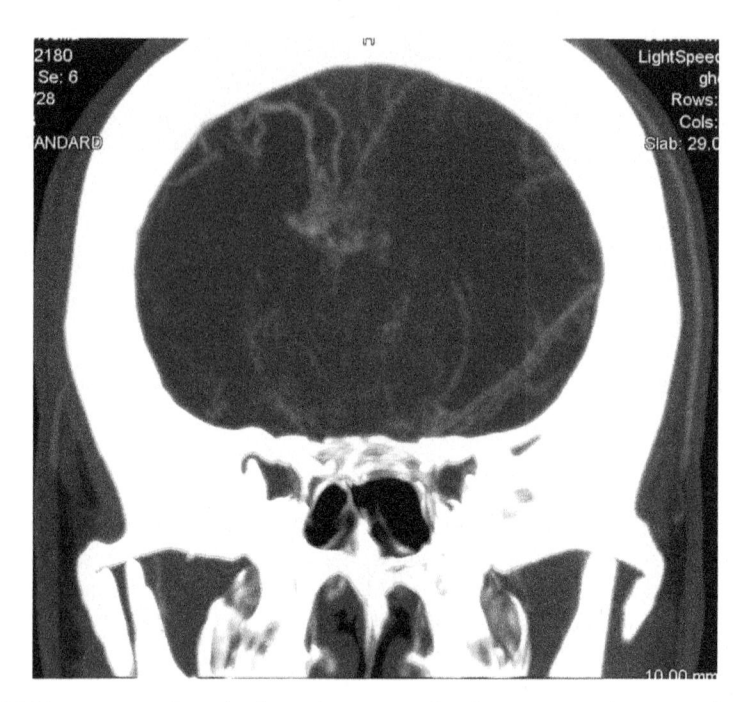

14 CHILD AND ADOLESCENT NEUROLOGY FOR PSYCHIATRISTS

■ **FIGURE 2.1** Moya moya collaterals. Coronal reconstruction from computed tomography angiography (CTA) demonstrates "puff of smoke" appearance of moya moya collaterals in a child with bilateral internal carotid artery (ICA) occlusion.

its relationship to the surrounding anatomy (Fig. 2.1). Children usually require conscious sedation because the contrast injection consists of a rapid bolus that is difficult to tolerate.

MAGNETIC RESONANCE IMAGING

Magnetic resonance imaging is the current gold standard for demonstrating neural tissue in vivo. The superior soft tissue contrast resolution of MRI allows for detailed characterization of the gray and white matter, which is the most necessary component in detecting brain abnormalities. Spatial resolution of MRI is slightly less than that which is available with CT scan. The magnetic field required to produce MR images precludes the use of MRI for patients with certain metallic surgical implants as well as implanted electronic devices (e.g., cochlear implants, pacemakers, and defibrillators). Imaging takes place inside a cylinder 3 feet in diameter and several feet in length in configured magnets. More "open" magnet designs may reduce some of the claustrophobic problems associated with "closed" bore magnets. Patient motion significantly degrades image quality. Excellent tissue visualization and no ionizing radiation make MRI the imaging test of choice in the pediatric population. Because MRI is useful in staging hemorrhage of different ages, it is often applicable to investigation of suspected nonaccidental trauma. There are only scarce nonemergent clinical scenarios where CT represents the neuroimaging modality of choice.

Generic MRI has several adjuncts, including magnetic resonance angiography (MRA), cerebrospinal fluid (CSF) flow studies, diffusion weighted imaging (DWI), diffusion tensor imaging (DTI), perfusion, functional MRI, and spectroscopy.

Magnetic resonance angiography is a specific imaging sequence designed to emphasize fluid flow within vessels. Thin-section axial or coronal images are acquired (without contrast) and are then reconstructed in three dimensions. These images provide near millimeter resolution and demonstrate most vascular abnormalities.

Cerebrospinal flow studies are one of the few MRI examinations tailored to maximize temporal resolution over spatial resolution or tissue contrast. In general, several sagittal images are rapidly acquired over the same midline space to produce a cine effect (i.e., a "mini-movie"). The flow of CSF through the ventricles and cisterns is emphasized by employing a phase-contrast pulse sequence. This problem-solving tool is frequently used to demonstrate the physiologic significance of low cerebellar tonsils in symptomatic patients or confirm flow diversion in patients with third ventriculostomies for hydrocephalus.

Diffusion weighted imaging measures molecular motion of extracellular water molecules and is particularly useful in the setting of acute ischemia. Cytotoxic edema is reflected as restricted diffusion. DWI is also useful in defining the diffusion characteristics of fluid collections (e.g., arachnoid cysts and epidermoid inclusion cysts) (Fig. 2.2).

SPECIALIZED TECHNIQUES

Perfusion imaging

Perfusion imaging involves dynamic imaging of the brain with CT or MRI after the administration of an intravenous contrast agent. This allows evaluation of blood perfusion to an area of interest, and assessment of other features such as capillary permeability and angiogenesis. Perfusion imaging plays a role in, among other things, the investigation of central nervous system (CNS) tumors, white matter diseases, and acute infarcts in defining penumbra.

Diffusion tensor imaging

Diffusion tensor imaging is an MRI technique that measures the degree of anisotropy (asymmetrical diffusion, also called fractional anisotropy) of water molecule motion in a region of

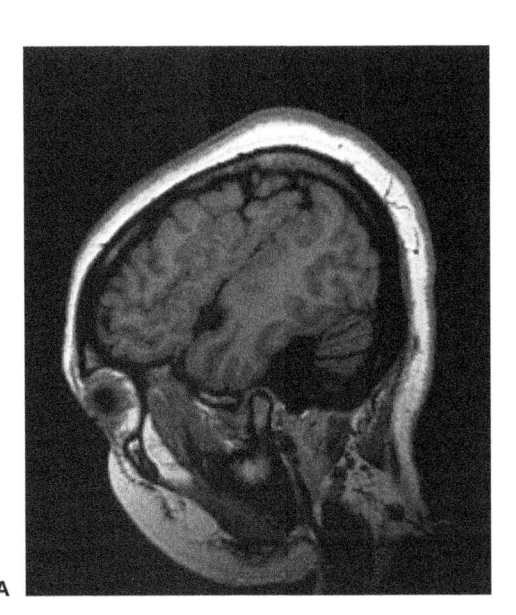

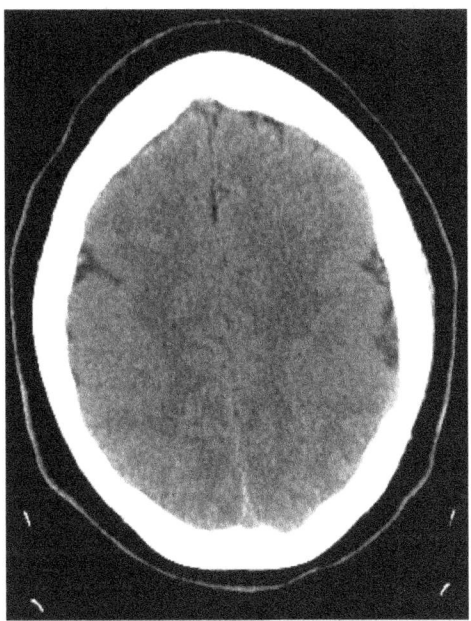

■ **FIGURE 2.2** Polymicrogyria. **A:** Sagittal T1 magnetic resonance imaging (MRI) demonstrates numerous small gyri in a patient with seizures. **B:** Axial noncontrast CT in the same patient shows apparent pachygyria, failing to define the gray-white detail.

interest. Capitalizing on its ability to detect the preferential diffusion of water molecules in white matter tracts, DTI is often used to study brain maturation, abnormalities underlying neurological deficits, and white matter injury following traumatic or toxic brain insults.

Magnetic resonance spectroscopy

Magnetic resonance spectroscopy (MRS) uses an MRI scanner to evaluate the chemical composition of a selected volume of tissue. This approach does not yield an image, but rather a spectrum, which is displayed as a series of peaks, whose positions correspond to different metabolites. MRS can be used to study biochemical alterations in neoplasms, infections, neurodegenerative diseases, infarcts, and metabolic disorders.

Functional magnetic resonance imaging

Functional imaging refers to the technique of using an image to display information about the biological activity of an organ or tissue, rather than its anatomical structure alone. Functional MRI (fMRI) is a type of functional imaging that uses the different magnetic properties of oxygenated and deoxygenated hemoglobin to detect and display the pattern of blood flow within the brain that varies according to its activity. Anatomical images obtained during the same examination allow correlation of structure with function. In pediatric patients, fMRI shows promise for the evaluation language disorders and language mapping prior to epilepsy surgery.

Positron emission tomography

Positron emission tomography (PET) is a nuclear medicine imaging technique that employs radioactively labeled, biologically active molecules to obtain functional information. The most commonly used agent is a glucose analogue, fluorine-18 fluorodeoxyglucose (F-18 FDG). A PET scanner detects F-18 FDG taken up by metabolically active cells. PET can be used to study neurological disorders, such as tumors, strokes, seizures, and dementia.

Molecular imaging

In contrast to most types of radiological imaging, which provide anatomical information, molecular imaging refers to the in vivo measurement, analysis, and depiction of biological processes at the cellular and molecular levels. This is a rapidly developing field that holds great promise for the characterization, monitoring, and treatment of disease and for pharmaceutical development. Because it facilitates the detection and characterization of gene and protein abnormalities, as well as the defining of cellular processes, such as signal transduction, molecular imaging will be increasingly central to the translation of basic science into clinical applications within many spheres of medicine (2).

CONSIDERATIONS WHEN IMAGING CHILDREN

Radiological imaging of children involves practical and ethical concerns that should be borne in mind when deciding whether imaging is indicated and, if so, which modality should be employed. Among these concerns are a child's ability to tolerate the examination, the clinical stability, a need for sedation, and exposure to ionizing radiation. Each of these factors may be more problematical when imaging children than adults.

A typical brain MRI scan with contrast takes approximately 40 minutes to complete, requires complete immobility, and is performed in a noisy, potentially claustrophobic machine. Many children, unable to tolerate this situation, require varying levels of sedation or anesthesia. In addition to their inherent risk, sedation or anesthesia increases the complexity, expense, and duration of the study. (To some extent, fast, motion-compensated, T2-weighted MRI sequences ameliorate these problems.) Alternatively, the difficulties associated with MRI scanning can be reduced or eliminated by the faster and less threatening environment of CT scanning.

Perhaps the greatest concern when imaging children is exposure to ionizing radiation and its potential for inducing malignancy. The chief source of radiation exposure in medical imaging is from CT, which accounts for nearly 70% of all medical radiation (3). The use of CT among pediatric patients has increased over the past decades in both absolute and relative numbers, with pediatric studies constituting up to 11% of all CT examinations by 1999 (3,4). Radiation exposure is of relatively greater concern in children compared with adults due to inherently greater radiosensitivity, larger organ doses for a given set of machine parameters, and their longer lifetime during which cancer may develop (4). Of particular note is the radiation dose to the ocular lenses because they are included in most head CT and all paranasal sinus CT examinations. The lenses may begin to develop cataracts after exposure to 0.5 to 2.0 Gy of radiation. However, the typical sinus scan using modern multislice CT scanners imparts a radiation dose of approximately 24.5 mGy to the lens, substantially below the threshold dose. This exposure can be further decreased by using low-dose scanning techniques. In addition, multislice CT scanners have the ability to reformat axial images into additional planes, eliminating the need for direct coronal scanning (5).

Brenner et al. (6) estimate that the lifetime cancer mortality risk attributable to the radiation from a single CT scan in a 1-year-old patient is 0.18% for an abdominal CT and 0.07% for a head CT. Although this radiation dose is not insignificant, it is important to note that these numbers represent a small (approximately 0.35%) increase over the background rate of lifetime cancer mortality (6). In addition, for any given properly selected patient, the benefits of a CT study likely far outweigh the potential risks (7), making it difficult to translate the previous data into appropriate recommendations. Therefore, probably the best advice to physicians who are ordering neuroimaging studies on pediatric patients is to adhere to the as low as reasonably achievable (ALARA) principle of radiation exposure. Indeed, there is anecdotal evidence that a significant proportion of CT scans are not clearly justified by medical necessity (1). Pediatric physicians and radiologists should work closely together to determine whether a CT scan is indicated for a given clinical question or whether another imaging modality, such ultrasound or MRI, could provide an acceptable alternative, thereby eliminating exposure to ionizing radiation. For example, fast MRI techniques, previously discussed, are increasingly used for monitoring pediatric patients with chronic neurological problems, such as hydrocephalus, that require repeated imaging. Even patients with programmable cerebrospinal fluid shunt valves, with the valve "reset" after the procedure, can be imaged this way.

Neuroimaging in Common Clinical Situations

HEADACHES

Headaches are extremely common in children and adolescents, with a prevalence of 37% to 51% in 7 year olds, increasing to 57% to 82% by age 15 (8). The prevalence of migraine headaches in adolescent boys relative to girls is approximately 1:1.5 (3.8% and 6.6%, respectively) (9). Headache symptoms are the presenting complaint in approximately 1.3% of pediatric emergency department visits (10). Although the possible causes of headaches in children are myriad and most often benign, many children with headaches undergo imaging examinations to exclude neurological diseases that require immediate medical or surgical intervention. However, the role and value of neuroimaging in the evaluation of headache in children remains controversial, in part, because of a paucity of well-designed, sufficiently sized studies (8).

A recent practice parameter published by the American Academy of Neurology (AAN) (8) reviewed the available evidence regarding the value of neuroimaging in children with recurrent headaches. Among children imaged with CT or MRI for recurrent headache, 16% had imaging abnormalities, but most of these were incidental or not necessarily surgical (including Chiari malformations, arachnoid cysts, and paranasal sinus disease) (Fig. 2.3). Only 2.3% of patients had lesions that required surgical treatment, such as tumors or vascular malformations. Notably, all patients with lesions requiring surgery had abnormal neurological examinations and no patient with a normal examination had a lesion requiring surgery. This practice parameter therefore concluded that routine neuroimaging is not indicated in children with recurrent headaches and normal neurological examinations.

Neuroimaging should be considered if patients have abnormal neurological findings, especially papilledema, nystagmus, and gait or motor abnormalities (9). Other symptoms or signs that may warrant imaging include the following: recent onset of severe, persistent headache; change in the type of headache; headaches that awaken a child or occur immediately upon wakening; absence of a family history of migraines; associated significant confusion, disorientation, or emesis; and the coexistence of seizures (8,9). In most cases, the imaging modality of choice is MRI.

It is worth mentioning that intracranial aneurysms are rare in children. Their incidence is one per million per year, which is one hundredth of the incidence in adults (11). In a large series, only 0.6% of ruptured aneurysms were found in patients younger than 19 years (12). If a patient presents with the "worst headache of life" and subarachnoid hemorrhage (SAH) is suspected, initial imaging should be with noncontrast CT. However, because CT can miss subacute or small amounts of hemorrhage, a negative CT scan in this clinical scenario should be followed by lumbar puncture. Subarachnoid hemorrhage may also be seen with trauma. When SAH is due to ruptured aneurysm, the hemorrhage is usually extensive and present in the sulci and basal cisterns. By comparison, traumatic SAH is most often seen in the posterior interhemispheric fissure, along the tentorium cerebelli, or within the sulci adjacent to the site of injury. A small amount of SAH in the setting of trauma should not necessarily prompt investigation for intracranial aneurysm.

SEIZURES

Febrile seizures—seizures in infants and children from 6 months to 5 years of age, with associated fever and no evidence of CNS infection or other neurological disease—occur in approximately 2% to 4% of children (13). Other than a slightly increased risk relative to the general population of subsequent epilepsy, simple febrile seizures are considered benign. A practice parameter released by the American Academy of Pediatrics recommends that neuroimaging not be performed in the evaluation of first simple febrile seizures (14).

The role of neuroimaging in the evaluation of children with first nonfebrile seizures without an apparent provocative cause is less well defined. A review and practice parameter published in 2000 by the AAN (15) found that CT and MR scans in these patients showed abnormalities in up to 33%, although significant abnormalities that influenced management were seen in only 0% to 7% of cases, with an average of 2%. Significant imaging findings were more often seen in patients with focal seizures or other specific focal clinical findings, and included lesions, such as tumors, hydrocephalus, subarachnoid or porencephalic cysts, and cysticercosis. MRI abnormalities, such as atrophy, structural brain malformations, and mesial temporal sclerosis, were relatively common but usually did not influence management. Therefore, this AAN practice parameter concluded that

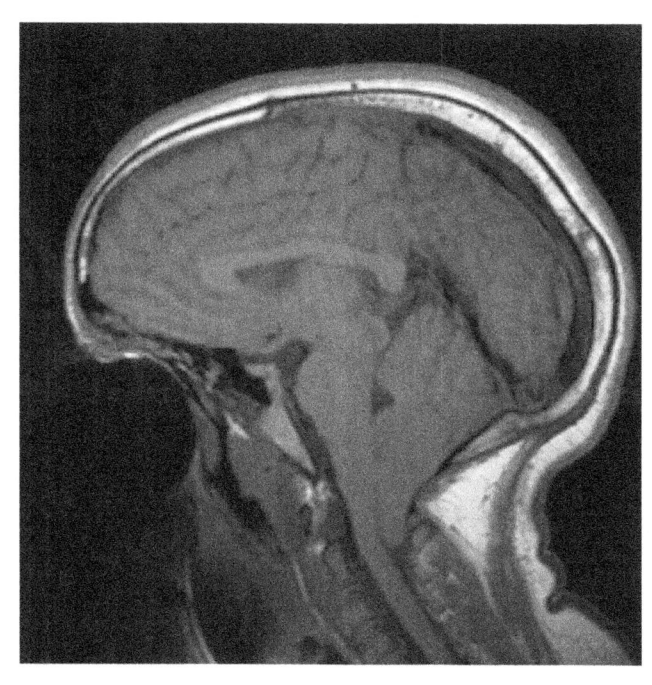

■ **FIGURE 2.3** Chiari I malformation. Sagittal T1 MRI in an adolescent with headache demonstrates tonsillar herniation at the foramen magnum.

there is insufficient evidence to recommend routine neuroimaging for first nonfebrile seizures in children. However, another review published by the AAN in 2007 found that in children presenting with first seizures, abnormal head CT findings are present in 0% to 21% of patients, and these findings influenced management in 3% to 8% of patients. This review concluded that emergent CT examination is "possibly useful for acute management" of such patients (16).

Most sources support the conclusion that emergency imaging is indicated for children who show prolonged focal postictal deficits or who do not return to baseline within several hours, infants younger than 6 months, and for patients with acquired immunodeficiency syndrome (AIDS) (15,16). Nonurgent imaging should be considered for children with seizures who are younger than 1 year or who have abnormal neurological examinations; for those with unexplained, significant cognitive or motor deficits; and for those with partial seizures or electroencephalographic (EEG) findings not consistent with benign partial epilepsy of childhood or primary generalized epilepsy. Although MRI is the modality of choice in most cases, CT may further characterize any lesions (15).

In the case of status epilepticus, imaging plays a role when the cause is unknown. It may identify structural abnormalities or exclude the need for neurosurgical treatment (17). Imaging should be performed only after the child is clinically stabilized and the seizures controlled. Again, MRI is more sensitive and specific than CT, although CT is often more readily available and may require less sedation (Fig. 2.4).

MINOR HEAD INJURY

Head trauma in children accounts annually for more than 500,000 visits to emergency departments and more than $1 billion in health care costs (18). Because most injuries are minor, the optimal neuroimaging is a matter of significant clinical concern. However, this

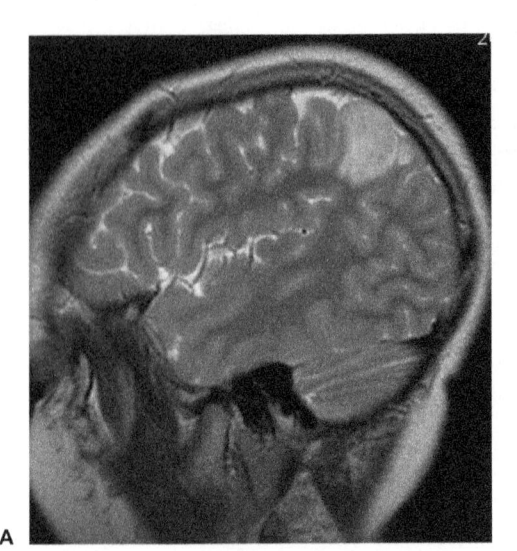

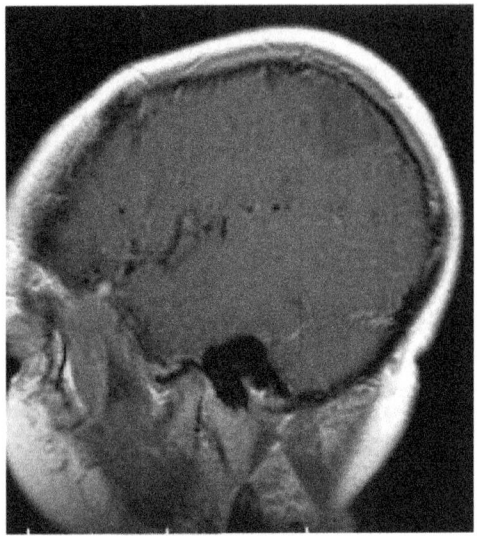

■ **FIGURE 2.4** Dysembryoplastic neuroectodermal tumor (DNET). Sagittal T2 **(A)** and contrast-enhanced **(B)** T1 scans in a 6-year-old with seizures demonstrate a nonenhancing parietal DNET.

topic is controversial because of the differing definitions of minor head trauma, difficulty of clinical evaluation, and lack of definitive studies comparing clinical outcomes between different management strategies, such as routine imaging and observation.

Some authors define minor head trauma as a closed head injury without altered mental status, abnormal or focal neurological examination findings, or evidence of skull fracture at the time of initial evaluation (19). Others employ the Glasgow Coma Scale (GCS), defining minor head trauma by ranges of scores from 13 to 15 (18). Many people use the term "concussion" synonymously for minor head trauma. The AAN defines concussion as "a trauma induced alteration in mental status that may or may not involve loss of consciousness" (20). Regardless of the definition used, the detection of intracranial injury on the basis of physical examination findings is notoriously difficult, and no clinical finding or combination of findings reliably identifies all significant intracranial injuries (21). This further underscores the important role of research in developing guidelines relating to the utility of imaging in the management of minor head trauma. Conversely, in the setting of imaging findings, there is a need to consider the fact that not every abnormality detected with neuroimaging may turn out to be clinically significant. The proportion of children with minor head trauma who will eventually need neurosurgical intervention is small; the exact number is a matter of some debate, although a recent article argued that the number is definitely less than 1% and likely less than 0.5% (22).

There is broad agreement that any patient with evidence of skull fracture should undergo neuroimaging. Signs of skull fracture include hemotympanum, the Battle sign (postauricular ecchymosis), "raccoon eyes" (periorbital hematoma), palpable depressed fracture, serosanguineous leakage from the nose or ear, and cranial nerve palsies. Imaging should be considered for patients with pre-existing disorders that may mask new processes or consequences of trauma, or that may be exacerbated by trauma, such as bleeding diatheses, arteriovenous malformations, and CSF shunts. Imaging is also indicated for patients with altered mental status, GCS of less than 15, a deteriorating clinical course, or focal neurological abnormalities (18,19,21,22). Some authors recommend that imaging be considered when trauma is associated with loss of consciousness or persistent vomiting (22), or with cases of posttraumatic amnesia, seizures, persistent or worsening headaches, or behavioral changes (18,21). Imaging is not recommended if a child is asymptomatic at the time of evaluation, with a GCS of 15, and if none of the previously mentioned clinical indicators is apparent.

If neuroimaging is performed, most sources recommend CT scanning, in large part because of its wide availability, speed, relatively low cost, and superior bony detail. Skull radiographs are generally of limited utility. CT is also the modality of choice for craniofacial fractures, hyperacute or acute intracranial hemorrhage, and especially subarachnoid hemorrhage. In general, CT imaging is sensitive for intracranial pathology that requires medical or surgical treatment, and patients with a normal head CT have a very low risk of later neurological deterioration (18). However, MRI is very sensitive for intracranial pathology and more sensitive than CT for injuries, such as small intracranial hematomas or contusions, diffuse axonal injury, and brainstem injuries (23-25). MRI should also be considered in cases in which an abnormal clinical examination exceeds the CT findings in severity (Fig. 2.5).

CHILD ABUSE

It has been estimated that up to 30% of children in the United States experience some form of child abuse prior to the age of 18 (26). Physical abuse is the leading cause of death in children. Although abuse accounts for only 10% of injury under the age of 2, up to 50% of such injury includes head injury. Eighty percent of fatal abusive injury is related to head injury. Nonaccidental head injury is responsible for a disproportionate percentage of serious traumatic brain injury, resulting in mortality in 30%, severe neurological deficit in 30% to 50%, and recovery in only 30% of cases (27-29).

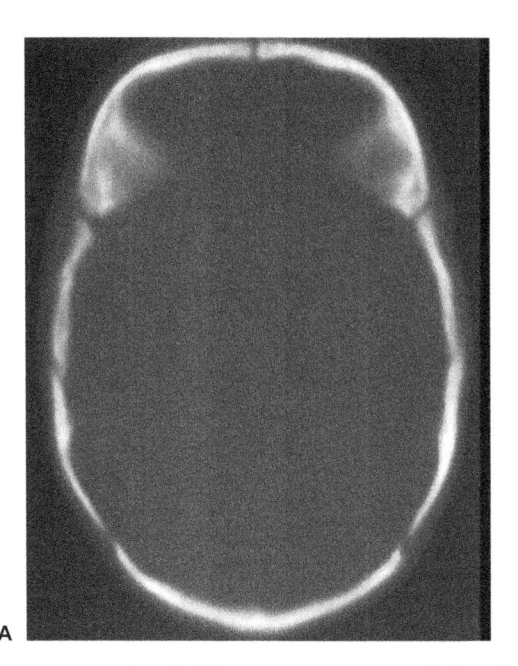

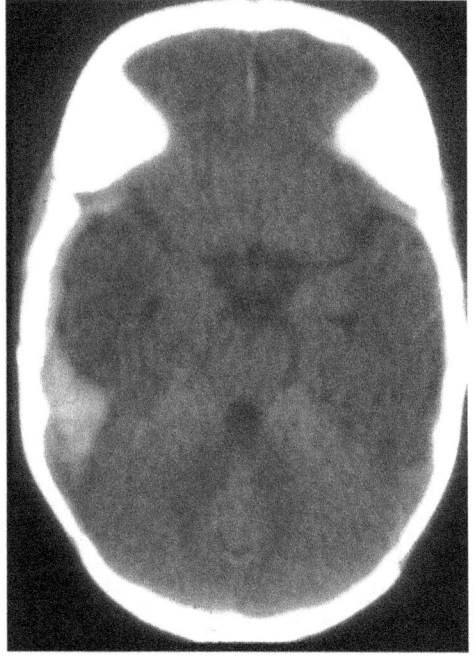

■ **FIGURE 2.5** Skull fracture, CT. **A:** Bone window demonstrates right temporal fracture. **B:** Brain window shows associated extra-axial hemorrhage.

Shaking and impact mechanisms both result in similar brain injury. Rotational forces generated by angular acceleration and deceleration of the head result in brain movement around its center of gravity, as well as shearing of vascular and axonal structures. These forces are accentuated in the infant, in whom the neck muscles are relatively weak and the head is relatively large, with a head to body weight ratio five times greater than that of the adult. In this same population, the immaturity of the myelin and fragile axonal structure within the brain predisposes its vulnerability to shear injury (30-32).

The spectrum of findings in nonaccidental head injury includes subdural hematoma (SDH), shear injuries, diffuse axonal injury (DAI), white matter contusions, SAH, and retinal hemorrhage (RH) (33). Several of these were included in Caffey's initial description of the "whiplash/shaking injury syndrome," in which SDH, SAH, and RH were coupled with metaphyseal extremity fractures as indicators of non-accidental trauma (34,35). At autopsy, SDH is found in 90% of cases of nonaccidental head injury, in which it is typically bilateral, along the posterior interhemispheric fissure and falx, due to shear injury. This same shear mechanism may result in SAH due to venous tears (36). The incidence of SDH in cases of accidental trauma is only 28%, compared with 81% in cases of nonaccidental trauma (37). In a reported series of 150 infants younger than 24 months hospitalized for head injury, roughly half of the patients (48.7%) had SDH; however, almost two thirds (64.4%) of the SDH in these patients was due to nonaccidental injury. Accidental versus nonaccidental SDH may be differentiated by its imaging appearance. On CT, focal, homogeneous, hyperdense SDH is more common with accidental injury, whereas multifocal, mixed-density SDH is more typical of nonaccidental injury (33,38). SDH is the most common finding in cases of nonaccidental head injury (48.7%); other imaging findings, in order of decreasing frequency, include skull fracture (13.3%), SAH (12%), depressed fracture (10.7%), epidural hematoma (7.3%) contusion (6%), and DAI (2%) (37). In general, skull fracture is uncommon with falls from less than 3 feet. When skull fracture is associated with SDH, or is multiple, complex, depressed, or diastatic, the possibility of nonaccidental trauma should be considered (38).

In the evaluation of nonaccidental trauma, various imaging modalities play a role, including skeletal survey, CT, MRI, and nuclear medicine scans. For head injury, CT best demonstrates fractures, and MRI is more sensitive in detecting and characterizing SDH and shear injury. No single finding is independently diagnostic of abusive head injury. Rather, a constellation of findings, including injuries of different chronicity, may suggest the diagnosis (Fig. 2.6).

Intracranial Neoplasms

GENERAL CONSIDERATIONS

All ages considered, pediatric brain tumors occur in roughly equal frequency within the posterior fossa and supratentorial compartment, although supratentorial tumors predominate in the first 2 years of life (39). Although CT is commonly used in the evaluation of pediatric brain tumors, MRI is the imaging modality of choice, because of its multiplanar capability and its ability to image the posterior fossa without the artifact (related to surrounding dense bone) that hinders CT evaluation of this region. Moreover, MRI is superior to CT for the assessment of subarachnoid metastatic disease (40,41). The intravenous administration of contrast with both CT and MRI is often useful, if not necessary, to further characterize lesions. MRS is a specialized MRI technique that may provide helpful information, by assessing tumor grade and differentiating tumor from granulation tissue

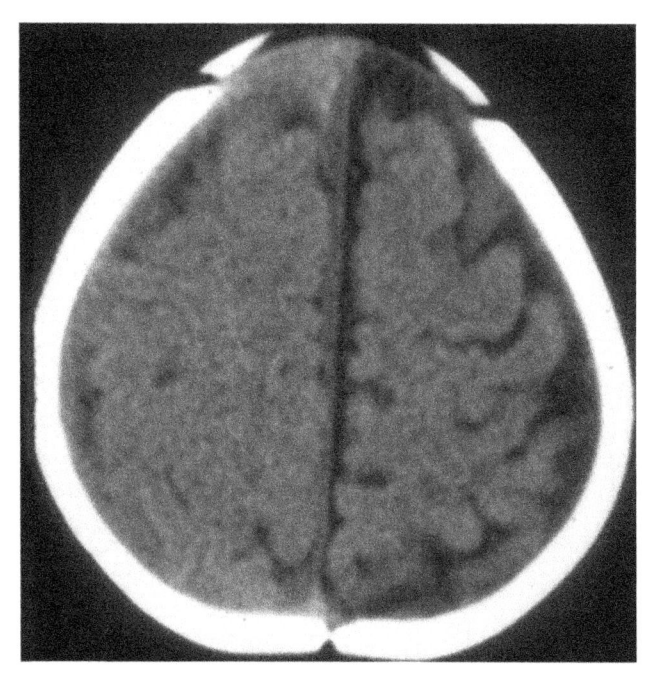

■ **FIGURE 2.6** Subdural hematoma. CT in a case of nonaccidental trauma shows subdural hematoma (SDH) of three different densities and, therefore, ages.

or necrosis. Magnetic resonance perfusion imaging may also contribute to evaluating tumor grade and distinguishing neoplasm from various other brain lesions.

POSTERIOR FOSSA NEOPLASMS

Clinical presentation

Posterior fossa tumors most often present clinically with symptoms related to hydrocephalus and increased intracranial pressure, such as headaches, nausea, vomiting, and increasing head circumference. Patients may also exhibit symptoms referable to cerebellar dysfunction, such as ataxia, nystagmus, and dysdiadochokinesia. Depending on the exact tumor location, cranial nerve deficits and long tract signs may be present, especially with brainstem tumors.

Medulloblastoma

Medulloblastoma is a highly malignant tumor of the posterior fossa and is the most common posterior fossa neoplasm in children. It affects males two to four times as commonly as females and is primarily seen in children (median age at diagnosis is 9 years), although it can occur infrequently in adults. This is an aggressive tumor, with invasion of the brainstem and CSF dissemination commonly seen (42,43).

Medulloblastomas are typically located within the midline cerebellar vermis, behind the fourth ventricle. On CT studies, the lesion classically appears hyperdense, surrounded by hypodense vasogenic edema, and demonstrates homogeneous contrast enhancement. Hydrocephalus is extremely common, due to mass effect on the fourth ventricle, and atypical features such as calcification, cysts, and necrosis may be present (43). The MRI

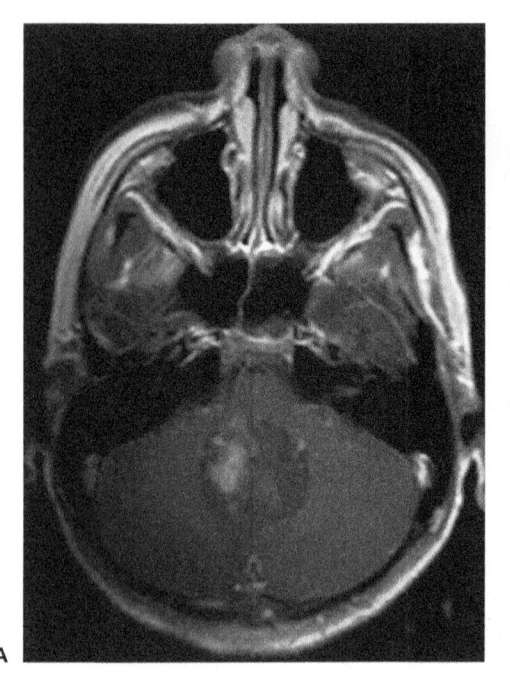

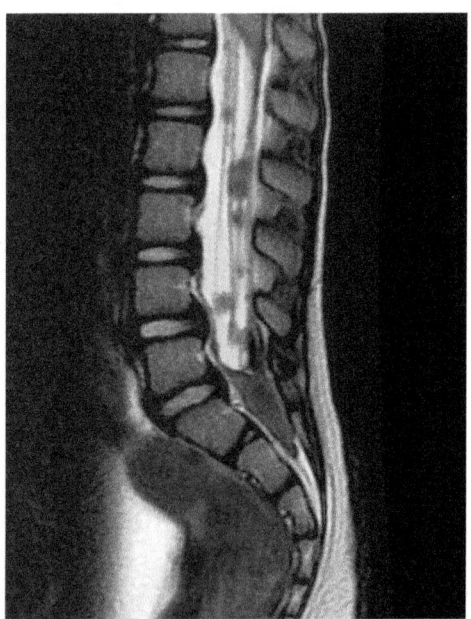

■ **FIGURE 2.7 A:** Medulloblastoma. Axial, T1 contrast-enhanced MRI demonstrates a midline, solid tumor of the vermis, medulloblastoma, compressing the fourth ventricle. **B:** In a different patient with medulloblastoma, sagittal T2 MRI shows cerebrospinal fluid seeding of tumor into the spinal subarachnoid space.

appearance of medulloblastoma is more variable, with isointense to hypointense signal on T1-weighted images, variable signal intensity on T2-weighted images, and heterogeneous contrast enhancement on post-gadolinium T1-weighted images (42). Contrast-enhanced MR examination of the entire brain and spine is obligatory in cases of medulloblastoma, as CSF dissemination is common and indicates a poorer prognosis (42) (Fig. 2.7).

Atypical teratoid/rhabdoid tumors

Atypical teratoid/rhabdoid tumor is a rare malignant neoplasm that predominantly affects children younger than 2 years. It resembles medulloblastoma histologically and radiologically but is now classified separately because of the tumor's resistance to standard therapies for medulloblastoma. The prognosis is dismal, with usual survival of less than 1 year after diagnosis (44). The tumor most often arises in the cerebellum, although it may occur supratentorially as well. It may spread through the subarachnoid spaces. Imaging characteristics are similar to those of medulloblastomas and ependymomas, but atypical teratoid/rhabdoid tumors are often more heterogeneous in appearance than typical medulloblastomas (43).

Cerebellar astrocytomas

Astrocytomas are the most common pediatric brain neoplasm overall, and approximately 40% of them occur in the cerebellum (43). Most cerebellar astrocytomas are of the low-grade pilocytic type and typically affect children and young adults. Pilocytic astrocytomas are usually treated with surgical resection, with an excellent prognosis (45).

Imaging reveals a well-marginated mass in the cerebellar midline or hemisphere, which is typically predominantly cystic or necrotic. Less than 10% are completely solid (43). Cystic lesions frequently have an enhancing tumor nodule in the wall. The solid portions of this tumor are generally hypodense or isodense to white matter on precontrast CT images, a useful imaging characteristic for distinguishing this tumor from medulloblastoma, which is usually hyperdense (43). MRI is variable but generally demonstrates solid portions of the tumor to be hypointense relative to normal brain on T1-weighted images and hyperintense on T2-weighted images (43,45) (Fig. 2.8).

Ependymomas

Ependymomas are the third most common pediatric brain tumor and comprise approximately 10% of posterior fossa tumors in children (46). These tumors arise from ependymal cells lining the ventricular system and central canal of the spinal cord and have a propensity to grow in an exophytic fashion into the ventricular lumen. In the posterior fossa, they may extend from the fourth ventricle into the cerebellopontine angle (CPA) cistern via the foramina of Luschka, or via the foramen of Magendie into the cisterna magna and through the foramen magnum into the cervical spinal canal (46). Hydrocephalus is common. On CT, posterior fossa ependymomas are isodense to hyperdense solid masses, with moderate heterogeneous contrast enhancement. Calcification is seen in up to 50%, and small cysts or hemorrhage may also be present (43). The MR appearance is nonspecific, with slightly decreased signal intensity on T1-weighted images, and isointensity with gray matter on T2-weighted images (43). Although less common than with medulloblastoma, spread of ependymomas via the CSF may occur, especially with higher grade tumors and younger patients (47), and therefore imaging of the entire neuraxis is appropriate.

Brainstem astrocytomas

Brainstem tumors account for 10% to 20% of pediatric CNS neoplasms, and the vast majority of them are astrocytomas (48,49). Brainstem astrocytomas are a heterogeneous group of tumors that vary in their location within the brainstem, growth pattern, and imaging appearance. They are classified as either focal or diffuse (49). Focal tumors are

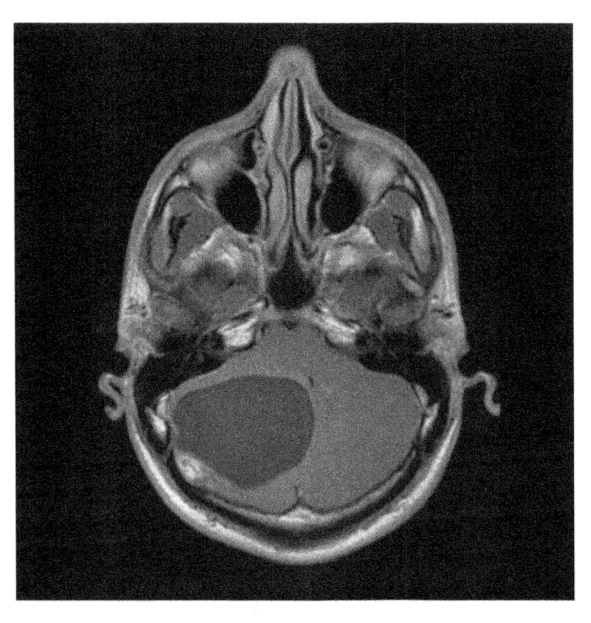

■ **FIGURE 2.8** Cerebellar pilocytic astrocytoma. Axial T1 contrast-enhanced MRI of a cystic tumor with an enhancing mural nodule, typical of pilocytic astrocytoma.

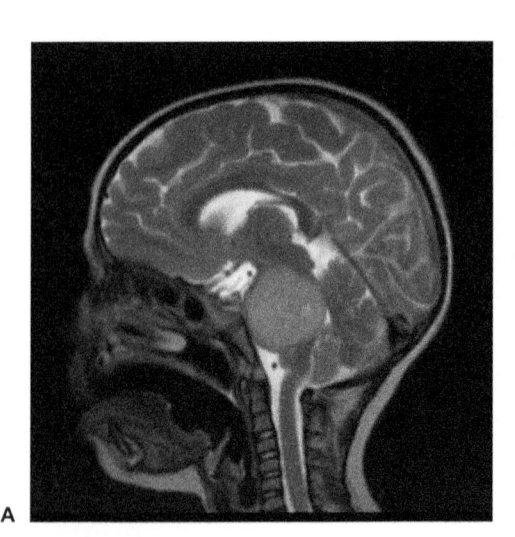

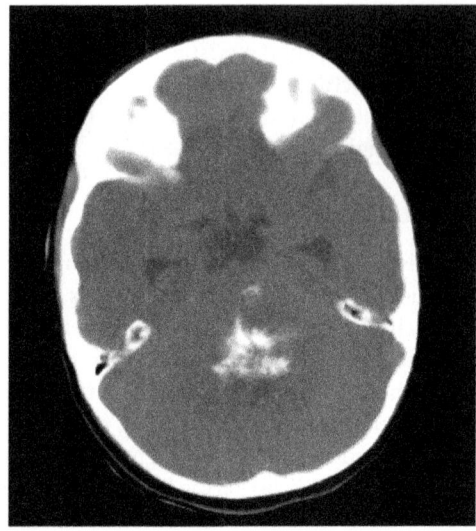

FIGURE 2.9 A: Brainstem glioma. Sagittal T2 MRI demonstrates abnormal enlargement and signal within the pons, with compression of the fourth ventricle by brainstem glioma. **B:** Axial, noncontrast CT scan, 6 months later, following radiation therapy, demonstrates calcification within the treated lesion.

discrete lesions, typically originating from the midbrain or medulla, which often grow in an exophytic fashion from the brainstem. Focal tumors in the tectal region portend a relatively favorable prognosis and may require only CSF diversion for treatment (43). Diffuse tumors are more common than focal tumors, accounting for up to 75% of brainstem tumors and have a very grave prognosis. They usually originate from the pons and diffusely infiltrate and enlarge the brainstem (49,50). Diffuse tumors are hypodense on CT scans, with indistinct margins. On MRI, they are most often hypointense on T1-weighted images, without significant contrast enhancement, and hyperintense on T2-weighted images (48,50) (Fig. 2.9).

SUPRATENTORIAL TUMORS

Astrocytomas

Astrocytomas are the most common supratentorial tumor in children, comprising approximately 30% of such tumors and affecting all age groups (43). Clinical symptoms are determined by the location of the tumor, but may include signs of increased intracranial pressure, headaches, focal deficits, or seizures. The imaging appearance is variable depending on tumor grade and histology, but lesions of the cerebral hemispheres often have imaging characteristics similar to those described above for cerebellar astrocytomas (see also Fig. 2.8). In general, the degree of tumor heterogeneity, amount of surrounding vasogenic white matter edema, and incidence of hemorrhage all increase with higher grade tumors (43). Astrocytomas may also be located in the hypothalamus or optic pathways, the latter location being characteristic of neurofibromatosis type 1.

Ependymomas

Approximately one third of intracranial ependymomas in children arise supratentorially (51). These tumors occur in the periventricular regions and have imaging features similar to the posterior fossa ependymomas described previously.

Craniopharyngiomas

Craniopharyngiomas constitute 6% to 9% of intracranial tumors in children and are most often found in the suprasellar region (52). Because of their location, presenting symptoms often include headaches, visual dysfunction, and endocrine abnormalities. Hydrocephalus may occur when the lesion is large (53). The classic CT appearance of pediatric craniopharyngiomas is that of a cystic mass with calcifications and contrast enhancement of the solid portions. MRI also shows an enhancing cystic mass with variable T1 signal in the cysts (sometimes hyperintense, due to elevated protein content) and hyperintensity on T2-weighted sequences (43) (Fig. 2.10).

Pineal region tumors

Tumors of the pineal region in children account for approximately 3% to 11% of childhood tumors (54). Patients most often present clinically with symptoms related to hydrocephalus, local growth, or Parinaud syndrome (a cluster of ocular abnormalities, including paralysis of upward gaze, caused by pressure on the tectum of the midbrain) (54,55).

Germ cell tumors are the most common pineal region tumors, and include germinomas, teratomas, yolk sac tumors, embryonal carcinomas, choriocarcinomas, and mixed tumors. Germinomas account for more than 50% of pineal region tumors. Their peak incidence is in adolescence, and there is a conspicuous male predominance (43). CT typically shows a homogeneous isodense to hyperdense mass. On MRI, these lesions can be variable but often are similar in intensity to gray matter on T1- and T2-weighted sequences (56) (Fig. 2.11). Germinomas may spread via the CSF, a situation best detected by contrast-enhanced MRI of the brain and spine. Teratomas are much less common than germinomas but may also occur in the pineal region. These are extremely heterogeneous lesions, which may show evidence of fat, soft tissue, cysts, and calcium (43).

Pineocytomas and pineoblastomas are neoplasms derived from pineal parenchymal cells; they constitute approximately 11% to 28% of pineal region tumors (57). Pineocytomas are

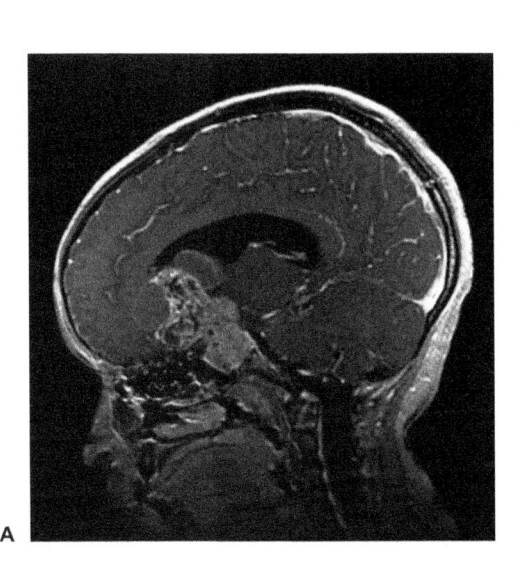

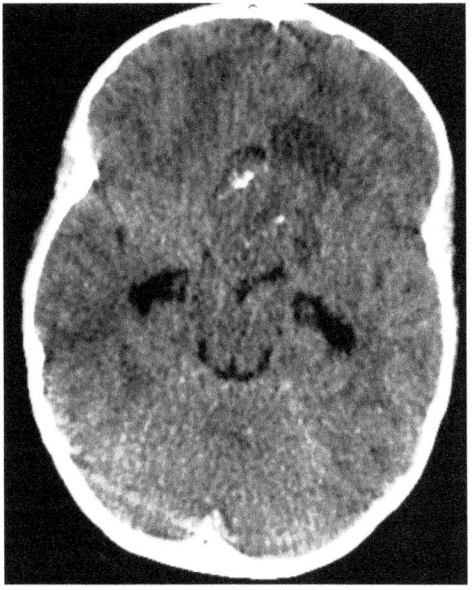

■ **FIGURE 2.10 A:** Craniopharyngioma. Sagittal T1 contrast-enhanced MRI demonstrates a suprasellar, enhancing cystic lesion, with evidence of calcification on axial noncontrast CT scan **(B)**.

benign, whereas pineoblastomas are highly malignant, invasive tumors that resemble medulloblastoma histologically (57). CT shows both tumors as isodense to hyperdense lesions with calcifications and marked enhancement. Pineoblastomas may be larger, more lobulated, and more heterogeneous than pineocytomas. The MRI appearance of these tumors is variable, although pineocytomas tend to be hyperintense on T2-weighted images, whereas pineoblastomas are more isointense to gray matter on the same sequences. Pineoblastomas are prone to CSF dissemination, and therefore contrast-enhanced MRI of the entire CNS is essential (43,56).

Small, benign cysts of the pineal gland are relatively common in adolescents and adults, found in up to 40% of routine autopsies (57). They are generally asymptomatic and have varied appearances on CT and MRI, depending on protein content. However, because pineal neoplasms may include cystic components, if a simple pineal cyst is suspected on the basis of a neuroimaging study, follow-up MRI scans with contrast are recommended at 6 and 12 months in order to assess for interval growth and exclude neoplasm.

Other pineal region tumors seen in children include gliomas, dermoids, epidermoids, choroid plexus papillomas, and vascular malformations (Fig. 2.11).

The Phakomatoses

The phakomatoses are a group of inherited disorders, also known as neurocutaneous syndromes, which affect organs of ectodermal origin, including the central and peripheral nervous systems, the skin, and the eyes (see Chapter 10). Clinically, these conditions may present with characteristic cutaneous, ocular, or skeletal signs; learning disabilities or mental retardation; seizures; or focal deficits. Four diseases usually included in this category are neurofibromatosis (NF), tuberous sclerosis (TS), Sturge-Weber syndrome (SWS), and Von Hippel-Lindau disease (VHL).

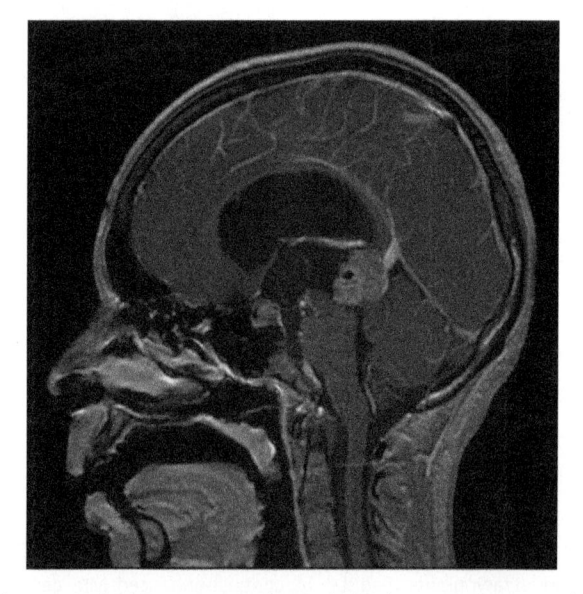

■ **FIGURE 2.11** Germinoma. Sagittal T1 contrast-enhanced MRI demonstrates a complex pineal region mass.

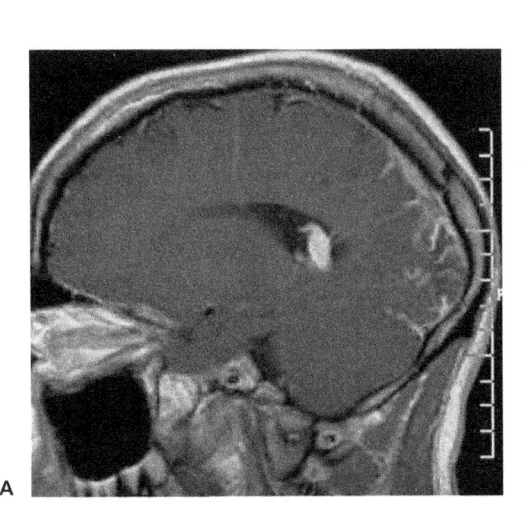

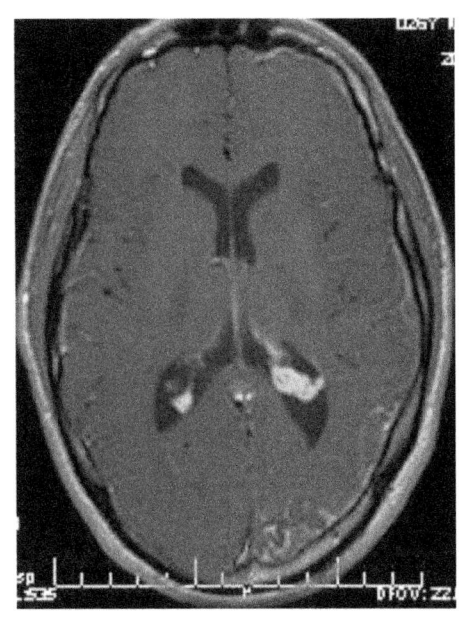

■ **FIGURE 2.12 A** and **B**: Sturge Weber. Sagittal and axial contrast enhanced T1-weighted MR images demonstrate occipito-parietal pial and intraventricular choroid angiomatosis in a patient with seizures and encephalotrigeminal angiomatosis.

NEUROFIBROMATOSIS

Two main forms of neurofibromatosis have been characterized (see Chapter 10). The most common form is neurofibromatosis type 1 (NF1), also called von Recklinghausen disease, with an incidence of 1 in 3,000 to 4,000 persons. It is caused by defects in the NF1 gene on chromosome 17 and is inherited in an autosomal dominant fashion, although 50% of cases are related to spontaneous mutations (58). This protean disorder has a multitude of clinical manifestations, and CNS lesions occur in up to 15% of cases (43). These include gliomas of the optic pathways, other intracranial gliomas, myelin vacuolization, cerebrovascular abnormalities, sphenoid wing dysplasia, plexiform neurofibromas, hydrocephalus, and macrocephaly. Spinal manifestations include kyphoscoliosis, dural ectasia, and paraspinal neurofibromas (59). MRI is the modality of choice for evaluating CNS pathology in neurofibromatosis patients.

Gliomas of the optic pathways are the most common intracranial tumor in NF1. These gliomas are typically low grade, can occur anywhere along the optic pathway, and can be unilateral or bilateral. They manifest as enlargement of the optic nerves and/or chiasm, and on MRI are hypointense on T1-weighted sequences, with variable contrast enhancement, and hyperintense on T2-weighted sequences (59). Gliomas may also occur in the brainstem, cerebellum, or elsewhere in the brain or spinal cord, and are most often of the low-grade pilocytic subtype (60). Foci of increased signal intensity on T2-weighted images constitute another common imaging finding in NF1 patients. Seen in 43% to 93% of patients, these lesions are found bilaterally in the cerebellum, basal ganglia, brainstem, and thalami. They do not enhance with contrast, and correspond pathologically to areas of intramyelinic vacuolar or spongiotic change (61,62). MRS may be useful in distinguishing these benign hyperintense foci from low-grade gliomas, which can have similar imaging characteristics (58,59).

Neurofibromatosis type 2 (NF2) is 10 times less common than NF1 and is related to defects on chromosome 22, which are transmitted in an autosomal dominant pattern (60).

The hallmark of this disease is the development of bilateral acoustic schwannomas, eventually seen in nearly all patients, presenting with hearing loss, tinnitus, or balance dysfunction. Multiple additional schwannomas, gliomas, meningiomas, and ependymomas can also occur in the brain and spine, and cataracts may be present. Indeed, the presence of meningioma in a child should prompt consideration of NF2 as a diagnosis. In contrast to NF1, skeletal dysplasias, learning disabilities, and skin manifestations are uncommon (59,60).

STURGE-WEBER SYNDROME

Sturge-Weber syndrome, or encephalo-trigeminal angiomatosis, is a rare congenital condition (1 in 40,000) of uncertain etiology or inheritance (58). It is characterized by intracranial leptomeningeal and choroid angiomatosis, abnormal deep venous drainage, and progressive atrophy of the affected cerebral hemisphere(s) (Fig. 2.12) (63). Most often there is an associated facial angioma, or port-wine stain, in the ophthalmic division of the trigeminal nerve distribution ipsilaterally. Ocular manifestations include choroidal angiomas and congenital glaucoma, or buphthalmos. Patients present clinically with intractable seizures, headaches, strokelike episodes, hemiparesis, mental retardation, and visual defects (64). The principal imaging findings include cerebral atrophy and cortical calcification underlying the leptomeningeal angioma. Calcification is best seen on CT and classically appears as parallel, "tram-track" cortical calcifications of the affected parietal and occipital lobes. Angiomatosis of the chorioid plexus within the ipsilateral lateral ventricle may be seen. MRI is superior to CT for demonstrating the extent of superficial enhancement related to the leptomeningeal angioma (43,58).

TUBEROUS SCLEROSIS

Tuberous sclerosis is an autosomal dominant disease related to genetic alterations on chromosomes 9 and 16 (see Chapter 10). Its prevalence is approximately 1 in 6,000 to 10,000 births, and the majority of cases are due to sporadic mutations (58). The "classic" clinical triad of tuberous sclerosis, consisting of seizures, mental retardation, and facial angiofibroma (sometimes referred to as adenoma sebaceum), is seen in only one third of patients. TS is a complex, multifarious disorder that can affect nearly any organ system. Intracranially, the characteristic lesions are cortical and subcortical hamartomas ("tubers") and subependymal nodules. Cortical hamartomas may appear as enlarged, abnormally shaped gyri, whereas subcortical hamartomas demonstrate abnormally increased signal on T2-weighted images in the subcortical white matter. Subependymal nodules line the ependymal surfaces and protrude into the ventricles. These lesions have a variable MRI appearance depending on patient age and lesion composition. They often calcify, which is best demonstrated by CT, or can be seen on MRI as areas of low signal intensity on T2-weighted images (58,63). Subependymal nodules may or may not enhance on MRI, a distinction bearing no clinical significance (63). Up to 15% of TS patients are at risk for developing a subependymal giant cell astrocytoma. These low-grade tumors usually develop near the foramen of Monro, progressively enlarge, and may cause obstructive hydrocephalus (43,63).

Neuroimaging plays an important role in the diagnosis and management of tuberous sclerosis. Current recommendations are for cranial imaging with CT or MRI every 1 to 3 years in children with TS, to detect complications (65). In addition, MRS and perfusion imaging can be helpful in distinguishing between benign hamartomas and neoplasms. Other specialized MRI techniques as well as PET imaging have shown promise for determining which brain lesions are epileptogenic so that they may be removed surgically (43,66).

VON HIPPEL-LINDAU DISEASE

Von Hippel-Lindau disease (VHL), also known as CNS angiomatosis, is an autosomal dominant disorder that has been traced to gene defects on chromosome 3. As with other phakomatoses, VHL affects multiple organ systems, but the hallmark feature in the CNS is the development of hemangioblastomas of the brain, spine, and retina. In the retina, a unique feature of these lesions is calcification. In the brain, hemangioblastomas are most frequently found in the cerebellum. On imaging, these benign tumors may appear as completely solid lesions, or more often as an enhancing tumor nodule within a large cyst in the cerebellar hemisphere (43). MRI may reveal evidence of hemorrhage as well as serpiginous structures of low signal intensity related to flow within enlarged blood vessels. Spinal hemangioblastomas have similar imaging characteristics and may be accompanied by significant edema as well as syringohydromyelia (63). Patients usually present clinically in the second to third decade of life, most often with symptoms caused by retinal angiomas, such as visual dysfunction, pain, or retinal detachment. Patients may also develop symptoms of cerebellar dysfunction or increased intracranial pressure secondary to cerebellar tumors, causing mass effect and hydrocephalus. Rarely, patients may present with deafness resulting from endolymphatic sac tumors that occur in up to 10% of VHL patients (43,58).

Vascular Malformations

Intracerebral vascular malformations may be categorized into four main types: arteriovenous malformations (AVMs), cavernous malformations, venous malformations, and capillary telangiectasias. Of these, AVMs are the most likely to cause neurological complications, due to mass effect and their propensity to bleed (43) (Fig. 2.13). Patients may present with seizures, headaches, focal neurological deficits, hydrocephalus, or hemorrhage. AVMs represent abnormal connections between arteries and veins without intervening capillaries, but with intervening normal brain parenchyma. As such, they appear on MRI as a tangle of serpiginous structures with signal void due to flow. There may be associated hemorrhage that acutely is hyperdense on noncontrast CT and has characteristic MRI appearances depending on its stage.

Cavernous malformations, or cavernomas, represent collections of dilated vascular sinusoids without intervening normal brain parenchyma. These slow-flow lesions are prone to repeated bouts of hemorrhage, although most episodes are subclinical and many cavernomas are discovered incidentally (43). The presence of different stages of blood within these lesions accounts for their variable, mixed signal intensity on noncontrast T1- and T2-weighed MRI pulse sequences.

Venous malformations, known as developmental venous anomalies (DVAs) or venous angiomas, are composed of abnormal medullary or subcortical veins that converge into a single prominent vein. This configuration gives them a distinctive appearance on MRI or catheter angiography which has been likened to a "caput medusa." They rarely bleed and are almost always asymptomatic and incidentally discovered. Capillary telangiectasias are clusters of dilated capillaries separated by normal brain parenchyma. These lesions most often occur in the brainstem and do not hemorrhage (43). They demonstrate increased signal on T2-weighted MRI and may faintly enhance.

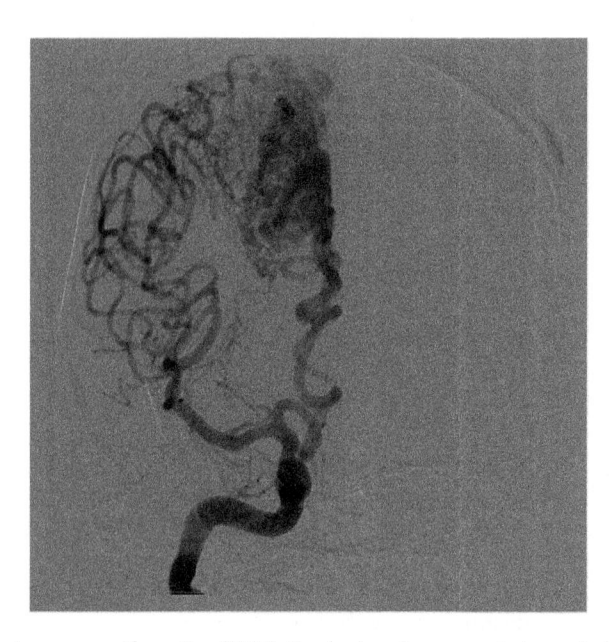

■ **FIGURE 2.13** Arteriovenous malformation (AVM). Cerebral angiogram, anterior-posterior (AP) view demonstrates frontal AVM supplied by the anterior cerebral artery, with arteriovenous (A-V) shunting into the superior sagittal sinus.

Vascular Occlusive Disease

Ischemic stroke in children has become increasingly recognized over the last several decades, likely due in part to improved awareness, better diagnostic techniques, and improved survival of children with predisposing conditions. The incidence is now reported to be between 3 and 8 per 100,000 children per year (67). Whereas in adults the overwhelming cause of arterial ischemic stroke is atherosclerosis, in children the risk factors are manifold and often multiple. The single most common underlying disorder is congenital heart disease (68). Other common causes include vasculopathies of many types, including transient cerebral arteriopathy of childhood, basal occlusive disease with (moya moya) or without telangiectasia, post-varicella angiopathy, and thrombophlebitis associated with meningitis or other infections. Vasculitis may also be associated with systemic diseases such as Takayasu arteritis, polyarteritis nodosa, juvenile rheumatoid arthritis, and inflammatory bowel disease. Intravascular disorders such as sickle cell disease, platelet disorders, iron deficiency anemia, and prothrombotic states are additional important risk factors (68,69). Arterial dissection can cause strokes and is frequently associated with trauma. Finally, cerebral infarction (often hemorrhagic) may occur secondary to cortical venous and dural sinus thrombosis. Risk factors for venous thrombosis include head and neck infections, trauma, dehydration, sepsis, and prothrombotic conditions.

Regardless of etiology, most cerebral infarctions in children (excluding neonates for the purposes of this discussion) share similar CT and MRI characteristics. On CT, an acute stroke is most often seen as an area of hypodensity conforming to a vascular distribution, involving both cortex and white matter, with obscuration of the gray-white interface due to edema in the affected area. Subtle mass effect with sulcal and/or ventricular effacement can be detected. MRI can detect an acute infarct within minutes or hours of its occurrence by applying DWI, which shows the infarct as an area of hyperintensity. As time goes on, the infarct will become increasingly hyperintense on T2-weighted and fluid-attenuated inversion recovery (FLAIR) images. In the subacute phase (i.e., approximately 5 days to 4 weeks), the infarct will show gyral enhancement, related to breakdown of the blood-brain barrier in the affected area. Prior to this, in the more acute phases, intravascular and meningeal enhancement is seen in the region of the infarct. Chronic infarcts appear as porencephaly with focal atrophy, and have signal characteristics approximating CSF (hypointense on T1-weighted and hyperintense on T2-weighted images). MRA and CTA, in addition to conventional catheter angiography, are important techniques for investigating vascular occlusive disease in children (Fig. 2.14).

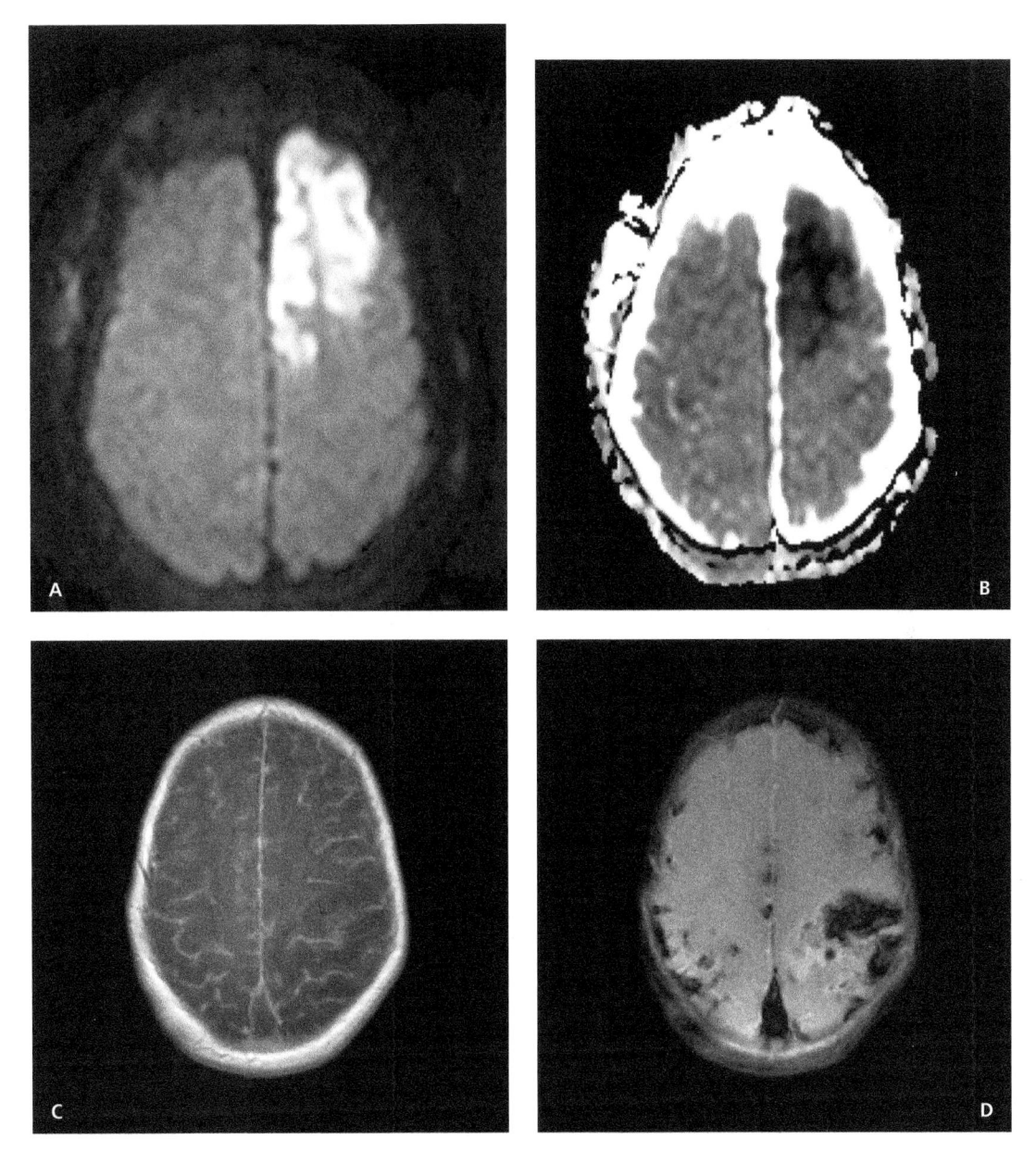

■ **FIGURE 2.14 A** and **B:** Arterial infarction. Axial MR diffusion weighted image (DWI) **(A)** demonstrates restricted diffusion within an acute anterior cerebral artery distribution infarct due to traumatic arterial occlusion in a 9-year-old. Low signal on the ADC map confirms the finding **(B)**. **C** and **D:** Venous infarction. Axial contrast-enhanced T1 MRI **(C)** demonstrates thrombosis of the sagittal sinus; bilateral hemorrhagic venous infarction is best seen on the gradient echo scan **(D)**.

Central Nervous System Infection

Neuroimaging plays an important role in the diagnosis and management of pediatric CNS infection and its complications. Meningitis, in the setting of otitis media, sinusitis, or other systemic infections, may result in communicating or obstructive hydrocephalus, subdural effusion (common with *Haemophilus influenzae*), empyema (subdural or epidural), cerebritis, cerebral abscess, ventriculitis, sinus thrombosis, and venous or arterial infarction. Brain imaging is often performed preliminary to a lumbar puncture and should be carefully reviewed for parameningeal sources of infection, as well as early complications. Regardless of modality, intravenous contrast is useful in the evaluation of infection (Fig. 2.15). Although CT is often more accessible, more amenable to critical care monitoring of the septic child, and more tolerant of sporadic motion, new, fast MRI sequences are available that allow for effective and efficient follow-up examinations for chronic conditions such as hydrocephalus. MRI is more sensitive to early or subtle edema and acute ischemia as well as vascular patency.

Some infections have characteristic, even if not specific, imaging findings. Tuberculous meningitis, for example, has a predilection for the basal cisterns. Herpes encephalitis involves the medial temporal lobes, cingulate gyrus. and insular cortex. Although petechial hemorrhage may be seen in pathological specimens, it is not always apparent on imaging studies. Human immunodeficiency virus (HIV) infection in children results in basal ganglia calcification and cerebral atrophy. Progressive multifocal leukoencephalopathy (PML) may occur in these and other immunocompromised children. In the HIV-positive pediatric population, intracranial masses are more commonly lymphoma than toxoplasmosis or cryptococcal infection. Cysticercosis lesions, which may result in seizures, typically measure approximately 1 cm and are cystic, with calcification present once the organism dies. The lesions may be parenchymal, intraventricular, or within the subarachnoid space or may present as racemose cysts at the skull base.

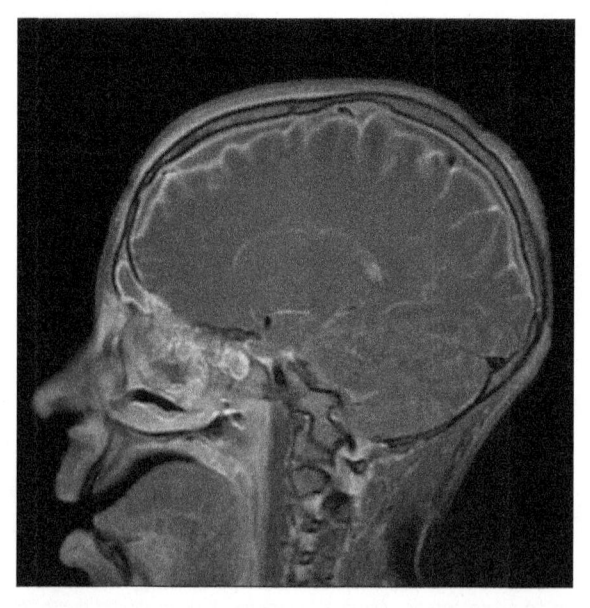

■ **FIGURE 2.15** Complications of frontal sinus infection. Sagittal T1 contrast-enhanced MRI (with fat saturation) demonstrates rim-enhancing frontal, ethmoid, and maxillary sinus infection with epidural empyema.

Metabolic and White Matter Disorders

WHITE MATTER DISEASES

White matter disease processes are typically classified as demyelinating, wherein normal myelin is formed, and is subsequently destroyed, and dysmyelinating, where there is failure of normal myelin formation. MRI best detects and differentiates among these diseases (70).

Demyelination may occur as a parainfectious process, typically following a viral illness. This entity, known as acute disseminated encephalomyelitis (ADEM), may involve the brain and spinal cord, as its name implies. ADEM is typically a monophasic illness in which symptoms resolve in the majority of cases (43). Multiple sclerosis (MS), by comparison, is a primary demyelinating process that is more common in adults than in childhood, wherein it occurs mainly in adolescents (71) (see Chapter 15). In this population it is more prevalent in females and frequently affects the infratentorial white mater and spinal cord (72,73) (Fig. 2.16). Neuromyelitis optica, also known as Devic disease, is distinct from MS and consists of optic neuritis in combination with extensive spinal cord involvement over three or more segments.

Dysmyelinating diseases include Alexander disease and Canavan disease, both of which present with macrocephaly, and are differentiated by brainstem involvement in Canavan disease and frontal predominance in Alexander disease. Normocephalic dysmyelinating diseases include Krabbe disease and metachromatic leukodystrophy. Adrenoleukodystrophy has both demyelinating and dysmyelinating features. It characteristically occurs in young males and involves the occipital white matter. The splenium of the corpus callosum, cerebral peduncles, and cerebellar white matter may also be affected. MRI is the imaging modality of choice in the evaluation of white matter disease. Gadolinium contrast is useful in monitoring active demyelination, as are advanced MRI techniques such as spectroscopy, DTI, and fMRI.

Posterior reversible encephalopathy syndrome (PRES) may occur in children and adolescents, particularly in the setting of immunosuppressive therapy or with renal failure in combination with hypertension. Seizure, headache, altered mental status, and cortical blindness are common presenting symptoms, related to the typical occipital and parietal location of lesions. Imaging findings consist of white and gray matter edema affecting the parietal and occipital lobes, and less frequently the frontal and temporal lobes, cerebellum, brainstem, and basal ganglia. The clinical signs and symptoms and the imaging findings are reversible (74).

METABOLIC DISORDERS

The hallmark of metabolic disorders on neuroimaging examinations is the symmetry of findings. These entities are usually diagnosed early, and include phenylketonuria (PKU) and certain mucopolysaccharidoses (types I, II, III, and VII).

Basal ganglia involvement is common in Leigh disease, Wilson disease, and mitochondrial encephalomyopathies. Whereas the CT finding of symmetrical basal ganglia hypodensity is similar in these diseases, MRI better differentiates among them based on the distribution of hyperintense signal on T2-weighted imaging. Leigh disease involves the putamen, globus pallidus, and caudate, in addition to the periaqueductal gray matter (75). Wilson disease may affect the thalami and, less often, the white matter. Mitochondrial disorders demonstrate atrophy and white matter lesions, beyond the basal ganglia involvement.

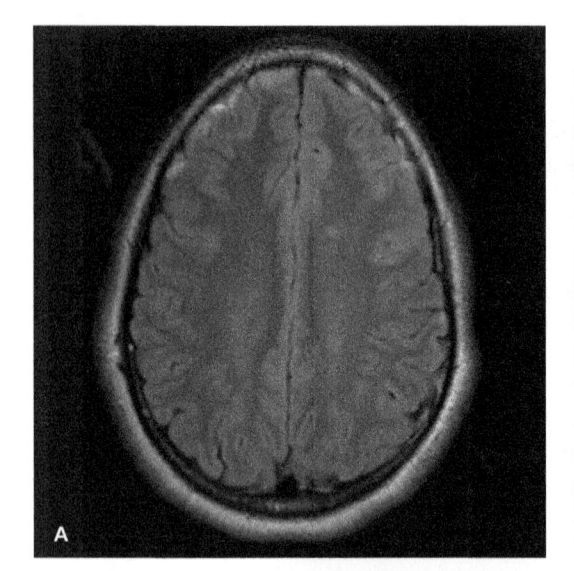

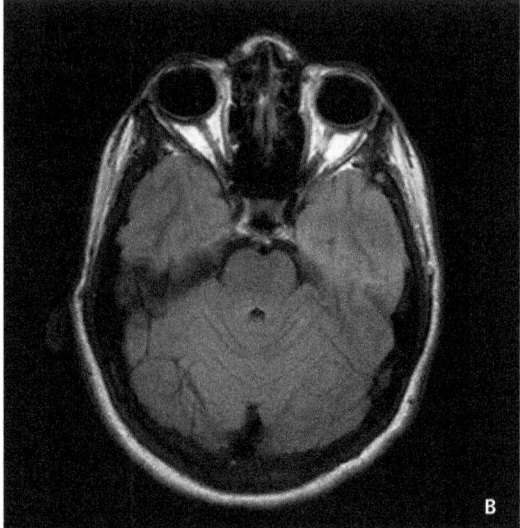

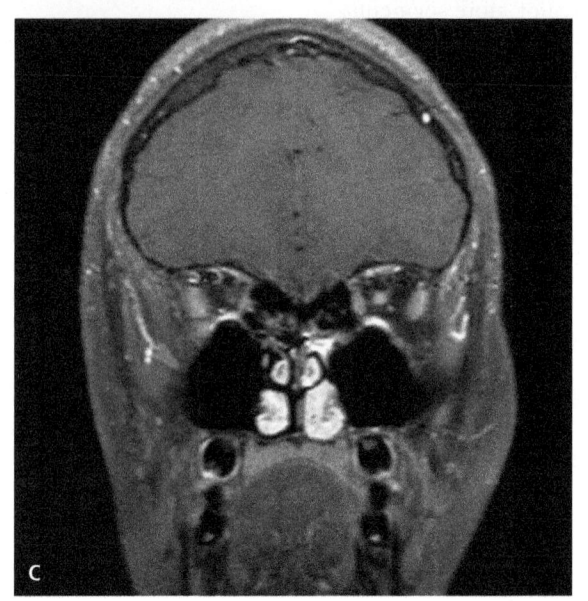

■ **FIGURE 2.16** Demyelinating disease. Axial fluid-attenuated inversion recovery (FLAIR) images demonstrate a punctate periventricular white matter lesion **(A)** and abnormal signal within the left optic nerve **(B)**, which enhances with contrast on the coronal T1 contrast-enhanced MRI **(C)**.

Congenital Anomalies

Congenital anomalies may result in developmental delay, mental retardation, or seizures. In defining most congenital anomalies, MRI is the imaging modality of choice, given its multiplanar capability and better contrast resolution between white and gray matter, which is particularly important in imaging migrational disorders. These disorders include gray matter heterotopia, schizencephaly, lissencephaly, pachygyria, and polymicrogyria. Heterotopic gray matter appears normal in signal and enhancement characteristics but is in an abnormal location, classified as subependymal, subcortical, and band

(76). Heterotopia may be seen in isolation or associated with other anomalies, such as schizencephaly and agenesis of the corpus callosum. Schizencephaly is defined by a gray-matter–lined cleft extending from the cortex to the ventricle through the affected hemisphere. It is classified as open or closed lip and may be bilateral. Agenesis of the corpus callosum is best detected by MRI, as are its associated anomalies, when present. In addition to gray matter heterotopia, these associated anomalies include Dandy Walker malformation and callosum lipoma.

Lissencephaly, or "smooth brain," may refer to cases of agyria (absent gyri) or pachygyria, with few, broad gyri present. In addition, the brain may have a "figure of eight" or hourglass shape (Fig. 2.17). Polymicrogyria may be confused with pachygyria on neuroimaging, due to the multiple, difficult-to-detect convolutions in the cortex.

Holoprosencephaly, resulting from incomplete division of the developing brain, is classified—in order of increasing severity—as lobar, semilobar, and alobar (Fig. 2.18). All types have a monoventricle in common, due to absence of the septum. Other midline anomalies, including facial clefts, may be present. The lobar form may be difficult to differentiate from septo-optic dysplasia, which is distinguished by optic nerve atrophy.

The Dandy Walker syndrome is defined by a posterior fossa cyst in communication with the fourth ventricle, due to absence of the cerebellar vermis. The term Dandy Walker variant refers to only partial absence of the vermis, inferiorly. This should not be confused with a large cisterna magna or with a posterior fossa arachnoid cyst.

Chiari malformations, type I, may present with headache, typically unrelated to hydrocephalus, which is more common in Chiari type II malformations. The fourth ventricle is normal in size and position in type I and is small and low lying in the type II malformation, in which hydrocephalus occurs frequently. MRI is the imaging modality of choice for providing CSF flow information for type I and for defining the cranial and spinal features (lumbosacral myelomeningocele) for type II, as needed.

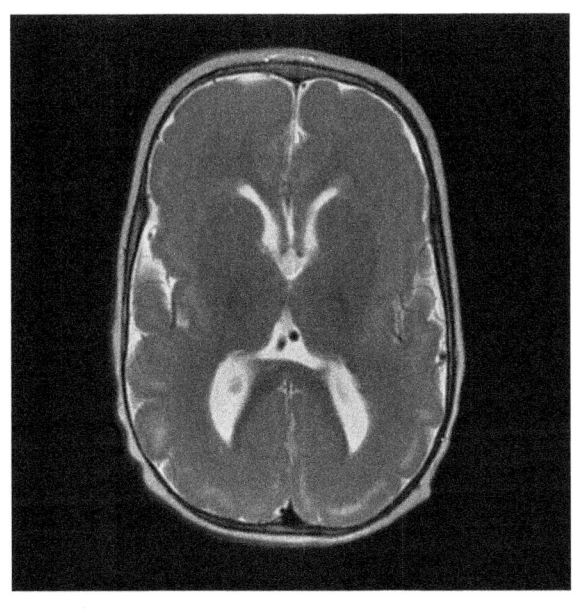

■ **FIGURE 2.17** Lissencephaly. Axial T2 MRI demonstrates "smooth brain" with almost no sulci in a 1-year-old child.

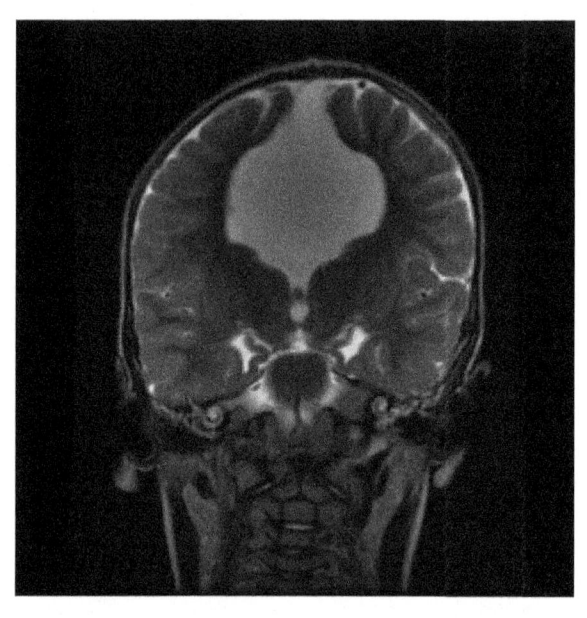

■ FIGURE 2.18 Holoprosencephaly. Coronal T2 MRI demonstrates a monoventricle, due to absent septum in a child with lobar holoprosencephaly.

Neuroimaging in Specific Neuropsychiatric Disorders

To date, most research on brain imaging in specific psychiatric disorders has taken place in adults. As previously discussed, radiological imaging of children, especially for research, entails practical and ethical considerations that have complicated investigations. Although many chronic psychiatric disorders are thought to have roots in childhood and adolescence, little is yet known about normal brain development. This lack of knowledge hinders attempts to identify abnormalities and untangle the complex interplay among cause, effect, and compensatory response (77). The interpretation of neuroimaging studies in children is complicated by significant differences in brain attributes based on gender and physiological maturation, by variation in body and brain structure size, and by the existence of variables such as handedness, intelligence, socioeconomic status, comorbid illness, and medical treatment (78,79). In addition, study design has suffered from small sample size, limited comparison with healthy controls, variation in image acquisition techniques, lack of standardized measurement methods, and differences in data interpretation and analysis (78). As a result of these challenges, reported findings are often confusing or contradictory, making it difficult to arrive at generalizations.

Therefore, neuroimaging research has not yet reached the point where it directly offers meaningful guidance in the diagnosis or clinical management of major childhood psychiatric disorders (80). Imaging research does, however, encourage basic scientists and clinicians to ground theories of disease in neuroscience and enables the refinement of animal models of disease, greatly facilitating further basic research and pharmaceutical development (80). Discovery of brain abnormalities associated with psychopathology may allow for the identification of biological subgroups, thereby suggesting targeted treatments, and functional imaging may permit precise measurement of treatment effects. These strategies are especially important when considering such heterogeneous conditions as attention deficit disorder and autism (81). Furthermore, as the molecular basis underlying disease processes becomes better understood, molecular imaging may take the lead in the diagnosis and management of neuropsychiatric syndromes.

CHILDHOOD-ONSET SCHIZOPHRENIA

Childhood-onset schizophrenia (COS) is more rare than the adult form and results in more severe symptoms and brain abnormalities but generally follows the same morphological trends. Studies of children and adolescents with COS have revealed differences in the size of various brain structures, with most studies showing decreases in right and left hemispheres as well as total brain volumes. The whole-brain volume decrease is of greater magnitude in COS than in adult schizophrenia, and larger reductions in volume appear to correlate with increased severity of negative symptoms as measured by the Scale for the Assessment of Negative Symptoms (81,82). Other structural findings include an increase in basal ganglia size, which may result from neuroleptic exposure, ventricular enlargement, decreased midsagittal thalamic area, and smaller volumes of the vermis and inferior posterior lobe of the cerebellum (79). In addition, a decrease in overall cortical thickness and cortical loss localizing to the prefrontal and temporal regions with increasing age has been reported (83). MRS has shown lower N-acetylaspartate/creatine ratios in the bilateral frontal lobes, specifically the dorsolateral prefrontal cortex, and the hippocampal area, suggesting neuronal damage or dysfunction in these regions (79).

ATTENTION DEFICIT HYPERACTIVITY DISORDER

Attention deficit hyperactivity disorder (ADHD) is thought to involve both structural and functional brain abnormalities, particularly within the frontostriatal structures. Functional imaging studies have supported this hypothesis, showing consistent patterns of hypofunction in the dorsal anterior cingulate cortex, lateral prefrontal cortex, and striatum (84,85). These abnormalities may be a consequence of extrinsic developmental events as well as related to aberrant brain development. Evidence suggests that abnormally low functional activity within the vermis, as demonstrated on fMRI, may be a consequence of psychological trauma in early development (86,87). More widespread structural changes have also been described, including smaller total cerebral volumes, smaller total white matter volumes in unmedicated children, and smaller volumes of the dorsolateral prefrontal cortex, the basal ganglia, corpus callosum, and cerebellum (88,89).

AUTISM

To date, neuroimaging studies of children with autism have yielded an assortment of discrepant results, likely due to the heterogeneity of the disorder, significant differences in study design, and the inclusion of adults and children within the same study groups (79,90). The most consistently reported finding is increased total brain volume and increased total lateral ventricle volume, although there is disagreement whether this is restricted to early childhood or is also seen in adults (91). Some investigators have described decreased volume in various parts of the corpus callosum and cerebellum, whereas others have not (81). Functional imaging studies have shown hypoperfusion of the bilateral temporal lobes in autistic children, as well as abnormal patterns of cortical activation (92). However, the clinical utility of these findings is limited, and the AAN has published a practice parameter stating that "[t]here is no clinical evidence to support the role of routine clinical neuroimaging in the diagnostic evaluation of autism, even in the presence of megalencephaly" (93).

RETT SYNDROME

Rett syndrome (RTT) is a progressive neurodevelopmental disorder predominantly affecting female children. These children develop normally from birth until they begin to regress. Classic features include cognitive impairment, deficits in communication, stereotypical movements, and growth failure. The disease is associated with a mutation of the MECP2 gene located on the X chromosome. However, of those affected by RTT, not all carry the MECP2 gene, and not all carriers of the gene are affected. Variable expression related to X-chromosome inactivation and association with other mutations is the prevailing explanation for this phenomenon. Dawna Duncan Armstrong, of Baylor College of Medicine, Houston, Texas, describes RTT as a disorder of development "in the function, structure, and chemistry of neurons . . . caused by MECP2 deficiency." Clinical, neuropathological, and neuroimaging studies have shown that there is an early and marked decrease in brain and cerebral size in RTT (94). Recent evidence suggests that selective reductions of dorsal parietal gray matter and preservation of the occipital cortex are basic neuroanatomical features of RTT, whereas preferential reduction of the anterior frontal lobe appears to be a correlate of clinical severity in this disorder. The most affected brain regions include those that may underlie key functional deficits observed in RTT (95).

AFFECTIVE DISORDERS

Children and adolescents with depressive disorders have demonstrated decreased frontal lobe volumes and increased lateral ventricle volumes relative to total cerebral volume (96). Functional imaging of depressed adolescents, using single photon emission computed tomography (SPECT), has shown alterations of regional cerebral blood flow (rCBF), with increased relative rCBF in the right mesial temporal cortex (including the amygdala) and parts of the bilateral temporal lobes, and decreased rCBF in the left parietal lobe, anterior thalamus, and right caudate (97). MRS studies have measured higher Ch/Cr ratios in the orbitofrontal cortex of depressed adolescents relative to healthy adolescents, and fMRI studies have demonstrated decreased amygdala responses to fearful faces in depressed children (97).

Studies of bipolar disorder in children are limited. There is evidence that pediatric bipolar disease is associated with white matter signal hyperintensity in cortical and subcortical regions, although this is a nonspecific finding. Some studies have found smaller amygdala sizes in bipolar children compared with adults (98). Asymmetry of the amygdala, hippocampus, and cingulate gyrus has been reported, in association with decreased fractional anisotropy in several subcortical regions, using DTI (99,100). fMRI studies suggest a range of abnormal patterns of brain activation, and MRS data indicate alterations in N-acetylaspartate creatine ratios, glutamate/glutamine ratios, and myoinositol levels in various parts of the brain (98). However, more work in these areas is needed before meaningful conclusions can be drawn.

OBSESSIVE-COMPULSIVE DISORDER

Positron emission tomography of patients with obsessive-compulsive disorder (OCD) demonstrates patterns of hypermetabolism in orbitofrontal, anterior cingulate, thalamic, and caudate regions. The hypermetabolism in some of these regions is attenuated when OCD symptoms are treated (101). Pediatric patients may also have a decrease in striatal volumes and an increase in total corpus callosum area, but results are not consistent across all studies (102).

TOURETTE SYNDROME

Structural neuroimaging studies of children with Tourette syndrome have shown an increase in area of several parts of the corpus callosum and enlarged prefrontal cortical volumes, particularly in younger children (103). Studies of normal controls have reported asymmetry of the basal ganglia (left greater than right), and several early studies suggested that Tourette syndrome patients demonstrated reduction or reversal of this normal asymmetry (104,105). However, a more recent, larger study by Peterson et al. (106) did not find aberrant basal ganglia asymmetry in Tourette syndrome patients; they did, however, show a significant reduction in caudate nucleus volume. A study of monozygotic twins with discordant severity of symptoms also found reduced caudate volumes in the more severely affected twin, raising the possibility of nongenetic factors contributing to observed morphological changes (81). Most functional studies have been limited to adult patients (103), but some PET evidence may implicate abnormal dopamine function in the caudate nucleus and midbrain in adolescents with Tourette syndrome (97).

Questions

1. Which imaging modality provides the best tissue contrast without exposure to ionizing radiation, making it the best pediatric neuroimaging modality in most cases?
   A. CT
   B. skull radiographs
   C. MRI
   D. ultrasound

2. Regarding a child with recurrent headaches, which of the following is true?
   A. Neuroimaging must be performed in all cases.
   B. The headaches are most likely due to a ruptured intracranial aneurysm.
   C. A negative CT scan excludes intracranial hemorrhage.
   D. Neuroimaging is unlikely to yield clinically significant findings if the neurological examination is normal.

3. Which of the following is true regarding child abuse?
   A. In the appropriate clinical setting, bilateral subdural hemorrhages of mixed density can be suggestive of abuse.
   B. Neuroimaging alone can be diagnostic of child abuse.
   C. MRI is superior to CT for demonstrating bony detail.
   D. Shear injuries to the brain are less likely to occur in children compared with adults.

4. What is the most common type of pediatric brain neoplasm overall?
   A. atypical teratoid/rhabdoid tumor
   B. pineoblastoma
   C. astrocytoma
   D. ependymoma

5. Which of the following statements is false?
   A. In general, CT scanning is faster and better tolerated than MR scanning.
   B. Exposure to ionizing radiation is less of a concern in children compared with adults, because children are relatively less radiosensitive and receive relatively lower doses for a given examination.
   C. Neuroimaging should be performed in cases of trauma when there is an abnormal neurological examination or evidence of skull fracture.
   D. MRI is superior to CT in the evaluation of posterior fossa lesions.

6. True or False: Generally speaking, current neuroimaging techniques yield results that are highly sensitive and specific for most neuropsychiatric disorders.
   A. True
   B. False

Answers

1. C
2. D
3. A
4. C
5. B
6. B

REFERENCES

1. Brenner DJ, Hall EJ. Computed tomography-an increasing source of radiation exposure. *N Engl J Med.* 2007;357:2277-2284.
2. Hoffman JM, Gambhir SS. Molecular imaging: the vision and opportunity for radiology in the future. *Radiology.* 2007;244:39-47.
3. Mettler FA Jr, et al. CT scanning: patterns of use and dose. *J Radiol Prot.* 2000;20:353-359.
4. Brenner DJ. Estimating cancer risks from pediatric CT: going from the qualitative to the quantitative. *Pediatr Radiol.* 2002;32:228-223; discussion 242-244.
5. Zammit-Maempel I, Chadwick CL, Willis SP. Radiation dose to the lens of eye and thyroid gland in paranasal sinus multislice CT. *Br J Radiol.* 2003;76:418-420.
6. Brenner D, Elliston C, Hall E, Berdon W. Estimated risks of radiation-induced fatal cancer from pediatric CT. *AJR Am J Roentgenol.* 2001;176:289-296.
7. Haaga JR. Radiation dose management: weighing risk versus benefit. *AJR Am J Roentgenol.* 2001;177:289-291.
8. Lewis DW, et al; Quality Standards Subcommittee of the American Academy of Neurology; Practice Committee of the Child Neurology Society. Practice parameter: evaluation of children and adolescents with recurrent headaches: report of the Quality Standards Subcommittee of the American Academy of Neurology and the Practice Committee of the Child Neurology Society. *Neurology.* 2002;59:490-498.
9. Medina LS, D'Souza B, Vasconcellos E. Adults and children with headache: evidence-based diagnostic evaluation. *Neuroimaging Clin North Am.* 2003;13:225-235.
10. Burton LJ, et al. Headache etiology in a pediatric emergency department. *Pediatr Emerg Care.* 1997;13:1-4.
11. Punt J. Surgical management of paediatric stroke. *Pediatr Radiol.* 2004;34:16-23.
12. Huang J, et al. Intracranial aneurysms in the pediatric population: case series and literature review. *Surg Neurol.* 2005;63:424-432.
13. Warden CR, et al. Evaluation and management of febrile seizures in the out-of-hospital and emergency department settings. *Ann Emerg Med.* 2003;41:215-222.
14. [No authors listed]. Practice parameter: the neurodiagnostic evaluation of the child with a first simple febrile seizure. American Academy of Pediatrics. Provisional Committee on Quality Improvement, Subcommittee on Febrile Seizures. *Pediatrics.* 1996;97:769-772.
15. Hirtz D, et al. Practice parameter: evaluating a first nonfebrile seizure in children: report of the quality standards subcommittee of the American Academy of Neurology, The Child Neurology Society, and The American Epilepsy Society. *Neurology.* 2000;55:616-623.
16. Harden CL, et al. Reassessment: neuroimaging in the emergency patient presenting with seizure (an evidence-based review): report of the Therapeutics and Technology Assessment Subcommittee of the American Academy of Neurology. *Neurology.* 2007;69:1772-1780.
17. Riviello JJ Jr, et al; American Academy of Neurology Subcommittee; Practice Committee of the Child Neurology Society. Practice parameter: diagnostic assessment of the child with status epilepticus (an evidence-based review): report of the Quality Standards Subcommittee of the American Academy of Neurology and the Practice Committee of the Child Neurology Society. *Neurology.* 2006;67:1542-1550.
18. Schutzman SA, Greenes DS. Pediatric minor head trauma. *Ann Emerg Med.* 2001;37:65-74.
19. [No authors listed]. The management of minor closed head injury in children. Committee on Quality Improvement, American Academy of Pediatrics. Commission on Clinical Policies and Research, American Academy of Family Physicians. *Pediatrics.* 1999;104:1407-1415.
20. [No authors listed]. Practice parameter: the management of concussion in sports (summary statement). Report of the Quality Standards Subcommittee. *Neurology.* 1997;48:581-585.
21. Savitsky EA, Votey SR. Current controversies in the management of minor pediatric head injuries. *Am J Emerg Med.* 2000;18:96-101.
22. Gordon KE. Pediatric minor traumatic brain injury. *Semin Pediatr Neurol.* 2006;13:243-255.
23. Ashwal S, Holshouser BA, Tong KA. Use of advanced neuroimaging techniques in the evaluation of pediatric traumatic brain injury. *Dev Neurosci.* 2006;28:309-326.
24. Sigmund GA, et al. Multimodality comparison of neuroimaging in pediatric traumatic brain injury. *Pediatr Neurol.* 2007;36:217-226.

25. Mannion RJ, et al. Mechanism-based MRI classification of traumatic brainstem injury and its relationship to outcome. *J Neurotrauma.* 2007;24:128-135.
26. Bremner JD. Neuroimaging of childhood trauma. *Semin Clin Neuropsychiatry.* 2002;7(2):104-112.
27. Keenan HT, et al. A population-based study of inflicted traumatic brain injury in young children. *JAMA.* 2003;290:621-626.
28. Bruce DA, Zimmerman RA. Shaken impact syndrome. *Pediatr Ann.* 1989;18:482-484, 486-489, 492-494.
29. Case ME. Abusive head injuries in infants and young children. *Leg Med (Tokyo).* 2007; 9(2):83-87.
30. Duhaime AC, et al. The shaken baby syndrome. A clinical, pathological, and biomechanical study. *J Neurosurg.* 1987;66:409-415.
31. Duhaime AC, et al. Nonaccidental head injury in infants—the "shaken-baby syndrome". *N Engl J Med.* 1998;338:1822-1829.
32. Gean AD. Pediatric trauma. In: *Imaging of Head Trauma.* New York: Raven Press; 1994.
33. Tung GA, et al. Comparison of accidental and nonaccidental traumatic head injury in children on noncontrast computed tomography. *Pediatrics.* 2006;118:626-633.
34. Caffey J. On the theory and practice of shaking infants. Its potential residual effects of permanent brain damage and mental retardation. *Am J Dis Child.* 1972;124:161-169.
35. Caffey J. The whiplash shaken infant syndrome: manual shaking by the extremities with whiplash-induced intracranial and intraocular bleedings, linked with residual permanent brain damage and mental retardation. *Pediatrics.* 1974;54:396-403.
36. Zimmerman RA, et al. Computed tomography of craniocerebral injury in the abused child. *Radiology.* 1979;130:687-690.
37. Vinchon M, et al. Accidental and nonaccidental head injuries in infants: a prospective study. *J Neurosurg.* 2005;102(4 suppl):380-384.
38. Stoodley N. Neuroimaging in non-accidental head injury: if, when, why and how. *Clin Radiol.* 2005;60:22-30.
39. Rosemberg S, Fujiwara D. Epidemiology of pediatric tumors of the nervous system according to the WHO 2000 classification: a report of 1,195 cases from a single institution. *Childs Nerv Syst.* 2005;21:940-944.
40. Kramer ED, et al. Comparison of myelography with CT follow-up versus gadolinium MRI for subarachnoid metastatic disease in children. *Neurology.* 1991;41:46-50.
41. Blews DE, et al. Intradural spinal metastases in pediatric patients with primary intracranial neoplasms: Gd-DTPA enhanced MR vs CT myelography. *J Comput Assist Tomogr.* 1990;14:730-735.
42. Koeller KK, Rushing EJ. From the archives of the AFIP: medulloblastoma: a comprehensive review with radiologic-pathologic correlation. *Radiographics.* 2003;23:1613-1637.
43. Barkovich JA. *Pediatric Neuroimaging.* 4th ed. Philadelphia: Lippincott Williams and Wilkins, 2005.
44. Bambakidis NC, et al. Atypical teratoid/rhabdoid tumors of the central nervous system: clinical, radiographic and pathologic features. *Pediatr Neurosurg.* 2002;37(2):64-70.
45. Koeller KK, Rushing EJ. From the archives of the AFIP: pilocytic astrocytoma: radiologic-pathologic correlation. *Radiographics.* 2004;24: 1693-1708.
46. Teo C, et al. Ependymoma. *Childs Nerv Syst.* 2003;19(5-6):270-285.
47. Rezai AR, et al. Disseminated ependymomas of the central nervous system. *J Neurosurg.* 1996;85:618-624.
48. Recinos PF, Sciubba DM, Jallo GI. Brainstem tumors: where are we today? *Pediatr Neurosurg.* 2007;43(3):192-201.
49. Fisher PG, et al. A clinicopathologic reappraisal of brain stem tumor classification. Identification of pilocystic astrocytoma and fibrillary astrocytoma as distinct entities. *Cancer.* 2000;89:1569-1576.
50. Jallo GI, Biser-Rohrbaugh A, Freed D. Brainstem gliomas. *Childs Nerv Syst.* 2004;20(3):143-153.
51. Allen JC, Siffert J, Hukin J. Clinical manifestations of childhood ependymoma: a multitude of syndromes. *Pediatr Neurosurg.* 1998;28(1):49-55.
52. Ohmori K, Collins J, Fukushima T. Craniopharyngiomas in children. *Pediatr Neurosurg.* 2007;43:265-278.
53. Garrè ML, Cama A. Craniopharyngioma: modern concepts in pathogenesis and treatment. *Curr Opin Pediatr.* 2007;19:471-479.
54. Drummond KJ, Rosenfeld JV. Pineal region tumours in childhood. A 30-year experience. *Childs Nerv Syst.* 1999;15(2-3):119-126.
55. Banks KP, Brown SJ. AJR teaching file: solid masses of the pineal region. *AJR Am J Roentgenol.* 2006;186(3 suppl):S233-235.
56. Korogi Y, Takahashi M, Ushio Y. MRI of pineal region tumors. *J Neurooncol.* 2001;54:251-261.
57. Hirato J, Nakazato Y. Pathology of pineal region tumors. *J Neurooncol.* 2001;54:239-249.
58. Lin DD, Barker PB. Neuroimaging of phakomatoses. *Semin Pediatr Neurol.* 2006;13(1):48-62.
59. Rodriguez D, Young Poussaint T. Neuroimaging findings in neurofibromatosis type 1 and 2. *Neuroimaging Clin North Am.* 2004;14:149-170.
60. Korf BR. The phakomatoses. *Neuroimaging Clin North Am.* 2004;14:139-148.
61. Mentzel HJ, et al. Pediatric brain MRI in neurofibromatosis type I. *Eur Radiol.* 2005;15:814-822.
62. DiPaolo DP, et al. Neurofibromatosis type 1: pathologic substrate of high-signal-intensity foci in the brain. *Radiology.* 1995;195:721-724.
63. Smirniotopoulos JG. Neuroimaging of phakomatoses: Sturge-Weber syndrome, tuberous sclerosis, von Hippel-Lindau syndrome. *Neuroimaging Clin North Am.* 2004;14:171-183.

64. Comi AM. Advances in Sturge-Weber syndrome. *Curr Opin Neurol.* 2006;19:124-128.
65. Roach ES, et al. Tuberous Sclerosis Consensus Conference: recommendations for diagnostic evaluation. National Tuberous Sclerosis Association. *J Child Neurol.* 1999;14:401-1407.
66. Luat AF, Makki M, Chugani HT. Neuroimaging in tuberous sclerosis complex. *Curr Opin Neurol.* 2007;20:142-150.
67. deVeber G. Stroke and the child's brain: an overview of epidemiology, syndromes and risk factors. *Curr Opin Neurol.* 2002;15:133-138.
68. deVeber G. Arterial ischemic strokes in infants and children: an overview of current approaches. *Semin Thromb Hemost.* 2003;29:567-573.
69. Lynch JK, Han CJ. Pediatric stroke: what do we know and what do we need to know? *Semin Neurol.* 2005;25:410-423.
70. Cheon JE, et al. Leukodystrophy in children: a pictorial review of MR imaging features. *Radiographics.* 2002;22:461-476.
71. Ness JM, et al; International Pediatric MS Study Group. Clinical features of children and adolescents with multiple sclerosis. *Neurology.* 2007;68(16 suppl 2):S37-45.
72. Ebner F, Millner MM, Justich E. Multiple sclerosis in children: value of serial MR studies to monitor patients. *AJNR Am J Neuroradiol.* 1990;11:1023-1027.
73. Osborn AG, et al. Multiple sclerosis in adolescents: CT and MR findings. *AJR Am J Roentgenol.* 1990;155:385-390.
74. Alehan F, et al. Posterior leukoencephalopathy syndrome in children and adolescents. *J Child Neurol.* 2007;22:406-413.
75. Medina L, et al. MR findings in patients with subacute necrotizing encephalomyelopathy (Leigh syndrome): correlation with biochemical defect. *AJR Am J Roentgenol.* 1990;154:1269-1274.
76. Barkovich AJ, Kuzniecky RI. Gray matter heterotopia. *Neurology.* 2000;55:1603-1608.
77. Frith CD. The value of brain imaging in the study of development and its disorders. *J Child Psychol Psychiatry.* 2006;47:979-982.
78. Santosh PJ. Neuroimaging in child and adolescent psychiatric disorders. *Arch Dis Child.* 2000;82:412-419.
79. Hendren RL, De Backer I, Pandina GJ. Review of neuroimaging studies of child and adolescent psychiatric disorders from the past 10 years. *J Am Acad Child Adolesc Psychiatry.* 2000;39:815-828.
80. Pine DS. A primer on brain imaging in developmental psychopathology: what is it good for? *J Child Psychol Psychiatry.* 2006;47:983-986.
81. Eliez S, Reiss AL. MRI neuroimaging of childhood psychiatric disorders: a selective review. *J Child Psychol Psychiatry.* 2000;41:679-694.
82. Alaghband-Rad J, et al. Childhood-onset schizophrenia: biological markers in relation to clinical characteristics. *Am J Psychiatry.* 1997;154:64-68.
83. Greenstein D, et al. Childhood onset schizophrenia: cortical brain abnormalities as young adults. *J Child Psychol Psychiatry.* 2006;47:1003-1012.
84. Dickstein SG, et al. The neural correlates of attention deficit hyperactivity disorder: an ALE meta-analysis. *J Child Psychol Psychiatry.* 2006; 47:1051-1062.
85. Bush G, Valera EM, Seidman LJ. Functional neuroimaging of attention-deficit/hyperactivity disorder: a review and suggested future directions. *Biol Psychiatry.* 2005;57:1273-1284.
86. Teicher MH, et al. The neurobiological consequences of early stress and childhood maltreatment. *Neurosci Biobehav Rev.* 2003;27(1-2):33-44.
87. Zang YF, et al. Altered baseline brain activity in children with ADHD revealed by resting-state functional MRI. *Brain Dev.* 2007;29(2):83-91.
88. Castellanos FX, et al. Developmental trajectories of brain volume abnormalities in children and adolescents with attention-deficit/hyperactivity disorder. *JAMA.* 2002;288:1740-1748.
89. Seidman LJ, Valera EM, Makris N. Structural brain imaging of attention-deficit/hyperactivity disorder. *Biol Psychiatry.* 2005;57:1263-1272.
90. Stanfield AC, et al. Towards a neuroanatomy of autism: a systematic review and meta-analysis of structural magnetic resonance imaging studies. *Eur Psychiatry.* 2007 Aug 30 [Epub ahead of print].
91. Palmen SJ, van Engeland H. Review on structural neuroimaging findings in autism. *J Neural Transm.* 2004;111:903-929.
92. Boddaert N, Zilbovicius M. Functional neuroimaging and childhood autism. *Pediatr Radiol.* 2002;32(1):1-7.
93. Filipek PA, et al. Practice parameter: screening and diagnosis of autism: report of the Quality Standards Subcommittee of the American Academy of Neurology and the Child Neurology Society. *Neurology.* 2000;55:468-479.
94. Kaufmann WE, Pearlson GD, Naidu S. The neuroanatomy of Rett syndrome: neuropathological and neuroimaging studies. *Rivista Medica.* 1998;4:187-199.
95. Carter JC, et al. Selective cerebral volume reduction in Rett syndrome: a multiple-approach MR imaging study. *AJNR Am J Neuroradiol.* 2007 Dec 7 [Epub ahead of print].
96. Steingard RJ, et al. Structural abnormalities in brain magnetic resonance images of depressed children. *J Am Acad Child Adolesc Psychiatry.* 1996;35:307-311.
97. Fu, et al. *Neuroimaging in Psychiatry.* London: *Informa Healthcare,* 2003.
98. Pavuluri MN, Birmaher B, Naylor MW. Pediatric bipolar disorder: a review of the past 10 years. *J Am Acad Child Adolesc Psychiatry.* 2005;44:846-471.
99. Lipton ML, et al. *Neuroimaging Findings Specific for Bipolar Disorder in Children: Quantitative Structural and Diffusion Tensor Imaging,* American Society for Neuroradiology, Toronto, ON, 2005.

100. Zampolin R, et al. *White Matter Deficits Correlate with Limbic Structural Asymmetry in Pediatric Bipolar Disorder: A Diffusion Tensor Imaging Study. Organisation for Human Brain Mapping,* Florence, Italy, 2006.
101. Saxena S, et al. Localized orbitofrontal and subcortical metabolic changes and predictors of response to paroxetine treatment in obsessive-compulsive disorder. *Neuropsychopharmacology.* 1999;21:683-693.
102. Friedlander L, Desrocher M. Neuroimaging studies of obsessive-compulsive disorder in adults and children. *Clin Psychol Rev.* 2006;26(1):32-49.
103. Gerard E, Peterson BS. Developmental processes and brain imaging studies in Tourette syndrome. *J Psychosom Res.* 2003;55(1):13-22.
104. Peterson B, et al. Reduced basal ganglia volumes in Tourette's syndrome using three-dimensional reconstruction techniques from magnetic resonance images. *Neurology.* 1993;43:941-949.
105. Singer HS, et al. Volumetric MRI changes in basal ganglia of children with Tourette's syndrome. *Neurology.* 1993;43:950-956.
106. Peterson BS, et al. Basal ganglia volumes in patients with Gilles de la Tourette syndrome. *Arch Gen Psychiatry.* 2003;60:415-424.

CHAPTER 3

Movement Disorders in Children and Adolescents

KELLY CONDEFER AND RACHEL SAUNDERS-PULLMAN

Movement disorders occupy a unique intersection between neurology and psychiatry. They may have comorbid psychiatric features that can be due to the same underlying process as the movement disorder or may be reactive to the stress, disability, or social stigma of the movement disorder. For example, depression and anxiety have a high incidence among patients with movement disorders and are sometimes a reactive phenomenon; alternatively, they also may be related to the underlying pathophysiology of the disorder. Less frequently, as in the case of psychogenic movement disorders, no underlying neurological etiology of the abnormal movements is found.

Although in most movement disorders, the psychiatric features present concurrent with or subsequent to the development of movements, psychiatric features may occasionally be the initial symptom. For example, child psychiatrists may be confronted with initial presentations of degenerative neuropsychiatric disorders, such as Wilson disease and Huntington disease (HD), in which irritability and withdrawal may appear before the abnormal movements (1). This chapter reviews the movement disorders encountered in childhood, with a special emphasis on the relevance of these disorders to psychiatrists.

Overview

Movement disorders are associated with abnormalities of the basal ganglia or their connections. The basal ganglia, a group of deep gray matter nuclei, including the caudate, putamen, globus pallidus, and subthalamic nuclei, along with their connections, constitute the extrapyramidal system. This system regulates and controls the motor corticospinal (pyramidal) system. Pyramidal system lesions may cause weakness and spasticity. Although this chapter briefly discusses these impairments because they may accompany movement disorders, particularly in children with cerebral palsy, its focus is on abnormalities of motor control.

Movement disorders are usually stratified as hypokinetic (too little movement) or hyperkinetic (uncontrolled excessive movement). The hyperkinetic disorders include tics, tremor, dystonia, chorea, and myoclonus. Although classification of abnormal movements is based on phenomenology rather than anatomical location, different anatomical sites within the basal ganglia have classic movement associations. For example, lesions of the substantia nigra typically result in bradykinesia and rest tremor; those of the caudate nucleus, chorea; and those of the putamen, dystonia.

The phenomenology of movement disorders is shared between children and adults, but pediatric movement disorders have several distinct clinical characteristics. With the exception of tics, movement disorders appearing in childhood are less common than those appearing in adulthood, are more likely to be a result of an underlying static or progressive disease process (2), and are more likely to have a metabolic or genetic etiology. Therefore a thorough examination, including skin examination, family history, and birth and developmental history, is imperative in the evaluation of every child presenting with a movement disorder. Because earlier-onset disease is more likely to be metabolic, imaging and laboratory evaluations also vary depending on the age at onset of a movement disorder. For example, children with dystonia should undergo magnetic resonance imaging (MRI) to rule out secondary disease (3). The clinical course depends on the time that the insult occurs during development. For instance, dopamine deficiency occurring at an early age is associated with prominent dystonia and some parkinsonism, whereas in adults, it results in parkinsonism with limited dystonia. Furthermore, dystonia starting in childhood is more likely to affect the limbs and progress to the trunk and neck, whereas in adults, it is more likely to start in the arm, neck, or face, and often does not spread (4). Because children's nervous systems are continually developing, a static injury to the brain can cause variable or progressive symptoms as a child grows (5). This principle becomes imperative when monitoring and treating children with dystonia or chorea resulting from a static encephalopathy.

Although worrisome, not all involuntary movements in children are abnormal. For example, stereotypy, a repetitive purposeless movement of the hands, frequently occurs in impaired children. However, neurologists may see stereotypy in neurodevelopmentally normal children, and in them, it may spontaneously resolve (6). This chapter divides movement disorders primarily by their major phenomenologic subgroups (i.e., parkinsonism, tremor, dystonia and myoclonus, with additional emphasis on Wilson disease, psychogenic movement disorders, and paroxysmal movement disorders).

Parkinsonism

The prototypical hypokinetic disorder is parkinsonism. In contrast to that in adults, parkinsonism occurs infrequently in children (7). The cardinal features of parkinsonism include bradykinesia, rigidity, rest tremor, and postural instability. Manifestations of bradykinesia are drooling, hypomimia, hypophonic speech, aprosody, loss of spontaneous gesturing, and micrographia. In children with these features, physicians should differentiate true parkinsonism from psychomotor slowing, which is the slowness of movements associated with depression, and assess for additional movements. Features that can be present in parkinsonism and not psychomotor slowing are postural instability and decrementing amplitudes during rapid alternating movements, such as repetitive hand opening and closing.

Whenever childhood parkinsonism is identified, a diagnosis of Wilson disease, a treatable neurodegenerative disorder, should be considered. This important disease is discussed in more detail later. The differential diagnosis of childhood parkinsonism also includes brainstem tumors and strokes, the akinetic juvenile form of HD (Westphal variant), young-onset Parkinson disease, neurodegeneration with brain iron accumulation, some spinocerebellar atrophies, dopa-responsive dystonia, and the juvenile form of neuronal ceroid lipofuscinosis. In each of these disorders, parkinsonism is usually not the sole neurological feature. For example, juvenile HD is associated with eye-movement abnormalities, and many of the others, including dopa-responsive dystonia and young-onset Parkinson disease, may also show dystonia along with parkinsonism (8). As childhood parkinsonism is extremely rare, and its etiologies are varied, its psychiatric comorbidities are not well described. However, higher rates of depression have been observed in patients with young-onset as opposed to older-onset Parkinson disease (9).

The remainder of the chapter focuses on hyperkinetic movement disorders, which are the most frequent movement disorders in children.

Tremor

Tremor, among the most common of all movement disorders, is defined as the rhythmical oscillation of part of the body around one or more joints (10–13). Tremors can be classified according to whether they occur (a) at rest, (b) while maintaining a posture, (c) with generalized activity, or (d) during the execution of a specific task. Examinations should include careful observation of patients with their eyes closed and arms resting in their laps, with their arms outstretched (posture holding), while reaching toward objects, such as in the finger–nose–finger task, and while writing and pouring.

Essential tremor (ET) is by far the most common form of action tremor. It is prominent with actions, such as pouring (14), writing and finger–nose–finger task, and with sustained posture. There is a lack of long-term prognostic data for children, but the mean age at onset of ET in a large childhood-onset series was 8.8 years (15). It has been estimated that only 5% of ET has onset in childhood, and it is not known whether childhood-onset ET is more severe or has a worse prognosis than the later-onset variety (16). Whereas adults with ET may exhibit hand, head, and voice tremor, children are much less likely to develop head tremor (17). Amplitude of tremor tends to increase with age (18). Approximately 50% of patients have evidence of other, mild cerebellar signs such as abnormal tandem gait (19). In adults with essential tremor, alcoholism is a frequent psychiatric comorbidity; however this has been less well studied in children (20).

Postural tremor, a 6- to 12-Hz tremor, occurs in both essential and enhanced physiological tremor (13). Enhanced physiological tremor can appear in the setting of the use of sympathomimetic drugs, lithium, steroids, and valproic acid, as well as with metabolic disorders, such as thyrotoxicosis and hypoglycemia. This tremor rarely requires treatment beyond discontinuation of the inciting medication, in those cases in which it may be removed. Children with hereditary and nonhereditary neuropathies may also demonstrate tremor, which is suggestive of enhanced physiologic tremor (21). Tremor occurring predominantly at rest is very rare in children and adolescents. When ET is very severe, it can also appear at rest but will still be more prominent with action (22). Intention tremor, a 2- to 4-Hz action tremor, elicited by finger–nose–finger testing, may be seen with cerebellar disease. Cerebellar tremor is different from ET in that the child has difficulty hitting the target and there is a widening arc in reaching for the target (dysmetria). The tremor is usually due to disease in the cerebellum or its outflow pathways. A directional tremor, tending toward a particular posture, termed *dystonic tremor*, is described in this chapter's section on dystonia. Jerky, fast, irregular tremor may be a manifestation of myoclonus. Psychogenic tremor may also present in childhood, and this also is discussed later in the section on psychogenicity.

Case One

In a 12-year-old boy, a slow, high-amplitude tremor developed in both of his arms over the course of 3 months. The tremor was at first mild and present mostly with action. In the past month, it had progressed, such that he was no longer able to write in school, and he began to have difficulty putting a fork to his mouth. In addition, rapid speech developed, and he sometimes slurred his words. His parents noted that he tended to drool. For the previous year, he had become increasingly defiant in his behavior, often losing his temper and going into violent rages at home. His schoolwork had deteriorated significantly.

His examination revealed no discoloration of the irises to inspection and no organomegaly. His facial expression revealed dystonic grinning (*risus sardonicus*) with some drooling, and his speech was dysarthric and hypophonic. Motor examination revealed a high-amplitude tremor that was most prominent proximally, when arms were elevated, and both hands were placed near the nose, and worsened with action.

Blood tests revealed normal liver functions, a normal antistreptolysin (ASO) titer, a normal serum copper level, and a ceruloplasmin level of 20 mg per deciliter (normal, 20–60 mg/dL). He was referred for ophthalmoscopic examination, which revealed bilateral Kaiser–Fleischer rings. A 24-hour urine copper excretion was 400 μg per 24 hours (normal, <50 μg/24 h).

Discussion: Wilson disease can present with cognitive changes and behavioral abnormalities before other neurological or hepatic dysfunction is evident. The most common personality changes seen are impulsiveness and antisocial behavior; frank dementia can also occur, but psychosis is rare (1). The characteristic wing-beating tremor of Wilson disease appeared in conjunction with neuropsychiatric symptoms in this patient. Serum ceruloplasmin levels are normal in about 5% of patients with neurological involvement.

When tremor significantly affects handwriting and other activities of a child's daily life, treatment is warranted. There is little evidence for the treatment of ET in children. First-line medications for ET in adults include propranolol and primidone. Propranolol is the most effective tremor-suppressing medication (23). Although they do not achieve central nervous system (CNS) penetration like propranolol, other β-blockers also are efficacious, suggesting that the therapeutic effect may be partially mediated by peripheral β-adrenergic receptors (24). Primidone is a barbiturate with antitremor activity (25). Starting with a very low dose and slowly titrating the dose to the lowest effective dose may prevent side effects, particularly sedation and nausea. When propranolol is contraindicated, as in asthmatics or children with depression, topiramate and clonazepam also may be effective (26).

Wilson Disease

Wilson disease, a rare disorder of copper metabolism, deserves special mention because it is treatable and hereditary. This disorder results from deficient excretion of copper into the bile, leading to toxic accumulations of copper in the liver, kidney, brain, and cornea (27). It is progressively degenerative unless identified and treated. In about 15% of cases, neuropsychiatric symptoms such as cognitive decline, impulsive behavior, antisocial behavior, and personality change occur before the onset of abnormal movements (1,28). Although symptoms may be subtle, features that meet criteria for anxiety disorder or manic–depressive disorder may develop. Approximately 40% of cases present with neurological symptoms, usually after age 12, whereas another 40% present with liver disease, usually before age 12 (29). The manifestations of Wilson disease are diverse, but three general clinical presentations are seen, each of which may overlap: (a) an akinetic-rigid syndrome resembling parkinsonism, (b) a generalized dystonic syndrome, and (c) "pseudosclerosis" with postural and action wing-beating tremor. Symptoms usually appear between ages 11 and 25 years but can appear as early as 4 years (30). Dystonia is a frequent feature and can affect the face and oropharynx, resulting in the characteristic *"risus sardonicus,"* or the appearance of a forced grin, as well as drooling.

Because of its treatability and protean spectrum of clinical manifestations, physicians should consider Wilson disease in any child with a movement disorder. Kaiser–Fleisher rings are visible in virtually all patients with neurological Wilson disease, and low ceruloplasmin levels occur in all but 5% of patients. Ceruloplasmin levels can be falsely low in protein-loss states and falsely elevated in pregnancy. Copper levels in 24-hour urine collections are more diagnostically reliable: rates less than 50 μg per 24 hours exclude the disease, and most patients with Wilson disease will have rates of greater than 100 μg per 24 hours. In inconclusive cases, a liver biopsy showing copper deposition is the definitive test.

Wilson disease is an autosomal recessive disorder due to mutations in a copper-transporting adenosine triphosphatase (ATPase) gene on chromosome 13 (31,32). It may be caused by either two copies of one mutation (homozygous) or one copy of two different mutations (compound heterozygote). Because a multitude of causal mutations occur, genetic testing is unwieldy (27).

Treatment of neurological Wilson disease had centered on *d*-penicillamine, but this drug can result in irreversible neurological worsening. Therefore current first-line treatment is the drug tetrathiomolybdate (33). This drug both blocks copper absorption and binds to copper in a nontoxic way, making it beneficial as an acute therapy. Usually this is coupled with zinc maintenance therapy, which also blocks absorption, and is a safe choice in children for chronic treatment (34). As tetrathiomolybdate is available only on an experimental basis, physicians should consider referring severe cases as an emergency to a center specializing in Wilson disease. Liver transplant also successfully reverses neurological manifestations of Wilson disease in about 80% of cases (35). With all forms of treatment, neurological symptomatic improvement normally occurs over a period of 6 months to a year.

Abnormal Tone: Spasticity, Rigidity, and Dystonia

SPASTICITY

Abnormalities of tone occur in a large proportion of childhood movement disorders because of their association with cerebral palsy. Sometimes termed "static encephalopathy," cerebral palsy is actually a spectrum of disorders caused by an ischemic or toxic injury to the brain, occurring pre- or perinatally. Spasticity falls outside the rubric of extrapyramidal movement disorders, being a sign of upper motor neuron, or pyramidal, dysfunction. Nevertheless, this chapter considers spasticity because it can contribute significant disability to children with movement disorders. *Spasticity* is hypertonia in which resistance to passive muscle stretch is increased with increased speed of the stretch. It tends to vary with direction of the stretch (5). Limbs tend to assume contracted, fixed, flexed positions, depending on the level of injury in the CNS. Most often in children, spasticity results from perinatal injury causing static encephalopathy when the primary motor cortex and descending motor pathways are involved. Examination will demonstrate hyperreflexia and clonus. In patients who do not ambulate, improvement in joint mobility is imperative for preventing contractures. Medical therapy with baclofen, clonidine, and tizanidine reduces spinal motor neuron excitability. In severe cases, intrathecal baclofen delivered via a pump may be necessary. Botulinum toxin injected into limb muscles may also improve tone and facilitate grooming (36).

Rigidity is hypertonia in which resistance to passive stretch does not depend on the speed or angle of stretch (5). With rigidity, as opposed to spasticity, patients do not assume a fixed posture. Rigidity is usually seen in conjunction with parkinsonism, as discussed earlier.

DYSTONIA

Dystonia is a syndrome characterized by sustained muscle contractions that produce twisting and repetitive movements or abnormal postures (37). The movements seen in dystonia tend to be *directional*. This stands in contrast to chorea, which can also appear as writhing and twisting but tends to be more random and dancelike. The twisting or torsional nature of the contractions may force the body into abnormal positions that may be intermittent or sustained. These positions are consistent and reproducible on examination. Dystonia is usually worse with action, and sometimes may be present only with particular actions, such as equinovarus posturing of the foot when walking forward but not backward, or abduction of the arm when writing. This very characteristic action specificity of dystonia sometimes tempts clinicians to misdiagnose these movements as psychogenic.

When dystonia results in tremor (*dystonic tremor*), a so-called *null point* may be identified on examination. The affected limb or neck shows little or no tremor in this position. In contrast, spasticity and rigidity do not vary depending on the action. Also, many children and young adults discover one or more "sensory tricks" (*geste antagoniste*) that help control their dystonia, such as lightly touching one's chin with a finger to straighten the neck when cervical dystonia is present. Even thinking of doing the sensory trick is often enough to improve the dystonia, highlighting the higher-order processing involved in modulating this movement disorder (38). The pathophysiology of dystonia is complex and involves abnormalities of both globus pallidal firing and intracortical inhibition (39,40).

Although the term *dystonia* was initially coined to describe a particular form of childhood onset, primary torsion dystonia (dystonia musculorum deformans, or Oppenheim disease) (41), physicians should consider dystonia a sign rather than a single disease entity. Dystonia can be classified by age at onset, anatomical distribution, and etiology. A strong relation exists between age at onset and distribution, with onset before age 23 years being more associated with lower-limb dystonia that often spreads to involve the trunk and arms. Adult-onset dystonia typically starts in the neck, face, or vocal cords and remains localized (4,42). Etiologically, dystonia can be classified as primary or secondary (43), as shown in Table 3.1. The primary dystonias encompass all dystonias for which no degenerative brain pathology can be identified. They are also characterized by the following (43): (a) dystonia as the sole abnormality (except tremor), (b) absence of laboratory or imaging data to suggest acquired or degenerative cause, (c) absence of a response to levodopa, and (d) absence of known history implicating an environmental, structural, or pharmacological cause such as neuroleptic exposure or stroke.

The archetypal genetic form of primary dystonia in children, DYT-1, is inherited as an autosomal dominant trait with incomplete penetrance. With only approximately 30% of gene carriers ever developing symptoms, the etiology of the incomplete penetrance is unclear, but it likely involves environmental or genetic modifiers (44). Onset is in childhood, usually in the leg or arm initially. It may generalize to involve both legs and trunk, remain in one arm, or become bibrachial. Although it may present in adulthood, DYT-1 usually does not appear in individuals older than 24 years (45). DYT-1 dystonia is due to a three-

TABLE 3.1 DIFFERENTIAL DIAGNOSIS OF DYSTONIA IN CHILDREN

Primary Childhood-onset Dystonias

DYT-1 (childhood-onset generalized, primarily begins in lower limb)
DYT-6 (childhood-onset generalized, primarily begins in arm or cranial)
Other unidentified forms of primary dystonia that are likely genetic.

Dystonia-plus Syndromes

Dopa-responsive dystonia (DYT-5)
Rapid-onset dystonia parkinsonism
Myoclonus-dystonia (DYT-11)

Secondary Dystonias

Vascular/Structural/Hypoxic	*Heredodegenerative Diseases (usually not pure dystonia)*
Dystonic cerebral palsy	Autosomal dominant:
Pachygyria	Juvenile parkinsonism, juvenile Huntington, neuroferritinopathy, spinocerebellar ataxia type 3, dentatorubropallidoluysian atrophy.
Stroke	
Arteriovenous malformation	
Infectious	*Autosomal recessive:*
Viral encephalitides	Wilson, Niemann-Pick type C, neuronal ceroid-lipofuscinosis, GM1 and GM2 gangliosidoses, metachromatic leukodystrophy, Lesch–Nyhan syndrome, homocystinuria, glutaric acidemia, methylmalonic acidemia, ataxia telangiectasia
HIV encephalitis	
Immune Related	
Antiphospholipid syndrome	
Rasmussen syndrome	
Drug and Toxin Induced	
Tardive dystonia due to dopamine blockers	*Mitochondrial Diseases*
Carbon monoxide, manganese, cyanide, methanol	Leigh disease
Psychogenic Dystonia	Leber hereditary optic neuropathy with dystonia

base pair (GAG) deletion in the gene coding for the *torsin A* protein (46). No structural abnormalities are visible on MRI, although abnormal basal ganglia metabolism is noted on functional imaging such as fluorodeoxyglucose–positron emission tomography (FDG-PET) (47). Early recurrent major depression has been found to be associated with the GAG deletion in DYT-1, independent of the presence of physical disability, suggesting that the depression may itself be an expression of the abnormal gene (48).

Secondary dystonias include genetic disorders in which dystonia is one of several manifestations of the disease and those due to environmental or acquired causes. Dystonia related to metabolic disorders, heredodegenerative diseases, mitochondrial disorders, and toxic environmental exposures often show abnormalities of the basal ganglia on neuroimaging. However, some patients with secondary dystonias have normal findings on neuroimaging. In this category with normal imaging are several rare disorders termed "dystonia-plus" syndromes, which are caused by genetic defects that result in dystonia in association with another movement disorder. These include dopa-responsive dystonia (DRD), myoclonus-dystonia (MD), and rapid-onset dystonia parkinsonism (RDP). All three of these rare genetic disorders have psychiatric manifestations and comorbidities that are only just beginning to be described, deepening questions about the role of the basal ganglia in mood disorders (49,50). Higher rates of depression and obsessive–compulsive disorder (OCD) have been identified both in patients with these syndromes and in non-manifesting mutation carriers, compared with the general public.

Dopa-responsive dystonia classically has its onset in childhood, although relatives may have adult-onset parkinsonism. Onset is usually characterized by bilateral leg dystonia, often with toe walking and spasticity. It is often associated with a diurnal variation (i.e., symptoms are better in the morning than in the evening) (51). This variability has sometimes led to the incorrect diagnosis of psychogenicity, although it should be noted that during any examination point, the signs will be consistently reproduced. Parkinsonism and postural instability may also be present in children, and the disorder may be confused with cerebral palsy (52,53).

A dominantly inherited deficiency in the guanosine triphosphate (GTP) cyclohydrolase enzyme (GCH-1) is usually the cause of DRD (51). GCH-1 is involved in the synthetic pathway for tetrahydrobiopterin (BH_4). BH_4 is a cofactor for tyrosine hydroxylase, the rate-limiting step in the synthesis of dopamine. BH_4 is also a coenzyme in the synthesis of tyrosine and serotonin. Cerebrospinal fluid measurements reflect low biopterin and low dopamine metabolites. Mutation sequencing does not identify all individuals with DRD (54). The diagnosis can be most reliably made by the dramatic and sustained reversal of symptoms with low-dose levodopa (55). Carriers of this enzyme defect have been found to have higher rates of major depressive disorder and OCD than the general population (49).

Myoclonus-dystonia, which is a distinct genetic disorder associated with mutations of the epsilon sarcoglycan gene (56) (*DYT11*), usually presents in childhood or adolescence with proximal myoclonic jerking and dystonia. Although these are usually seen together, some individuals may demonstrate only myoclonus, and others, only isolated dystonia. Symptoms are responsive to alcohol, and the higher rate of alcohol dependence is thought to be secondary to self-palliation. M-D is also associated with obsessive–compulsive disorder (49).

The treatment of dystonia in childhood depends in part on etiology. Atypical features on examination or history—drug exposures, dystonia at rest rather than action, hemidystonia, early speech abnormalities, cranial dystonia in a child, abnormal neurological examination, or any imaging or laboratory abnormalities—suggest a secondary rather than a primary dystonia. If physicians identify a secondary cause, the underlying disorder is the primary therapeutic target if a treatment is available. In particular, a levodopa trial should be instituted in every child with dystonia who has normal brain imaging to rule out that the dystonia is DRD. When dystonia is primary, or when the underlying disorder is untreatable, symptomatic treatment of dystonia includes anticholinergic medications, benzodiazepines, and muscle relaxants. The anticholinergic medication trihexyphenidyl may be used alone (57) or in combination with baclofen or clonazepam or both to treat primary generalized dystonia. Although it may be associated with memory impairment in adults, trihexyphenidyl may be tolerated in children in doses exceeding 40 mg daily. The peripheral anticholinergic side effects of trihexyphenidyl, such as dry eyes, constipation, and stomach pain, can be countered with low doses of pyridostigmine, an acetylcholinesterase inhibitor. Anticonvulsants such as topiramate and levetiracetam have also shown some benefit as adjunctive therapies (58,59). Botulinum toxin may be used for prominent limb dystonia (60).

Deep-brain stimulation (DBS) involves the implantation of electrodes into subcortical structures in the brain, through which continuous electrical stimulation may be applied to the targeted brain structure. This therapy has shown promise in the alleviation of such diverse neurological problems as dystonia, tremor, and cluster headache. DBS targeting the subthalamic nucleus has been Food and Drug Administration (FDA) approved since 1996 for the treatment of adults with idiopathic Parkinson disease. However, it was not until 2005 that the efficacy of stimulating the globus pallidus internal segment was clearly established in children with DYT-1 primary dystonia (61). In this controlled trial, patients with primary dystonia ranging in age from 14 to 54 years old experienced a 30% to 50% improvement in their dystonia symptoms. Risk of a significant intra- or perioperative event such as stroke, hemorrhage, and death may be 1% to 2%, depending on the implanting center. Therefore DBS is still reserved for medically refractory cases of generalized dystonia. Reports also are emerging of the efficacy of DBS in some forms of symptomatic dystonia in children, such as dystonia related to pantothenate kinase–associated neurodegeneration (62).

> ## Case Two
>
> A 6-year-old girl had greater difficulty walking over the course of several months. Her parents noted that her left foot would turn in when she walked, and her running had a galloping quality. She started falling, sometimes losing balance out of the blue, and cramping in her hand occurred when she was drawing. She could walk almost normally in the mornings, but by 4 PM, she could barely walk and fell frequently. She was the product of a normal term pregnancy and met all developmental milestones on time. Her father had writer's cramp, and her paternal grandfather had Parkinson disease.
>
> On examination, she had normal intelligence. Skin examination revealed no signs of neurocutaneous disease, and irises had no discoloration. Neurological examination revealed dystonia in both feet and legs, most evident when she was walking and running, and hyperreflexia at the knees and ankles. Pull test was positive for retropulsion, and she needed to be caught to prevent falling.
>
> An MRI scan of the brain was normal, and complete blood count (CBC), liver-function tests (LFTs), and metabolic panel were normal. An ASO titer was normal, and genetic testing for DYT-1 was negative. A trial of a low dose of levodopa was instituted. With 1 tablet of carbidopa/levodopa, 25/100 per day, the dystonia in her legs disappeared, and her walking normalized. Genetic testing for mutations in the GTP cyclohydrolase I gene (*GCH1*) revealed a mutation.
>
> **Discussion:** DRD often presents in childhood with leg dystonia that is worse later in the day. Signs of parkinsonism, such as the postural instability seen in this example, are often present. Spasticity can also occur, and some children with this condition have been misdiagnosed for years as having cerebral palsy. Genetic testing for mutations in GCH1 is negative in up to 30% of DRD cases. Patients can be maintained with very low doses of levodopa indefinitely, with low risk of side effects, and efficacy seems to be maintained over the long term. A trial of levodopa should be considered in every child with an undiagnosed dystonia or parkinsonism.

Tics and Stereotypies

TICS

Tics are the most commonly encountered movement disorder in children, comprising about 40% of all pediatric cases seen at a tertiary-care movement disorders clinic (7). Tics are a heterogeneous group of spontaneous, brief, simple or complex movements or vocalizations that abruptly interrupt normal actions or speech. Unlike almost all other abnormal movements, tics of all kinds tend to be preceded by an inner feeling, sensation, or urge that is relieved by doing the tic. Examples of this characteristic urge include "burning" in the eyes before an eye blink or a "dry throat" before throat clearing. Another unique characteristic of tics is suppressibility. Patients can often partially suppress tics in certain social situations, only to release them more violently later when free of social constraints. Periods of stress, excitement, boredom, fatigue, or heat exposure can increase tics (63). Tics may wax and wane over time and may change in appearance or anatomical distribution.

Tics are characterized as motoric or phonic. Simple motor tics include eye blinking, nose twitching, head jerks, bruxism, mouth opening, and abdominal muscle tensing. Complex motor tics involve multiple muscle groups and may appear to be a semipurposeful action. Examples include gesturing (when obscene, termed *copropraxia*), trunk bending, and head shaking. Motor tics of all kinds can be clonic, characterized by quick jerking movements, or dystonic, characterized by more sustained posturing. Simple phonic tics include sniffing, throat clearing, grunting, squeaking, or coughing. Finally, complex phonic tics include echolalia (repeating another's words), coprolalia (uttering obscene words or phrases), and palilalia (repeating one's own sentences, particularly the last part of the sentence or word). Coprolalia, although infamous in its association with Tourette syndrome (TS), actually occurs very rarely, in about 10% of cases, according to one large series (64).

Tics occurring in an otherwise neurologically and developmentally normal child are usually considered primary or part of TS, as discussed later. Secondary causes of tics to consider include infection, trauma, cocaine use, and neuroleptic exposure (65). In a subset of children, tics or OCD or both develop in temporal correlation with group A β-hemolytic streptococcal infections. This association, termed PANDAS (pediatric autoimmune neuropsychiatric disorders associated with streptococcal infection), carries with it treatment implications, as patients fitting this description have responded well to immune-modulating therapies (66,67). The concept is controversial, however, because streptococcal infections are common, and tic disorders can have acute onsets in the absence of infections (68).

Tourette syndrome is the archetypal tic disorder. Because no biological marker exists for TS, the diagnosis rests on the patient's symptoms and signs, and fulfillment of diagnostic criteria. Criteria for TS according to the Tourette Syndrome Classification Study Group (68a) are listed in Table 3.2. The *Diagnostic and Statistical Manual of Mental Disorders–IV* (DSM-IV) criteria are similar but also require that disability attributable to the tics be present. Although the criteria state that onset of TS should be before 21 years of age, 96% of cases actually manifest before age 11 years (69).

Tourette syndrome clusters within families, but specific genes have not been identified. The disorder tends not to be progressive. According to one study, half of patients in whom

TABLE 3.2 THE TOURETTE SYNDROME CLASSIFICATION STUDY GROUP DIAGNOSTIC CRITERIA

1. Both multiple motor and one or more phonic tics are present during the illness, but not necessarily concurrently.
2. Tics must occur many times per day, nearly every day, or intermittently throughout a period of more than 1 y.
3. The anatomical location, number, frequency, type, complexity, or severity of tics must change over time.
4. Onset must be before age 21.
5. Involuntary movements and noises cannot be explained by another medical condition.
6. Motor and/or phonic tics must be directly witnessed by a reliable examiner during the illness.

- *Definite TS meets all six criteria*
- *Probable TS type 1 meets all criteria except 3 and/or 4*
- *Probable TS type 2 meets all criteria except 1 (includes either single motor tic plus phonic tics, or multiple motor tics plus possible phonic tic)*

TS, Tourette syndrome.

Data from Tourette Syndrome Classification Study Group. Definitions and classification of tic disorders. *Arch Neurol.* 1993;50:1013–1016.

TS developed in childhood were tic free by 18 years old (70). However, other studies have shown tics to be persistent into adulthood, albeit less disabling and severe (71,72).

In addition to tics, TS manifests significant neurobehavioral symptoms that often affect treatment greatly. Children with TS have been shown to have a higher incidence of attention-deficit hyperactivity disorder (ADHD), OCD, separation anxiety, overanxious disorder, simple phobia, social phobia, agoraphobia, mania, major depressive disorder, and oppositional defiant disorder (73). In one database of 3,500 TS patients, only 12% had tics in isolation (74). The unifying feature of these comorbid problems seems to be poor impulse control. The coexistence of ADHD and TS, which occurs in approximately 48% of TS patients (75), poses a distinct therapeutic challenge because stimulant drugs have been reported to trigger or worsen tics (76). ADHD occurring in the setting of TS appears to have the same character as ADHD occurring in isolation (77,78). However, it appears that distinctive aggravating factors of ADHD are found in TS, such as intrusive thoughts, compulsive fixation of gaze, sedating effects from anti-tic medications, and the mental exertion required to suppress tics.

When treating attention deficit in TS, the most likely contributing factor should be sought after and targeted. Stimulant medications work as well on ADHD whether associated or not with TS (79). ADHD is often present before the onset of tics in TS, and therefore studies that demonstrate the onset of tics after stimulant-medication treatment are difficult to interpret. A recent review of the literature regarding the use of psychostimulants in TS concluded that group data as a whole do not indicate that stimulants significantly worsen tics; however, in individual patients, tics may worsen in response to stimulants (80). Stimulant medications are not contraindicated in patients with tics, and the decision to use stimulants in the presence of tics should be assessed on an individual basis.

Obsessive–compulsive disorder also is an important part of the neurobehavioral spectrum of TS. Obsessional slowness and bradyphrenia contribute significantly to poor school performance in some TS patients (81). Unlike ADHD, OCD associated with TS takes a different form from primary OCD, in which cleanliness and hygiene dominate symptoms. In TS, OCD primarily involves obsessions with symmetry, fear of harming oneself or others, and the need to say or do things just right (82). In patients with TS and OCD, premonitory sensory phenomena associated with tics and compulsions tend to be stronger, and therefore their tics can be more difficult to control (83).

The first step in treating tics and TS is to decide whether treatment is necessary. Many patients who respond to counseling and behavioral modification do not require medication. Working with schools to modify learning environments, such as providing break periods to release tics and allowing extra time on tests, can be very helpful.

When tics interfere with functioning, however, medication is usually necessary. Dopamine-receptor blockers are the most effective tic suppressors and have historically been considered first-line therapy (84). However, the risk of tardive symptoms and side effects such as weight gain, sedation, and depression limit the usefulness of these drugs. Pimozide and haloperidol are the only two neuroleptics approved by the FDA for the treatment of TS, but the efficacy of risperidone has also been reported (85). Data are mixed as to the efficacy of other atypical neuroleptics, such as clozapine, olanzapine, quetiapine, and ziprasidone. A pilot study, however, showed that ziprasidone decreased tic severity by 35% (7% placebo) (86). Ziprasidone has the advantage of possibly causing less weight gain than the other atypicals. Some groups anecdotally recommend starting with fluphenazine because the incidence of dose-limiting side effects seems to be lower with this drug. To limit the occurrence of extrapyramidal side effects, patients must be very closely monitored. Whenever possible, doses should be decreased and the medication stopped during periods of remission. Tetrabenazine is a dopamine depleter and partial dopamine blocker that is probably as effective as neuroleptics at reducing tics, and it does not cause extrapyramidal side effects (87). It is not readily available and not yet FDA approved in the United States, but can be obtained through approved academic centers.

Alternatively, the α-2 agonists clonidine and guanfacine, which are generally well tolerated, may be used as initial therapy. In a head-to-head single-blinded pilot study, clonidine was equally effective as risperidone at suppressing tics (88). Guanfacine has been shown in a double-blinded placebo-controlled trial to decrease tic severity by about 30% (compared with 7% placebo) (89). Importantly, these medications may also improve symptoms of ADHD. Dopamine blockers and α-2 agonists can be very effective in patients with complex tics and behavioral comorbidity. However, in patients with simple motor tics, and especially clonic tics, small open-label studies support the use of clonazepam (90,91). Clonazepam may also be useful as an adjunct in children with both tics and ADHD who are being treated with clonidine (92). Botulinum toxin type A has also been effective in treating simple motor tics, and interestingly, it also seems to decrease the sensory phenomena preceding the tics (93). Botulinum toxin injections to the vocal cords have also been successfully used to treat severe coprolalia (94).

Case Three

In a 9-year-old boy, excessive eye blinking developed and tended to be worse toward the end of the day and when he was overtired. Several months later, intermittent head jerking to the side and abdominal tensing movements developed, which sometimes caused him to flex forward. When emotionally excited, he tended to let out repetitive high-pitched squeals. Eye blinking eventually resolved, but the other movements and vocalizations continued and worsened over the course of a year. He described a strong sensation of "tensing" in his neck and abdomen that was relieved when he did the tics. His mother also noted that he is a "neat freak" and always tends to spin once to the right when he enters a room. His school performance deteriorated. Although he did not have tics during class, he was unable to sustain attention on his schoolwork. He was unable to sit in a chair for the duration of class, and he described the intense effort needed to suppress his tics during school.

Birth and development were normal. Neurological examination was normal, aside from the presence of multiple simple motor and phonic tics. Brain imaging was normal, as were ASO titers, thyroid function, and liver function.

Clonidine was chosen as first-line therapy for his tics in the hope that it would also improve his attention deficit. The dose was slowly titrated up to a dose of 0.1 mg three times daily, at which point, the severity of his tics decreased somewhat. An effort was made to allow him regular breaks during class, during which he could leave the room and release his tics. With these interventions, his attention during classes improved, and grades improved.

Discussion: Most patients with TS have significant disability related to comorbid attention deficit and obsessive–compulsive behaviors. Although dopamine-receptor blockers are the most potent tic-suppressing drugs, α-2 agonists like clonidine and guanfacine may be useful in children with both ADHD and tics. Although controlled trials that support the use of these nonstimulant drugs in ADHD are lacking, these agents show promise in improving both attention deficit and tics.

Stereotypies

Stereotypies are repetitive, nonpurposeful gestures or movements of the hands that may be partially suppressible. Physicians find them in association with autistic-spectrum disorders, OCD, schizophrenia, and in states of sensory deprivation, such as blindness. Frequently occurring stereotypies include arm flapping, finger drumming, body rocking, neck extension, and leg shaking. For example, the hand-wringing stereotypy is characteristically seen in association with Rett syndrome (95), a progressive neurodegenerative disorder inherited in X-linked dominant fashion. Its CNS manifestations are diverse and generally progress through four stages, beginning with deceleration of head growth and hypotonia by 1.5 years of age, followed by stereotypy development and loss of language by age 4 years. Several years after the onset, symptoms progress to include ataxia, breathing dysfunction, rigidity, and bradykinesia.

In general, stereotypies have an earlier age at onset than do tics, and the movements tend to be more rhythmical, fixed in pattern, distractible, and prolonged. Unlike children with tics, which tend to vary in character and anatomical distribution with time, those with stereotypy tend to make the same movements as they get older. Because stereotypy usually does not interfere with functioning, specific treatment is not usually necessary. In any case, stereotypies characteristically do not respond well to pharmacological therapy.

Chorea

Chorea is a hyperkinetic movement disorder characterized by involuntary, continuous, abrupt, rapid, unsustained, irregular movements that flow randomly from one body part to another. Chorea is sometimes difficult to distinguish from the abnormal athetoid, or twisting, movements that can occur with dystonia. A general rule of thumb is that chorea tends to flow randomly and unpredictably from one body part to another, whereas dystonic movements tend to be directional and predictable. Generalized chorea can have a dancelike quality; hence the term "St. Vitus dance" is used for Sydenham chorea (SC). Children sometimes partially suppress or camouflage the movements. For example, they may turn an involuntary arm movement into adjusting their clothes or running a hand through their hair. This is termed *parakinesia*. Another classic feature of chorea is *motor impersistence*, or the inability to sustain muscle tone, which can cause significant motor impairment. Examples of motor impersistence include the "milk-maid's grip" (inability to sustain a constant grip) and the darting tongue (inability to maintain tongue protrusion), which can often be demonstrated in adult HD patients.

Unlike dystonia, in which primary idiopathic forms exist, chorea in children is often due to an underlying pathological condition. However, a few rare, familial primary forms of chorea are found, and chorea can sometimes be seen in normal infants but should disappear by 8 months of age.

Whereas HD is the most notorious choreiform illness in adults, juvenile-onset HD is initially seen with a parkinsonian syndrome rather than chorea. In children, the most common cause of chorea is SC, a postinfectious complication of group A β-hemolytic streptococcal infection and a disease-defining criterion for rheumatic fever (96). The disorder is thought to have an autoimmune basis, and anti–basal ganglia antibodies have been demonstrated in the sera of patients with active SC (97,98). A definite causal relation between these antibodies and the appearance of chorea has not been demonstrated, but evidence suggests that these antibodies have a pathological effect on the basal ganglia (99). The chorea develops acutely, usually 4 to 8 weeks after a bout of streptococcal pharyngitis. Onset may be delayed for up to 8 months, long after ASO titers have decreased, sometimes masking the streptococcal connection. The usual age at onset is 8 to 9 years, with a female predominance (100). The chorea is normally generalized, but in 20% of cases, it may affect only one side of the body (101). The clinical spectrum of SC ranges from mild transient chorea to persistent disabling chorea associated with dysarthria, hypotonia, weakness, and behavioral changes (102). Frank dysarthria may be accompanied by a "disinclination to speak," with a specific pattern of decreased phonemic verbal output described in one series (103). From 60% to 80% of patients display cardiac involvement, usually in the form of mitral valve dysfunction. About 30% of patients have arthritis along with the chorea, whereas a full 20% may have chorea as the sole manifestation of acute rheumatic fever (102).

Neurobehavioral symptoms such as obsessions and compulsions have long been recognized as part of the clinical spectrum of SC. Obsessions and compulsions are present in higher than expected frequencies in patients with SC, but not in patients with rheumatic fever without chorea (104). Another recent series demonstrated that obsessive–compulsive behaviors, OCD, and ADHD are all more frequent among SC patients than in healthy controls or patients with rheumatic fever without chorea (105). These links between SC and neurobehavioral symptoms led to the concept that an autoimmune basis may underlie an entire subgroup of neurobehavioral syndromes first seen in childhood, such as OCD, tics, and TS (67,106). This concept of PANDAS, which was discussed earlier in the section on tics, remains controversial. Streptococcal infections are common in children, and in some cases, the association between onset of infection and onset of tics or OCD may be coincidental (68). Controversy still exists as to whether a postinfectious form of OCD, independent of the presence of a movement disorder, may exist. A recent review by Pavone et al. (107) concluded that the PANDAS spectrum likely represents a heterogeneous and overlapping group of neurobehavioral disorders similar conceptually to the connective tissue disorders, and that group A β-hemolytic streptococcal infections may lead to a wide range of neuropsychiatric symptoms.

Because ASO titers may be normal by the time chorea appears and anti–basal ganglia antibodies are not diagnostic of the disorder, diagnosing SC often depends on ruling out other secondary causes of chorea. Table 3.3 lists etiologies of chorea in children. An MRI scan of the brain should be obtained to exclude an ischemic or mass lesion. When chorea is due to stroke, often a delayed onset is found, suggesting that the pathological processes that contribute to chorea, such as remyelination, inflammatory changes, and oxidative stress, take time to occur (108). MRI findings, which are not diagnostic for SC, may range from normal to nonspecific white-matter changes (102).

Drug-induced chorea, also high on the list of differential diagnoses, can be seen with oral contraceptive use, neuroleptic medications, anticonvulsants, and amphetamines. Infections, such as human immunodeficiency virus (HIV), and bacterial encephalitides, such as mycoplasma, have also been associated with chorea (109,110). Therefore, a lumbar puncture should be considered to rule out an active infection. Nonketotic hyperglycemia has long been recognized as a cause of hemichorea, most often in women older than 60 years, but it has also been reported in children (111). Systemic lupus erythematosus (SLE) should also be considered, although rarely is chorea the sole manifestation of lupus. For example, in one series of 90 patients with childhood-onset SLE, 4 had hemichorea, and of these, 2 had elevated anticardiolipin antibodies (112).

In the treatment of SC, secondary prophylaxis with penicillin should be maintained until the age of 21 years (113). Although the disorder is often self-limited and resolves with time, symptomatic treatment is often required. Unfortunately, no controlled trials support the use of medications that improve involuntary movements in SC. Although extensive trial data are lacking, valproic acid may be used as first-line, and atypical neuroleptics such

TABLE 3.3 DIFFERENTIAL DIAGNOSIS OF CHOREA IN CHILDREN

Infectious / Immune related	Metabolic
Sydenham chorea Postinfectious chorea Systemic lupus erythematosus Antiphospholipid antibody syndrome Henoch–Schönlein purpura	*Neurometabolic:* Lesch–Nyhan syndrome Lysosomal storage diseases (Krabbe, metachromatic leukodystrophy) Amino acidopathies Mitochondrial disorders (Leigh syndrome) *Systemic metabolic* Hypoparathyroidism Electrolyte imbalances (hypernatremia, hyponatremia, hypomagnesemia, hypocalcemia) Hyperglycemia
Drug and Toxin Related	**Heredodegenerative diseases**
Anticonvulsants Cocaine Amphetamines Tricyclics Neuroleptics (tardive dyskinesias or withdrawal-emergent dyskinesias) Carbon monoxide Heavy metals (manganese, mercury, thallium)	Ataxia–telangiectasia Friedreich ataxia Spinocerebellar ataxias Dentatorubropallidoluysian atrophy (DRPLA) Wilson disease Neurodegeneration with brain iron accumulation (including pantothenate-kinase–related neurodegeneration) Tuberous sclerosis
Endocrine	**Vascular / Structural / Hypoxia**
Hyperthyroidism Hypoparathyroidism Perinatal anoxia–cerebral palsy	Stroke, hemorrhage, arteriovenous malformation Moyamoya disease
	Benign choreas
	Benign familial chorea Physiologic chorea of infancy

as risperidone may be tried as second-line agents, but there is a risk of the development of tardive dyskinesias. Carbamazepine appears to be as effective as valproic acid at suppressing chorea and may be used in patients who cannot tolerate valproate (114). In patients with illness refractory to these therapies, a course of methylprednisolone may reduce chorea (115).

Case Four

A 6-year-old girl who was healthy and developmentally normal acutely developed flinging and dancing movements involving both arms and legs. The movements, which were not suppressible, were random and unpatterned. They disappeared only during sleep. After 2 weeks, hoarseness of her voice developed, and she had difficulty swallowing liquids. Her personality changed, such that she became more aggressive and impulsive, biting people around her and having frequent temper tantrums. Her parents recalled that 3 months earlier, she had a sore throat and cough, and a month before the abnormal movements, a raised red geographic-appearing rash developed; it migrated from her abdomen to all four extremities before disappearing.

Examination revealed a developmentally normal child with no skin lesions and dysarthric speech. Her irises had no discoloration. Cranial nerves were normal, aside from a sluggish gag reflex and motor impersistence of her tongue. Motor examination revealed hypotonia in all extremities, normal strength, and abnormal dancelike involuntary movements involving both arms, both legs, and her trunk. Reflexes were 2+ throughout. Serum glucose, electrolytes, thyroid-function, and liver-function tests were normal. An ASO titer was normal. An MRI scan of the brain with contrast revealed no abnormality. Lumbar puncture revealed a normal opening pressure and normal cell counts and protein. An echocardiogram demonstrated mild mitral valve insufficiency but no vegetations. Anti-DNase-B titers were later obtained and were elevated, but ANA was normal.

Because her chorea persisted for more than 1 month, carbamazepine at 15 mg/kg/day was instituted. A course of prednisone at 2 mg/kg/day was instituted for 4 weeks, followed by a taper. Within 2 months, the chorea had diminished, but it persisted, and the medication was continued. Behavior improved somewhat, but the patient became more hyperactive, had difficulty sitting in one place, and could not finish tasks.

Discussion: Making the diagnosis of SC can be difficult. Although ASO titers usually normalize 8 weeks after infection, anti-DNAase-B titers may remain elevated for up to 1 year. Symptomatic treatment with carbamazepine, valproic acid, and D_2 blockers, like risperidone, have been tried, but no randomized trials support their use (114). The raised red rash seen in this patient was likely erythema marginatum, which usually disappears by the time chorea appears. Behavioral problems, obsessive–compulsive spectrum disorders, and ADHD occur in a higher frequency in patients with persistent SC, but a causal relation between these disorders has not been clearly defined (105,116).

Myoclonus

Myoclonus, a brief lightning-like jerk, can take the form of either a muscle contraction ("positive myoclonus") or a sudden muscle relaxation, as in asterixis ("negative myoclonus") (117). Many patients have a combination of positive and negative myoclonus. It may occur at rest or may be stimulus-induced by light, sound, touch, or action. Although myoclonus may appear similar to tics because both can seem clonic and lightning-like, tics are suppressible and may have a premonitory urge associated with them. Anatomically, myoclonus may be divided into the following categories: (a) generalized (whole-body jerks at once); (b) multifocal (involving multiple parts of the body at different times); and (c) focal or segmental (involving one region of the body). The anatomical distribution of the myoclonus sometimes suggests its nervous system origin. For instance, cortical myoclonus presents as focal rhythmic jerking of the distal part of a limb that may progress to a seizure, or as the startle-induced generalized myoclonus that is seen in prion diseases (118). Myoclonus is usually symptomatic of an underlying condition, but it may also be physiologic, such as *hypnic myoclonus* occurring at sleep onset. Myoclonus may also transiently occur in normal children with fever (119). Myoclonus can also be induced

TABLE 3.4 DIFFERENTIAL DIAGNOSIS OF MYOCLONUS IN CHILDREN

Myoclonic Epilepsies	Symptomatic Myoclonus
Primary childhood myoclonic epilepsy syndromes	*Drugs and Toxins*
Juvenile myoclonic epilepsy	Opiates, selective serotonin reuptake inhibitors (SSRIs)
Cryptogenic myoclonic epilepsy	
Eyelid myoclonus with absences	Bismuth, heavy metals, methyl bromide
Infantile spasms	*Metabolic*
Absence epilepsy with myoclonus	Hepatic or renal failure
Lennox–Gastaut syndrome	Hyponatremia, hypoglycemia
Progressive myoclonic epilepsy syndromes	*Vascular*
Baltic myoclonus (Unverricht–Lundborg)	Posthypoxic myoclonus (Lance–Adams syndrome)
Lafora body disease	*Infectious/Immune*
Sialidosis	Viral encephalitides (subacute sclerosing panencephalitis, arbovirus, herpes simplex encephalitis)
Neuronal ceroid lipofuscinosis	
Myoclonic epilepsy with ragged red fibers (MERRF, mitochondrial)	
Dentatorubro-pallidoluysian atrophy (DRPLA)	Postinfectious encephalitis
Essential, physiologic	Opsoclonus–myoclonus syndrome
Sleep jerks, hiccups	Whipple disease
	Other neurodegenerative disorders
	Neurodegeneration with brain iron accumulation (PKAN)

by drugs, most notably the opiates. Numerous metabolic, toxic, and neurodegenerative disorders can result in myoclonus. Many of them are not reversible, including degenerative diseases, such as Rett syndrome; metabolic disorders, such as organic acidurias; lysosomal storage diseases; mitochondrial disorders, such as Leigh syndrome; and neurocutaneous disorders, such as tuberous sclerosis (120) (Table 3.4). In most of these disorders, myoclonus is one of many neurological features.

In children and adolescents, the most recognizable conditions in which myoclonus is a prominent and disabling clinical feature are the myoclonic epilepsy syndromes and the opsoclonus–myoclonus syndrome. The myoclonic epilepsies can be divided into progressive and nonprogressive forms. The prototypical nonprogressive myoclonic epilepsy is juvenile myoclonic epilepsy, which usually presents in adolescents with focal myoclonus and generalized tonic–clonic seizures. Good seizure control can usually be obtained with valproic acid or newer-generation antiepileptic drugs (AEDs), such as lamotrigine or topiramate (121,122). The progressive myoclonic epilepsies are a heterogeneous group of generalized seizure disorders associated with cognitive decline and myoclonus that usually present in childhood or adolescence, and are summarized in Table 3.4. The opsoclonus–myoclonus syndrome is a paraneoplastic syndrome characterized by dancing eye movements and myoclonus. Presentation is usually in early childhood, and 50% of cases are associated with a neuroblastoma (123). This rare disorder is also associated with significant neurobehavioral abnormalities, such as sleep disturbance and irritability (124). Pranzatelli et al. (125) postulated the cause is secondary cross-reactivity of an autoantibody against the tumor with as yet unidentified CNS antigens. Other autoimmune and immune-related causes of myoclonus include subacute sclerosing panencephalitis (SSPE), associated with measles virus, as well as other viral encephalitides. SSPE may present as a progressive dementia with myoclonus, and its incidence has decreased significantly because of widespread use of the measles vaccine.

When possible, treatment of myoclonus should be directed at the underlying cause. In most cases, however, the underlying disorder is not treatable, and treatment is aimed at symptomatic relief. Levetiracetam, valproic acid, and clonazepam are good choices for myoclonus of cortical origin (126), but levetiracetam should be avoided in the presence of concurrent mood or behavior disorders.

Paroxysmal Movement Disorders

About 20% of movement disorders seen in children and adolescents, excluding tics, are transient rather than sustained (127). Kotagal (128) recently catalogued the paroxysmal nonepileptic events seen in 134 children referred to a pediatric epilepsy-monitoring unit. In this series, the most common nonpsychiatric disorders were daydreaming, hypnic jerks, stereotyped movements, parasomnias, and movement disorders.

Paroxysmal movement disorders comprise a rare but treatable group of disorders known collectively as the paroxysmal dyskinesias. These disorders are often misdiagnosed as psychogenic disorders because of their episodic quality, tendency to begin suddenly, and occasional bizarre manifestations. The movements that occur in these disorders range from chorea to sustained contractions and dystonia, and to incoordination and ataxia. Migraine and epilepsy tend to occur with higher frequencies in families with paroxysmal dyskinesias, but the movements themselves are not epileptic. Video electroencephalographic (EEG) monitoring can capture, characterize, and differentiate these events from seizures. Although the episodic nature of these disorders suggests channelopathy as the underlying defect, for some of these disorders, the pathophysiology is not yet certain.

Paroxysmal dyskinesias respond variably to treatment with anticonvulsants or acetazolamide. They can be divided into two categories: (a) paroxysmal kinesiogenic (PKD) and nonkinesiogenic dyskinesias (PNKD), and (b) the episodic ataxias. PKD can be sporadic or inherited in an autosomal dominant fashion (129). Attacks tend to last seconds to minutes and can be precipitated by sudden movement, startle, hyperventilation, or exercise (130,131). Patients often report an aura before the dyskinesia, usually in the form of tingling in an affected limb. The movements usually respond well to treatment with AEDs, such as phenytoin, valproic acid, or carbamazepine, and the attacks tend to diminish in severity with age (130). Newer AEDs, such as lamotrigine and oxcarbazepine, have also been used successfully in this disorder (132,133). Typically, the EEG is normal during attacks, but forms of stimulus-induced seizures do exist that can appear similar to PKD (134).

Paroxysmal nonkinesiogenic dyskinesias can also be sporadic or familial (135). Attacks tend to last longer than those in PKD, from minutes to hours, and can be precipitated by caffeine, fatigue, or alcohol. It is sometimes difficult to differentiate PNKD from a psychogenic movement disorder because, unlike PKD, PNKD attacks can appear and resolve without provocation (136). These disorders in general do not respond well to the AEDs. Clonazepam has been found anecdotally to be the most effective therapy. Although several genetic localizations have been proposed, the classic familial form of this disorder as described by Mount and Reback has been linked to defects in the myofibrillogenesis regulator-1 (*MR-1*) gene on chromosome 2(137). Both PKD and PNKD, like other movement disorders, can be symptomatic of an underlying cause, such as demyelinating disease (138).

The episodic ataxias are a group of disorders that manifest as episodic incoordination and usually present before age 15. Type 1 is associated with myokymia and neuromyotonia, or abnormal muscle contractions, and is associated with defects in the voltage-gated potassium channel gene on chromosome 12 (139,140). Type 2 is usually associated with attacks of vertigo, migraine, nystagmus, and dysarthria, lasting hours to weeks (141).

Type 2 is linked to the calcium channel *CACNL1A4* gene (142). It is considered allelic to the disorder familial hemiplegic migraine and is treated with acetazolamide.

Psychogenic Movement Disorders

Psychogenic movement disorders arise in the context of unconscious emotional conflict or psychological stress, and in the absence of an organic etiology for the movements. It is not always possible, however, to identify a clear underlying conflict. These disorders are manifestations of somatoform disorders, factitious disorder, or malingering. Depression, anxiety, and other mood disorders are typically comorbid. Sparse literature is found on psychogenic movement disorders in childhood, but one series recently characterized the types of psychogenic events recorded in a pediatric epilepsy-monitoring unit in children of different age groups (128). In this study, conversion disorder was most commonly diagnosed in children older than 5 years, and its incidence increases with age (128). In addition, conversion was more common in boys among school-age children, and in girls in the adolescent age group. In children, in contrast to adults, the dominant side of the body is more likely to be affected by conversion (143). It is often more possible in children than in adults to identify specific precipitating life stressors that underlie the conversion (144).

Diagnosing a movement disorder as psychogenic is one of the most difficult tasks facing movement-disorder neurologists and requires a familiarity with all of the known organic movement disorders. Therefore the diagnosis is best left to a neurologist who specializes in movement disorders. The diagnostic process does not simply involve ruling out all possible organic causes of the movement. Rather, it is a dynamic synthesis of a detailed history and physical examination, in which key features of psychogenicity are actively sought (37).

The neurological examination can be very revealing. Excessive slowness and fatigue, giving way or false weakness, false sensory loss, *la belle indifférence,* and inconsistent movements that disappear with distraction suggest psychogenicity (145). Entrainment of a repetitive movement can sometimes be demonstrated on examination. This occurs when the psychogenic movement changes in speed or amplitude or both in relation to repetitive movements that the examiner asks the patient to mimic. The history of abrupt onset or resolution of movements, as well as variation in severity or quality of movements over time, is also suggestive. Important exceptions to these guidelines include SC, which can vary widely in severity over time, and tics, which can abruptly begin or resolve and can randomly vary in character and anatomical location over time.

Certain types of movements also are suggestive of psychogenicity in both children and adults. For example, rhythmical shaking that is equally severe at rest, with posture, and with action suggests psychogenicity (37). Bizarre gaits, knee-buckling without falling, deliberate slowness, excessive startle responses, and twisting movements of the jaw or face from side to side are common manifestations of psychogenic movement disorders.

Once a diagnosis of a psychogenic movement disorder is reached, the next step is a psychiatric evaluation aimed at establishing the psychodynamics at play for the individual patient. Very important in this process is identifying the degree of insight and establishing a relationship for ongoing psychotherapy. Favorable prognostic signs include acute onset, duration of less than 2 weeks, good premorbid functioning, absence of coexisting psychopathology, and the presence of an identifiable stressor (146). It should be noted that in children and adults alike, an underlying psychiatric diagnosis of mood or psychotic disorders need not be present. In a large adult series, the most common underlying psychiatric diagnosis encountered was somatoform disorder, particularly conversion disorder, often with accompanying depression (145). In general, psychotherapy has achieved the best results, with meaningful benefit achieved in 58% of patients treated this way in one series; however, relapse occurred in more than 20% of patients (145). Somatoform disorders appear to have the best prognosis, whereas factitious disorders and malingering are much more refractory to treatment. Patients with psychogenic movement disorders are often subjected to exhaustive batteries of tests with multiple physicians before the correct diagnosis is reached. When appropriate psychiatric treatment is instituted early, prognosis for achieving remission can be quite good. Treating a psychogenic disorder as organic with inappropriate medications often delays appropriate psychiatric treatment and may perpetuate the reward mechanism that is often at play in the child, contributing to chronic disability.

Case Five

In a 12-year-old girl with normal development and intelligence, tremors acutely developed in both hands after an asthma attack in gym class. The tremors were intermittent, always occurring in situations of stress or anxiety, and occurred equally at rest, with posture, or with action. They sometimes interfered with her writing and school work. After 6 months, the tremors abruptly stopped, and she remained tremor free and otherwise normal for a period of 1 year. Then, 1 year later, the tremors again abruptly developed after the girl started a new school. This time, a sinus infection triggered the tremors. In addition to hand tremors, she now had violent whole-body shaking with retained consciousness, and leg shaking that affected her walking. Again symptoms tended to wax and wane. She reported two separate instances of palpitations, dyspnea, and a feeling of doom that came over her while riding the subway.

On examination, she had no discoloration of the irises, and skin examination was normal. Neurological examination was normal, aside from an irregular high-amplitude tremor involving both arms, her trunk, and both legs that occurred throughout the examination and changed in character, distribution, and frequency with distraction. Her gait was stiff-legged and excessively slow, with frequent bobbing up and down, and veering right and left, but without falling. She seemed undistressed by the movements and often laughed during the examination.

Ceruloplasmin and 24-hour urine copper testing was normal. An MRI scan of the brain was normal. The 24-hour closed-circuit television (CCTV) EEG monitoring revealed no EEG correlate to her movements.

The diagnosis of a psychogenic movement disorder was made, and she was referred for psychiatric evaluation. Important life stressors were uncovered during the interview; for instance, she had recently moved to a much smaller apartment because her father lost his job, and in attending a new school, for the first time she had been separated from her sister, who was close in age. A regimen of psychotherapy and pharmacotherapy aimed at treating panic symptoms was instituted. Within 6 weeks, she achieved remission from her abnormal movements.

Discussion: Psychogenic movement disorders often begin and remit abruptly. In children, it is often possible to uncover triggering life stressors that set off the movements. Although triggers in this case were obvious, it was still important to rule out treatable neuropsychiatric conditions such as Wilson disease and seizure activity. Once appropriate psychiatric care was instituted, this patient was able to gain control over the shaking and return to productivity in school.

Drug-induced Movement Disorders

Like adults, children are susceptible to drug-induced movement disorders. Psychostimulants, selective serotonin reuptake inhibitors (SSRIs), mood stabilizers, and dopamine receptor–blocking agents (DRBAs) all carry a risk of the development of a movement disorder. Notably, the use of these medications in children is increasing.

Drug-induced movement disorders can be categorized as *acute reactions, continuous reactions,* and *tardive dyskinesias.* Acute reactions include neuroleptic malignant syndrome (NMS) and serotonin syndrome (SS), which have systemic features coupled with rigidity and tremor, and the acute dystonic reactions, which tend to be pure movement disorders. In children, NMS more often occurs after beginning DRBAs, whereas in adults, it can also occur on DRBA discontinuation (147). Tremor, myoclonus, and dystonia are sometimes seen with NMS and SS, and these disorders are reviewed in detail elsewhere (148,149).

If acute dystonic reaction occurs, it develops in 90% of cases within 1 to 5 days of starting either a neuroleptic medication or a dopamine-blocking antiemetic medication, such as chlorpromazine or metoclopramide (150). Young age and male gender are risk factors for developing this reaction, which usually manifests as some combination of orofacial dystonia, trunk and neck arching or extension, eye deviation, and, more severely, laryngospasm (151,152). The reaction is idiosyncratic, and previous exposure to a DRBA without resultant dystonia does not indicate immunity from developing ADR. When DRBAs must be administered to children, pretreatment for 7 days with an anticholinergic medication like benztropine can prevent this complication (153). Treatment of acute dystonic reaction is achieved by intravenous administration of anticholinergics such as diphenhydramine or benztropine, followed by oral diphenhydramine.

Continuous drug-induced movement disorders arise at any point during treatment with a medication and resolve on discontinuation of the medication. Examples in this category include tremor induced by mood stabilizers like valproic acid, and drug-induced parkinsonism or akathisia. Often, the movement disorder is mild and tolerated as a medication side effect. In the case of parkinsonism induced by DRBAs, in which symptoms can be disabling, the offending drug should be discontinued if possible. If this does not result in improvement, or in cases in which the drug cannot be discontinued, anticholinergic therapy or amantadine can sometimes be helpful. Akathisia is a sensory symptom, described as an intense sense of inner restlessness, discomfort, and the need to move. Often patients with akathisia have involuntary vocalizations like grunting and sighing associated with the abnormal movements. The movements tend to be stereotyped and can include hand wringing, pacing, and foot tapping. Akathisia, which can be very disabling, can arise during treatment with a number of classes of medications, most commonly dopamine blockers and, less often, SSRIs (154). Less commonly, it has been reported in association with calcium channel blockers, carbamazepine, tricyclics, buspirone, and ethosuximide (155). Again, the problem is best handled by discontinuing or reducing the dosage of the offending medication. When this is not possible, propranolol is first-line therapy for symptomatic relief (156). Clonidine and anticholinergic medications can also provide symptomatic benefit (155).

Tardive dyskinesias (TDs) usually occur after at least 3 months of treatment with DRBAs. To be diagnosed with TD, the patient must have been exposed to a DRBA within 6 months from the onset of symptoms, although occasionally the movements occur up to a year after exposure (157). TD can arise during treatment with a DRBA, or after discontinuation of the agent. Risk of TD increases with increasing time on the medication, and begins to increase from the first few months of treatment with DRBAs (158). Although rare in children, and more common in postmenopausal women, it is also possible to develop tardive dyskinesias after short-term use of metoclopramide (159,160). In general, the higher the drug's affinity for the D_2 receptor, the higher the likelihood it will result in TD. The exact pathophysiology of TD is still unclear, however, and is likely more complicated than simple D_2 hypersensitivity. As for affinities for the D_2 receptor, risperidone and haloperidol have the highest, whereas olanzapine and quetiapine have intermediate, and clozapine has the lowest affinity.

Children are particularly at risk for another tardive phenomenon termed *withdrawal-emergent dyskinesia (WD)*, which typically appears 2 weeks to 2 months after a dopamine blocker is abruptly withdrawn. Slow tapering of the medication does not always prevent this from occurring (161). Both TD and WD are more likely to occur in neurologically abnormal children treated with dopamine blockers, such as those with autistic-spectrum disorders or a history of pre- and perinatal complications (161).

Clinically, both classic TD and WD manifest with repetitive, rhythmic, orofacial movements like chewing and tongue protrusion, but more generalized dystonia and chorea involving the arms and trunk can also occur. The term "tardive dyskinesia" actually refers to the classic syndrome with repetitive mouth movements. However, it is well recognized that tardive forms of every conceivable movement disorder exist, including dystonia, akathisia, myoclonus, tremor, tics, chorea, and oculogyric crises. When a question arises as to the etiology of dystonia appearing in childhood, the presence of retrocollis and back arching can suggest TD, and a history of DRBA exposure should be sought. It is important to remember that tardive phenomena can result from any dopamine-blocking medication, including antinausea medications, such as metoclopramide. Only an extensive medical history may uncover an exposure to these apparently innocuous medicines. Physicians should keep in mind that the development of a movement disorder in a psychiatric patient is not always drug induced. Diseases like Wilson disease and HD, which may cause similar movements, should also be considered and appropriately investigated.

Withdrawal-emergent dyskinesia normally remits spontaneously, but TD generally persists and may even worsen with dopamine-blocker discontinuation. However, gradual withdrawal of the DRBA should be considered first-line therapy for TD. One prospective study in adults showed a 33% remission of TD within 2 years of drug discontinuation (162). Drug discontinuation is not always possible, especially in the treatment of chronic psychotic disorders. Although drug discontinuation is the ideal, data suggest that continuing antipsychotic medications does not always exacerbate TD, and some patients' dyskinesias even improve in the long term while they are taking stable doses of DRBAs (163).

When TD symptoms are still disabling, and psychiatric symptoms are stable on the lowest possible dose of DRBA, a number of pharmacological options for treatment exist. Some options work best for classic TD; others are better for tardive dystonia; and still others, for tardive akathisia. The dopamine depleters reserpine and tetrabenazine effectively decrease movements of classic TD (164,165). Because they reduce all dopaminergic synaptic activity, some believe that they may allow the brain to "heal" in addition to lessening TD symptoms. This stands in contrast to the atypical antipsychotics quetiapine and clozapine, which also can reduce TD symptoms but still expose the brain to some D_2 blockage, which may perpetuate the underlying pathophysiology of TD. Tetrabenazine has a quicker onset than reserpine and tends to cause less depression and parkinsonism. Jain et al. (166) have shown that it is safe and effective for use in children with hyperkinetic movement disorders. However, because tetrabenazine can precipitate severe depression, pretreatment with SSRIs may be considered. This medication has not yet been approved in the United States.

As second-line therapies, quetiapine and clozapine can also help alleviate movements. Vitamin E is a controversial treatment for TD. Risk of side effects is low, and several studies have demonstrated its effectiveness in reducing TD, but the largest double-blind placebo-controlled study on this topic did not show benefit (167). When the tardive movements are predominantly dystonia, anticholinergic medications, such as trihexyphenidyl, are as effective as the dopamine depleters (158). One report suggests the effectiveness of melatonin in treating TD (168). Finally, multiple case reports in the literature describe non-sustained improvement in TD after electroconvulsive therapy (ECT) (169,170). As controlled trials of ECT are lacking, this therapy should be reserved for patients requiring ECT for psychiatric care.

Future Directions

The treatment of movement disorders has enjoyed a renaissance in the past decade or so, largely because of advances in molecular genetics and the development of DBS as an effective and exciting therapy for a variety of movement disorders.

In addition to the use of DBS in primary and secondary dystonia, several reports in the literature have demonstrated efficacy of DBS in TS, including one recent report that also showed improvement in obsessions and compulsions in a severe TS patient (171). DBS will undoubtedly continue to play a central role in treating a variety of childhood movement disorders.

Advances in molecular genetics have also revolutionized our understanding of movement disorders, as new molecular targets for disease-modifying therapy are identified. For example, DYT-1 dystonia is associated with aggregates of the protein *torsin*. Once the protein structure of this abnormal protein was identified, animal models of the disease were developed. The mutated torsin abnormally aggregates in one such worm model, thus providing a useful way to screen potential disease-modifying drugs that may alter the aggregation (172). The first disease-modifying treatments for primary dystonia may well appear in the next few years based on advances like these.

Summary

In summary, movement disorders represent a diverse and fascinating group of disorders that occupy a unique crossroads between neurology and psychiatry. Their diagnosis and treatment in children and adolescents are challenging but often very rewarding for the treating physician and patient alike. Child psychiatrists are sometimes faced with initial and chronic presentations of these disorders, and an understanding of movement disorders can definitively enhance psychiatric patient care.

Questions

1. Which of the following findings is supportive of a diagnosis of neurological Wilson disease?
   A. normal ceruloplasmin level
   B. 24 hour urine copper level less than 50 mcg/24 hours
   C. normal MRI of the brain
   D. presence of Kaiser-Fleischer rings on formal slit lamp examination

2. Velocity dependent resistance to passive stretch is termed:
   A. rigidity.
   B. spasticity.
   C. dystonia.
   D. clonus.

3. Juvenile onset Huntington disease normally presents with:
   A. chorea.
   B. an akinetic-rigid, parkinsonian syndrome.

C. wing-beating tremor.
D. spasticity with ataxia.

4. Withdrawal emergent dyskinesias:
   A. develop within a month after stopping treatment with SSRIs.
   B. are more likely to occur in neurologically and developmentally normal children.
   C. always occur within days after withdrawal of a dopamine-blocking medication.
   D. usually manifests as repetitive, rhythmic orofacial movements with chewing or tongue protrusion.

5. A 9-year-old, developmentally normal girl developed turning in of her left foot and toe curling that tended to worsen toward the end of the day. MRI brain was normal, and testing for DYT-1 dystonia was negative. What is the most appropriate next step in management?
   A. treatment with an anticholinergic medication
   B. treatment with baclofen
   C. botulinum toxin injections into the leg
   D. a therapeutic trial of levodopa

6. Generalized torsion dystonia related to the DYT-1 gene is inherited as:
   A. an autosomal recessive trait.
   B. an autosomal dominant trait with complete penetrance.
   C. an autosomal dominant trait with incomplete penetrance.
   D. an X-linked recessive trait.

7. Tics are characterized by all of the following EXCEPT:
   A. partial suppressibility.
   B. tend not to vary in character over time.
   C. sensory premonitory symptoms.
   D. brief sense of relief after releasing the tic.

8. Tourette Syndrome is most often accompanied by which of the following?
   A. antisocial personality disorder
   B. obsessive compulsive behaviors
   C. psychosis
   D. somatoform disorder

9. Sydenham Chorea
   A. tends to develop gradually within one month of a streptococcal infection.
   B. may develop following a streptococcal skin infection.
   C. may be associated with severe hypotonia, weakness, behavioral changes, and dysarthria.
   D. among school age children, it is more common in boys.

10. Good prognostic indicators related to psychogenic movement disorders include all of the following EXCEPT:
    A. a developmentally normal child with good premorbid functioning.
    B. acute onset of the movement.
    C. long duration of the symptoms.
    D. the presence of an identifiable provoking stressor.

Answers

1. D. Low ceruloplasmin levels, high excretion of urine copper, and abnormalities in the basal ganglia on brain MRI are characteristic of neurological Wilson disease. Almost all patients with neurological Wilson disease have K-F rings identifiable on slit lamp examination, though rare case reports exist of patients in whom they were absent.

2. B. Spasticity is a velocity-dependent and directional resistance to passive stretch usually due to dysfunction of the pyramidal tracts, and it may be associated with clonus. Rigidity is an extrapyramidal sign characterized by nonvelocity dependent passive stretch resistance. Dystonia is involuntary co-contractions of agonist and antagonist muscles producing abnormal posturing and movement.

3. B. While adult onset HD presents with chorea, juvenile onset HD usually presents with a parkinsonian syndrome (Westfal variant).

4. D. WD usually occur 2 weeks to 2 months following dopamine blocking medication withdrawal. Although they may occur in normal children, they are more likely, like tardive dyskinesias, to develop in neurologically and developmentally abnormal children. Unlike TD, WD are usually self-limited. They appear clinically similar to classic TD with orofacial movements, but they can also manifest as various forms of dystonia.

5. D. This case describes a typical presentation of dopa-responsive dystonia (DRD). A levodopa trial is indicated in all children with an unexplained movement disorder in order to assess dopamine responsiveness.

6. C. The DYT-1 GAG deletion is inherited in an autosomal dominant fashion with incomplete penetrance.

7. B. Tics are partially suppressible, usually associated with a premonitory "urge," accompanied by a sense of relief afterwards, and tend to vary in character and anatomic distribution with time.

8. B. ADHD, OCD, separation anxiety, overanxious disorder, simple phobia, social phobia, agoraphobia, mania, major depressive disorder, and oppositional defiant disorder are all seen in higher frequency in association with Tourette Syndrome than in the general population.

9. C. SC develops acutely 4 to 8 weeks (sometimes longer) following strep pharyngitis. It has not been associated with strep skin infections. A wide clinical spectrum exists and symptoms may include hypotonia, weakness, dysarthria, tantrums and aggressive behavior. It is more common in girls.

10. C. Good premorbid functioning, acute onset, short duration, and the presence of an identifiable stressor are all good prognostic indicators in psychogenic movement disorders in children.

REFERENCES

1. Dening TR, Berrios GE. Wilson's disease: psychiatric symptoms in 195 cases. *Arch Gen Psychiatry.* 1989;46:1126–1134.
2. Sanger TD. Pediatric movement disorders. *Curr Opin Neurol.* 2003;16:529–535.
3. Albanese A, Barnes MP, Bhatia KP, et al. A systematic review on the diagnosis and treatment of primary (idiopathic) dystonia and dystonia plus syndromes: report of an EFNS/MDS-ES Task Force. *Eur J Neurol.* 2006;13:433–444.
4. O'Riordan S, Raymond D, Lynch T, et al. Age at onset as a factor in determining the phenotype of primary torsion dystonia. *Neurology.* 2004;63:1423–1426.
5. Sanger TD, Delgado MR, Gaebler-Spira D, et al. Classification and definition of disorders causing hypertonia in childhood. *Pediatrics.* 2003;111:e89–e97.
6. Tan A, Slagado M, Fahn S. The characterization and outcome of stereotypic movements in nonautistic children. *Mov Disord.* 1997;12:47–52.
7. Fernandez Alvarez E, Aicardi J. *Movement disorders in children.* London: MacKeith Press, 2001.
8. Saunders-Pullman R, Braun I, Bressman S. Pediatric movement disorders. *Child Adolesc Psychiatr Clin North Am.* 1999;8:747–765.
9. Schrag A, Schott JM. Epidemiological, clinical, and genetic characteristics of early-onset parkinsonism. *Lancet Neurol.* 2006;5:355–633.
10. Critchley E. Clinical manifestations of essential tremor. *J Neurol Neurosurg Psychiatry.* 1972;35:365–372.
11. Elble RJ, Koller WC. *Tremor.* Baltimore: The Johns Hopkins Press, 1990.
12. Findley LJ, Koller WC. Essential tremor: a review. *Neurology.* 1984;37:1194–1197.
13. Marsden CD. Origins of normal and pathological tremor. In: Findley LJ, Capildeo R, eds. *Movement disorders: tremor.* New York: Oxford University Press, 1984:7–84.
14. Soland VL, Bhatia KP, Volonte MA, Marsden CD. Focal task-specific tremors. *Mov Disord.* 1996;11:665–670.
15. Jankovic J, Madisetty J, Vuong KD. Essential tremor among children. *Pediatrics.* 2004;114:1203–1205.
16. Hornabrook RW, Nagurney JT. Essential tremor in Papua New Guinea. *Brain.* 1976;99:659–672.
17. Louis ED, Dure LS, Pullman S. Essential tremor in childhood: a series of nineteen cases. *Mov Disord.* 2001;16:921–923.

18. Elble RJ. Essential tremor frequency decreases with time. *Neurology.* 2000;55:1547–1551.
19. Singer C, Sanchez-Ramos J, Weiner WJ. Gait abnormality in essential tremor. *Mov Disord.* 1994;9:193–196.
20. Hess CW, Saunders-Pullman R. Movement disorders and alcohol misuse. *Addict Biol.* 2006;67:117–125.
21. Paulson GW, Reider CR. Movement disorders in childhood. In: Watts RL, Koller WC, eds. *Movement disorders: neurologic principles and practice.* New York: McGraw-Hill Co., 1997:661–666.
22. Jankovic J. Essential tremor and Parkinson's disease. *Ann Neurol.* 1989;25:211.
23. Calzetti S, Sasso E, Baratti M, Fava R. Clinical and computer-based assessment of long-term efficacy of propranolol in essential tremor. *Acta Neurol Scand.* 1990;81:392–396.
24. Guan X-M, Peroutka SJ. Basic mechanisms of actions of drugs used in the treatment of essential tremor. *Clin Neuropharmacol.* 1990;13:210–223.
25. Koller WC, Royse VL. Efficacy of primidone in essential tremor. *Neurology.* 1986;36:121–124.
26. Ondo WG, Jankovic J, Connor GS, et al., Topiramate Essential Tremor Study Investigators. Topiramate in essential tremor: a double-blind, placebo-controlled trial. *Neurology.* 2006;66:672–677.
27. Pfeiffer RF. Wilson's disease. *Semin Neurol.* 2007;27:123–132.
28. Lin J-J, Lin K-J, Wang H-S, Wong M-C. Psychological presentations without hepatic involvement in Wilson disease. *Pediatr Neurol.* 2006;35:284–286.
29. Brewer GJ. Recognition, diagnosis, and management of Wilson's disease. *Proc Soc Exp Biol Med.* 2000;223:39–46.
30. Stremmel W, Meyerrose KW, Niderau C, et al. Wilson disease: clinical presentation, treatment, and survival. *Ann Intern Med.* 1991;115:720–726.
31. Petrukhin K, Fischer SG, Pirastu M, et al. Mapping, cloning and genetic characteristics of the region containing the Wilson disease gene. *Nat Genet.* 1993;5:338–343.
32. Tanzi RE, Petrukhin K, Chernov I, et al. The Wilson disease gene is a copper transporting ATPase with homology to the Menkes disease gene. *Nat Genet.* 1993;5:344–350.
33. Brewer GJ, Dick RD, Yuzbasiyan-Gurkan V, et al. Initial therapy of Wilson's disease: patients with tetrathiomolybdate. *Arch Neurol.* 1991;48:42–47.
34. Brewer GJ, Dick RD, Johnson VD, et al. Treatment of Wilson's disease with zinc XVI: treatment during the pediatric years. *J Lab Clin Med.* 2001;137:191–198.
35. Stracciari A, Tempestini A, Borghi A, Guarino M. Effect of liver transplantation on neurological manifestations in Wilson disease. *Arch Neurol.* 2000;57:384–386.
36. Graham HK, Boyd RN, Fehlings D. Does intramuscular botulinum toxin A injection improve upper-limb function in children with hemiplegic cerebral palsy? *Med J Aust.* 2003;178:95–96.
37. Fahn S, Williams DT. Psychogenic dystonia. *Adv Neurol.* 1988;50:431–455.
38. Greene P, Bressman S. Exteroceptive and interoceptive stimuli in dystonia. *Mov Disord.* 1998;13:549–551.
39. Hashimoto T. Neuronal activity in the globus pallidus in primary dystonia and off-period dystonia. *J Neurol.* 2000;247:49–52.
40. Sohn YH, Hallett M. Disturbed surround inhibition in focal hand dystonia. *Ann Neurol.* 2004;56:595–599.
41. Oppenheim H. Uber eine eigenartige Krampfkrankheit des kindlichen und jugendlichen Alters (Dysbasia lordotica progressive, Dystonia musculorum deformans). *Neurol Centrabl.* 1911;30:1090–1107.
42. Greene P, Kang UJ, Fahn S. Spread of symptoms in idiopathic torsion dystonia. *Mov Disord.* 1995;10:143–152.
43. Bressman SB. Dystonia: genotypes, phenotypes and classification. *Adv Neurol.* 2004;94:101–107.
44. Saunders-Pullman R, Shriberg J, Shanker V, Bressman S. Penetrance and expression of dystonia genes. *Adv Neurol.* 2004;94:121–125.
45. Bressman SB, Raymond D, Wendt K, et al. Diagnostic criteria for dystonia in DYT1 families. *Neurology.* 2002;59:1780–1788.
46. Ozelius LJ, Hewett JW, Page CE, et al. The early-onset torsion dystonia gene (DYT1) encodes an ATP-binding protein. *Nat Genet.* 1997;17:40–48.
47. Carbon M, Su S, Dhawan V, et al. Regional metabolism in primary torsion dystonia: effects of penetrance and genotype. *Neurology.* 2004;62:1384–1390.
48. Heiman GA, Ottman R, Saunders-Pullman RJ, et al. Increased risk for recurrent major depression in DYT1 dystonia mutation carriers. *Neurology.* 2004;63:631–637.
49. Van Hove JL, Steyaert J, Matthijs G, et al. Expanded motor and psychiatric phenotype in autosomal dominant Segawa syndrome due to GTP cyclohydrolase deficiency. *J Neurol Neurosurg Psychiatry.* 2006;77:18–23.
50. Hess CW, Raymond D, de Carvalho A, et al. Myoclonus, dystonia, obsessive compulsive disorder, and alcohol dependence in SGCE mutation carriers. *Neurology.* 2007;68:522–524.
51. Segawa M, Nomura Y, Nishiyama N. Autosomal dominant guanosine triphosphate cyclohydrolase I deficiency (Segawa disease). *Ann Neurol.* 2003;54(Suppl 6):S32–S45.
52. Nygaard TG, Waran SP, Levine RA, et al. Dopa-responsive dystonia simulating cerebral palsy. *Pediatr Neurol.* 1994;11:236–240.
53. Jan M. Misdiagnoses in children with Dopa-responsive dystonia. *Pediatr Neurol.* 2004;31:298–303.
54. Hagenah J, Saunders-Pullman R, Hedrich K, et al. High mutation rate in dopa-responsive dystonia

with comprehensive GCHI screening. *Neurology.* 2005;64:908–911.
55. Saunders-Pullman R, Blau N, Hyland K, et al. Phenylalanine loading as a diagnostic test for DRD: interpreting the utility of the test. *Mol Genet Metab.* 2004;83:201–212.
56. Zimprich A, Grabowski M, Asmus F, et al. Mutations in the gene encoding epsilon-sarcoglycan cause myoclonus-dystonia syndrome. *Nat Genet.* 2001;29:66–69.
57. Burke RE, Fahn S, Marsden CD. Torsion dystonia: a double-blind, prospective trial of high dosage trihexyphenidyl. *Neurology.* 1986;36:160–164.
58. Papapetropoulos S, Singer C. Improvement of cervico-trunco-brachial segmental dystonia with topiramate. *J Neurol.* 2006;253:535–536.
59. Tarsy D, Ryan RK, Ro SI. An open-label trial of levetiracetam for treatment of cervical dystonia. *Mov Disord.* 2006;21:734–735.
60. Pullman SL, Greene P, Fahn S, Pedersen SF. Approach to the treatment of limb disorders with botulinum toxin A: experience with 187 patients. *Arch Neurol.* 1996;53:617–624.
61. Vidailhet M, Vercueil L, Houeto JL, et al. Bilateral deep brain stimulation of the globus pallidus in primary generalized dystonia. *N Engl J Med.* 2005;352:459–467.
62. Castelnau P, Cif L, Valente EM, et al. Pallidal stimulation improves pantothenate kinase-associated neurodegeneration. *Ann Neurol.* 2005;57:38–41.
63. Lombroso PJ, Mack G, Scahill L, et al. Exacerbation of Gilles de la Tourette syndrome associated with thermal stress: a family study. *Neurology.* 1991;41:1984–1987.
64. Goldenberg JN, Brown SB, Weiner WJ. Coprolalia in younger patients with Gilles de la Tourette syndrome. *Mov Disord* 1994;9:622–625.
65. Chouinard S, Ford B. Adult onset tic disorders. *J Neurol Neurosurg Psychiatry.* 2000;68:738–743.
66. Leonard HL. New developments in the treatment of obsessive-compulsive disorder. *J Clin Psychiatry.* 1997;58(Suppl 14):39–45.
67. Swedo SE, Leonard HL, Mittleman BB, et al. Identification of children with pediatric autoimmune neuropsychiatric disorders associated with streptococcal infections by a marker associated with rheumatic fever. *Am J Psychiatry.* 1997;154:110–112.
68. Kurlan R, Kaplan EL. The PANDAS etiology for tics and obsessive-compulsive symptoms: hypothesis or entity? Practical considerations for the clinician. *Pediatrics.* 2004;113:883–886.
68a. Tourette Syndrome Classification Study Group. Definitions and classification of tic disorders. *Arch Neurol.* 1993;50:1013–1016.
69. Robertson MM. The Gilles de la Tourette syndrome: the current status. *Br J Psychiatry.* 1989;154:147–169.
70. Leckman JF, Zhang H, Vitale A, et al. Course of tic severity in Tourette syndrome: the first two decades. *Pediatrics.* 1998;102:14–19.
71. Goetz CG, Tanner CM, Stebbins GT, et al. Adult tics in Gilles de la Tourette syndrome: description and risk factors. *Neurology.* 1992;42:784–788.
72. Pappert EJ, Goetz cg, Louis ED, et al. Objective assessments of longitudinal outcome in Gilles de la Tourette syndrome. *Neurology.* 2003;61:936–940.
73. Kurlan R, Como PG, Miller B, et al. The behavioral spectrum of tic disorders: a community-based study. *Neurology.* 2002;59:414–420.
74. Freeman RD, Fast DK, Burd L, et al. Tourette Syndrome International Database Consortium: an international perspective on Tourette syndrome selected findings from 3500 individuals in 22 countries. *Dev Med Child Neurol.* 2000;42:436–447.
75. Comings DE, Comings BG. Tourette's syndrome and attention-deficit disorder. In: Cohen DJ, Bruun RD, Leckman JF, eds. *Tourette's syndrome and tic disorders.* New York: John Wiley & Sons, 1988:119–135.
76. Price RA, Leckman JF, Pauls DL, et al. Gilles de la Tourette syndrome: tics and central nervous system stimulants in twins and non-twins. *Neurology.* 1986;36:232–237.
77. Sherman EM, Shepard L, Joschko M, et al. Sustained attention and impulsivity in children with TS: comorbidity and confounds. *J Clin Exp Neuropsychol.* 1998;20:644–657.
78. Sukhodolsky DG, Scahill L, Zhang H, et al. Disruptive behavior in children with Tourette's syndrome: association with ADHD comorbidity, tic severity, and functional impairment. *J Am Acad Child Adolesc Psychiatry.* 2003;42:98–105.
79. Gadow KD, Sverd J, Sprafkin J, et al. Long-term MPH therapy in children with comorbid ADHD and chronic multiple tic disorder. *Arch Gen Psychiatry.* 1999;56:330–336.
80. Erenberg G. The relationship between Tourette syndrome, ADHD, and stimulant medication: a critical review. *Semin Pediatr Neurol.* 2006;12:217–221.
81. Singer HS, Schuerholz LJ, Denckla MB. Learning difficulties in children with Tourette's syndrome. *J Child Neurol.* 1995;10:558–561.
82. Eapen V, Robertson MM, Alsobrook JP, Pauls DL. Obsessive-compulsive symptoms in Gilles de la Tourette syndrome and obsessive compulsive disorder: differences by diagnosis and family history. *Am J Med Genet.* 1997;74:432–438.
83. Miguel EC, do Rosario-Campos MC, Prado HS, et al. Sensory phenomena in obsessive-compulsive disorder and Tourette's disorder. *J Clin Psychiatry.* 2000;61:150–156.
84. Jimenez-Jimenez FJ, Garcia-Ruiz PJ. Pharmacological options for the treatment of Tourette's disorder. *Drugs.* 2001;61:2207–2220.
85. Bruggeman R, van der Linden C, Buitelaar JK, et al. Risperidone versus pimozide in Tourette's disorder: a comparative double-blind parallel-group study. *J Clin Psychiatry.* 2001;62:50–56.

86. Sallee FR, Kurlan R, Goetz CG, et al. Ziprasidone treatment of children and adolescents with Tourette's syndrome: a pilot study. *J Am Acad Child Adolesc Psychiatry.* 2000;39:292–299.
87. Jankovic J, Orman J. Tetrabenazine therapy of dystonia, chorea, tics, and other dyskinesias. *Neurology.* 1988;38:391–394.
88. Gaffney GR, Perry PJ, Lund BC, et al. Risperidone versus clonidine in the treatment of children and adolescents with Tourette's syndrome. *J Am Acad Child Adolesc Psychiatry.* 2002;41:330–336.
89. Scahill L, Chappell PB, Kim YS, et al. A placebo-controlled study of guanfacine in the treatment of children with tic disorders and attention deficit hyperactivity disorder. *Am J Psychiatry.* 2001;158:1067–1074.
90. Gonce M, Barbeau A. Seven cases of Gilles de la Tourette's syndrome: a partial relief with clonazepam: a pilot study. *Can J Neurol Sci.* 1977;4:279–283.
91. Goetz CG. Clonidine and clonazepam in Tourette's syndrome. *Adv Neurol.* 1992;58:245–251.
92. Steingard RJ, Goldberg M, Lee D, DeMaso DR. Adjunctive clonazepam treatment of tic symptoms in children with comorbid tic disorders and ADHD. *J Am Acad Child Adolesc Psychiatry.* 1994;33:394–399.
93. Jankovic J. Botulinum toxin in the treatment of dystonic tics. *Mov Disord.* 1994;9:347–349.
94. Scott BL, Jankovic J, Donovan DT. Botulinum toxin into vocal cord in the treatment of malignant coprolalia associated with Tourette's syndrome. *Mov Disord.* 1996;11:431–433.
95. Nomura Y, Segawa M. Characteristics of motor disturbances of the Rett syndrome. *Brain Dev.* 1990;12:27–30.
96. Jummani R, Okun M. Sydenham chorea. *Arch Neurol.* 2001;58:311–313.
97. Husby G, Van De Rijn U, Zabriskie JB, et al. Antibodies reacting with cytoplasm of subthalamic and caudate nuclei neurons in chorea and acute rheumatic fever. *J Exp Med.* 1976;144:1094–1110.
98. Church AJ, Cardoso F, Dale RC, et al. Anti-basal ganglia antibodies in acute and persistent Sydenham's chorea. *Neurology.* 2002;59:227–231.
99. Teixeira AL Jr, Cardoso F, Souza AL, Teixeira MM. Increased serum concentrations of monokine induced by interferon-gamma/CXCL9 and interferon-gamma-inducible protein 10/CXCL-10 in Sydenham's chorea patients. *J Neuroimmunol.* 2004;150:157–162.
100. Cardoso F, Silva CE, Mota CC. Sydenham's chorea in 50 consecutive patients with rheumatic fever. *Mov Disord.* 1997;12:701–703.
101. Nausieda PA, Grossman BJ, Koller WC, et al. Sydenham chorea: an update. *Neurology.* 1980;30:331–334.
102. Zomorrodi A, Wald ER. Sydenham's chorea in western Pennsylvania. *Pediatrics.* 2006;117:e675–e679.
103. Cunningham MC, Maia DP, Teixeira AL Jr, Cardoso F. Sydenham's chorea is associated with decreased verbal fluency. *Parkinsonism Relat Disord.* 2006;12:165–167.
104. Asbahr FR, Negrao AB, Gentil V, et al. Obsessive-compulsive and related symptoms in children and adolescents with rheumatic fever with and without chorea: a prospective 6-month study. *Am J Psychiatry.* 1998;155:1122–1124.
105. Maia DP, Teixeira AL Jr, Quintao Cunningham MC, Cardoso F. Obsessive compulsive behavior, hyperactivity, and attention deficit disorder in Sydenham chorea. *Neurology.* 2005;64:1799–1801.
106. Swedo SE, Leonard HL, Kiessling LS. Speculations on antineuronal antibody-mediated neuropsychiatric disorders of childhood. *Pediatrics.* 1994;93:323–326.
107. Pavone P, Parano E, Rizzo R, Trifiletti RR. Autoimmune neuropsychiatric disorders associated with streptococcal infection: Sydenham chorea, PANDAS, and PANDAS variants. *J Child Neurol.* 2006;21:727–736.
108. Scott BL, Jankovic J. Delayed-onset progressive movement disorders after static brain lesions. *Neurology.* 1996;46:68–74.
109. Beskind DL, Keim SM. Choreoathetotic movement disorder in a boy with *Mycoplasma pneumoniae* encephalitis. *Ann Emerg Med.* 1994;23:1375–1378.
110. Decaux G, Szyper M, Ectors M, et al. Central nervous system complications of *Mycoplasma pneumoniae*. *J Neurol Neurosurg Psychiatry.* 1980;43:883–887.
111. Lapidoth T, Galun E. Hyperglycemia as a cause of chorea. *Arch Intern Med.* 1989;149:1905.
112. Olfat MO, Al-Mayouf SM, Muzaffer MA. Pattern of neuropsychiatric manifestations and outcome in juvenile systemic lupus erythematosus. *Clin Rheumatol.* 2004;23:395–399.
113. Cardoso F. Infectious and transmissible movement disorders. In: Jankovic J, Tolosa E, eds. *Parkinson's disease and movement disorders.* 4th ed. Baltimore: Williams & Wilkins, 2002:930–940.
114. Genel F, Arslanoglu S, Uran N, Saylan B. Sydenham's chorea: clinical findings and comparison of the efficacies of sodium valproate and carbamazepine regimens. *Brain Dev.* 2002;24:73–76.
115. Teixeira AL Jr, Maia DP, Cardoso F. Treatment of acute Sydenham's chorea with methyl-prednisolone pulse-therapy. *Parkinsonism Relat Disord.* 2005;11:327–330.
116. Hounie AG, Pauls DL, do Rosario-Campos MC. Obsessive-compulsive spectrum disorders and rheumatic fever: a family study. *Biol Psychiatry.* 2007;61:266–272.
117. Tassinari CA, Rubbioli G, Parmeggiani L, et al. Epileptic negative myoclonus. *Adv Neurol.* 1995;67:181–197.
118. Hallett M, Chadwick D, Marsden CD. Cortical reflex myoclonus. *Neurology.* 1979;29:1107–1125.

119. Rajakumar K, Bodensteiner JB. Febrile myoclonus: a survey of pediatric neurologists. *Clin Pediatr (Phila)*. 1996;35:331–332.
120. Pranzatelli MR. Myoclonus in childhood. *Semin Pediatr Neurol.* 2003;10:41–51.
121. Gericke CA, Picard F, de Saint-Martin A, et al. Efficacy of lamotrigine in idiopathic generalized epilepsy syndromes: a video-EEG–controlled, open study. *Epilept Disord.* 1999;1:159–165.
122. Biton V, Bourgeois BF, YTC/YTCE Study Investigators. Topiramate in patients with juvenile myoclonic epilepsy. *Arch Neurol.* 2005;62:1705–1708.
123. Mitchell WG, Davalos-Gonzalez Y, Brumm VL, et al. Opsoclonus-ataxia caused by childhood neuroblastoma: developmental and neurologic sequelae. *Pediatrics*. 2002;109:86–98.
124. Hayward K, Jeremy RJ, Jenkins S, et al. Long-term neurobehavioral outcomes in children with neuroblastoma and opsoclonus-myoclonus-ataxia syndrome: relationship to MRI findings and anti-neuronal antibodies. *J Pediatr.* 2001;139:552–559.
125. Pranzatelli MR. Paraneoplastic syndromes: an unsolved murder. *Semin Pediatr Neurol.* 2000;7:118–130.
126. Caviness JN, Brown P. Myoclonus: current concepts and recent advances. *Lancet Neurol.* 2004;3:598–607.
127. Fernandez-Alvarez E. Transient movement disorders in children. *J Neurol.* 1998;245:1–5.
128. Kotagal P, Costa M, Wyllie E, Wolgamuth B. Paroxysmal nonepileptic events in children and adolescents. *Pediatrics.* 2002;110:46–50.
129. Gancher ST, Nutt JG. Autosomal dominant episodic ataxia: a heterogeneous syndrome. *Mov Disord.* 1986;1:239–253.
130. Demirkiran M, Jankovic J. Paroxysmal dyskinesias: clinical features and a new classification. *Ann Neurol.* 1995;38:571–579.
131. Kertesz A. Paroxysmal kinesiogenic choreoathetosis: an entity within the paroxysmal choreoathetosis syndrome: description of 10 cases including 1 autopsied. *Neurology.* 1967;17:680–690.
132. Gocay A, Gocay F. Oxcarbazepine therapy in paroxysmal kinesiogenic choreoathetosis. *Acta Neurol Scand.* 2000;101:344–345.
133. Pereira AC, Loo WJ, Barnford MM, et al. Use of lamotrigine to treat paroxysmal kinesiogenic choreoathetosis. *J Neurol Neurosurg Psychiatry.* 2000;68:796–797.
134. Hirata K, Katayama S, Saito T, et al. Paroxysmal kinesiogenic choreoathetosis with abnormal electroencephalogram during attacks. *Epilepsia.* 1991;32:492–494.
135. Mount LA, Reback S. Familial paroxysmal choreoathetosis. *Arch Neurol Psychiatry.* 1940;44:841–847.
136. Bressman SB, Fahn S, Burke RE. Paroxysmal non-kinesiogenic dystonia. *Adv Neurol.* 1988;50:403–413.
137. Rainier S, Thomas D, Tokarz D, et al. Myofibrillogenesis regulator 1 gene mutations cause paroxysmal dystonic choreoathetosis. *Arch Neurol.* 2004;61:1025–1029.
138. Berger JR, Sheremata WA, Melamed E. Paroxysmal dystonia as the initial manifestation of multiple sclerosis. *Arch Neurol.* 1984;41:747–750.
139. Bhatia KP. Episodic movement disorders as channelopathies. *Mov Disord.* 2000;15:429–433.
140. Litt M, Kramer P, Browne D, et al. A gene for episodic ataxia/myokymia maps to chromosome 12p13. *Am J Hum Genet.* 1994;55:702–709.
141. Baloh RW, Yue Q, Furman JM, Nelson SF. Familial episodic ataxia: clinical heterogeneity in four families linked to chromosome 19p. *Ann Neurol.* 1997;41:8–16.
142. von Brederlow B, Hahn A, Koopman WJ, et al. Mapping of the gene for acetazolamide responsive hereditary paroxysmal cerebellar ataxia to chromosome 19p. *Hum Mol Genet.* 1995;4:279–284.
143. Regan J, LaBarbera J. Lateralization of conversion symptoms in children and adolescents. *Am J Psychiatry.* 1984;141:1279–1280.
144. Zeharia A, Mukamel M, Carel C, et al. Conversion reaction: management by the paediatrician. *Eur J Pediatr.* 1999;158:160–164.
145. Williams DT, Ford B, Fahn S. Phenomenology and psychopathology related to psychogenic movement disorders. *Adv Neurol.* 1995;65:231–257.
146. Marjama J, Troster A, Koller W. Psychogenic movement disorders. *Neurol Clin.* 1995;13:283–297.
147. Rodnitzky RL. Drug-induced movement disorders in children. *Semin Pediatr Neurol.* 2003;10:80–87.
148. Ener RA, Meglathery SB, Van Decker WA, Gallagher RM. Serotonin syndrome and other serotonergic disorders. *Pain Med.* 2003;4:63–74.
149. Caroff SN, Mann SC. Neuroleptic malignant syndrome. *Psychopharmacol Bull.* 1988;24:24–29.
150. Garver DI, Davis JM, Dekermejian H, et al. Dystonic reactions following neuroleptics: time, course, and proposed mechanisms. *Psychopharmacology.* 1976;47:199–201.
151. Rupniak NM, Jenner P, Marsden CD. Acute dystonia induced by neuroleptic drugs. *Psychopharmacology.* 1986;88:403–419.
152. Russell SA, Hennes HM, Herson KJ, et al. Upper airway compromise in acute chlorpromazine ingestion. *Am J Emerg Med.* 1996;14:467–468.
153. Winslow RS, Stillner V, Coons DJ, Robison MW. Prevention of acute dystonic reactions in patients beginning high-potency neuroleptics. *Am J Psychiatry.* 1986;143:706–710.

154. Baldassano CF, Truman CJ, Nierenberg A, et al. Akathisia: a review and case report following paroxetine treatment. *Comprehens Psychiatry.* 1996;37:122–124.
155. Blaisdell GD. Akathisia: a comprehensive review and treatment summary. *Pharmacopsychiatry.* 1994;27:139–146.
156. Adler L, Angrist B, Peselow E, et al. A controlled assessment of propranolol in the treatment of neuroleptic-induced akathisia. *Br J Psychiatry.* 1986;149:42–45.
157. Stacy M, Jankovic J. Tardive dyskinesia. *Curr Opin Neurol Neurosurg* 1991;4:343–349.
158. Kang UJ, Burke RE, Fahn S. Natural history and treatment of tardive dystonia. *Mov Disord.* 1986;1:193–208.
159. Putnam PE, Orenstein SR, Wessel HB, Stowe RM. Tardive dyskinesia associated with use of metoclopramide in a child. *J Pediatr.* 1992;121:983–985.
160. Mejia NI, Jankovic J. Metoclopramide-induced tardive dyskinesia in an infant. *Mov Disord.* 2005;20:86–89.
161. Campbell M, Armenteros JL, Malone RP, et al. Neuroleptic-related dyskinesias in autistic children: a prospective, longitudinal study. *J Am Acad Child Adolesc Psychiatry.* 1997;36:835–843.
162. Kane JM, Woerner M, Borenstein M, et al. Integrating incidence and prevalence of tardive dyskinesia. *Psychopharmacol Bull.* 1986;22:254–258.
163. Gardos G, Cole JO, Haskell D, et al. The natural history of tardive dyskinesia. *J Clin Psychopharmacol.* 1988;8:31S–37S.
164. Jankovic J, Beach J. Long-term effects of tetrabenazine in hyperkinetic movement disorders. *Neurology.* 1997;48:358–362.
165. Ondo WG, Hanna PA, Jankovic J. Tetrabenazine treatment for tardive dyskinesia: assessment by randomized videotape protocol. *Am J Psychiatry.* 1999;156:1279–1281.
166. Jain S, Greene PE, Frucht SJ. Tetrabenazine therapy of pediatric hyperkinetic movement disorders. *Mov Disord.* 2006;21:1966–1972.
167. Adler LA, Rotrosen J, Edson R, et al. Vitamin E treatment for tardive dyskinesia. *Arch Gen Psychiatry.* 1999;56:836–841.
168. Shamir E, Barak Y, Shalman I, et al. Melatonin treatment for tardive dyskinesia: a double blind placebo controlled crossover study. *Arch Gen Psychiatry.* 2001;58:1049–1052.
169. Sienaert P, Peuskens J. Remission of tardive dystonia (blepharospasm) after electroconvulsive therapy in a patient with treatment-refractory schizophrenia. *J ECT.* 2005;21:132–134.
170. Nobuhara K, Matsuda S, Okugawa G, et al. Successful electroconvulsive treatment of depression associated with a marked reduction in the symptoms of tardive dyskinesia. *J ECT.* 2004;20:262–263.
171. Shahed J, Poysky C, Kenney R, et al. GPi deep brain stimulation for Tourette syndrome improves tics and psychiatric comorbidities. *Neurology.* 2007;68:159–160.
172. Caldwell GA, Cao S, Sexton EG, et al. Suppression of polyglutamine-induced protein aggregation in *Caenorhabditis elegans* by torsin proteins. *Hum Mol Genet.* 2003;12:307–319.

SUGGESTED READINGS

Brewer GJ, Terry CA, Aisen AM, Hill GM. Worsening of neurologic syndrome in patients with Wilson's disease with initial penicillamine therapy. *Arch Neurol.* 1987;44:490–493.

Dening TR. Psychiatric aspects of Wilson's disease. *Br J Psychiatry.* 1985;147:677.

DiMario FJ. Childhood head tremor. *J Child Neurol.* 2000;15:22–25.

Factor SA, Podskalny GD, Molho ES. Psychogenic movement disorders: frequency, clinical profile, and characteristics. *J Neurol Neurosurg Psychiatry.* 1995;59:406–412.

Fahn S, Marsden C. The treatment of dystonia. In: Marsden CD, Fahn S, eds. *Movement disorders 2.* London: Butterworths, 1997:359–382.

Gilbert DL, Sethuraman G, Sine L, et al. Tourette's syndrome improvement with pergolide in a randomized, double-blind, crossover trial. *Neurology.* 2000;54:1310–1315.

Hallet M. Classification and treatment of tremor. *JAMA.* 1991;226:115.

Lou JS, Jankovic J:. Tremors. In: Appel SH, ed. *Current neurology,* Vol 11. Chicago: Mosby-Yearbook, 1991:232.

Louis ED, Vonsattel JP, Honig LS, et al. Essential tremor associated with pathologic changes in the cerebellum. *Arch Neurol.* 2006;63:1189–1193.

Marras C, Andrews D, Sime EA, Lang AE. Botulinum toxin for simple motor tics: a randomized, double blind, controlled clinical trial. *Neurology.* 2001;56:605–610.

Prasad A, Kuzniecky RI, Knowlton RC, et al. Evolving antiepileptic drug treatment in juvenile myoclonic epilepsy. *Arch Neurol.* 2003;60: 1100–1105.

Saunders-Pullman R, Shriberg J, Heiman G, et al. Myoclonus-dystonia: possible association with obsessive-compulsive disorder and alcohol dependence. *Neurology.* 2002;58:242–245.

Silvestri R, DeDomenico P, DiRosa AE, et al. The effects of nocturnal physiologic sleep on various movement disorders. *Mov Disord.* 1990;5:8–14.

CHAPTER 4

Tourette Syndrome and Tic Disorders in Children and Adolescents

ROBERT A. KING AND TAMAR STEINBERG

Tics are sudden, involuntary, repetitive, but nonrhythmical movements or vocalizations. They range in number, frequency, persistence, and associated comorbidity from the isolated transient symptoms found in transient tic disorder to the chronic, multiple motor and vocal tics of Tourette syndrome (TS) that are often accompanied by various forms of psychopathology (see Definitions and Natural History and Clinical Phenomenology, further on).

TS stands as a model developmental neuropsychiatric disorder in several respects (1). Although clearly neurological in origin (with a complex genetic and neurobiological substrate), the clinical phenomenology and course of the disorder are influenced by the interplay between genetic and environmental protective and risk factors (including perinatal adversity and hormonal exposure, infection, and psychological factors such as stress). Over and above the direct psychosocial burden that significant tics pose for the child and family, TS is associated in many cases with increased autonomic lability, vulnerability to anxiety and/or depression, and a spectrum of attentional and neurocognitive difficulties (2). Thus, a comprehensive approach to understanding and treating the tic disorders requires an appreciation of multiple explanatory frames of reference (genetics, neurobiology, immunology) and clinical modalities (pharmacological, cognitive behavioral, psychodynamic, family, neuropsychological, educational). Not surprisingly, then, children with tic disorders are often seen by both pediatric neurologists and child psychiatrists, as their comprehensive evaluation and management requires a broad biopsychosocial approach.

Estimates of the prevalence of tics vary widely depending on age (prevalence decreases with age), methods of ascertainment (parental report, direct observation, clinical records), and definition. [In contrast to earlier versions of the DSM, DSM-IV-TR (3) dropped impairment as a diagnostic criterion for TS.]

Transient tics are common in school-aged children, with estimated prevalences ranging from 4% to 24% (4–6). For example, direct classroom observation on multiple occasions of community school-aged children found that 18% of 5- to 12-year-olds had a single tic or transient tics, whereas an additional 6% had multiple or persistent tics (5). Prevalence estimates for school-aged children with TS also vary widely, from about 5 to 100 per 10,000, with community samples showing substantial higher rates than clinical samples, suggesting that many cases remain undiagnosed or untreated (4,7). Boys are more likely than girls to manifest tics, with a gender ratio of about 2:1. TS has been described in most ethnic groups studied, with differences in reported rates in clinical settings most likely reflecting propensity to seek help, rather than true ethnic variations in prevalence. In a community epidemiologic survey, the Great Smoky Mountains Youth Study found no differences in prevalence rates for tic disorder or TS between white and African-American children or across income groups (4).

Definitions

MOTOR TICS

Simple motor tics are sudden, fleeting, or fragmentary movements such as blinking, grimacing, head jerking, or shoulder shrugs. *Complex motor tics* consist of several simple motor tics occurring in an orchestrated sequence or semipurposeful movements, such as touch or tapping; these may also have a more sustained, twisting, dystonic character.

PHONIC TICS

Simple phonic tics consist of simple, unarticulated sounds such as throat clearing, sniffing, grunting, squeaking, or coughing. *Complex phonic tics* consist of out-of-context syllables, words, phrases, or paroxysmal changes of prosody.

Complex tics may involve socially inappropriate or obscene gestures (copropraxia) or utterances (coprolalia), as well as echo phenomena, such as echolalia or echopraxia (repeating others' words or gestures), which exemplify the suggestibility of tics. Infrequently, complex tics may include self-injurious behavior (cheek chewing, eye poking, self-hitting).

Diagnostic Criteria

The following diagnostic criteria are from reference 3.

DSM-IV-TR diagnostic criteria for transient tic disorder

A. Single or multiple motor and/or vocal tics (i.e., sudden, rapid, recurrent, nonrhythmical, stereotyped motor movements or vocalizations).
B. The tics occur many times a day, nearly every day for at least 4 weeks, but for no longer than 12 consecutive months.
C. The onset is before age 18 years.
D. The disturbance is not due to the direct physiological effects of a substance (e.g., stimulants) or a general medical condition (e.g., Huntington disease or postviral encephalitis).
E. Criteria have never been met for TS or chronic motor or vocal tic disorder.

Diagnostic criteria for chronic motor or vocal tic disorder

A. Single or multiple motor or vocal tics (i.e., sudden, rapid, recurrent, nonrhythmical, stereotyped motor movements or vocalizations), but not both, have been present at some time during the illness.
B. The tics occur many times a day, nearly every day or intermittently throughout a period of more than 1 year, and during this period there was never a tic-free period of more than 3 consecutive months.
C. Criteria C, D same as above.
E. Criteria have never been met for TS.

Diagnostic criteria for Tourette syndrome

A. Both multiple motor and one or more vocal tics have been present at some time during the illness, although not necessarily concurrently.
B. The tics occur many times a day (usually in bouts) nearly every day or intermittently throughout a period of more than a year, and during this period there was never a tic-free period of more than 3 consecutive months.
C. Criteria C, D same as above.

It is not clear to what extent these DSM frequency and duration criteria truly demarcate distinctive syndromes with differing etiologies, symptomatic concomitants, or clinical courses, rather than points on a spectrum of symptomatic severity in the expression of a common underlying genetic vulnerability.

Natural History and Clinical Phenomenology

The most common age of onset for tics is between 4 and 6 years of age. Initial sniffing or blinking tics may be mistaken for allergies or eye problems. It is only with their waxing and waning and the subsequent appearance of other tics that the diagnosis becomes clear. There is also often an anatomic progression, with head and facial tics being the first to appear and more caudal and more complex tics appearing later.

Stress (8), fatigue, exciting events (trips, beginning of school), or even childhood colds (9) can exacerbate tics. Tics are often transiently suppressible, which may lead adults to draw the mistaken conclusion that they are voluntary, because they may appear in one setting but not another. Tics may also diminish or disappear during tasks that require focused attention and fine motor control, such as music or sports. They often diminish or disappear during sleep but can recur during rapid eye movement (REM) and other sleep phases. The characteristic pattern is for tics to wax and wane in bouts over the course of the day and weeks, with the disappearance of one tic to be replaced by different ones.

By middle childhood, many youngsters with chronic tics are able to describe and localize premonitory sensations or urges that precede the tics (10). These sensations or urges may be described as an "itch" or "tickle" that is transiently relieved by performing the tic and that grows worse if the tic is suppressed or resisted. In this sense, many children report, in essence, that their tics straddle the boundary between "voluntary" and "involuntary," "physical" and "mental." For some children, the constant bombardment of premonitory urges may be as distracting or debilitating as the tics themselves.

Once considered a disabling and lifelong disorder, it is now clear that most cases of TS are mild, with marked improvement or remission of tics in the majority of cases by late adolescence (6,11,12). The period of "worst-ever" tic severity usually spans 7 to 12 years of age, following which tics often improve spontaneously in terms of frequency and subjective distress. By later adolescence or young adulthood, three quarters of childhood cases, tics disappear or decrease substantially, 15% remain stable, and 15% worsen (11,13). [Video and direct observation may reveal more residual tics than does self-report (14).] Unfortunately, comorbid symptoms of attention deficit hyperactivity disorder (ADHD), obsessive-compulsive disorder (OCD), and anxiety may not show the same improvement with age (12). Indeed, the presence of comorbid OCD, phobias, or ADHD in childhood or early adolescence may be predictors of more persistent tics (6).

COMMON COMORBID DISORDERS

In addition to the pathognomonic tics of TS, many patients also suffer from symptoms of OCD, ADHD, impulsivity, proneness to anxiety and depression, uneven neuropsychological profiles, and learning difficulties (2). When present, these comorbid conditions may be more distressing or impairing than the tics themselves, and hence are important targets of assessment and intervention. Youngsters with TS plus comorbid OCD and/or ADHD usually have more adaptive difficulties than those with tics alone (15,16). Sleep problems and migraine may also be more common in individuals with TS. Trichotillomania or body dysmorphic disorder may also be more common in probands with TS and their relatives.

Obsessive-compulsive disorder

The prevalence of obsessive-compulsive symptoms ranges from 11% to 80% in clinical and community samples, depending on the sample, means of assessment, and criteria used (2). Viewed in isolation, simple compulsions may be difficult to distinguish from complex tics (e.g., forced repetitive touching, which may include dangerously hot objects). (Some patients differentiate tics prompted or accompanied by a physical sensation from compulsions prompted by mental phenomena.) Although patients with TS may manifest the usual harm-avoidant obsessions and compulsions found in OCD patients without tics, concerns about symmetry, ordering, and exactness, as well as intrusive aggressive, sexual, or religious images, appear to be more common in tic-related OCD. TS-related compulsions are often driven by the need to get some appearance or physical sensation "just right," rather than by anxiety reduction or harm avoidance. (For example, a youngster may need to set down a cup repeatedly until he or she feels or hears the right "clunk"; repeat an action in odd- or even-numbered sets; or go through a doorway precisely through the middle or by leading with the right foot.)

Attention deficit hyperactivity disorder

ADHD, as well as oppositional behavior, is found in at least one half of clinically referred children and adolescents, with considerably lower rates in nonreferred samples (6), suggesting that comorbid ADHD may be an important predisposing factor for seeking clinical help. It is also not uncommon to see children with ADHD who have developed transient or persistent tics after being started on stimulant medication, posing a sometimes difficult therapeutic dilemma (see Treatment of Comorbid Attention Deficit Hyperactivity Disorder, further on.)

Differential Diagnosis of Tic Disorder

The diagnosis of tic disorder for TS is straightforward in most cases. Tics can usually be distinguished from other movement disorders in that they are semivoluntary (partially suppressible), often preceded by an urge or premonitory sensation, and reproducible on request; they occur in repetitive patterns (over the short run) and may persist, albeit diminished, in sleep (17). To make the diagnosis, a detailed history, with special attention to these features, and a thorough physical examination are necessary. When conducting a physical examination, it should be taken into consideration that a patient may have a mixture of movement disorders. For example, a patient treated with neuroleptics may suffer from tics, akathisia, tardive or withdrawal dyskinesia, and/or drug-induced acute dystonia simultaneously (18). (Some children have both tic disorder and motor stereotypies.) Children with uncomplicated tic disorder have a normal neurological examination, although formal neuropsychological testing may reveal subtle difficulties in fine visuomotor coordination (19).

In most typical cases, the diagnosis can be made without electroencephalogram (EEG), magnetic resonance imaging (MRI), or laboratory studies, such as serum copper or ceruloplasmin.

STEREOTYPICAL MOVEMENTS

Distinguishing true tics from *stereotypies* or *self-stimulating behaviors*, such as rocking, head banging, flapping, or spinning, is a common diagnostic problem in young children. Compared with tics, stereotypies usually have an earlier onset (often by age 3 years), greater complexity, and relatively fixed form and locus, and they appear more voluntary in nature. When old enough, children usually describe their tics as intrusive, bothersome, disruptive, and largely involuntary. In contrast, stereotypies are often bothersome to parents, but not to the child who often appears to find them pleasurable and resists adult attempts to interrupt them. These apparently self-stimulating movements occur largely at times of boredom, excitement, or, less commonly, distress but rarely disrupt coordinated movements and usually persist over months and years without much change in form or location. Although common in children with pervasive developmental disorders (20), they can also be seen in developmentally normal children with normal intelligence quotients (IQs) (21) and may run in families.

CHOREA

Chorea is a syndrome characterized by a continuous flow of abrupt, involuntary muscle contractions producing irregular, unpredictable, brief, jerky movements that migrate randomly from one part of the body to another. Unlike tics, choreic movements are not preceded by an urge or premonitory sensations.

Postinfectious forms of chorea

The commonest cause of childhood chorea is Sydenham chorea (SC), presumably an autoimmune poststreptococcal disorder associated with rheumatic fever (see Chapter 3) (22). The typical age at onset of SC is 8 to 9 years and is very rarely seen in children younger than age 5 years. Typically, children develop the disease 4 to 8 weeks after streptococcal pharyngitis, but longer intervals may occur. As noted in the section on *p*ediatric *a*utoimmune *n*europsychiatric *d*isorders *a*ssociated with *s*treptococcus (PANDAS), children with SC commonly display other de novo neuropsychiatric symptoms, such as tics, attentional disorders, and OCD. SC is usually a self-limiting disorder lasting 8 to 9 months, but up to 50% of children may show persistent chorea at 2-year follow-up. Other infections may also cause chorea (see Chapter 3).

In contrast to children with SC, those with tic disorder or OCD hypothesized to be due to PANDAS by definition do not have a history of full-blown chorea but may show fine "choreiform" movements, pronator drift, or motor impersistence in stressed postures. Children with putative PANDAS have also been found to have normal echocardiograms.

Drug-induced chorea

Various drugs, including antiepileptic drugs, psychostimulants, dopamine receptor blocking agents, and oral contraceptives, can also induce chorea.

Genetic forms of chorea

Benign hereditary chorea, ataxia telangiectasia, paroxysmal kinesogenic choreoathetosis, Wilson disease, and Huntington disease (HD) can all cause movement disorders with choreiform movements. Although chorea is the prototypical movement disorder in HD, patients can also present with eye movement abnormalities, dystonia, myoclonus, ataxia, dysarthria, dysphagia, or tics (23). In early-onset cases of HD in children and adolescents, parkinsonism or dystonia, rather than chorea, may predominate (see Chapter 3).

MYOCLONUS AND SEIZURES

Myoclonic jerks

Myoclonic jerks are brief (<200 ms) shocklike muscular contractions that lack the continuous random flow of movements typical of chorea and, unlike tics, are completely involuntary. Myoclonic jerks of the shoulders and arms appearing shortly after awakening are typical of juvenile myoclonic epilepsy (JME); the large majority of these patients also experience grand mal or absence seizures. Segmental spinal myoclonus may be associated with several spinal cord disorders, including various forms of progressive ataxia.

Epilepsies with typical absence (petit mal)

Absence seizures are characterized by a brief lapse of consciousness lasting 5 to 10 seconds. With hyperventilation or photic stimulation, the EEG study demonstrates 3-Hz spike and wave discharges (24). Minor movements occur in 70% of patients during episodes, including lip smacking or twitching of the eyelids or face; transient slight loss of body tone can cause the child to drop objects. Some absence attacks are more complex, with behavioral automatisms or prolonged symmetric myoclonic movements of the head or extremities. In contrast to the brief lapses of consciousness found in absence seizures, individuals with tics remain fully conscious during their movements.

Epilepsies with complex partial seizures, temporal lobe seizures

These seizures arise from a focal origin, most commonly in the temporal lobe, and produce a period of impaired consciousness accompanied by staring or a dazed expression, oral movements or drooling, muttering or mumbling, stiffening of body or limbs, searching or orienting movement, or other behavioral changes. In general, the younger the patient, the less complex is the seizure. Typically, younger children have automatisms characterized by lip smacking, chewing, or other automatisms. Some patients can describe an aura preceding the seizure, which consists of visceral sensations and anxiety (25). In contrast to complex partial seizures, tics are usually at least transiently suppressible and are not accompanied by an alteration in consciousness, postictal confusion or tiredness, or amnesia for the event.

DYSTONIA

Dystonia is characterized by sustained muscle contractions causing repetitive twisting movements or abnormal postures caused by simultaneous contraction of agonist and antagonist muscles (26). Dystonia can be either primary or secondary to another disorder. Examples include cervical dystonia, which causes the head to turn in a consistent direction, or *blepharospasm,* which produces involuntary closure of the eyes. The movements are prolonged and patterned, and they involve the same muscle group over time, in contrast to the usual pattern of multiple fluctuating tics found in TS. Unlike tics, dystonic movements are not preceded by an urge, and there is no relief when the movement is executed. Many patients discover a tactile or proprioceptive sensory trick that reduces the dystonia. For instance, patients with cervical dystonia may be able to keep their head upright by touching their chin.

Dystonia is aggravated by voluntary movements. Task-specific dystonia occurs only during a specific action such as writing (writer's cramps). Dystonia is worsened by fatigue and stress and abates with relaxation or sleep. Dystonia can be focal, most commonly involving the neck, oromandibular, or periorbital muscles. It can also be segmental, multifocal hemidystonia or generalized.

Early-onset dystonia appears around age 9 years, is characterized by involvement of limbs, and rarely involves the neck or cranial nerves. About 50% of early-onset dystonias become generalized and, compared with adult-onset cases, are more often primary.

Commercial clinical screening is available for the commonest genetic form of primary dystonia, a deletion in the DYT1 gene located on chromosome 9q34.21.

NEUROACANTHOCYTOSIS

The term *neuroacanthocytosis* is used to describe a group of rare disorders associated with neurological symptoms and acanthocytes, erythrocytes with an unusual starlike appearance with spiky- or thorny-appearing projections that can be seen on blood smear.

One such disorder that causes chorea and tics is Levine-Critchley syndrome, produced by a mutation in a specific gene called chorein (also called *VPS13A*). In contrast to TS, the onset of the disorder, usually in the third or fourth decade of life, is first manifested by lip and tongue biting, which is followed by orolingual dystonia, chorea, and motor and vocal tics, as well as personality changes, cognitive decline, seizures, dysphagia, and dysarthria. Specific genes have also been identified for several other genetic syndromes involving movement disorder with choreiform or Parkinson-like features, various other neurological abnormalities, and acanthocytosis (27). Laboratory findings include more than 3% acanthocytes on the peripheral blood smear and elevated creatine phosphokinase (CPK) as a result of muscle wasting (28). Brain MRI demonstrates caudate atrophy and increased signal in caudate and lentiform nuclei.

TARDIVE DYSKINESIAS

Tardive dyskinesias (TDs) are involuntary movements of the tongue, lips, face, trunk, and extremities that occur in patients treated with long-term dopamine antagonist medications. This disorder is quite rare in children and is much more commonly found in elderly patients with prolonged neuroleptic use. Although most often associated with the use of the typical neuroleptics, tardive dyskinesias may occur from other types of exposure; individuals with schizophrenia appear especially vulnerable to developing TDs after exposure to anticholinergics, substances of abuse, toxins, and other agents.

The dopamine-receptor antagonists that are frequently used to treat patients with tics may themselves cause movement disorders, including "tardive tourettism" (29), a form of tardive dyskinesia that includes motor and vocal tics. The diagnosis of acute and chronic dyskinesia is based on precise medical and pharmacological history documentation. TDs may improve with increased doses of dopamine antagonists, making the differential diagnosis more complex. This disorder, as opposed to TS, is much more common in elderly patients with prolonged neuroleptic use and is quite rare in children.

CONVERSION DISORDER

Adolescents with dramatic whole-limb movements, unusual gait, shaking, or other dramatic movements may sometimes be misdiagnosed as having a tic disorder, rather than receiving the correct diagnosis of conversion disorder. Unlike tic disorder, conversion disorder often does not appear until adolescence, usually without any convincing history of significant earlier simple motor or phonic tics. (It is very rare to have significant complex tics without a history of simple tics.) Save in cases of well-established tic disorder in which prolonged bouts may sometimes be seen, most bouts of tics are fleeting; in contrast, conversion disorder movements may continue uninterrupted for minutes. Youngsters with flurries of dramatic true tics are usually quite distressed by them, in contrast to those with conversion disorder, who may appear relatively unconcerned at the degree of seeming functional impairment. Finally, a family history of tics or OCD is common in tic disorder but may be absent in conversion disorder.

Etiological Factors

NEUROBIOLOGICAL SUBSTRATE

Multiple lines of evidence point to dysregulation of corticostriatothalamocortical circuits as the neurobiological basis of TS (30–32), with the likelihood of primary abnormalities in both frontal cortical and striatal structures.

GENETIC

Twin studies suggest a strong genetic component to TS, with monozygotic twins having 86% concordance rate for chronic tic disorder versus a 20% rate for dizygotic twins (31). The same studies also suggest the importance of perinatal factors, with the monozygotic (MZ) co-twin with lower birth weight usually having greater tic severity.

Increased rates of TS, chronic motor tics, and/or OCD are found in first-degree relatives of TS probands. When these diagnoses are considered together, it is common to find affected individuals on both parents' sides of the pedigree in families of TS probands. The genetics of TS appears to be complex with likely genetic heterogeneity, polygenetic influences, and environmental interactions complicating the picture. The largest linkage study to date of individuals and extended pedigrees with TS or chronic tics found strong evidence of linkage for a region on chromosome 2p, with several other regions providing more modest evidence of susceptibility loci for TS (33). Cytogenetic abnormalities in isolated TS patients and their relatives have pointed to other regions of interest, including a candidate gene at 13q31.1 coding for SLITRK 1, a protein highly expressed in the brain and influencing neuron development (34).

PERINATAL FACTORS

Although findings across studies have been inconsistent, various forms of perinatal adversity have been associated with increased risk of TS, including maternal smoking, low birth weight, low Apgar score, increased parental age, and maternal complications (35). Tic severity has been associated with lower birth weight, increased first-trimester nausea and vomiting, and birth complications. How such environmental risk factors might interact with genetic factors to impact the basal ganglia and related structures is an important area for continued study.

INFECTIOUS/AUTOIMMUNE FACTORS AND THE PANDAS CONTROVERSY

The observation that SC is often accompanied by de novo OCD (even prior to the onset of involuntary movements), anxiety, and tics, prompted Swedo et al. (36) to hypothesize that some cases of tics and/or OCD represent PANDAS, which they suggested were characterized by prepubertal onset, sudden onset, and/or dramatic exacerbations occurring in close temporal association with group A beta-hemolytic streptococcal infection (GABHS) and minor neurological abnormalities such as choreiform movements (motor impersistence, irregular, small jerky, asymmetric movements, but not frank chorea) or clumsiness. Other apparently poststreptococcal neurological conditions have recently been described (22). Furthermore, the observation that sera from putative PANDAS cases can induce antibody-mediated activation of calcium-calmodulin–dependent protein (CaM) kinase II activity in neuronal cells (37) suggests the kinds of mechanisms that might link autoantibodies with changes in neuronal signal transduction.

Despite much clinical and immunological research, the PANDAS hypothesis has remained controversial (30,38,39), in part because there is no diagnostic test to establish in any given case whether the co-occurrence of recent GABHS infection and the onset or exacerbation of tics/OCD are causally related rather than merely coincidental (GABHS, tics, and OC symptoms all being common in this age group). Studies of circulating autoantibodies and other immune markers have been equivocal in differentiating putative PANDAS cases, non-PANDAS cases of tic disorder, and controls (30). Several ambitious prospective studies, which are nearing publication, promise to shed further light on this controversial subject (40).

In support of the PANDAS hypothesis, however, analysis of population-based epidemiological data from a large health maintenance organization (HMO) found that children receiving their first diagnosis of TS, tic disorder, or OCD were significantly more likely to have had a GABHS infection during the preceding 3-month and 12-month period than were matched controls; having had multiple GABHS infections in the preceding year increased the likelihood of a new diagnosis of TS by 13.6-fold (41).

Clinical Assessment

Because the goals of treatment extend beyond tic reduction to include supporting the youngster's overall social, academic, and emotional development, a detailed assessment of all these areas, as well as family history and adaptive strengths, is essential.

REALMS OF ASSESSMENT

Tic severity

A detailed history of the onset and subsequent vicissitudes of tics should be obtained from both the parent and the child, with attention to the degree of associated distress, physical discomfort, functional impairment, or social stigma. Young children may be unaware of or may deny various tics, whereas older children may report subtle premonitory urges or tics of which their parents are unaware. Youngsters should also be asked about the degree to which they can voluntarily suppress or delay different tics (e.g., at school) and with what degree of attendant discomfort. It is also useful to determine when was the worst-ever period for motor and phonic tics, respectively, (as they may run different courses), and to ask the parents and child to rate the current subjective severity of tics on a 0 to 10 (none to worst ever) scale.

Tics may not always be observable during the clinical examination itself, either because of the natural fluctuations of tics or the child's spontaneously suppressing them in an unfamiliar situation. Hence, it is useful to observe the child for tics while beginning the interview around some neutral topic, such as the child's recreational activities, hobbies, school, or peer interests, before focusing the discussion on the tics themselves. Because tics are often suggestible, inquiring about prior tics that have faded may spontaneously re-elicit them.

The PANDAS hypothesis implies that the clinical history should also include a review of whether the child has had frequent GABHS infections; whether the onset and any exacerbations have been gradual or abrupt; and what, if any, is the temporal relationship of the onset and subsequent exacerbations of the tic/OCD symptoms to GABHS infections.

Presence and severity of comorbid disorders

As noted, the comorbid disorders that accompany tics may be functionally or developmentally more disabling than the tics themselves. Specific inquiry needs to be made about current or past ADHD symptoms, the various categories of obsessions and compulsions, anxiety symptoms (generalized anxiety, phobias, separation anxiety, panic attacks), or depression.

Youngsters with TS may be prone to depression or anxiety for a variety of reasons (2). Although the risk of anxiety (other than OCD) or depression in the relatives of TS probands does not appear to be increased, some evidence exists that individuals with TS have greater autonomic lability, perhaps predisposing to anxiety, and, like individuals with other basal ganglia disorders, a vulnerability to depression. Constitutional vulnerability aside, the fear or actual experience of teasing or stigmatization can undermine self-esteem and increase anxious self-consciousness. The constant barrage of tics and premonitory urges, as well as the frequently comorbid ADHD, OCD, and learning difficulties can induce feelings of hopelessness and learned helplessness in children. Like children with ADHD uncomplicated by tics, children with comorbid TS and ADHD experience greater academic and social difficulties with deleterious effects on their self-esteem (42). Finally, the various medications used in treating TS, OCD, and/or ADHD can all cause sedation, dysphoria, or increased anxiety as unintended side effects.

Thus, one specific role for the child psychiatrist in the management of TS lies in assessing the presence of anxiety and/or depression, clarifying potential contributing factors, and planning appropriate therapeutic interventions, whether psychotherapeutic, environmental, educational, and/or psychopharmacological.

School and social adjustment

Children with TS often have difficulties with fine motor coordination, impulsivity, concentration, and executive functioning, as well as uneven neuropsychological profiles and problems with visuomotor integration (19,43). True ADHD, present from preschool years on and often preceding the onset of tics, must be distinguished from the situation of the child with a history of good concentration and impulse control who becomes distractible in the face of an onslaught of tics and premonitory urges during a tic exacerbation. Detailing the child's academic strengths and weaknesses and assessing the adequacy of the child's educational placement and instructional programming is an important component of the initial evaluation. The potential impact of tics on classmates, teachers, and the classroom environment should be assessed.

Family factors

TS symptoms influence and, in turn, are influenced by the family system, and it is essential to recognize this reciprocal relationship. The family's attitudes and reactions to the child's disorder must be assessed, as well as the family's overall stresses and coping resources, because stress is an important nonspecific exacerbant of tics (8).

The family's attitudes and preconceived notions about the child's tics must be assessed. A detailed family psychiatric and medical history is important, as anxiety, OCD, and tics are all common in the relatives of children with TS. When a parent has also had similar symptoms, this may be a useful source of empathy for the parent in understanding the child's experience. If an affected parent has done well personally and occupationally, the parent's example can provide a reassuring model for the child that one can thrive despite having had a tic disorder. On the other hand, a parental history of tics or OCD can also occasion counterproductive parental overidentification and apprehension, because the child's experience of growing up with tics may be quite different from the parent's.

Overall psychological and developmental functioning

The presence of tics or a tic disorder must not overshadow the parents', child's, and clinician's appreciation of the child's overall personality, interests, aspirations, and strengths. The youngster's individual talents, interests, and social networks provide important buffers for a sense of self-esteem and efficacy in the face of the unpredictability of bothersome tics and must be supported. The impact of tics (and associated difficulties) varies over the course of development. Adolescents, for example, may be particularly concerned about the impact on peer acceptance and romantic opportunities.

STANDARDIZED ASSESSMENT MEASURES

Standardized instruments for assessing the clinical severity of tics, obsessions, and compulsions are useful for documenting baseline severity, ensuring a comprehensive survey of symptoms at the time of the initial evaluation, and tracking subsequent symptom evolution or treatment response. (See reference 1 for a compilation of such instruments.)

Instruments for assessing tics

The most widely used scale for assessing tic severity in clinical studies is the Yale Global Tic Severity Scale (YGTSS) (44). Based on a clinician interview, the YGTSS rates the number, frequency, intensity, complexity, and interference for motor and phonic tics separately and yields a total tic score, an overall impairment rating, and a global severity score. Ratings based on videotaping under standardized conditions have also been used to rate tic severity and may detect tics of which the patient is unaware; however, this method is time consuming and requires considerable rater training and appropriate equipment (45).

Instruments for assessing obsessions and compulsions

The Yale Brown Obsessive Compulsive Scale (Y-BOCS) and its adaptation for children (CY-BOCS) (46) are clinician-rated, semistructured, interview-based scales whose reliability and validity have been well studied; they yield scores for obsession severity, compulsion severity, and combined total score. Rather than viewing obsessions and compulsions as separate phenomena, factor analytic studies of OCD symptoms consistently find several dimensions of thematically related obsessions and compulsions that are associated with apparently distinctive patterns of comorbidity (e.g., presence or absence of tics), genetic transmission, treatment response, and neurobiological substrate (47). The Dimensional Y-BOCS (DY-BOCS) is an instrument that assesses the presence and severity of six distinct dimensions of obsessions and compulsions concerning (a) harm due to aggression/injury/violence; (b) moral/sexual/religious issues; (c) symmetry or "just-right" perceptions, counting, or arranging; (d) contamination and cleaning; (e) hoarding; and (f) miscellaneous (including somatic concerns) (48).

Treatment

OVERALL PRINCIPLES

Because tic disorders and their associated conditions often persist for many years, the clinician should have an ongoing relationship with the child and family through which he or she can address the vicissitudes of the child's symptoms and their impact on the various phases of development. In addition to offering expertise regarding diagnosis and judicious pharmacological decision making, the clinician has the task of helping the parents and patient focus on the whole child and ensuring that an appreciation of the child's adaptive strengths does not get lost behind the diagnostic labels and symptoms.

Many parents fear the diagnosis of TS as implying a severe, disabling, life-long condition of cursing and bizarre behaviors. Educating the parents and child about the disorder is thus crucial, as the majority of cases are mild, coprolalia is uncommon, and tics improve spontaneously in the majority of youngsters by the end of adolescence (6,12,13). The Tourette's Syndrome Association (www.tsa-usa.org) is an invaluable source of educational materials and resources. In this Internet age, parents are often overwhelmed by a flood of information, both accurate and spurious. Given the wide diversity of cases in terms of severity and comorbid difficulties, the clinician's guidance is crucial in helping parents navigate and understand how this vast body of information applies to their particular child.

ESTABLISHING THE TARGETS OF TREATMENT

The focus of any intervention should depend on which symptoms are most impairing on the basis of a comprehensive assessment. Children who have only tics, without marked OCD or ADHD, usually fare the best, and mild, nonimpairing tics may not require any specific intervention. In more severe or complicated cases, although tics may be problematic, the first priority for intervention may involve addressing other areas of difficulty, such as ADHD, impulsive behaviors, learning problems, OCD, anxiety, or depression. Which comorbidities are most problematic may change over time. Hence, there must be an ongoing dialogue between clinician, family, and child regarding which symptoms require intervention and their relative priorities. This assessment is especially important in that medications useful for one symptom area may cause difficulty in other symptoms or areas of functioning [e.g., neuroleptics causing problematic sedation, or stimulants or selective serotonin reuptake inhibitors (SSRIs) causing tic exacerbations]. In children with multiple comorbid disorders, it is sometimes difficult to avoid polypharmacy, and the trade-offs between potential benefits and side effects must always be explicitly discussed.

TREATMENT OF TICS

Medication

General principles of psychopharmacology for tics

There is no evidence that medication affects the long-term course of tics. Thus, a trial of medication is indicated only when the tics are causing sufficient distress, physical discomfort, social stigmatization, or interference with classroom participation that the potential benefits of medication outweigh the potential side effects. The goal is to reduce tics to a tolerable level, because attempting to eliminate tics altogether is usually unsuccessful and risks sedation, cognitive blunting, or other dose-related side effects.

A careful discussion with parents (and, when appropriate, adolescent) to identify the target symptoms, level of current impairment and distress, potential side effects, and realistic expectations for benefits is thus a prologue to beginning pharmacotherapy. A trial of medication is best conducted in the context of an ongoing relationship with patient and family in which there is open communication regarding symptom changes, possible side effects, and other concerns.

Several important principles guide the pharmacological treatment of tics (49):

1. Patients should be started on a low dose, and the dose should be gradually titrated upward, in small increments, after waiting long enough to judge response.
2. The lowest effective maintenance dose should be used to prevent or minimize side effects.
3. Although polypharmacy cannot always be avoided when comorbid problems are prominent, it should be minimized to the extent possible.
4. Only one medication should be added or discontinued at a time.
5. If medications are to be decreased or discontinued, they should be tapered very slowly to avoid rebound exacerbation of tics.

It is sometimes advisable to delay beginning or immediately increasing medication when there is a flare-up of tics (e.g., around the beginning of the school year) because many flare-ups subside spontaneously. Because intermittent transient exacerbations can occur on even an optimal anti-tic medication regimen, physicians must guard against inadvertently ratcheting up to higher and higher doses of medication, with attempts to decrease the dose hampered by bothersome rebound exacerbations. Several recent reviews have surveyed the pharmacological treatment of TS (49–52).

Alpha-adrenergic agents

As the first choice for mild to moderate tics, many clinicians prefer one of the alpha-adrenergic agonists (guanfacine or clonidine). Although these medications do not have as robust a tic-suppressing effect as the neuroleptics and are not effective in as many patients, they have the advantage of fewer side effects. They have the additional advantage of being mildly effective for symptoms of comorbid ADHD. Although clonidine has been in longer use for tics, many clinicians prefer guanfacine as less sedating, longer acting, and more effective for comorbid ADHD, perhaps by virtue of its greater specificity for prefrontal postsynaptic alpha 2_A receptors (53).

In contrast to the neuroleptics, which are best given at bedtime to accommodate their side effect of sedation, guanfacine or clonidine for treatment of tics is best administered in divided doses (usually 2 to 3 times a day for guanfacine, 3 to 4 times a day for clonidine). Clonidine is started with a single 0.05-mg morning dose (0.025 mg for younger children). If well tolerated, additional doses of 0.025 to 0.05 mg are added at intervals of 5 to 7 days, first at lunch or early afternoon and then after school. If tics are troublesome in the evening, an additional suppertime dose may be added. If necessary, the strength of each dose is gradually increased in small increments, up to a daily total of about 0.3 mg in divided doses; side effects often become a problem beyond this level. Clonidine can also be administered by means of a transdermal patch, but this often causes skin irritation. The corresponding starting dose for guanfacine is 0.5 mg, with 0.25-mg increments up to a total of 2 to 3 mg, if necessary, in three divided doses. The response to clonidine or guanfacine is usually gradual, sometimes requiring a few weeks to become apparent. These agents may also be modestly helpful for irritability, impulsivity, and ADHD.

The principal side effect of the alpha-adrenergic agents is dose-related sedation which may decrease with time. Other side effects include irritability, dry mouth, and light-headedness or orthostatic hypotension. Although clonidine may be helpful for insomnia, both agents can occasionally cause midsleep disruption. Combining the two drugs can produce hypotension and should be avoided.

Discontinuing clonidine or guanfacine must be done gradually to avoid rebound tic exacerbations and, in the case of abrupt discontinuation of clonidine, rebound increases in blood pressure.

Dopamine-blocking and dopamine-depleting agents

The neuroleptics are the first-choice agents for moderate to severe tics, or when the alpha-adrenergic agents are not sufficiently effective. Although TDs are extremely rare in children on low doses of typical neuroleptics, many clinicians and parents feel more comfortable using the newer atypical neuroleptics, which have a lower risk of TD. Haloperidol, pimozide, risperidone, and ziprasidone, the neuroleptics that have been best studied in controlled trials, appear to have comparable effect sizes of about 0.8 to 1.0 after several weeks compared with the more modest effects of clonidine and guanfacine. Hence the choice of neuroleptic is best made on the basis of tolerability and potential side effects. Ziprasidone is not commercially available in a low enough dose formulation to be tolerated by most preadolescent children. Of the older neuroleptics, fluphenazine has also been widely used in clinical practice. Case reports or open-label trials are also available for aripiprazole and quetiapine. Anti-tic efficacy appears to be related to the relative potency of dopamine D2 blockade. Hence, it cannot be assumed that all atypical neuroleptics are effective for tics, because the paradigmatic atypical neuroleptic clozapine, which, like quetiapine, is a poor D2 blocker, is not effective for tics.

Sedation and cognitive blunting are common, dose-related side effects of all the neuroleptics. In our experience, if the equivalent of 2 to 4 mg of haloperidol, risperidone, fluphenazine, or pimozide does not produce sufficient improvement, escalation to higher doses is more likely to produce more incremental side effects than benefit; furthermore, because of the phenomena of rebound exacerbations, weaning a patient off high doses of neuroleptic, even if the drug is ineffective for tics, is often a protracted and arduous process.

All of the neuroleptics, new and old, have the potential for acute neurological side effects such as parkinsonism, akathisia, and acute dystonic reactions (e.g., torticollis, oculogyric crisis). Although readily reversible with either a reduction in dose or an anticholinergic, these acute dystonic reactions can be alarming to patients and families if not forewarned. Other common side effects of the neuroleptics include de novo school phobia and depression; akathisia and hyperprolactinemia, which is associated with dopamine blockade and may produce galactorrhea.

Recent concerns about the atypical neuroleptics have been raised regarding weight gain secondary to appetite stimulation and related metabolic abnormalities of lipid and glucose regulation. Olanzapine, quetiapine, and risperidone appear to be the worst offenders.

Hence, careful tracking of weight, height, and fasting lipid/cholesterol and glucose levels is important with these drugs.

Prolonged cardiac conduction time (increased QTc) is also a concern with pimozide and, to a lesser extent, ziprasidone. A baseline electrocardiogram, repeated annually and with dose increases, is prudent for children taking either of these two drugs. Parents and pediatricians of children on pimozide should be particularly aware of the hazard of drugs, such as the macrolide antibiotics, that inhibit cytochrome P450 3A4, as fatal arrhythmias can result when these drugs are combined with pimozide (54).

Tiapride and sulpride, two specific D2-blocking agents, are commonly used in Europe for tics but are not available in the United States. Tetrabenazine, a dopamine-depleting drug, is also not on the market in the United States but has proven useful for tics in open-label studies. Side effects include sedation, depression, sleep disturbance, and parkinsonism.

Other pharmacological agents

Beyond the alpha-adrenergic agents and anti-dopaminergic agents discussed previously, a plethora of medications of various classes have been tried in small open trials (50,51,52), either alone or in conjunction with the neuroleptics. These reports are difficult to interpret because of small sample size, placebo effects (which can be substantial), and the probably great heterogeneity of subjects, many of whom had failed to respond to the standard agents. Nonetheless, some of these agents deserve mention.

Several antiepileptics (topiramate, valproate, and levetiracetam) have proven useful in some open trials of patients with TS. The utility of topiramate is often limited by dose-related sedation and cognitive blunting, and acute angle-closure glaucoma has been reported. In an open study of children with TS, levetiracetam, in doses of 1 to 2 g per day, produced a 20% reduction in tics. The use of valproate in girls with obesity may possibly increase the risk of polycystic ovary disease.

Baclofen, a $GABA_B$ (gamma-aminobutyric acid) receptor agonist used for treating spasticity, has produced equivocal results in an open trial and one controlled trial (55).

Botulinum toxin injection can be very useful for reducing specific problematic localized tics, such as strenuous blinking or loud vocal tics, but does not affect tics unrelated to the injected sites; care must be taken to avoid muscle weakness or dysphonia because the effects can persist up to 90 days (56,57).

Emerging treatments

Habit reversal therapy

Habit reversal therapy (HRT) for tics is an adaptation of the original work of Azrin and Nunn. HRT focuses on (a) teaching children to increase their awareness of premonitory urges preceding troublesome tics, (b) developing and implementing competing responses that are incompatible with performing the tic, (c) employing relaxation techniques, and (d) contingency management of situations that elicit or reinforce tics (58). A controlled trial of HRT versus supportive psychotherapy found that HRT significantly reduced tic severity over the course of treatment and that these gains were maintained at 6-month follow-up (59). Positive treatment response was predicted by performance on a neuropsychological measure of response inhibition, the Visuospatial Priming Task. Multisite studies of HRT in children and adults with TS are under way to clarify patient selection, optimal treatment design, predictors of response, generalizability across tics, and the attentional burden for the patient of employing the technique. Many patients report spontaneously suppressing their tics during work, school, or social situation, but at the cost of concomitant increased inner tension and difficulty in concentrating.

Repetitive transcranial magnetic stimulation (rTMS)

Although several earlier studies of rTMS over various cortical regions found it ineffective for tics, Mantovani et al. (60) recently found that 1-Hz stimulation over the supplementary motor area produced a clinically significant improvement (67% reduction in tic severity) in five TS patients. If confirmed, rTMS may prove a safe, effective, albeit labor-intensive. intervention for severe tics.

Deep brain stimulation

Deep brain stimulation (DBS) has been successfully used to treat a small number of severely impaired, medication-refractory adult cases of TS. The selection of cases most likely to benefit from DBS and the optimal targets for electrode placement and stimulus parameters require systematic study (61). DBS has been used on rare occasions in adolescents with severe, intractable TS (62) but raises difficult ethical and selection issues, in light of the trend toward spontaneous amelioration of tics with age in a majority of youngsters (63).

TREATMENT OF COMORBID OBSESSIVE-COMPULSIVE DISORDER

OC symptoms are common in individuals with tic disorders and can be a major source of distress and functional impairment, even when the tics themselves are not troublesome.

Medication

Selective serotonin reuptake inhibitors

The SSRIs, such as sertraline (64), fluoxetine (65), paroxetine (66), and fluvoxamine (67), have been shown to be effective in children with OCD (68). Because the presence of a comorbid tic disorder has been an exclusionary criterion for many clinical trials for pediatric OCD, data about their efficacy for tic-related OCD in children are sparse (69). The SSRIs are generally well tolerated in youngsters with comorbid tics and OCD (70), with the commonest side effect in children being behavioral activation. Occasionally SSRIs may cause tic exacerbation or de novo tics (71).

Recent Food and Drug Administration (FDA) black-box warnings have raised concerns over a potential increase in suicidal ideation/suicide attempts in children and adolescents treated with SSRIs. A recent meta-analysis of double-blind placebo-controlled pediatric trials of SSRIs found a twofold increase in relative risk (compared with placebo) of suicidal ideation/attempts in youngsters receiving SSRIs for OCD or non-OCD anxiety disorders, a relative increase comparable to that found in youngsters receiving second-generation antidepressants for depression (72). However, because the base rate of suicidal ideation/attempts is much lower in placebo-treated children with OCD than in placebo-treated depressed children, the absolute magnitude of increased suicidal ideation/attempts is significantly lower in youngsters receiving SSRIs for OCD (4 of 362 children on SSRIs versus 1 of 339 children on placebo).

Neuroleptic augmentation strategies

Tic-related forms of OCD differ from non–tic-related OCD in several respects, including phenomenology and responsiveness to SSRIs (73). Tic-related OCD is less responsive to SSRI monotherapy than is non–tic-related OCD, in both children (69,74) and adults, and may require augmentation with a neuroleptic to obtain an optimal response. Controlled clinical trials have found augmentation of SSRIs with haloperidol, risperidone, or quetiapine to be effective for tic-related OCD; only open trials or case study data are available for other neuroleptics (75,76). Adverse drug interactions must be avoided when co-administering neuroleptics and SSRIs.

Cognitive-behavioral therapy

Cognitive behavioral therapy (CBT) has been extensively developed and studied for children and adolescents with OCD (77). A comparative trial in a mixed group of youngsters with OCD either with or without tics found that a combination of sertraline and CBT was superior (effect size 1.3) to CBT alone (effect size 1.0), which in turn was superior to sertraline alone (effect size 0.7). In the 15% of youngsters who also had a comorbid tic disorder, sertraline alone was no more effective than placebo, whereas combined treatment was more effective than CBT alone, which in turn was superior to placebo (74).

These data suggest that youngsters with substantial tic-related OCD symptoms should have a combination of both SSRI medication and CBT. When the OC symptoms involve a preponderance of "just right" phenomena rather than anxiety-driven, harm-avoidant obsessions and compulsions, the usual exposure/response prevention CBT techniques may require modification to include more habit-reversal techniques (73).

TREATMENT OF COMORBID ATTENTION DEFICIT HYPERACTIVITY DISORDER

General principles of psychopharmacology for tic-related attention deficit hyperactivity disorder

A large proportion of children ultimately diagnosed with TS initially present with ADHD symptoms, even prior to the onset of tics, and these symptoms often first bring such children to medical attention. Comorbid ADHD is thus a common feature in many youngsters with tic disorders and is often more impairing than the tics themselves (15,16,42,78).

Controversy over stimulants in tic disorder

The use of stimulants in youngsters with tic disorder has been an area of considerable controversy.

On one hand, clinical experience and some clinical trials (79) and discontinuation studies (80) suggest that some children and youngsters on the stimulants may develop either a de novo tic disorder or an exacerbation of existing tics. For example, in a placebo-controlled, double-blind cross-over study (81) of the effects of d-amphetamine or methylphenidate (MPH) on tic severity, a majority of children with TS and comorbid ADHD experienced improvement of ADHD symptoms while taking stimulants, with acceptable side effects; however, one third of the youngsters had stimulant-associated exacerbations of tics that outweighed the clinical benefits of the stimulants on their ADHD symptoms. In addition to tic exacerbations, a small number of children also showed largely transient obsessive-compulsive symptoms on the stimulants. In general, adverse effects on tics were worse at higher stimulant dosage levels; d-amphetamine produced more side effects than did MPH; and adverse effects of stimulants on tics attenuated somewhat with time.

On the other hand, several studies have supported the notion that many children with comorbid ADHD and tics can benefit from MPH at moderate doses (0.1 to 0.5 mg/kg) without substantial adverse effects on tics (82,83).

Alpha-adrenergic agents

For children with mild ADHD symptoms, or when parents or clinicians are reluctant to try a stimulant for fear of tic exacerbation, the alpha-adrenergic agents are a reasonable first choice, because they may have the dual benefit of both moderating tics and improving ADHD symptoms. As discussed previously in the section on treatment of tics, although data on the use of clonidine are more extensive, many clinicians prefer guanfacine because of its longer action, lesser sedating effects, and apparently greater effectiveness for ADHD symptoms (53).

A multisite randomized study (83) compared MPH alone, clonidine alone, MPH and clonidine combined, and placebo alone in children with ADHD and tics. Both clonidine alone and MPH alone were more effective than placebo in reducing ADHD symptoms. The combination of clonidine and MPH produced the greatest benefit. Clonidine appeared to be most helpful for impulsivity and hyperactivity, whereas MPH appeared most useful for inattention. The study found that MPH, alone or in combination, did not increase tics over the short-term period of the trial.

Other agents

For youngsters whose ADHD symptoms do not sufficiently improve on an alpha-adrenergic drug, or who cannot tolerate a stimulant, a variety of secondary agents may prove useful, including atomoxetine, the tricyclic antidepressants, or bupropion.

A recent controlled study of atomoxetine in youngsters with comorbid ADHD and tics found significantly greater improvement in ADHD symptoms, as well as a decrease in tics and tic-related impairment, with atomoxetine, compared with placebo (84). Isolated cases of tic exacerbations, however, have been reported with atomoxetine (85).

Of the tricyclics, desipramine has been the most studied in children with comorbid tics and ADHD (86), although there are also limited studies of imipramine and nortriptyline. In general, these tricyclics have been found to significantly improve ADHD symptoms, with either positive or no effects on tic severity. A careful individual and family cardiac history, baseline electrocardiogram and blood pressure (periodically repeated in accordance with FDA guidelines), and attention to metabolic interference from other medications are important because of the potential for increased heart rate and conduction time changes in children taking these agents and a possible increase in the risk of sudden cardiac death (87).

PSYCHOSOCIAL INTERVENTIONS

Although TS and related tic disorders are neurological conditions, their course and impact on adaptive functioning and development are strongly influenced by psychosocial factors. Having been told that tics are largely involuntary and that pressing youngsters to suppress them is usually counterproductive, some parents may draw the fallacious corollary that it is inadvisable to actively discourage other inappropriate impulsive behaviors and therefore fail to set suitable consistent limits and consequences. This is especially problematic in the many children with TS who have comorbid ADHD or another disruptive behavior disorder. Helping the youngster and family distinguish which behaviors are true tics and which are more voluntary and controllable is sometimes a difficult task, but an important one in helping to restore some sense of mastery to parents and child, rather than allowing them to simply feel at the mercy of seemingly unpredictable, uncontrollable forces.

Disruptive behaviors in children with tic disorder are amenable to the same parent management and cognitive behavioral techniques that have proven effective in children without tic disorder. For example, a randomized trial of parent management training in children with comorbid tic disorder and disruptive behavior showed a significant decrease in irritable and noncompliant behavior, compared with a "treatment as usual" control group (88).

School is a challenging setting for many youngsters with TS. When tics are prominent, the child may face teasing or ostracism by peers. Informational literature and video materials suitable for educators and school nurses are available from the Tourette's Syndrome Association (www.tsa-usa.org). When appropriate, the clinician should work with the child, parents, and school to find the optimal way to educate classmates about the child's symptoms in such a way as to enlist support and discourage stigmatization. When the movements or noises are disruptive to the classroom milieu, school personnel need guidance in planning and implementing suitable, nonpunitive accommodations that do not further isolate or stigmatize the child. Like parents, school personnel may also have difficulty, especially in children with comorbid ADHD, in distinguishing between true tics and potentially controllable impulsive behavior that requires appropriate limit setting.

In addition to social and behavioral difficulties in the school setting, many youngsters also have impairments in executive functioning, poor handwriting, and uneven cognitive profiles that impact learning (43). The clinician has an important role in helping ensure that children with TS who are experiencing school problems receive an adequate psychoeducational assessment, appropriate classroom and curricular accommodations, and, where needed, special educational interventions.

PANDAS CONTROVERSY: IMPLICATIONS FOR ASSESSMENT AND TREATMENT

While awaiting further clarification from the many research studies under way, what are the implications of the PANDAs hypothesis for practical management?

Children with sudden onset or exacerbations of tic/OCD symptoms warrant a careful throat culture, which, if positive for GABHS, should be treated with an appropriate course of antibiotics, with a follow-up culture a week or so later. Although highly specific, rapid strep tests are not as sensitive as a careful throat culture read at 48 hours. The misapprehension is widespread that elevated antistreptococcal titers (antistreptolysin O or antistreptococcal DNAase B) are somehow diagnostic of PANDAS. There is no evidence that these antibodies are pathogenic, and all they show is that a child had a strep infection some weeks earlier. Only positive throat cultures, and not antibody titers, are appropriate indications for antibiotic treatment. Because the initial co-occurrence of GABHS infection and tic/OCD symptoms may be coincidental or nonspecific, Swedo et al. (39) caution:

> A single positive throat culture or elevated anti-streptococcal antibody titer is not sufficient to determine that a child's neuropsychiatric symptoms are associated with streptococcal infections. Instead, the determination that a child fits the PANDAS profile is made through prospective evaluation and documentation of the presence of streptococcal infections in conjunction with at least 2 episodes of neuropsychiatric symptoms, as well as demonstrating negative throat culture or stable titers during times of neuropsychiatric symptom remission (pp. 908–909).

Because of the equivocal findings of antibiotic prophylaxis trials and the risks of antibiotic resistance for both the individual child and the community as a whole, this intervention should be reserved for those cases in which symptom exacerbations appear to be clearly linked to GABHS reinfection.

Summary

In addition to the stigma, distress, and functional challenges that tics pose for youngsters with TS and their families, this complex neuropsychiatric disorder often entails substantial comorbidity in the form of OCD, ADHD, and vulnerability to anxiety, depression, and learning difficulties (2). Although there is now an appreciation that tics per se often improve by early adulthood, the frequent persistence of these associated difficulties throughout childhood and adolescence requires a comprehensive approach to evaluation and management best accomplished in the context of a long-term partnership between clinicians, family, and patient. Beyond the relief of specific target symptoms, the overall clinical priority is supporting the child's and family's overall development, optimizing the development of adaptive strengths and talents, and safeguarding self-esteem and interpersonal relationships (1).

Youngsters with tic disorders are often seen by both pediatric neurologists and child psychiatrists. Both groups prescribe many of the same medications, although differences in practice style exist. On the other hand, some diagnostic and treatment approaches are likely to fall more within the expertise of one subspecialty rather than the other. For example, in complex cases, the neurologic differential diagnosis regarding other movement or seizure disorders is likely the purview of the pediatric neurologist, as are specialized interventions such as botulinum toxin injection. Similarly, comprehensive psychosocial assessment and treatment of interpersonal difficulties and psychiatric comorbidities such as depression, anxiety, or OCD may be more familiar territory for the child psychiatrist. Both specialists also need expertise in working with school personnel on the child's behalf and a close collaborative relationship with experienced clinical psychologists who can provide the detailed neuropsychological and educational assessment many children with TS require, as well as the growing armamentarium of useful specific cognitive behavioral techniques (88–90).

Although various anti-tic medications can be helpful, sedation, weight gain, and other side effects often limit their usefulness (52). Similarly, side effects often complicate the use of the antidepressants, anxiolytics, and stimulants used for OCD, anxiety, ADHD, and depressive symptoms associated with TS (49,50).

Developing newer, more satisfactory medications thus remains an important area of research. At the same time, nonpharmacological approaches, such as CBT, also deserve clinical and research emphasis, as their effectiveness may often be as great as, and more durable than, that of medication for certain symptoms (74).

Deeper insights into the genetic and neurobiological causes and subtypes of TS may in turn yield more effective means of treatment and prevention. One valuable clinical advance would be the identification of specific biological or immunological markers for streptococcal-related forms of tic disorder or OCD. Such markers would help clarify pathogenic mechanisms as well as distinguish those cases where streptococcal (or other) infections play a truly causal, as opposed to coincidental, role.

Finally, a more thorough understanding of the aberrant neurocircuitry and pathophysiology of tics and OCD may help to refine electrophysiological interventions (32). Although it seems likely that DBS will continue to be reserved for only the most chronic and debilitating cases, it remains to be seen whether there is a role for less intrusive modalities, such as rTMS, in helping to re-regulate the disordered patterns of activation and disinhibition that appear to underlie TS and related disorders.

Questions

1. Compared with alpha-adrenergic agents such as guanfacine or clonidine, neuroleptics
   A. are superior for problems of inattention or hyperactivity.
   B. have a lower risk of weight gain.
   C. are generally more potent anti-tic agents.
   D. pose less of a risk of sedation.

2. Stereotypies (stereotypic movement disorder)
   A. run a more fluctuating course than tics.
   B. usually respond well to anti-tic medications.
   C. are experienced by the child as more pleasurable and less bothersome than tics.
   D. occur almost exclusively in children with retardation or autism spectrum disorders.

3. In using neuroleptics to treat tics:
   A. The dose should be rapidly increased until tics are eliminated.
   B. If tic control is not achieved, the neuroleptic should be promptly discontinued.
   C. Sedation is rarely a problem.
   D. Reducing or stopping the medication should be done slowly to avoid withdrawal or rebound exacerbations.

4. Based on the natural history of TS:
   A. Childhood tics usually produce persistent impairment into adulthood.
   B. Spontaneous improvement of tics occurs in most cases by young adulthood.
   C. The severity of comorbid ADHD and OCD symptoms over time is usually directly related to tic severity.
   D. Long-term adaptation is unaffected by psychosocial interventions.

5. Coprolalia
   A. is common in TS.
   B. often occurs in the absence of simple motor or phonic tics.
   C. occurs primarily in situations that provoke anger or frustration.
   D. is ego-dystonic and occurs out of context.

6. In cases of comorbid tic disorder and ADHD:
   A. Stimulants can be safely used without fear of increasing tics.
   B. Stimulants should never be used for fear of increasing tics.
   C. A cautious trial of stimulants may be warranted if ADHD impairment is substantial.
   D. The risk of stimulant-related tics appears to be independent of dose.

7. In children with tic disorders and comorbid OCD, specific SSRIs
   A. are usually effective in treating OCD symptoms.
   B. can be used without fear of exacerbating tics.
   C. may require augmentation with a low dose of neuroleptic.
   D. are contraindicated because of the dangers of suicidality.

8. In treating children with TS:
   A. The primary goal of pharmacotherapy is tic eradication.
   B. Prompt drug treatment is essential to minimize morbidity.
   C. Psychosocial interventions are rarely effective.
   D. Anti-tic medication is indicated only for tics that are bothersome or impairing.

9. A 7-year-old boy presents with recent onset of tics. Laboratory findings include an elevated anti-streptolysin O and anti-streptococcal DNAase B titers:
   A. The elevated anti-streptococcal titers are diagnostic of PANDAS.

B. Antibiotic treatment should be begun promptly.
C. Antibiotic prophylaxis is indicated.
D. Antibiotics are usually indicated only in the case of a positive throat culture.

10. A diagnosis of PANDAS
    A. can be made on the basis of the abrupt appearance of tics or OCD soon after a strep infection.
    B. is warranted by the finding of elevated anti-streptococcal antibody titers in a child with tics.
    C. can be made only on the basis of a recurrent pattern of abrupt onset or dramatic exacerbations of tics or OCD in close proximity to a group A beta-hemolytic strep infection.
    D. is an indication for either plasmapheresis or intravenous immunoglobulin.

Answers

1. C
2. C
3. D
4. B
5. D
6. C
7. C
8. D
9. D
10. C

REFERENCES

1. Leckman JF, Cohen DJ, eds. *Tourette's Syndrome—Tics, Obsessions, Compulsions: Developmental Psychopathology and Clinical Care.* New York: John Wiley and Sons; 1999.
2. King RA, Scahill L. Emotional and behavioral difficulties associated with Tourette's syndrome. *Adv Neurol.* 2001;85:78–88.
3. American Psychiatric Association. *Diagnostic and Statistical Manual of Mental Disorders.* 4th ed, text revision ed. Washington, DC: American Psychiatric Association; 2000.
4. Costello E, et al. The Great Smoky Mountains Study of Youth. Goals, design, methods, and the prevalence of DSM-III-R disorders. *Arch Gen Psychiatry.* 1996;53:1129–1136.
5. Snider LA, et al. Tics and problem behaviors in schoolchildren: prevalence, characterization, and associations. *Pediatrics.* 2002;110(2 Pt 1):331–336.
6. Peterson BS, et al. Prospective, longitudinal study of tic, obsessive-compulsive, and attention-deficit/hyperactivity disorders in an epidemiological sample. *J Am Acad Child Adolesc Psychiatry.* 2001;40:685–695.
7. Scahill LD, et al. Public health significance of tic disorders in children and adolescents. *Adv Neurol.* 2005;96:240–248.
8. Lin H, et al. Psychosocial stress predicts future symptom severities in children and adolescents with Tourette syndrome and/or obsessive-compulsive disorder. *J Child Psychol Psychiatry Allied Disciplines.* 2007;48(2):157–166.
9. Hoekstra PJ, et al. Association of common cold with exacerbations in pediatric but not adult patients with tic disorder: a prospective longitudinal study. *J Child Adolesc Psychopharmacol.* 2005;15:285–292.
10. Leckman JF, Walker DE, Cohen DJ. Premonitory urges in Tourette's syndrome. *Am J Psychiatry.* 1993;150:98–102.
11. Leckman JF, et al. Course of tic severity in Tourette syndrome: the first two decades. *Pediatrics.* 1998;102(1 Pt 1):14–19.
12. Bloch MH, et al. Adulthood outcome of tic and obsessive-compulsive symptom severity in children with Tourette syndrome.[see comment]. *Arch Pediatr Adolesc Med.* 2006;160:65–69.
13. Singer HS. Discussing outcome in Tourette syndrome. *Arch Pediatr Adolesc Med.* 2006;160:103–105.
14. Pappert EJ, et al. Objective assessments of longitudinal outcome in Gilles de la Tourette's syndrome. *Neurology.* 2003;61:936–940.
15. Sukhodolsky DG, et al. Disruptive behavior in children with Tourette's syndrome: association with ADHD comorbidity, tic severity, and functional impairment. *J Am Acad Child Adolesc Psychiatry.* 2003;42(1):98–105.
16. Hoekstra PJ, et al. Relative contribution of attention-deficit hyperactivity disorder, obsessive-compulsive disorder, and tic severity to social and behavioral problems in tic disorders. *J Develop Behav Pediatr.* 2004;25:272–279.

17. Jankovic J. Differential diagnosis and etiology of tics. *Adv Neurol.* 2001;85:15–29.
18. Kompoliti K, et al. Hyperkinetic movement disorders misdiagnosed as tics in Gilles de la Tourette syndrome. *Movement Disord.* 1998;13:477–480.
19. Bloch MH, et al. Fine-motor skill deficits in childhood predict adulthood tic severity and global psychosocial functioning in Tourette's syndrome. *J Child Psychol Psychiatry Allied Disciplines.* 2006;47:551–559.
20. Carcani-Rathwell I, Rabe-Hasketh S, Santosh PJ. Repetitive and stereotyped behaviors in pervasive developmental disorders. *J Child Psychol Psychiatry.* 2006;47:573–581.
21. Miller JM, et al. Behavioral therapy for treatment of stereotypic movements in nonautistic children. *J Child Neurol.* 2006;21:119–125.
22. Snider LA, et al. Post-streptococcal autoimmune disorders of the central nervous system. *Curr Opin Neurol.* 2003;16:359–365.
23. Walker FO. Huntington's disease. *Lancet.* 2007;369(9557):218–228.
24. Menkes JH, Sarnat HB, Maria BL. *Child neurology.* 7th ed. Philadelphia: Lippincott Williams & Willkins; 2005.
25. Pacia SV, et al. Clinical features of neocortical temporal lobe epilepsy. *Ann Neurol.* 1996;40:724–730.
26. Geyer H, Bressman SB, The diagnosis of dystonia. *Lancet Neurol.* 2006;5:780–788.
27. Spitz MC, Jankovic J, Killan JM. Familial tic disorder, parkinsonism, motor neuron disease, and acanthocytosis: a new syndrome. *Neurology.* 1985;35:366–370.
28. Hardie RJ, et al. Neuroacanthocytosis. A clinical, haematological and pathological study of 19 cases. *Brain.* 1991;114(Pt 1A):13–49.
29. Bharucha KJ, Sethi KD. Tardive tourettism after exposure to neuroleptic therapy. *Movement Disord.* 1995;10:791–793.
30. Harris K, et al. Tic disorders: neural circuits, neurochemistry, and neuroimmunology. *J Child Neurol.* 2006;21:678–689.
31. Olson LL, et al. Tourette syndrome: diagnosis, strategies, therapies, pathogenesis, and future research directions. *J Child Neurol.* 2006;21:630–641.
32. Leckman JF, et al. Annotation: Tourette syndrome: a relentless drumbeat—driven by misguided brain oscillations. *J Child Psychol Psychiatry Allied Disciplines.* 2006;47:537–550.
33. Tourette Syndrome Association International Consortium for Genetics, Genome scan for Tourette disorder in affected-sibling-pair and multigenerational families. *Am J Hum Genet.* 2007;80:265–272.
34. Abelson JF, et al. Sequence variants in SLITRK1 are associated with Tourette's syndrome. *Science.* 2005;310:317–320.
35. Mathews CA, et al. Association between maternal smoking and increased symptom severity in Tourette's syndrome. *Am J Psychiatry.* 2006;163:1066–1073.
36. Swedo SE, et al. Pediatric autoimmune neuropsychiatric disorders associated with streptococcal infections: clinical description of the first 50 cases.[see comment][erratum appears in *Am J Psychiatry.* 1998;155:578]. *Am J Psychiatry.* 1998;155:264–271.
37. Kirvan CA, et al. Antibody-mediated neuronal cell signaling in behavior and movement disorders. *J Neuroimmunol.* 2006;179(1–2):173–179.
38. Kurlan R, Kaplan EL. The pediatric autoimmune neuropsychiatric disorders associated with streptococcal infection (PANDAS) etiology for tics and obsessive-compulsive symptoms: hypothesis or entity? Practical considerations for the clinician. *Pediatrics.* 2004;113:883–886.
39. Swedo SE, Leonard HL, Rapoport JL. The pediatric autoimmune neuropsychiatric disorders associated with streptococcal infection (PANDAS) subgroup: separating fact from fiction. *Pediatrics.* 2004;113:907–911.
40. Murphy TK, et al. Relationship of movements and behaviors to Group A Streptococcus infections in elementary school children. *Biological Psychiatry.* 2007;61:279–284.
41. Mell LK, Davis RL, Owens D. Association between streptococcal infection and obsessive-compulsive disorder, Tourette's syndrome, and tic disorder. *Pediatrics.* 2005;116:56–60.
42. Stokes A, et al. Peer problems in Tourette's disorder. *Pediatrics.* 1991;87:936–942.
43. Como P. Neuropsychological function in Tourette's syndrome. In: Kurlan R, ed. *Handbook of Tourette's Syndrome and Related Tic and Behavioral Disorders.* New York: Marcel Dekker; 2005:237–252.
44. Leckman JF, et al. The Yale Global Tic Severity Scale: initial testing of a clinician-rated scale of tic severity. *J Am Acad Child Adolesc Psychiatry.* 1989;28:566–573.
45. Goetz CG, et al. Rating scales and quantitative assessment of tics. *Adv Neurol.* 2001;85:31–42.
46. Scahill L, et al. Children's Yale-Brown Obsessive Compulsive Scale: reliability and validity. *J Am Acad Child Adolesc Psychiatry.* 1997;36:844–852.
47. Mataix-Cols D, et al. A multidimensional model of obsessive-compulsive disorder.[see comment]. *Am J Psychiatry.* 2005;162:228–238.
48. Rosario-Campos MC, et al. The Dimensional Yale-Brown Obsessive-Compulsive Scale (DY-BOCS): an instrument for assessing obsessive-compulsive symptom dimensions. *Molec Psychiatry.* 2006;11:495–504.
49. King RA, et al. Psychopharmacological treatment of chronic tic disorder. In: Martin A, et al., eds. *Pediatric Psychopharmacology: Principles and Practice.* New York: Oxford University Press; 2003.
50. Scahill L, et al. Contemporary assessment and pharmacotherapy of Tourette syndrome. *NeuroRx.* 2006;3(2):192–206.

51. Gilbert D. Treatment of children and adolescents with tics and Tourette syndrome. *J Child Neurol.* 2006;21:690–700.
52. Swain JE, et al. Tourette disorder and tic disorders: a decade of progress. *J Am Acad Child Adolesc Psychiatry.* 2007;46:947–968.
53. Scahill L, et al. A placebo-controlled study of guanfacine in the treatment of children with tic disorders and attention deficit hyperactivity disorder. *Am J Psychiatry.* 2001;158:1067–1074.
54. Desta Z, et al. Effect of clarithromycin on the pharmacokinetics and pharmacodynamics of pimozide in healthy poor and extensive metabolizers of cytochrome P450 2D6 (CYP2D6). *Clin Pharmacol Ther.* 1999;65(1):10–20.
55. Singer HS, et al. Baclofen treatment in Tourette syndrome: a double-blind, placebo-controlled, crossover trial.[see comment]. *Neurology.* 2001;56:599–604.
56. Kwak CH, Hanna PA, Jankovic J. Botulinum toxin in the treatment of tics. *Arch Neurol.* 200057:1190–1193.
57. Marras C, et al. Botulinum toxin for simple motor tics: a randomized, double-blind, controlled clinical trial. *Neurology.* 2001;56:605–610.
58. Himle MB, et al. Brief review of habit reversal training for Tourette syndrome. *J Child Neurol.* 2006;21:719–725.
59. Wilhelm S, et al. Habit reversal versus supportive psychotherapy for Tourette's disorder: a randomized controlled trial. *Am J Psychiatry.* 2003;160:1175–1177.
60. Mantovani A, et al. Repetitive transcranial magnetic stimulation (rTMS) in the treatment of obsessive-compulsive disorder (OCD) and Tourette's syndrome (TS). *Int J Neuropsychopharmacol.* 2006;9(1):95–100.
61. Mink JW, et al. Patient selection and assessment recommendations for deep brain stimulation in Tourette syndrome. *Mov Disord.* 2006;21:1831–1838.
62. Shahed J, et al. GPi deep brain stimulation for Tourette syndrome improves tics and psychiatric comorbidities. *Neurology.* 2007;68:159–160.
63. Gilbert DL. Deep brain stimulation for a teen with tics? *Neurology.* 2007;68:85.
64. The Pediatric OCD Treatment Study Team. Cognitive-behavior therapy, sertraline, and their combination for children and adolescents with obsessive-compulsive disorder: the Pediatric OCD Treatment Study (POTS) randomized controlled trial. *JAMA.* 2004;292:1969–1976.
65. Geller DA, et al. Fluoxetine treatment for obsessive-compulsive disorder in children and adolescents: a placebo-controlled clinical trial.[see comment]. *J Am Acad Child Adolesc Psychiatry.* 2001;40:773–779.
66. Geller DA, et al. Paroxetine treatment in children and adolescents with obsessive-compulsive disorder: a randomized, multicenter, double-blind, placebo-controlled trial. *J Am Acad Child Adolesc Psychiatry.* 2004;43:1387–1396.
67. Riddle MA, et al. Fluvoxamine for children and adolescents with obsessive-compulsive disorder: a randomized, controlled, multicenter trial. *J Am Acad Child Adolesc Psychiatry.* 2001;40:222–229.
68. Geller DA, et al. Which SSRI? A meta-analysis of pharmacotherapy trials in pediatric obsessive-compulsive disorder.[see comment]. *Am J Psychiatry.* 2003;160:1919–1928.
69. Geller DA, et al. Impact of comorbidity on treatment response to paroxetine in pediatric obsessive-compulsive disorder: is the use of exclusion criteria empirically supported in randomized clinical trials? *J Child Adolesc Psychopharmacol.* 2003;13(suppl 1):S19–S29.
70. Scahill L, et al. Fluoxetine has no marked effect on tic symptoms in patients with Tourette's syndrome: a double-blind placebo-controlled study. *J Child Adolesc Psychopharmacol.* 1997;7(2):75–85.
71. Fennig S, et al. Emergence of symptoms of Tourette's syndrome during fluvoxamine treatment of obsessive-compulsive disorder. *Br J Psychiatry.* 1994;164:839–841.
72. Bridge JA, et al. Clinical response and risk for reported suicidal ideation and suicide attempts in pediatric antidepressant treatment: a meta-analysis of randomized controlled trials. *JAMA.* 2007;297:1683–1696.
73. King R, et al. Obsessive-compulsive disorder in Tourette's syndrome. In: Kurlan R, ed. *Handbook of Tourette's Syndrome and Related Tic and Behavioral Disorders.* New York: Marcel Dekker; 2005:427–453.
74. March JS, et al. Tics moderate treatment outcome with sertraline but not cognitive-behavior therapy in pediatric obsessive-compulsive disorder. *Biological Psychiatry.* 2007;61:344–347.
75. Bloch MH, et al. A systematic review: antipsychotic augmentation with treatment refractory obsessive-compulsive disorder. [erratum appears in *Mol Psychiatry.* 2006;11:795]. [Review] [49 refs]. *Mol Psychiatry.* 2006;11:622–632.
76. Denys D, et al. Quetiapine addition in obsessive-compulsive disorder: is treatment outcome affected by type and dose of serotonin reuptake inhibitors? *Biological Psychiatry.* 2007;61:412–414.
77. March JS, et al. Cognitive-behavioral psychotherapy for pediatric obsessive-compulsive disorder. *J Clin Child Psychol.* 2001;30(1):8–18.
78. Spencer T, et al. Tourette disorder and ADHD. *Adv Neurol.* 2001;85:57–77.
79. Castellanos FX, et al. Controlled stimulant treatment of ADHD and comorbid Tourette's syndrome: effects of stimulant and dose. *J Am Acad Child Adolesc Psychiatry.* 1997;36:589–596.
80. Riddle MA, et al. Effects of methylphenidate discontinuation and re initiation in children with

Tourette's syndrome and ADHD. *J Child Adolesc Psychopharmacol.* 1995;5:205–214.
81. Castellanos FX, et al. Controlled stimulant treatment of ADHD and comorbid Tourette's syndrome: effects of stimulant and dose. *J Am Acad Child Adolesc Psychiatry.* 1997;36:589–596.
82. Gadow KD, Sverd J. Attention deficit hyperactivity disorder, chronic tic disorder, and methylphenidate. *Adv Neurol.* 2006;99:197–207.
83. Tourette Syndrome Study Group. Treatment of ADHD in children with tics: a randomized controlled trial. *Neurology.* 2002;58:527–536.
84. Allen AJ, et al. Atomoxetine treatment in children and adolescents with ADHD and comorbid tic disorders. *Neurology.* 2005;65:1941–1949.
85. Lee TS, et al. Atomoxetine and tics in ADHD. [see comment]. *J Am Acad Child Adolesc Psychiatry.* 2004;43:1068–1069.
86. Spencer T, et al. A double-blind comparison of desipramine and placebo in children and adolescents with chronic tic disorder and comorbid attention-deficit/hyperactivity disorder. *Arch Gen Psychiatry.* 2002;59:649–656.
87. Amitai Y, et al. Excess fatality from desipramine in children and adolescents. *J Am Acad Child Adolesc Psychiatry.* 2006;45:54–60.
88. Scahill L, et al. Randomized trial of parent management training in children with tic disorders and disruptive behavior. *J Child Neurol.* 2006;21:650–656.
89. Piacentini JC, Chang SW. Behavioral treatments for tic suppression: habit reversal training. *Adv Neurol.* 2006;99:227–233.
90. Franklin M, et al. The pediatric obsessive-compulsive disorder treatment study: rationale, design, and methods. *J Child Adolesc Psychopharmacol.* 2003;13(suppl 1):S39–51.

CHAPTER 5

Epilepsy

JOHN M. PELLOCK

Seizure is the manifestation of a sudden, uncontrolled surge of neuronal firing. After a first seizure, approximately 50% of the patients will have a second one within 6 months. After two seizures, children have an approximately 80% chance of recurrence (1). Epilepsy, recurrent unprovoked seizures, is the most common neurological disorder in children.

Epilepsy affects 0.5% to 1% of children through age 16 years. Each year, 20,000 to 45,000 children are diagnosed with epilepsy. Of children 5 to 14 years of age, 325,000 are affected with epilepsy (2). Child neurologists spend at least 50% of their clinical time caring for patients with epilepsy because of seizures and their comorbidity. Epilepsy is more common in children with mental retardation and other underlying neurological and psychiatric disorders (3). Epilepsy of early childhood onset is more likely to indicate an underlying brain disorder than is epilepsy of middle childhood onset, which is likely to have an unknown or genetic cause (4,5).

Neurologists and psychiatrists have common ground not only in diagnosis but also in their prescribing of antiepileptic drugs (AEDs). In addition, psychiatrists might be asked to evaluate and treat epilepsy's comorbidities—depression, attention deficit hyperactivity disorder (ADHD), and anxiety—before or in conjunction with neurologists (3).

This chapter reviews (a) epilepsy and seizures, including their incidence, classification, etiology, and differential diagnosis; (b) AEDs and their effects on seizures and psychiatric disorders; and (c) psychiatric comorbidities of epilepsy.

Seizure Classification

The International League against Epilepsy has proposed a classification based on the clinical manifestations of the seizure and the electroencephalogram (EEG) (6). It differentiates partial from generalized seizures.

Partial seizures begin locally within a specific brain region, whereas generalized seizures have no clear focal onset. Partial seizures are further divided into those expressed by confusion or mild alteration of consciousness (complex partial) and those without alteration of consciousness (simple partial). Generalized seizures are defined by the presence or absence of the motor activity that accompanies the events, and are typically associated with impairment or a loss of consciousness (Table 5.1).

Seizures previously referred to as "grand mal" are convulsive, and include tonic, clonic, and tonic-clonic seizures, and seizures that have partial onset with secondary generalization.

TABLE 5.1 CLASSIFICATION OF EPILEPSY

I. Partial (focal, local) seizures
Definition: The first clinical and/or EEG changes indicate initial involvement of part of one hemisphere. Partial seizures are classified on the basis of an impairment of consciousness.
    A. Simple, partial seizures (no impairment of consciousness)
    B. Complex partial seizures (with impairment of consciousness)
    C. Partial seizures with secondary generalization
II. Generalized seizures
Definition: The first clinical and/or EEG changes indicate initial involvement of both hemispheres. Consciousness is impaired.
    A. Absence/atypical absence
    B. Myoclonic
    C. Clonic
    D. Tonic
    E. Tonic-clonic
    F. Clonic-tonic-clonic
    G. Atonic

The term *grand mal* may include seizures that have partial onset with secondary generalization. Thus, defining a seizure as grand mal or convulsive does not help determine a possible focal onset. However, documenting a partial (focal) onset is crucial in diagnosing localized pathology, such as mesial temporal sclerosis or a tumor. The term *petit mal* had been applied to "small seizures" that could include myoclonic seizures or staring spells, which could be either generalized absence or complex partial seizures. The clinical behavior associated with a partial seizure depends on the area of the brain that is affected; a behavioral or focal motor event will correlate with the cortical area involved. In adolescents, the most common focus for partial seizures is the temporal lobe. Those seizures often begin with an aura, such as fear or *déjà vu*. In young children, extratemporal partial seizures are more common.

NONEPILEPTIC EVENTS

On the other hand, what appears to be a seizure is occasionally a nonepileptic event, sometimes termed a "pseudoseizure." Although these events are paroxysmal and feature altered behavior, they do not produce an alteration on the EEG. Moreover, they often have no identifiable physiological cause and are frequently associated with psychiatric disturbances. In some children and adolescents, sexual or physical abuse has preceded these episodes.

Kotagal et al (7) reported paroxysmal nonepileptic events in 134 (15.2%) of 883 children and adolescents during a six-year period in the Cleveland Clinic Epilepsy Monitoring Unit (EMU). In that study, of children 5 to 12 years old, 61 had a diagnosis of nonepileptic events, including conversion disorder (psychogenic seizures), inattention, daydreaming spells, stereotypic movements, hypnic jerks, or paroxysmal movements. Of those children, 25% had concomitant epilepsy. Of adolescents, 12 to 18 years old, 48 had nonepileptic events. Of these adolescents, 83% had a conversion disorder and 19% had concomitant epilepsy. Thus, the demonstration of a nonepileptic behavior does not rule out the presence of epilepsy.

Having a family review the video-recorded event is a good way to document that the behavior in question represents the "seizure" reported. In cases of different types of episodes, management is quite difficult.

When both the clinical evaluation and the EEG suggest pseudoseizures, psychiatric consultation is advisable because of the high incidence of underlying psychiatric disorders (8,9). Frequently diagnosed nonepileptiform paroxysmal disorders in children and adolescents are listed in Table 5.2.

Children and adolescents with mental retardation, autism, or other pervasive developmental disorder (PDD) are subject to another diagnostic pitfall. Clinicians may misinterpret

TABLE 5.2 SYMPTOMS OF NONEPILEPTIFORM PAROXYSMAL DISORDERS

Unusual movement	Jitteriness	Self-stimulation
	Masturbation	Tics (Tourette's syndrome)
	Shuddering	Paroxysmal choreoathetosis or dystonia
	Benign sleep myoclonus	Pseudoseizures
	Startle responses	Eye movement
	Paroxysmal torticollis	Head nodding
Episodic features of specific disorders	Tetralogy spells	Hyperthyroidism
	Hydrocephalic spells	Gastroesophageal reflux
	Cardiac arrhythmias	Rumination
	Hypoglycemia	Drug poisoning
	Hypocalcemia	Cerebrovascular events
	Periodic paralysis	
Loss of tone or consciousness	Syncope	Narcolepsy/cataplexy
	Drop attacks	Attention deficit
Respiratory derangements	Apnea	Hyperventilation
	Breath holding	
Perceptual disturbances	Dizziness	Headache
	Vertigo	Abdominal pain
Behavior disorders	Head banging	Acute psychotic symptoms
	Night terrors	fugue
	Sleepwalking	phobia
	Nightmares	panic attacks
	Rage	hallucinations
	Confusion	autism
	Fear	

From Pellock JM. Other nonepileptic paroxysmal disorders. In: Wylie E, Gupta A, Lachhwani DK, eds. *The treatment of epilepsy, principles and practice.* 4th ed. Philadelphia: Lippincott Williams & Wilkins; 2006:632, with permission.

recurrent movements or behaviors (stereotypies) as seizures. In any case, a comprehensive diagnostic assessment from a neurologist may be indicated because children with these disorders may have a high rate of seizures. Similarly, children who are blind or deaf or both also have stereotypies, some of which are self-stimulating. Overall, the prognosis of nonepileptic events is better in children than in adults (10).

Etiology and Diagnosis of Childhood Epilepsy

The etiology of childhood epilepsy is often population-specific. For example, neurocysticercosis commonly causes epilepsy in citizens of Central America, where cysticercosis is endemic. The age of onset of epilepsy is also important. For example, children with inborn errors of metabolism, congenital malformations, and perinatal injuries tend to present with epilepsy at a young age. Genetic factors and head trauma are more common causes in the older child and adolescent. Although various type-specific gene abnormalities cause certain varieties of epilepsy, it is still unclear why specific mutations, which are associated with epilepsy, have variable expression, including different ages of onset in members of the same family (11).

The history and clinical characteristics of the events serve as the basis of the preliminary diagnosis. During a medical history, the physician should inquire whether activities such as staring spells or myoclonic jerks, which might represent seizures, also occur. In a similar fashion, the physician should ask about possible localized symptoms of seizures. For example, the parents may have noted momentary jerking of one limb or conjugate eye deviation prior to the onset of a seizure.

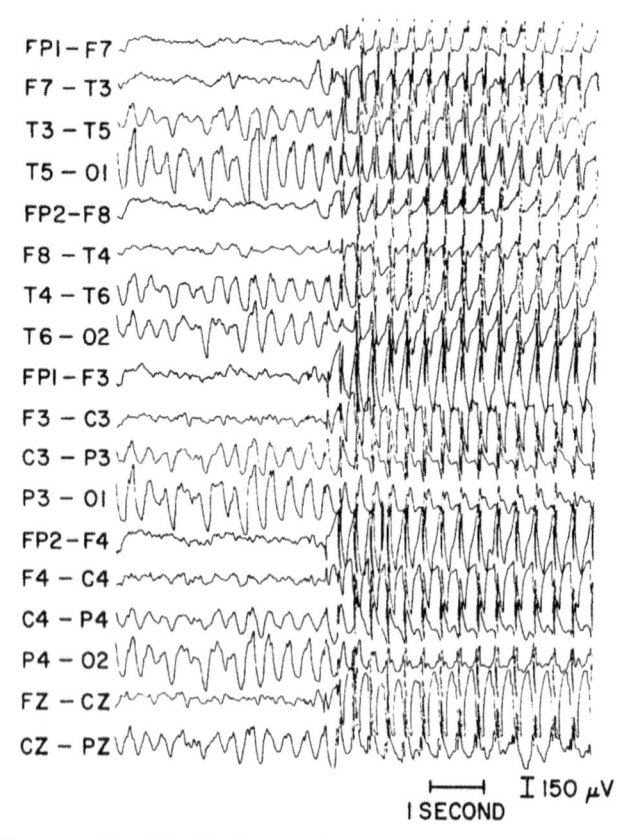

■ **FIGURE 5.1A** EEG as seen in a child with absence seizures.

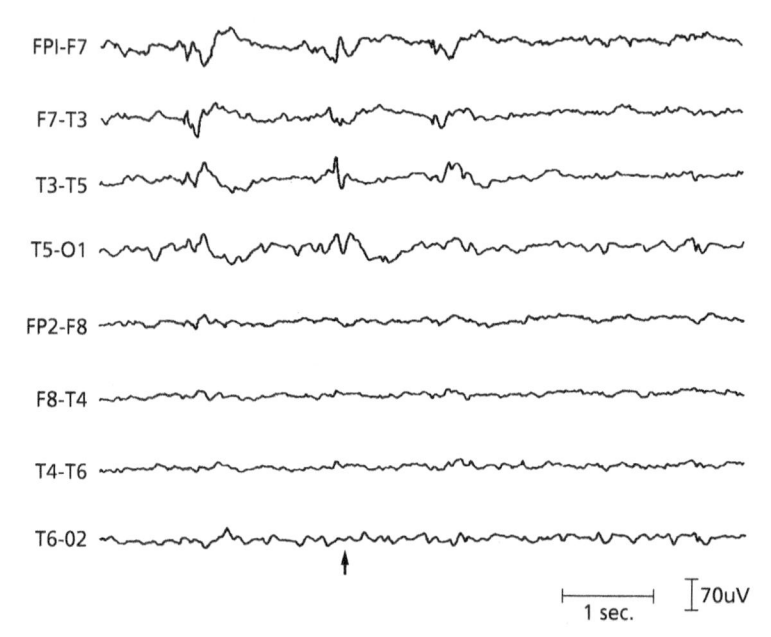

■ **FIGURE 5.1B** Electroencephalogram (EEG) as seen in a child with complex partial seizures. (Parts A and B from Rothner AD. Epilepsy. In: Kaufman DM, Solomon GE, Pfeffer CR, eds. *Child and adolescent neurology for psychiatrists*. Baltimore: Williams & Wilkins, 1992:98; with permission.)

The EEG during the typical episode provides a reliable documentation of the presence, classification, and origin of a seizure. In the usual clinical situation, a routine EEG is performed between events, that is, in the interictal period (12). The interictal EEG may be completely normal or may demonstrate abnormalities, such as generalized spike-and-waves or focal spikes, suggestive of generalized or focal onset epilepsy (Figs. 5.1A,B). An EEG may show focal slowing of background rhythms over a particular region, suggesting a structural lesion. EEGs should include photic stimulation and hyperventilation to activate potential epileptiform activity. When clinical events continue despite normal interictal EEGs, neurologists order prolonged (24 hours) EEG studies or an EEG at the time of day when spells usually develop, such as early morning or with sleep deprivation.

Notably, a normal EEG does not exclude a diagnosis of epilepsy. Moreover, identification of nonspecific abnormalities during a routine EEG does not confirm the diagnosis of epilepsy. Children's EEG records have numerous normal variants. For example, young children have prominent, central, sharp vertex activity during drowsiness and sleep that is frequently misinterpreted as being indicative of epilepsy but is normal.

Prolonged video-EEG monitoring in an EMU for 3 to 7 days is now standard for determining whether seizures are present and establishing an electroclinical correlation. In other words, it determines if a child's behavior coincides with a paroxysm of abnormal EEG activity. This monitoring confines children to a specially designed room, but within it they are free to move about and a parent can stay with them. EEG electrodes are glued to their scalp rather than secured with pins. In addition to the scalp electrodes, technicians may apply ones to measure other physiological functions, such as respiration, cardiac activity, and ocular movement, which would reflect sleep stages. The monitoring consists of continual digital recordings of closed circuit video observations of children's behavior and the simultaneous EEG. While the child is in the EMU, physicians often withdraw AEDs to allow seizure activity to emerge. Although exceptions appear in the literature, the results of video-EEG monitoring are generally accepted as the gold standard.

Neurologists order brain imaging in children in whom cerebral pathology is suspected. However, certain "benign epilepsy syndromes," such as childhood absence (see further on), do not require imaging. When imaging is performed, magnetic resonance imaging (MRI) is the modality of choice (12). Advanced imaging techniques, such as functional MRI (fMRI), positron emission tomography (PET), and other specialized imaging techniques, are currently appropriate only for those undergoing evaluation for epilepsy surgery.

Epilepsy in Children and Adolescents

EPILEPSY SYNDROMES

Epilepsy is not a single disease but rather a neurological disorder with variable clinical presentations and etiologies. The epilepsy syndromes are defined by their seizure type, age at onset, history and neurological examination, ictal and interictal EEG, family history, etiology, anatomical localization, and, perhaps most importantly, prognosis and heritability (13). These syndromes are generally divided into those characterized by focal (partial) pathology and those that have generalized seizures from the onset. Etiologies may be symptomatic (proven cause), cryptogenic (presumed but unproven), and idiopathic (frequently genetic in otherwise normal individuals).

The age of onset and whether the child is otherwise neurologically normal help differentiate the epilepsy syndrome and comorbid psychiatric features. Table 5.3 demonstrates

TABLE 5.3 AGE-RELATED EPILEPSY SYNDROMES[a]

Age Group	Normal Examination	Abnormal Examination
Preschool	Myoclonic-astatic (myoclonic-astatic, vibratory tonic/GSW rhythmic theta)	Lennox-Gastaut (tonic seizures, atypical absence, partial/slow, i.e., 2.5-Hz spike wave)
School age	Benign, rolandic, benign occipital (sensory, clonic/stereotyped IEDs) Childhood absence (absence/3-Hz spike-wave)	Landau-Kleffner, CSWS (rare seizures/ continuous spike waves in sleep Myoclonic absence (myoclonic absence/3-Hz spike-wave) Epilepsia partialis continua syndromes (Kojewnikoff, Rasmussen) (epilepsia partialis continua/polymorphic spikes)
Juvenile	Juvenile myoclonic Juvenile absence GTCS on awakening (as described/ generalized fast polyspike waves, PPR)	Progressive myoclonus (myoclonus, other/ slowed background)

[a]Diagnostic approach is based on seizure semiology/electroencephalographic (EEG) findings; age-related presentations of some common epilepsy syndromes are listed with seizure semiology and interictal EEG findings.

CSWS, continuous spike-wave during slow-wave sleep; GTCS, generalized tonic-clonic seizures; IED, interictal epileptiform discharges; PPR, photoparoxysmal responses.

From Nordli DR, Jr. Diagnostic difficulty in infants and children. *J Child Neurol.* 2002;17(suppl 1):S28–35 with permission.

the diagnostic approach to the differentiation of epilepsy syndromes based on the child's age at the onset of epilepsy and the neurological evaluation (14).

COMPLEX PARTIAL EPILEPSY

Complex partial epilepsy usually originates in the temporal lobe and its connections with the limbic system. Less often, it originates in the frontal or occipital lobe. Classically, the child or adolescent with complex partial epilepsy will first experience a conscious sensation, thought, perception, or emotion—the *aura*. This first part of the seizure localizes the origin of the seizure itself (*ictus*). Overwhelming fear is the most common aura; others that begin in the limbic system are a rising feeling in the epigastrium or an unpleasant olfactory hallucination (like burning rubber) emanating from the uncus. *Déjà vu, jamais vu*, or a repetitive thought may also constitute an aura. The aura is followed by an alteration of consciousness as discharges travel through the limbic system. Automatisms occur in at least 75% of patients (15). Examples of automatisms are lip smacking, uncontrollable laughing (gelastic epilepsy), and running in a circle (cursive epilepsy). If the discharges travel to the reticular formation, patients lose consciousness. A secondary generalized tonic-clonic seizure followed by postictal confusion and drowsiness can occur. Such ictal and postictal behaviors are often misinterpreted as psychiatric disturbances. During the ictal automatism or postictal period, children and adolescents may appear to be aggressive if someone tries to restrain them. Although less common in children than adults, patients may have complex partial status epilepticus, a form of nonconvulsive status epilepticus. Complex partial status epilepticus consists of prolonged seizures with automatisms that can masquerade as a fugue state. An EEG during an event is diagnostic.

In about 40% of adolescents and adults with complex partial epilepsy, the interictal EEG demonstrates temporal spikes in the awake state. If both wake and sleep states are recorded, EEGs are abnormal in about 80%. In children with partial complex epilepsy, the

TABLE 5.4 DIFFERENTIAL DIAGNOSIS OF STARING SPELLS

Clinical Data	Absence	Complex Partial	Daydreaming
Frequency/day	Multiple	Rarely >1–2	Multiple, situation dependent
Duration	Frequently below 10 sec; rarely >30 seconds	Average duration over 1 min, rarely <10 sec	Seconds to minutes
Aura	Never	Frequently	No
Eye blinking	Common	Occasionally	No
Automatisms	Common	Frequently	No
Postictal impairment	None	Frequently	No
Seizures activated			
By hyperventilation	Very frequently	Occasionally	No
Photic stimulation	Frequently	Rarely	No
EEG			
Ictal	Generalized spike and wave	Usually unilateral or bilateral temporal or frontal discharges	Normal
Interictal	Usually normal	Variable; may be spikes or sharp waves in frontal or temporal lobes	Normal

EEG, electroencephalogram.

From Holmes G. *Diagnosis and management of seizures in children.* Philadelphia: WB Saunders; 1987:177; with permission.

interictal EEG may show bilateral, usually asymmetrical spike-and-wave discharges from the temporal lobes.

Children and adolescents with complex partial epilepsy, compared with age-matched populations, carry a high incidence of psychiatric comorbidity, including behavior disturbances, depression, anxiety, and suicidality (15).

Complex partial epilepsy must be differentiated from absence epilepsy (petit mal), which has its onset in childhood (16) (Table 5.4). Complex partial epilepsy can begin at any age; however, about 50% of patients with complex partial epilepsy experienced their first seizure before the age of 25 years (17). In children and adolescents, as well as adults, complex partial epilepsy may originate in the frontal lobes.

Bizarre behavior may appear to be a panic attack, although the behaviors may appear unusual, undirected, confusional, followed by amnesia for the event, and, in the individual patient, relatively stereotypical. Some seizures will evolve to convulsive episodes, whereas others may remain characterized by abnormal behavior or dystonic posturing.

The diagnostic evaluation, treatment, and prognosis are different for absence and partial complex epilepsies. Complex partial epilepsy is often caused by a structural abnormality, whereas absence epilepsy is frequently inherited in an autosomal dominant pattern with incomplete penetrance and with no underlying structural lesion. The AED of choice and the possibility of surgery for partial complex epilepsy are also different.

BENIGN EPILEPSY SYNDROMES

The benign epilepsy syndromes occur in children who are otherwise neurologically normal. These children have no structural brain abnormality and have a good prognosis (17–20). The two most commonly occurring syndromes, presenting in school-aged children to both child neurologists and psychiatrists, are (a) childhood absence (petit mal) epilepsy and (b) benign epilepsy with centrotemporal spikes (BECTS) also referred to as benign rolandic epilepsy.

GENERALIZED BENIGN EPILEPTIC SYNDROMES
Childhood absence

Childhood absence, previously known as petit mal, is characterized by multiple daily seizures that appear as staring spells in 4- to 10-year-old children. Hyperventilation and sometimes photic stimulation with flashing lights precipitate the seizures. The EEG in childhood absence is characterized by symmetrical 3-Hz spike-and-wave activity. This EEG pattern is inherited as an autosomal dominant trait with incomplete penetrance. In addition, as video-EEG recording shows, automatisms, such as eye blinking and repetitive mouth movements, are quite common, especially in absence seizures lasting longer than a few seconds. Some children with absence have been misdiagnosed as having complex partial seizures because automatisms were thought to differentiate the two. A small proportion of children with absence epilepsy have associated tonic-clonic convulsions.

Children with absence seizures are treated with an AED, such as ethosuximide, valproate, or lamotrigine. With appropriate AED therapy, seizures significantly improve. During adolescence, these children seem to "grow out" of their seizures and neurologists can taper and discontinue their AED. When absence seizures occur multiple times daily, children may appear inattentive and experience a decline in their schoolwork. In fact, staring spells are often first noted by the teacher, who may interpret them as a sign of attention deficit disorder (ADD). Moreover, some of these children, even when seizures are under control, may also have attentional difficulties.

Absence seizures may cluster in prepubertal children and adolescents. For example, after going many days without seizures, affected children sometimes have numerous absences in the span of few days. These children also have a propensity for convulsive generalized tonic-clonic seizures. Therapy with ethosuximide, which controls only absence seizures, is frequently not completely effective. Instead, valproate, lamotrigine, levetiracetam, and topiramate may cover the spectrum of these juvenile absence seizures.

Approximately 9% of children with absence epilepsy have absence status (nonconvulsive status epilepticus). This condition typically produces a spell of complex behavior resembling complex partial epilepsy or a psychiatric fugue state that can last for 24 hours or more. A child in absence status appears stuporous but may be able to eat and answer questions, although slowly. During this period, the child or adolescent often may have speech arrest and even automatisms. Occasionally, a generalized tonic-clonic seizure terminates the absence status. The EEG in absence status consists of almost continuous generalized spike-and-wave discharges, but not always at 3 Hz. Nevertheless, the EEG shows intermittent 2- to 3-second periods of normal EEG activity. Absence status usually affects older children or adolescents.

The clues that distinguish absence status from psychiatric conditions include the following (16):

1. Abrupt onset
2. History of childhood absence epilepsy
3. No previous psychiatric diagnosis and normal behavior without psychological problems between attacks
4. Speech arrest during the attack

Juvenile myoclonic epilepsy

Juvenile myoclonic epilepsy (JME), sometimes known as Janz syndrome, is another generalized benign epilepsy syndrome seen in adolescents and young adults. JME may begin in late childhood as absences that are followed in adolescence by myoclonic jerks. Generalized tonic-clonic seizures occur in about 90% of patients. Typically, the onset of generalized tonic-clonic convulsions brings the patient to neurological attention. Although absences occur only in about one third of children, myoclonic jerks occur in all. Valproate, lamotrigine topiramate, zonisamide, and levetiracetam usually control JME, but other AEDs may exacerbate the myoclonus (17,20,21). Patients require lifelong medication because discontinuation almost always leads to seizure recurrence. EEGs of patients with JME demonstrate intermittent brief bursts of generalized 3.5- to 4.0-Hz spike-and-waves, with prolonged discharges during the actual seizures. Sleep deprivation and alcohol use frequently precipitate these seizures in susceptible adolescents. The seizures, especially the myoclonic jerks, are most commonly seen early in the morning or when these adolescents become fatigued later in the day.

Various authors have commented on the personality of adolescents with JME. As adolescents and adults, many of these individuals tend to take more risks and have difficulty complying with both AED regimens and the behavior necessary to control their epilepsy (22).

BENIGN PARTIAL EPILEPSY SYNDROMES

Benign epilepsy with centrotemporal spikes, or rolandic epilepsy

Benign epilepsy with centrotemporal spikes is typically associated with nocturnal or early morning seizures that may appear to the child's parents as a focal onset or generalized tonic-clonic seizure. Sometimes focal facial twitching or diurnal perioral sensations will be reported as paresthesias affecting the tongue and lips. Depending on the location of the seizure focus, motor aphasia may occur during the ictus or as a postictal phenomenon. Occasionally, children with BECT will also have staring spells or complex partial seizures during the day (18).

Children with BECTS generally have a time-limited course to their epilepsy: both their seizures and their EG abnormalities (centrotemporal spikes) typically abate by midadolescence. The EEG abnormality is most prominent during sleep. Overall, these children remain neurologically normal, continue to develop, and do well in school; however, they are occasionally found to have learning disabilities and primarily language-processing deficiencies. The seizures usually respond to carbamazepine (CBZ), oxcarbazepine, or valproic acid. If they do not respond to AEDs, the diagnosis of BECTS should be reconsidered (23–25).

BENIGN OCCIPITAL EPILEPSIES OF CHILDHOOD

The benign partial epileptic syndromes seen in childhood include benign occipital epilepsies. There are two types of the syndrome in this category. The more common syndrome has its onset at about 5 years of age. In it, seizures consist of ictal vomiting with eye and head deviation, which can progress onto a generalized tonic clonic seizure. Physicians sometimes mistake the ictal vomiting for that seen with a migraine variant. One variety of occipital epilepsy, with an average age of onset at 8 years into adolescence, is characterized by visual symptoms, such as transient visual loss or visual hallucinations. Visual symptoms are followed by automatisms or focal seizures that can secondarily generalize. The EEG findings—occipital spikes attenuated by eye opening—may be diagnostic. Children usually outgrow this disorder by the end of their teens (18).

EPILEPTIC ENCEPHALOPATHY

Lennox-Gastaut syndrome

In young children (ages 2 to 5 years), Lennox-Gastaut syndrome (LGS) is the most common epileptic encephalopathy; it is a severe type of epilepsy with seizures that are difficult to control, mental retardation, and further deterioration with refractory seizures.

Coexistent behavioral abnormalities include developmental delay and behavioral dyscontrol. In addition to having various convulsive seizures—drop (atonic, akinetic), tonic, or myoclonic seizures—children may have prolonged fugue-like periods. Prolonged or repetitive, nonconvulsive atypical absences alter the patient's mental state. The EEG is essential to demonstrate the characteristic slow spike-and-wave pattern and abnormal background.

Other conditions may cause similar behavior: medication (including AEDs and neuroleptics) intoxication, metabolic derangements, intercurrent infections, trauma, neurodegenerative disorders, and progressive encephalopathy (26). Psychiatrists will be asked to assist in the care of many of these patients with "dual diagnoses." A full evaluation for possible progressive encephalopathic etiologies must be considered in this and related childhood epilepsies. Although retarded, these children should not demonstrate deterioration when seizures are reasonably controlled.

SELECTED SYNDROMES THAT MAY PRESENT TO PSYCHIATRISTS
Landau-Kleffner syndrome

During the preschool or early school years, a child may present with a syndrome of acquired epileptic aphasia, which consists of language regression and an abnormal EEG with or without clinical seizures. This disorder, commonly called Landau-Kleffner syndrome (LKS), may resemble word deafness or verbal auditory agnosia. The language impairment may prompt the misdiagnosis of pervasive developmental disorder (PDD). Seizures in LKS, which are not the predominant symptom, are usually easily controlled. As LKS evolves, hyperactivity and autistic behavior, along with the language difficulties, may mimic a degenerative disease. There is overlap in some features, including the seizures. Children with autism and PDD syndromes have a higher incidence of epilepsy than other children. EEG abnormalities have been reported in more than 30% of children with these disorders (27,28).

The EEG in children with LKS may resemble a benign centrotemporal spike pattern, or it can demonstrate continuous spike-and-waves in sleep. Because of a rare association with intracranial pathology, children who seem to have LKS require a complete neurophysiological, metabolic, neuroimaging, and neuropsychological evaluation (29).

Treatment of Epilepsy

GENERAL PRINCIPLES

Antiepileptic drugs are the primary treatment modality for seizures. For acute control of prolonged seizures, benzodiazepines, such as diazepam, lorazepam, and midazolam, may be administered intravenously or rectally. Newer preparations for nasal and buccal administration are in development. After benzodiazepine administration, phenobarbital and phenytoin have been most commonly used for more lasting effect (20); however, the introduction of intravenous preparations of valproate and levetiracetam may change the treatment of children with acute seizures.

A single seizure episode does not always necessitate chronic AED treatment (12). Especially because all chronic AED treatment carries a risk of side effects, the decision to treat is based on a risk-benefit assessment. Approximately 50% or more of individuals receiving AEDs will report some adverse effect, at least on some occasions, most frequently at the time of initiating or escalating the dose.

In several circumstances, neurologists may prescribe an AED after what appears to be a single seizure. For example, in children who have global developmental delay or those found to have symptomatic seizures, because the risk of epilepsy is increased, a neurologist may prescribe an AED after a single seizure. Similarly, if a detailed history uncovers prior seizure-like events, even though the child was thought to have just had a "first seizure," neurologists frequently prescribe an AED. For example, staring spells in school or myoclonic jerks on awakening may, in retrospect, have been brief seizures.

Certain AEDs used primarily for treatment of partial seizures, with or without secondary generalization, may exacerbate absence or myoclonic seizures (9). For example, carbamazepine (CBZ) and oxcarbazepine (OXC) can exacerbate absence or myoclonic seizures. Another important fact is that ethosuximide (ETX) is useful only for absence seizures. Moreover, almost all AEDs can exacerbate seizures when given in too high a dose, especially if they produce lethargy (21). Among the AEDs that have a broad spectrum that can be used in partial, primary, and secondarily generalized epilepsy are valproate (VPA), lamotrigine (LTG), topiramate (TPM), zonisamide (ZNS), and levetiracetam (LEV).

Although CBZ treatment of partial onset epilepsy and valproate treatment of generalized epilepsy have been standard, newer agents, which have fewer side effects, may eventually supplant these AEDs (30). Still, not all of the new AEDs have received Food and Drug Administration (FDA) approval for use in children with epilepsy (31). Neurologists typically initiate treatment with a single AED (monotherapy). They slowly titrate the AED upward to achieve seizure control without producing undue adverse effects. If the first AED is unsuccessful, they select an alternative one. As they introduce the second medication, they usually gradually withdraw the first. When using multiple AEDs (polypharmacy), adverse effects tend to occur more frequently and drug interaction becomes more severe. The most frequent AED side effects are various forms of psychological difficulties, such as irritability, hyperactivity, concentration difficulties, and aberrant behavior. The side effects may be more pronounced in children with preexisting behavior difficulties and epileptic encephalopathy (26). Phenobarbital most commonly leads to adverse cognitive and behavioral side effects (32). The following section briefly reviews AEDs commonly used to treat children with epilepsy (20). Detailed reviews are available elsewhere (33).

ESTABLISHED ANTIEPILEPTIC DRUGS

Carbamazepine (Tegretol, Carbatrol)

Carbamazepine is indicated for partial seizures with or without secondary generalization and remains the drug of choice for many practitioners (30). CBZ's mechanism of action is through decreasing repetitive firing of sodium channels. Initial dosing of 5 to 10 mg/kg/day is gradually increased to 15 to 20 mg/kg/day or higher. CBZ metabolism involves the hepatic cytochrome P450 pathway. If the child is also taking another medication that influences P450 metabolism, interactions can occur. For example, if a child or adolescent has epilepsy well controlled with CBZ, the addition of fluoxetine may raise the level of CBZ to toxic levels. In this case, the dose of one or both medications would have to be adjusted. Because CBZ also induces its own metabolism, increasing doses paradoxically may result in a falling serum concentration even with CBZ monotherapy. Determining serum concentrations of AEDs is helpful in monitoring the pharmacokinetics and in checking patient compliance (34).

Because the half-life of CBZ is relatively short, three times daily dosing is recommended unless a sustained- or extended-release product is given. The most frequent side effects, which are typically dose-related, include lethargy, diplopia, dizziness, and gastrointestinal intolerance. Rash may occur in up to 10% of children. Life-threatening side effects, such as the Stevens-Johnson syndrome, aplastic anemia, bone marrow suppression, and hyponatremia, may rarely occur. There is an increased potential for teratogenesis in women of childbearing age.

Valproate (Depakote)

The active ingredient in all valproate products is valproic acid, which was the first "broad-spectrum" AED. Valproate is effective against both partial and generalized seizures, including absence, tonoclonic, myoclonic and atonic seizures, JME, and LGS. Valproate is frequently used as treatment for migraine and bipolar disorder, as well as for epilepsy. Valproate, which is highly protein-bound, has a short half-life and undergoes hepatic metabolism. The enteric-coated extended-release preparation can be administered once daily, but other formulations require more frequent administration. Although valproate is generally considered an enzyme inhibitor, other AEDs, such as phenytoin, CBZ, and phenobarbital, can induce its metabolism. Weight gain, hair loss, menstrual irregularities, polycystic ovary syndrome, and potential for teratogenesis are its potential side effects. Physicians should carefully consider all factors before prescribing valproate to adolescent women. Tremor and thrombocytopenia develop on a dose-dependent basis. Hyperammonemia, which is characterized by tremor and change in mental status, with or without liver toxicity, may occur, but it generally responds to decreasing the dose and the addition of carnitine. Idiosyncratic reactions include hepatotoxicity and pancreatitis (35).

Phenobarbital

The use of phenobarbital as an AED has decreased because of its side effect profile. However, because of its availability in parenteral form, phenobarbital is used as a second or third-line drug in the treatment of status epilepticus (30). It is a strong inducer of cytochrome P450 and its mechanism of action is through enhanced gamma-aminobutyric acid (GABA)-ergic activity. Its adverse effects include sedation, irritability, hyperactivity, and mental dulling. Symptoms of depression have been noted when children are treated with phenobarbital (26,32). Systemic rash may occur, but Stevens-Johnson syndrome is rare. Chronic use may enhance bone loss, especially in debilitated patients. Phenobarbital is associated with a risk for teratogenesis.

Phenytoin (Dilantin)

Phenytoin, the first nonsedating AED developed, remains popular in the treatment of acute, prolonged partial or generalized tonic-clonic seizures. Fosphenytoin, a prodrug, has the advantages of rapid parenteral administration in acute situations and absence of localized tissue injury. Phenytoin is used to treat partial and secondary seizures; however, it may exacerbate absence, tonic, and myoclonic seizures (21). It has nonlinear pharmacokinetics and is highly protein-bound. Adverse effects—predominantly neurotoxic—include nystagmus, ataxia, and confusion. Idiosyncratic effects include dermatological and hepatic hypersensitivity syndromes. The fetal hydantoin syndrome is a known teratogenic effect.

With chronic phenytoin use, children may develop gingival hyperplasia and hypertrichosis. Osteopenia complicates phenytoin treatment because of its enzyme-inducing properties. Interactions with other drugs are also common because of its cytochrome P450 induction, its own ability to be induced, and its being highly protein bound.

Ethosuximide (Zarontin)

Ethosuximide, which has little effect on convulsive or partial seizures, is primarily used for the treatment of absence seizures. Although it has a long half-life, dosages are usually divided because of gastrointestinal side effects, including abdominal pain, nausea, and vomiting. Some psychological and behavioral disturbances have also complicated its use. Severe rash and a lupus syndrome are uncommon idiosyncratic reactions.

Clonazepam (Klonopin)

Clonazepam, a benzodiazepine, is useful as a second-line therapy for myoclonic, atonic, and absence seizures, in conjunction with other AEDs, for children with epileptic encephalopathy. Its use is complicated by tachyphylaxis (need for increased dosing) and subsequent lethargy. Clonazepam rescues children having clusters of seizures. This AED works by enhancing GABA. As with other benzodiazepines, clonazepam must be slowly discontinued to avoid status epilepticus.

NEWER ANTIEPILEPTIC DRUGS
Oxcarbazepine (Trileptal)

Oxcarbazepine, which is chemically related to CBZ, has a therapeutic spectrum that includes only partial seizures. It is approved as an adjunctive medication and as monotherapy for children and adolescents beginning from the age of 4 years. The side effects are similar to those for CBZ except that it carries no "black box" warning for agranulocytosis or aplastic anemia. However, because hyponatremia occurs in about 2.5% of patients, serum sodium should be monitored. In addition, a serious rash has been reported, although less commonly than with CBZ. The usual side effects, which are similar to those of the other AEDs, include drowsiness, tiredness, and dizziness.

Gabapentin (Neurontin)

Although its greatest use is in the treatment of pain syndromes, gabapentin, like CBZ, is effective against partial seizures. Structurally related to GABA, gabapentin's action is multimodal and probably associated with a novel binding site. Its principal advantage is safety and lack of pharmacokinetic interactions. Side effects in some children are irritability, aggressiveness, and hyperactivity, but they dissipate with dose reduction or drug discontinuation. Drowsiness, fatigue, lethargy, and weight gain are more frequently reported in older children than adults.

Lamotrigine (Lamictal)

Lamotrigine is a broad-spectrum AED with a mechanism of action that includes sodium channel blockade. It is effective in treating both convulsive and nonconvulsive generalized seizures and seizures that have a partial onset. Although lamotrigine may completely control seizures in children and adolescents with LGS and JME, some patients will have an exacerbation of myoclonic seizures. Lamotrigine has few interactions with other drugs, but co-medications significantly alter its metabolism. A serious life-threatening rash, which is particularly likely to occur with rapid introduction of the drug or the coadministration of valproate, is an idiosyncratic reaction. The overall incidence of a rash may be as high as 10%, but a serious rash occurs in 1% or less of children treated with lamotrigine (36).

Levetiracetam (Keppra)

Levetiracetam, a new AED, also has broad-spectrum activity and very few pharmacokinetic interactions. Its mechanism of action is unknown. Although generally well tolerated, a few cases of agitation, aggression, irritability, and psychosis have occurred. Some of these behavioral symptoms may respond to pyridoxine (vitamin B_6) treatment, if not to drug reduction or discontinuation (37–40). Levetiracetam was initially approved for the treatment of partial epilepsy but more recently also for the treatment of JME because it is effective for myoclonic seizures (41).

Topiramate (Topamax)

Topiramate, another of the broad-spectrum AEDs, has multiple mechanisms of action. Inducers increase its metabolism. Although the most common side effects are similar to those of the other AEDs, impaired concentration, confusion, and word-finding difficulties have been noted at higher dosages. Using monotherapy at low doses seems to be associated with the fewest effects on cognition and behavior. Rare cases of psychosis and mood disorder have been reported. Other side effects include paresthesias, renal stones, glaucoma, weight loss, and appetite suppression. Topamax may produce acidosis and lower the CO_2 in children, which requires treatment with Bicitra (citric acid/sodium citrate) to counteract the acidosis.

Zonisamide (Zonegran)

Zonisamide, a broad-spectrum AED, is effective against both partial and generalized seizures, including myoclonic seizures. Its metabolism is inducible and its mechanism includes action on sodium channels. Its side effects include neurotoxicity. Some children become irritable in a dose-related fashion. Nephrolithiasis and an idiosyncratic rash have occurred. An unusual syndrome of oligohidrosis and hyperthermia has been reported. Its treatment is hydration and drug discontinuation.

ALTERNATIVE THERAPY

Additional therapies for patients with refractory epilepsy include ketogenic diet, vagus nerve stimulation, and epilepsy surgery. The ketogenic diet and, more recently, the Atkins diet have been recommended for children and families who are able to comply with a very strict regimen and altered lifestyle. The usual length of treatment with the ketogenic diet is 2 years. The ketogenic diet frequently leads to a decrease in the number of medications required to control epilepsy; however, the diet rarely allows complete elimination of AEDs (42). Children and adolescents eligible for epilepsy surgery have a localization-related epilepsy (epilepsy emanating from an identifiable focus in the brain), documented by video-EEG, MRI, and often PET. This type of epilepsy, especially when due to mesial temporal sclerosis, has the best surgical outcome. Several authors have recommended early surgery for patients with localization-related epilepsy who have an MRI scan showing an appropriate lesion (43). Removal of eloquent cerebral cortex limits some surgery, but young children may recover cognitive and motor function because of the plasticity of the young brain. Patients undergoing epilepsy surgery must generally remain on at least one AED for some time, but some of them may become seizure-free without any AED. Most can reduce the number and dose of AEDs—at least to levels with fewer side effects.

Vagus nerve stimulation (VNS), approved for children older than 11 years with refractory epilepsy, is an option for those who do not have an identifiable single epileptic focus in a silent area. VNS does not replace focal epilepsy surgery in epilepsy patients who are good candidates for surgery. VNS has led to significant improvement in approximately 30% of children with refractory epilepsy (44). Although the exact mechanism is unknown, intermittent stimulation of inhibitory deep brain structures is delivered from a battery pack placed beneath the skin on the chest, with leads secured to the left vagus nerve. This treatment modality has recently been approved for adult patients with refractory depression.

Neuropsychiatric Comorbidities of Epilepsy

Epilepsy, a chronic neurological disorder, has a major impact on the life of the child and the family. Significant neuropsychiatric comorbidity is associated with epilepsy. Children with epilepsy who are multihandicapped often have behavioral disturbances associated with encephalopathy, mental retardation, and motor dysfunction. However, among the comorbidities, there are more subtle associations, such as with depression, bipolar disorder, anxiety, ADHD, conversion reaction, and other neuropsychiatric diagnoses. Recent studies suggest that 50% to 60% of children with complex partial epilepsy or primary generalized epilepsy have a comorbid psychiatric diagnosis, compared with 12% to 18% of control subjects (32). Of the various psychiatric diagnoses, disruptive disorders including ADHD, oppositional defiant disorders (ODD), and conduct disorders are the most common. Multiple studies have suggested that physicians screen children with epilepsy for affective disorders because of their increased prevalence (3).

Attention deficit hyperactivity disorder and symptoms of inattention are perhaps the most commonly diagnosed comorbidity in pediatric epilepsy. In the past, this association was thought to be a consequence of ongoing seizures or AED therapy. The prevalence of comorbid ADHD and epilepsy in children ranges from 14% to 37%, with most studies reporting prevalence in the 30% range (45). Studies involving children with epilepsy treated with AEDs concur that nearly all of the seizure medications may produce some symptoms of inattention, hyperirritability, or hyperactivity (46). There also is a higher incidence of depression, mood instability, and suicidality in children and adolescents with partial complex epilepsy than in those with chronic disease.

COMORBID BEHAVIORAL MANIFESTATIONS

The typical treatment of children with ADHD includes the administration of psychostimulants in addition to social and educational enhancements and behavior modification. Whether stimulants promote seizures remains controversial, but there is little evidence that psychostimulants, when used in therapeutic doses in well-controlled seizure patients, produce seizures. Nevertheless, there have been rare individuals who seem sensitive to treatment. Perhaps most important, these children should be assessed to see if their inattention syndromes truly represent ADHD, subtle absence seizures, or other learning or behavioral abnormalities, such as processing deficiency, conduct disorder, or even depression.

Although psychosis appears to be an uncommon comorbidity of pediatric epilepsy, it may occur in children with complex partial epilepsy and, in rare instances, may be exacerbated by epilepsy surgery (32). The presence of focal EEG discharges, particularly with pathology in the temporal lobe, suggests that psychosis and epilepsy stem from similar underlying pathophysiology (47). Neuropsychological evaluation is imperative before epilepsy surgery in older children and adolescents.

Successful therapy for children and adolescents with epilepsy and psychiatric comorbidities requires not only appropriate AED treatment but also additional care, including psychiatric consultation, psychosocial support, and patient education. The positive and negative psychotropic effects of AEDs, which have recently been reviewed (48,49), are presented in Table 5.5. In addition to these effects, pharmacokinetic interactions, such as P450 pharmacokinetics, must be considered when these medications or others are used to treat behavioral disorders (Table 5.6). Pharmacodynamic effects, such as sedation, insomnia, tremor, and weight gain, may also result from either class of agents. Antipsychotic medications and antidepressants may decrease seizure thresholds. Seizure frequency must be carefully monitored while these medications are added or discontinued. In fact, increased sedation may be the sole reason for seizure exacerbation. Stimulants, such as methylphenidate and amphetamines, rarely exacerbate epilepsy in patients on appropriate AED therapy—unless they produce insomnia or interfere with sleep. Of the antidepressants, high-dose bupropion is known to increase seizures. Certain tricyclic antidepressants, especially clomipramine, and tricyclic antidepressants at toxic serum concentrations carry a

TABLE 5.5 PSYCHOTROPIC EFFECTS OF AEDS

Antiepileptic Drug	Negative	Positive
Barbiturates	Depression, hyperactivity	Anxiolytic, hypnotic
Phenytoin	Encephalopathy	
Ethosuximide	Behavioral abnormalities, psychosis	
Carbamazepine-oxcarbazepine		Mood stabilizing, antimanic
Valproate	Encephalopathy	Mood stabilizing, antimanic (anxiolytic)

AEDs, antiepileptic drugs.

Modified from Brodtkorb E, Mula M. Optimizing therapy of seizures in adult patients with psychiatric comorbidity. *Neurology.* 2006;67(suppl 4):S39–44; with permission.

moderately increased risk of seizures. Low-risk antidepressants include the selective serotonin reuptake inhibitors (SSRIs), trazodone, and nefazodone (26). Among the antipsychotics, clozapine and chlorpromazine carry the greatest convulsive risk. Moderately increased risk is seen with thioridazine, olanzapine, and quetiapine; low risk is seen with haloperidol and risperidone (26,49).

The quality of life issues associated with epilepsy have lifelong ramifications. Epilepsy at school age negatively affects learning; however, there seems to be no relationship

TABLE 5.6 RELEVANT INTERACTIONS BETWEEN ANTIEPILEPTIC AND PSYCHOTROPIC DRUGS

	CBZ	PB	PHT	VPA
Antidepressants				
Amitriptyline	↓	↓	↓	↑
Clomipramine	↑	↓	↓	↑
Imipramine	↓	↓	↓	↑
Desipramine	↓	↓	↑	↓
Fluoxetine	=↑		=	=
Paroxetine	=		=	=
Citalopram	↓	=	=	
Sertraline	↓	=		
Fluvoxamine	=			
Nefazodone	↓	↑		
Mirtazapine	↓	=		
Bupropion	↓		↑	↑
Antipsychotics				
Chlorpromazine	↓	↑	↓ ↑	↓
Thioridazine	↓	↓	↑ ↓	↑ ↑
Haloperidol	↓	=↑	↓ ↓	= =
Clozapine	↓	↓	↓	=↑
Olanzapine	↓	↓	↓	↑
Risperidone	↓	=↑	↓	=
Ziprasidone	↓	↓	↓	
Quetiapine	↓	↓ =	↓	=

Symbol at left refer to the psychotropic drug and symbols at right to the anticonvulsant drug, when prescribed in combination (blank fields—data not available).

↑, increased plasma concentration; ↓, decreased plasma concentration; =, unchanged plasma concentration; CBZ, carbamazepine; PB, phenobarbital; PHT, phenytoin; VPA, valproate.

From Brodtkorb E, Mula M. Optimizing therapy of seizures in adult patients with psychiatric comorbidity. *Neurology.* 2006;67(suppl 4):S39–44 with permission.

between school achievement and epilepsy onset after age 18 years. Seizures and AEDs are associated with low self-esteem and social stigma (50). Furthermore, epilepsy patients, including adults, adolescents, and children, may consider their illness separate from their general health and report that they have normal general health rather than include epilepsy as a medical disorder. In adulthood, many epilepsy patients are underemployed and some, particularly those with intractable epilepsy, do not marry and live at home with their parents, in foster homes, or in institutions (50). Although older studies indicated that only those epilepsy patients with significant neurological disability and uncontrolled seizures had significant comorbidities, recent data show significant adverse influences on overall quality of life because of neuropsychiatric comorbidities in many of them. Medical and supportive therapy, with a clear diagnosis and recognition of the entire scope of the neuropsychiatric disorder, is imperative for children and adolescents with epilepsy, to achieve their fullest potential.

Questions

1. In children and adolescents with psychogenic seizures (pseudoseizures), there is often a history of which of the following?
   A. sexual or physical abuse
   B. documented epilepsy
   C. family history of epilepsy
   D. all of the above

2. For which type of epilepsy do children and adolescents usually have to continue AEDs during adulthood?
   A. absence (petit mal) epilepsy
   B. juvenile myoclonic epilepsy
   C. benign rolandic epilepsy
   D. benign occipital epilepsy

3. Which of the following conditions is not comorbid with epilepsy?
   A. depression
   B. ADHD
   C. tics
   D. anxiety

4. The EEG is usually abnormal in what proportion of children with PDD and autistic spectrum disorder?
   A. 5%
   B. 10%
   C. 30%
   D. 50%

5. A 16-year-old girl with partial complex epilepsy, which was well controlled on CBZ (Tegretol), developed depression. Her psychiatrist prescribed fluoxetine (Prozac). One week later she developed headache, lethargy, and diplopia. Which is the most likely explanation?
   A. P450 inhibition
   B. seizure breakthrough
   C. head trauma
   D. encephalitis

6. Which of the following AEDs often leads to weight loss?
   A. levetiracetam (Keppra)
   B. valproate (Depakote)
   C. lamotrigine (Lamictal)
   D. topiramate (Topamax)

Answers

1. **D**

2. **B.** Although children and adolescents with certain types of epilepsy—partial complex and juvenile myoclonic epilepsy—usually must continue to take AEDs in adulthood, those who have had absence, benign rolandic, or benign occipital epilepsy seem to "grow out" of their epilepsy as they mature and are generally able to discontinue their AED.

3. **C.** At any age, either antidepressants or stimulants can be administered along with AEDs when the seizures are well controlled.

4. C

5. A. Fluoxetine-induced P450 inhibition leads to increased CBZ serum concentrations, which can cause signs of toxicity, including headache, lethargy, and diplopia.

6. D. Topiramate leads to weight loss, but the others, especially valproate, lead to a variable degree of weight gain. Moreover, valproate in young women may lead to oligomenorrhea, facial hair, and acne (hirsutism)—the polycystic ovary (Stein-Leventhal) syndrome.

REFERENCES

1. Engel J Jr. Classification of epileptic disorders. *Epilepsia.* 2001;42:316.
2. Shinner S, Pellock JM. Update on the epidemiology and prognosis of pediatric epilepsy. *J Child Neurol.* 2002;17(suppl1):S4–17.
3. Kanner AM. Recognition of the various expressions of anxiety, psychosis, and aggression in epilepsy. *Epilepsia.* 2004:45(suppl 2):22-27.
4. Hauser WA. Epidemiology of epilepsy in children. In: Adelson PD, Black RM, eds. *Surgical Treatment of Epilepsy in Children*. Philadelphia: WB Saunders; 1995:419
5. Hauser WA, Kurland LT. The epidemiology of epilepsy in Rochester, Minnesota, 1935 through 1967. *Epilepsia.* 1975;16:1–66.
6. Commission on Classification and Terminology of the International League Against Epilepsy: Proposal for revised electroencephalographic classification of epileptic seizures. *Epilepsia.* 1981;22:489–501.
7. Kotagal P, Costa M, Wyllie E, Wolgamuth B. Paroxysmal nonepileptic events in children and adolescents. *Pediatrics.* 2002;110:46–50.
8. Alper K, Devinsky O, Perrine K. Nonepileptic seizures and childhood sexual and physical abuse. *Neurology.* 1993;43:1950–1953.
9. Pellock JM. Other nonepileptic paroxysmal disorders. In: Wyllie E, ed. *The Treatment of Epilepsy: Principles and Practice*. 4th ed. Baltimore: Lippincott Williams & Wilkins; 2006.
10. Wyllie E, et al. Psychogenic seizures in children and adolescents: Outcome after diagnosis by ictal video and electroencephalographic recording. *Pediatrics.* 1985;85;480–485.
11. Gupta A, Scheffer IE. Genetic aspects of epilepsy and genetics of idiopathic generalized epilepsy. In: Wyllie E, ed. *The Treatment of Epilepsy: Principles and Practice*. 4th ed. Baltimore: Lippincott Williams & Wilkins; 2006.
12. Hirtz D, et al. Practice parameter: treatment of the child with a first unprovoked seizure: Report of the Quality Standards Subcommittee of the American Academy of Neurology and the Practice Committee of the Child Neurology Society. *Neurology.* 2003;60:166–175.
13. Commission on Classification and Terminology of the International League Against Epilepsy: Proposal for revised electroencephalographic classification of epileptic seizures. *Epilepsia.* 1981;22:489.
14. Nordli DR Jr. Diagnostic difficulty in infants and children. *J Child Neurol.* 2002;17(suppl 1):S28–35.
15. Feindel W, Penfield W, Jasper H. Localization of epileptic discharge in temporal lobe automatism. *Trans Am Neurol Assoc.* 1952;56, 14–17.
16. Solomon GE, Kutt H, Plum F. *Clinical Management of Seizures: A Guide for the Physician*. 2nd ed. Philadelphia: WB Saunders; 1983.
17. Currie S, et al. Clinical course and prognosis of temporal lobe epilepsy. A survey of 666 patients. *Brain.* 1971:94:173–190.
18. Panayiotopoulos CP. Idiopathic generalized epilepsies: a review and modern approach. *Epilepsia.* 2005;46(suppl) 9:1–6.
19. Roger J, et al, eds. *Epileptic Syndromes in Infancy, Childhood and Adolescence*. 4th ed. London: John Libbey Eurotext; 2006.
20. Pellock JM, Dodson WE, Bourgeois B, eds. *Pediatric Epilepsy, Diagnosis and Therapy*. 3rd ed. New York: Demos; 2007.
21. Sazgar M, Bourgeois, BF. Aggravation of epilepsy by antiepileptic drugs. *Pediatr Neurol.* 2005;33:227–234.
22. Trinka E, et al. Psychiatric co-morbidity in juvenile myoclonic epilepsy. *Epilepsia.* 2006;47:2086–2091.
23. Chahine L, Mikati MA. Benign pediatric localization-related epilepsies. Part II syndromes in childhood. *Epileptic Disord.* 2006;8:243–258.
24. Gobbi G, Boni A, Filippini M. The spectrum of idiopathic rolandic epilepsy syndromes and idiopathic occipital epilepsies: from the benign to the disabling. *Epilepsia.* 2006;47(suppl 2): 62–66.
25. Holtmann M, et al. Rolandic spikes increase impulsivity in ADHD-A Neuropsychological Pilot Study. *Brain Dev.* 2006;28:633–640.
26. Pellock JM. Managing behavioral and cognitive problems in children with epilepsy. *J Child Neurol.* 2004;19(suppl 1):S73–74.
27. Landau W, Kleffner FR: Syndrome of acquired aphasia with convulsive disorder in children. *Neurology.* 1957;7:523–530.
28. Tuchman RF, Rapin I. Regression in pervasive developmental disorders. *Pediatrics.* 1997;99:560–566.
29. Solomon G, et al. Intracranial EEG monitoring in Landau-Kleffner syndrome associated with left temporal lobe astrocytoma. *Epilepsia.* 1993;34:557–560.

30. Wheless JW, Clarke DF, Carpenter D. Treatment of pediatric epilepsy: expert opinion, 2005. *J Child Neurol.* 2005;20(suppl 1):S1–56.
31. Pellock JM. Bridging the gap: clinical guidelines versus individualized treatment. *Prog Epileptic Disord.* Surrey, UK: John Libby; 2007.
32. Pellock JM. The challenge of neuropsychiatric issues in pediatric epilepsy. *J Child Neurol.* 2004;19(suppl 1):S1–S5.
33. Wyllie E, ed. *The Treatment of Epilepsy: Principles and Practice.* 4th ed. Baltimore: Lippincott Williams & Wilkins; 2006.
34. Pellock JM, Willmore, J, Privitera M. Routine monitoring for safety and tolerability during chronic treatment with antiepileptic drugs. In: Engel J, Pedley TA, eds. *Epilepsy: A Comprehensive Textbook.* 2nd ed. New York: Lippincott Williams & Wilkins. 2007; 1311–1316.
35. Willmore LJ, Pickens IV, Pellock JM. Monitoring for adverse effects of antiepileptic drugs. In: Wyllie E, ed. *The Treatment of Epilepsy: Principles and Practice.* 4th ed. Baltimore: Lippincott Williams & Wilkins; 2006.
36. Hirsch LJ, et al. Predictors of Lamotrigine-associated rash. *Epilepsia.* 2006;47:318–322.
37. Ettinger AB. Psychotropic effects of antiepileptic drugs. *Neurology.* 2006;67:1916–1925.
38. Miller GS. Pyridoxine ameliorates adverse behavioral effect of levetiracetam in children. *Epilepsia.* 2002;43(suppl 7):62.
39. Chez MG, Murescan M, Kerschner S. Retrospective review of the effect of vitamin B6 (pyridoxine) as add-on therapy for behavioral problems associated with levetiracetam (Keppra) therapy. *Epilepsia.* 2005;46(suppl 8):146.
40. Huerter V, Thiele EA. The role of levetiracetam in pediatric epilepsy and tuberous sclerosis complex. *Epilepsia.* 2003;44(suppl 9):134.
41. Specchio LM, et al. Open label, long term, pragmatic study on levetiracetam in the treatment of juvenile myoclonic epilepsy. *Epilepsy Res.* 2006;71:32–39.
42. Freeman JM, Kossoff EH, Hartman AL. The ketogenic diet: one decade later. *Pediatrics.* 2007;119:535–543.
43. Wyllie E, Bingaman WE. Epilepsy surgery in infants and children. In: Wyllie E, Gupta A, Lachhwani DK, eds. *The Treatment of Epilepsy: Principles and Practice.* 4th ed. Baltimore: Lippincott Williams & Wilkins; 2006.
44. Wheless J. Vagus nerve stimulation. In: Pellock JM, Dodson WE, Bourgeois BFD, eds. *Pediatric Epilepsy: Diagnosis and Therapy.* 3rd ed. New York: Demos Medical Publishing; 2008.
45. Austin JK, Caplan R. Behavioral and psychiatric comorbidities in pediatric epilepsy: toward an integrative model. *Epilepsia.* 2007;48:1639–1651.
46. Aldenkamp AP, et al. Optimizing therapy of seizures in children and adolescents with ADHD. *Neurology.* 2006;67(12 suppl 4):S49–51.
47. Caplan R, et al. Formal thought disorder and psychopathology in pediatric primary generalized and complex partial epilepsy. *J Am Acad Child Adolesc Psychiatry.* 1997;36:1286–1294.
48. Brodtkorb E, Mula M. Optimizing therapy of seizures in adult patients with psychiatric comorbidity. *Neurology.* 2006;67(suppl 4):S39–44.
49. Pisani F, et al. Effects of psychotropic drugs on seizure threshold. *Drug Saf.* 2002;25:91–110.
50. Shackleton DP, et al. Living with epilepsy; long-term prognosis and psychosocial outcomes. *Neurology.* 2003;61:64–70.

CHAPTER 6

Developmental Characteristics of Sleep and Sleep Disorders in Children

JOSEPHINE ELIA AND THORNTON B. A. MASON II

Sleep is a fascinating phenomenon, and the study of sleep and sleep disorders has expanded exponentially in the past two decades. Sleep medicine is an interdisciplinary field, and advances in our understanding of sleep medicine have been made by molecular biologists as well as behaviorists. Although the exact function of sleep remains undefined, disturbed sleep can impair daytime functioning and can be associated with major adverse health effects. Sleep differs across the lifespan, and this chapter highlights the types of sleep studies that can and have been used to explore normal variation in childhood and adolescence. There are many relevant sleep disorders, including disruptions in circadian patterns, parasomnias of non–rapid eye movement (NREM) and rapid eye movement (REM) sleep, sleep-disordered breathing, periodic limb movements/restless legs syndrome (RLS), and narcolepsy. As this chapter demonstrates, complex and intriguing relationships exist between attention deficit hyperactivity disorder (ADHD) and sleep, as well as between seizures and sleep. Furthermore, ADHD medications and anticonvulsants may also directly affect sleep. Importantly, there are bidirectional relationships between sleep and internalizing disorders such as depression, anxiety, and behavioral problems, all of which are summarized here.

Overview of Sleep

Broadly, sleep may be classified into REM sleep and NREM sleep. In turn, NREM sleep consists of sleep stages 1 through 4. Stages 1 and 2 are "lighter" sleep, from which a child may be awakened relatively easily. Stage 1 sleep may be intermixed with wakefulness as a child transitions to sleep. By electroencephalogram (EEG), stage 2 sleep is marked by K-complexes (high-amplitude deflections, with a negative component followed by a positive component) and sleep spindles (bursts of brief, 12- to 14-Hz activity); for both, the paroxysmal discharges stand out from the background EEG activity. The remaining NREM sleep stages (3 and 4) are sometimes referred to collectively as slow wave sleep or delta sleep. These stages are characterized by high-amplitude (<75 uV) slow waves (with frequencies less than 2 Hz), with stage 4 sleep having a higher prevalence of these waves (1). Slow wave sleep tends to predominate in the first half of the night (Fig. 6.1). With inadequate prior sleep or prolonged wakefulness, there is a greater pressure for slow wave sleep, so that the percentage of total sleep spent in slow wave sleep increases. REM sleep is particularly associated with dreaming, although dreaming can occur in other sleep stages. The

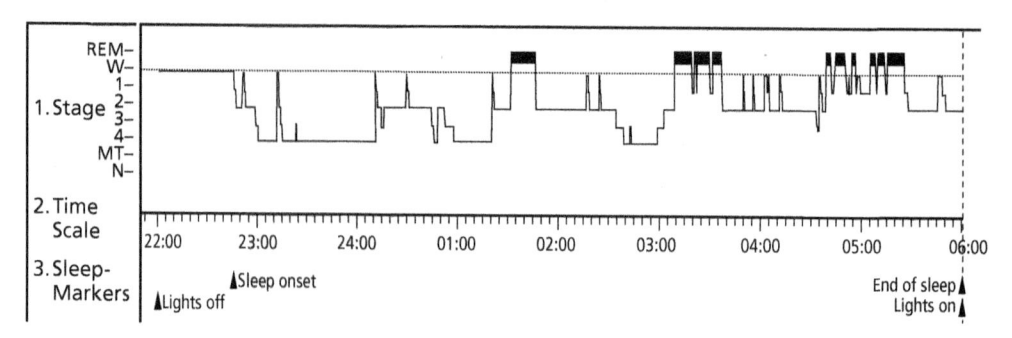

■ **FIGURE 6.1** The hypnogram shows the pattern of wake (W), non–rapid eye movement (REM) sleep stages 1–4, and REM sleep during an overnight polysomnography recording in a sleep laboratory. Note the prolonged sleep latency of greater than 1 hour on the time scale (lights off to sleep onset), the preponderance of slow wave sleep (stage 4) in the first half of the study, and the REM sleep prominence in the second half of the study.

EEG in REM sleep resembles wakefulness. REM sleep has both phasic features (eye movements; brief, small amplitude limb movements) and tonic components (without these movements). Overall, motor tone is strikingly decreased in REM sleep. REM sleep predominates in the second half of the night in older children and adults (Fig. 6.1).

Several types of studies have been developed to assess sleep. The gold standard for sleep analysis is overnight polysomnography. Polysomnography employs multiple leads to record important parameters simultaneously. By convention, four EEG leads are placed to measure central and occipital brain wave activity bilaterally. Two leads are placed on the outer canthus regions of the eyes to detect eye movements (blinking; REM sleep–associated movements). Airflow from the nose and mouth can be recorded by a thermistor that is sensitive to temperature differences between inhaled air (cooler) and exhaled air (warmer); nasal pressure transducers give a better indication, however, of the amount of air exchanged with breathing. In pediatrics, end-tidal carbon dioxide is frequently monitored by nasal cannula, and these data can be supplemented by transcutaneous carbon dioxide measurements if desired. Respiratory effort is measured by calibrated bands at the chest and abdomen. Electromyograms indicate muscle activity (movement) at several sites (chin region, legs). A single-lead electrocardiogram allows assessment of heart rate and screening for cardiac arrhythmias during sleep. A pulse oximeter is usually placed on a finger or toe to follow oxyhemoglobin saturations throughout the study. Currently, polysomnograms are recorded digitally, thereby allowing easy storage and facilitating analysis. Some polysomnography recordings are expanded with additional EEG leads for enhanced detection of epileptiform discharges or with a pH probe to detect gastroesophageal reflux. Concurrent video recordings are very helpful in detecting and characterizing a patient's movements during a sleep study. The polysomnography data are scored into sleep stages based on established criteria (1). Similarly, the data are scored for sleep-disordered breathing (2,3), arousals/awakenings, and leg movements (4).

When excessive daytime sleepiness is a concern, a multiple sleep latency test (MSLT) is sometimes performed on the day following an overnight polysomnogram. The set-up for an MSLT includes some but not all of the leads from an overnight study. Beginning 1½ to 2 hours after awakening from the overnight study, the patient will have a series of nap opportunities every 2 hours, with four to five naps total. The duration of the nap opportunities is standardized, and for each nap there is a determination of whether the child sleeps or not and, if so, the latency to sleep and the presence of REM sleep are noted. By averaging the results of all the naps, a mean sleep latency is determined (5).

Actigraphy has been used in both research and clinical settings for the assessment of sleep disorders in children and adults. Typically worn on the wrist of the nondominant hand, an actigraph resembles a watch and records the frequency and magnitude (acceleration/deceleration) of movement, which can in turn be used to generate rest-activity patterns; these patterns have been shown to be valid indications of sleep-wakefulness, respectively (6). Actigraphy recording over 1 to 2 weeks should allow for variation in weekday versus weekend schedules and, when paired with a concurrent sleep diary, can reflect a patient's typical (at home) sleep pattern. Some of the parameters that can be determined by routine actigraphy include sleep latency, total sleep time, the number of defined night wakings, the total duration of night wakings, and sleep efficiency (time spent asleep divided by total time in bed) (7,8).

Parents and older children can be asked to give details about their sleep and wake patterns through a sleep diary. The parents can indicate when a child is in bed ready for sleep; when the child actually falls asleep; the timing, duration, and number of night-time awakenings; the morning rise time; and the presence of any naps. Sleep diaries can effectively highlight insufficient sleep, weekday versus weekend variation, and erratic sleep patterns. A number of sleep questionnaires have also been developed to assess pediatric sleep and may serve as other valuable means of gathering clinical data (e.g., see references 9–11).

Sleep Duration Across Childhood and Adolescence

Total sleep duration is typically longest during infancy and decreases consistently from childhood through adolescence: total sleep duration is 14.2 (± 1.9) hours in 6-month-olds, 11 (± 0.8) in 6-year-olds, 9.3 (± 0.6) in 12-year-olds, and 8.1 (± 0.7) in 16-year-olds (12). Infants' and young children's naptime is included in calculating total sleep duration. Newborns are not entrained to light-dark cycles and spend the majority of each 24-hour period asleep, with a total of about 7 sleep and wake periods in 24 hours. Sleep is consolidated at 4 months of age into about three or four sleep periods, with two thirds of sleep occurring at night. With increasing age, the number of naps decreases. By around 18 months of age, children transition to a single nap per day. By age 3 years, only about half of children take a daytime nap, and naps chiefly disappear by school age (12). Indeed, it is abnormal for a prepubescent school-aged child to exhibit daytime sleepiness.

Regarding sleep architecture, in infants less than a year of age there is frequently a transition from wake to REM (active) sleep, and then to NREM (quiet) sleep. The incidence of these direct wake-to-REM transitions decreases between 3 and 9 months of age, but REM latency (the time from sleep onset to REM onset) is still very short (13). There is a relative prolongation of REM latency during childhood. Indeed, Montgomery-Downs et al. (14) studied normal children ages 3 to 8 years and reported that REM latency increased linearly across age in this window, with significant changes from ages 4 to 5 years and 5 to 6 years. The number of REM/NREM cycles also changes with development. Children aged 3 to 5 years have been found to have six cycles (mode), whereas children 6 to 7 years have five cycles. For both age groups, a significant linear trend has been reported for increased minutes of REM sleep across the night within cycles (14).

Behavioral Insomnia of Childhood

As reviewed by Mindell et al. (15), behavioral insomnia in children frequently presents with bedtime resistance or night-time awakenings or both. It occurs in 20% to 30% of young children. Mild and transient symptoms are common and constitute a disorder only if they are persistent and impair the child and/or the family. The two broad categories include sleep-onset association disorder and limit-setting disorder. Bedtime behavioral insomnia is often associated with children whose temperaments may be more irritable or require more adult intervention to calm down (16,17).

Sleep-onset association disorder refers to specific conditions that facilitate a child's falling asleep but when absent may result in prolonged sleep latency or nightly awakenings. Examples include positive associations that are controlled by the child (e.g., thumb sucking, cuddling a stuffed animal) and negative associations that are controlled by others (e.g., rocking, feeding, chauffeuring by parent). Given that children normally have brief arousals during the night (two to six times) (18), prolonged awakenings can result when the sleep association that they cannot control is not immediately available and can be disruptive when accompanied by crying and getting out of bed (19). Sleep association disorders affect infants and toddlers (ages 6 months to 3 years) and are not considered before 6 months of age, before an infant has reached a neurodevelopmental stage at which adequate sleep consolidation and regulation allow sleep for an extended amount of time (19). Sleep-onset association disorder can also affect the older child who may, for example, require a parent to lie in the same bed in order to fall asleep; when the child wakes during the night and the parent is no longer in the bed, the child may be unable to return to sleep.

Limit-setting sleep disorder refers to bedtime delay tactics (e.g., requesting additional bedtime stories, asking for a drink of water, posing multiple questions, debating), refusal to go to bed, or refusal to stay in bed. It occurs predominantly when parents do not set and enforce consistent limits. The delays result in shorter total sleep time but not in diminished sleep quality. Combined type sleep-onset association and limit-setting behavioral insomnia may also occur simultaneously in some children.

Effective treatments for behavioral insomnia include parental education and behavioral management techniques, such as extinction, graduated extinction, and positive routines. As reviewed by Mindell et al. (15) extinction procedures necessitate that the child is in bed at a designated time and parents refuse to respond to any requests or crying for as many nights as it may take to stop the behavior. A modified version in which parent(s) stay in the child's room but ignore the behavior may be more acceptable to some parents. Graduated extinction involves increasing the time interval between successive checks during which time the parent comforts the child for 15 to 30 seconds. Positive routines initially focus on developing a bedtime routine associated with quiet activities enjoyable to the child. Bedtime is delayed intentionally so that sleep cues become associated with positive experience, and once this is established, bedtime is gradually moved to an earlier time. The child may respond to small rewards for falling asleep independently. Behavioral treatments are preferred to pharmacotherapy.

Delayed Sleep Phase Syndrome

A circadian rhythm sleep disorder, delayed sleep phase syndrome type (DSPS) is characterized by difficulty with both falling asleep and awakening at conventional times (20). Sleep itself was thought to be normal (21); however, a controlled study has shown increases in stage 1 and 2 of sleep and decreases in slow wave sleep (22). The cause is complex: although cultural factors play a role, delays in circadian rhythms, including body temperature and melatonin rhythms, point to biological intrinsic factors in adults (23,24) as well as adolescents (25). Circadian gene variants have also been linked to DSPS, including Per3 (26), 3111 Clock (27), arylalkalamine N-acetyltransferase (28), and HDLA-DR1 (29).

A shift toward delayed sleep onset emerges as children enter adolescence (25,30), when offset of melatonin secretion has been shown to correlate with age and Tanner stage (31). This pubertal associated phase delay in circadian rhythms appears to continue in adolescence; melatonin secretion was actually delayed in 10th graders who started their day 65 minutes earlier, suggesting an impairment in adjusting sleep patterns to optimize sleep (32). DSPS with an early rise time can result in significant sleep deprivation that can impair daily functioning, worsen school performance, and increase moodiness (11). In young adults, car crashes are a significant risk (33).

Effective treatments include chronotherapy, exposure to early morning light, and exogenous melatonin. Chronotherapy involves delaying sleep onset for approximately 3 hours every day until sleep occurs at the designated conventional time (34). This treatment has practical limitations and the potential risk of inducing a non–24-hour sleep-wake cycle (35). An alternative to delaying the sleep-wake phase is advancing it with light-dark exposure and medication. Controlled light-dark exposure can shift circadian phase in adolescents (31). Exposure to light therapy in the morning with evening light restriction may restore a conventional time schedule (36–38). Melatonin administered in the late afternoon or early evening also has been found effective in advancing the circadian sleep clock (39).

Case One

During the parent-teacher conference, J.J.'s parents learn that their 14-year-old son is dozing off during the first and second periods. Bedtime on weeknights is 10:00 p.m., but frequently he is emailing friends and not falling asleep until 11 to 12 midnight. Aside from English (second period class) he has excellent grades, is well liked, and is cooperative at home. Therefore, his parents feel that he has earned the right to stay up later on weekends. He also sleeps later in the morning, allowing him to catch up on any missed sleep. What steps should be taken to improve this child's sleep?

Discussion: Weekend schedules that permit later bedtime and awakening can exacerbate a young adult's natural tendency to delay sleep onset. Computers serve as light sources, further delaying sleep onset. Minimizing these could be helpful. In addition, advocating for school days that start later for adolescents is also important.

Arousal Disorder Parasomnias

An important subset of pediatric parasomnias includes the disorders of arousal. These parasomnias may be considered part of a continuum, as they share overlapping features: sleepwalking, confusional arousals, and sleep terrors. Although most often occurring in slow wave sleep (stages 3 and 4 of NREM sleep), these parasomnias can also arise from stage 2 NREM sleep (40). Common among these disorders include incomplete transition from slow wave sleep, automatic behavior, altered perception of the environment, and variable degrees of amnesia for the event. The child's sleep stage transition from slow wave sleep is abnormal, often when shifting into lighter NREM sleep (e.g., stage 2) just prior to the first REM sleep episode. The patient in a sense becomes "stuck" between deep sleep and wakefulness (41). The EEG during these episodes demonstrates an admixture of theta, delta, and alpha frequencies. The disorder of arousal parasomnias are all more frequent in childhood than in adolescence or adulthood. Prevalence estimates in childhood for sleep terrors range from 1% to 6%; for sleepwalking, up to 17% with a peak at 8 to 12 years; and for confusional arousals, up to 17.3% (42).

Sleepwalking (somnambulism) in childhood shares features with that in adults. Sleepwalking may be either calm or agitated, with varying degrees of complexity and duration (43). The frequency of sleepwalking may be underestimated because of episodes that are unobserved or unremembered (44). Children with somnambulism are usually calm and do not demonstrate fear. They may walk into a parent's room, bathroom, or different parts of the house. Children with sleepwalking are at risk for injury. They may climb through windows, wander in bathrooms, attempt to walk downstairs, and sometimes leave the house. Injuries may include trauma from falls, lacerations from broken windows or patio glass doors, and even hypothermia from exposure.

Confusional arousals, which occur mainly in infants and toddlers, have more associated agitation than what would be expected with sleepwalking. A typical episode may begin with movements and moaning, and then evolves to confused and agitated behavior with calling out, crying, or thrashing (45). Attempts to wake the child fully are unsuccessful. The child appears confused, with eyes open or closed, and is very agitated or even combative. Physical injury is rarely seen (46). The child resists the parents' efforts at consolation, and more forceful attempts to intervene may result in increased resistance and further agitation. A confusional arousal episode may last 5 to 15 minutes (although sometimes longer) before the child calms and returns to a restful sleep.

Sleep terrors are dramatic partial arousals from slow wave sleep. The child may sit up suddenly and scream, with an intense, blood-curdling "battle cry." The episode is a fight-flight phenomenon. Autonomic activation is present, with mydriasis, diaphoresis, and tachycardia (47). Respiratory tidal volume is increased, and there is an intense look of fear on the face. Moreover, there is a "curious paradox" of endogenous arousal coexistent with external unarousability (48). With sleep terrors, children may report indistinct recollections of threats (monsters, spiders, snakes) from which they have to defend themselves (45,49). The differential diagnosis of sleep terrors includes nightmares, nocturnal panic attacks, epileptic events, and cluster headaches.

Multiple factors may influence arousal parasomnias. Age is an important issue, as many parasomnias are much more likely to occur in childhood than later in life. Other contributing factors include the homeostatic drive to sleep (with more frequent or more severe parasomnia episodes being associated with prolonged sleep deprivation), medications (e.g., neuroleptics, sedative hypnotics, stimulants, and antihistamines), a noisy or stimulating sleep environment, fever, stress, and intrinsic sleep disorders [such as obstructive sleep apnea and periodic limb movements in sleep (PLMS)] (50). In children, sleep-disordered breathing or PLMS-RLS may trigger sleep walking or sleep terrors, as these parasomnias have been reported to disappear after obstructive sleep apnea or PLMS-RLS treatment (49). In childhood, psychopathology is thought to be extremely rare as an influencing factor for arousal parasomnias (51). Several studies support a genetic predisposition (52,53).

Treatment of disorders of arousal in childhood includes reassuring parents that parasomnias are common and can be managed effectively. The parents should be counseled, when appropriate, on instituting important safety measures, that is, placing the mattress on the floor, securing the windows and outside doors, covering the windows with heavy curtains, and using alarm systems and bells to alert parents if the child leaves the room. Other nonpharmacological treatments include maintaining a sleep diary, which will foster routine notation of sleep times and may help to reinforce the principle of minimizing sleep deprivation, and eliminating caffeine-containing beverages. Medications are indicated for those rare, protracted cases with no associated sleep disorder, with frequent parasomnias, and with a threat of injury to the patient or others. Benzodiazepines and tricyclic antidepressants have been used successfully (54).

Case Two

A mother brings her 4-year-old daughter to the office because of frequent "nightmares." The girl falls asleep between 9:30 and 10 p.m. nightly and two to three times per week awakens suddenly between 11 p.m. and midnight. Her daughter screams with amazing intensity and then appears sweaty and moderately agitated, often pacing in her room. She reports that the girl does not respond to her ("looks right through her"), and her mother cannot do anything to stop an episode. In total, an episode can last 10 to 30 minutes. On the mornings following, her daughter has no recollection of the events and appears to be her normal, well-rested self. What is the likely diagnosis and the recommended treatment?

Discussion: These impressively intense events are consistent with sleep terrors. Key features include their typical onset 90 minutes to 2 hours after sleep onset, prominent agitation, the parent's inability to calm the child, and the girl's amnesia for the event. Her mother should first be reassured that sleep terrors are akin to sleep walking, are relatively common, are not routinely associated with psychiatric disorders, and usually disappear by adolescence. Sleep deprivation makes sleep terrors (and other arousal parasomnias) more likely, so the initial management should be focused on increasing total sleep duration. For this child, the bedtime should be gradually advanced to 8 p.m.; this will likely result in fewer, milder sleep terror episodes, if not eliminating them altogether. Medication is not indicated at this time.

Nightmares

Nightmares are characterized by terrifying dreams followed by awakening with vivid recall of the content and difficulty returning to sleep. An occasional nightmare occurs in more than 55% of children and adolescents, whereas 5% experience these several times per week (55). Nightmares occur more frequently in girls than in boys (56). They typically emerge after a very frightening or traumatic experience or a severe medical illness (57). Medications that can affect the central nervous system can also precipitate nightmares, but this occurs primarily in adults (58).

Children with nightmares have higher rates of sleep terrors, sleep walking, anxiety at bedtime, daytime somnolence (56), and snoring (59). Nightmares are also associated with daytime behavioral and emotional difficulties (55). In a 14-month follow-up study of 5- to 8-year-olds, nightmares persisted in 30% but parents did not express a need to seek remedies (56).

Sleep-disordered Breathing

Obstructive sleep apnea (OSA) is a term used to describe airway obstruction that results in decreased air exchange during sleep. Overnight polysomnography can demonstrate obstructive apneas (little or no air movement despite ongoing and sometimes increased respiratory effort) and obstructive hypopneas (shallow breathing), often in the setting of loud snoring and paradoxical breathing (thoracoabdominal asynchrony) (Fig. 6.2). In children, obstructive events tend to cluster during REM sleep, with breathing relatively unaffected often during NREM sleep. Moreover, despite moderate to severe obstructive sleep apnea in some children, sleep architecture tends to be preserved. Estimates of the prevalence of obstructive sleep apnea in children vary, based on the sensitivity and specificity of responses to questionnaires, a range of different sleep study techniques (not limited to overnight polysomnography), and the particular criteria applied for establishing obstructive sleep apnea (60). Snoring is extremely frequent in children and is associated with obstructive sleep apnea, as snoring represents a symptom of increased upper airway resistance. Snoring is found in 18% to 20% of infants, 7% to 13% of children ages 2 to 8 years, and 3% to 5% of older children (61).

In general, the prevalence of pediatric obstructive sleep apnea is approximately 2% (62). Obstructive sleep apnea in childhood is important because it may result in growth failure, cor pulmonale, developmental delay, and poor school performance (63,64).

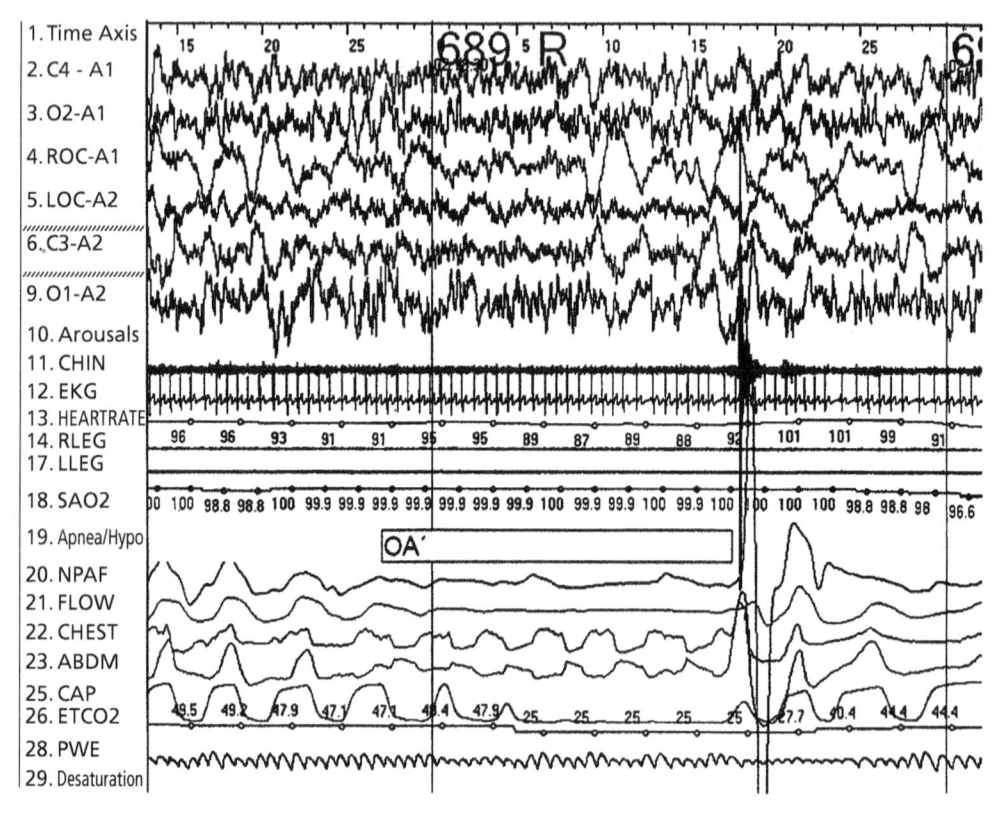

■ **FIGURE 6.2** This recording from an overnight polysomnogram shows an obstructive sleep apnea episode (OA) during REM sleep. Note that the chest (22. CHEST) and abdominal (23. ABDM) effort channels show in-phase or synchronous movements initially, then paradoxical (out-of-phase, asynchronous) movement during the apnea. The apneic episode is shown by the marked decrement in airflow in the nasal pressure transducer lead (20. NPAF), the thermistor lead (21. FLOW), and the end-tidal CO2 capnography channel (25.CAP). Brief movement and a short gasp terminate the apneic event.

Adenotonsillar hypertrophy plays a major contributory role; others include craniofacial structure, obesity, and neural control mechanisms of the upper airway (61,65–67). Genetics may also be important, as studies in adults have demonstrated a familial aggregation of sleep apnea (68–70), and a few studies have suggested such aggregation exists for pediatric sleep apnea (71,72).

Obstructive sleep apnea can be treated effectively (62). Because of the association with enlarged tonsils and adenoids, adenotonsillectomy has been recommended as first-line treatment, particularly for children in the 2-to 6-year age range. Weight loss, although helpful in decreasing lateral airway narrowing in obesity, is difficult to achieve and therefore may only complement other treatments. Continuous positive airway pressure (CPAP) therapy essentially uses a column of air to splint the airway open; bilevel positive airway pressure (BLPAP) allows lower pressures during expiration, and a backup or timed delivery of breaths if needed.

Central sleep apnea, which is fundamentally different from obstructive sleep apnea, is characterized by a diminished to absent drive to breathe (Fig. 6.3). Central apnea,

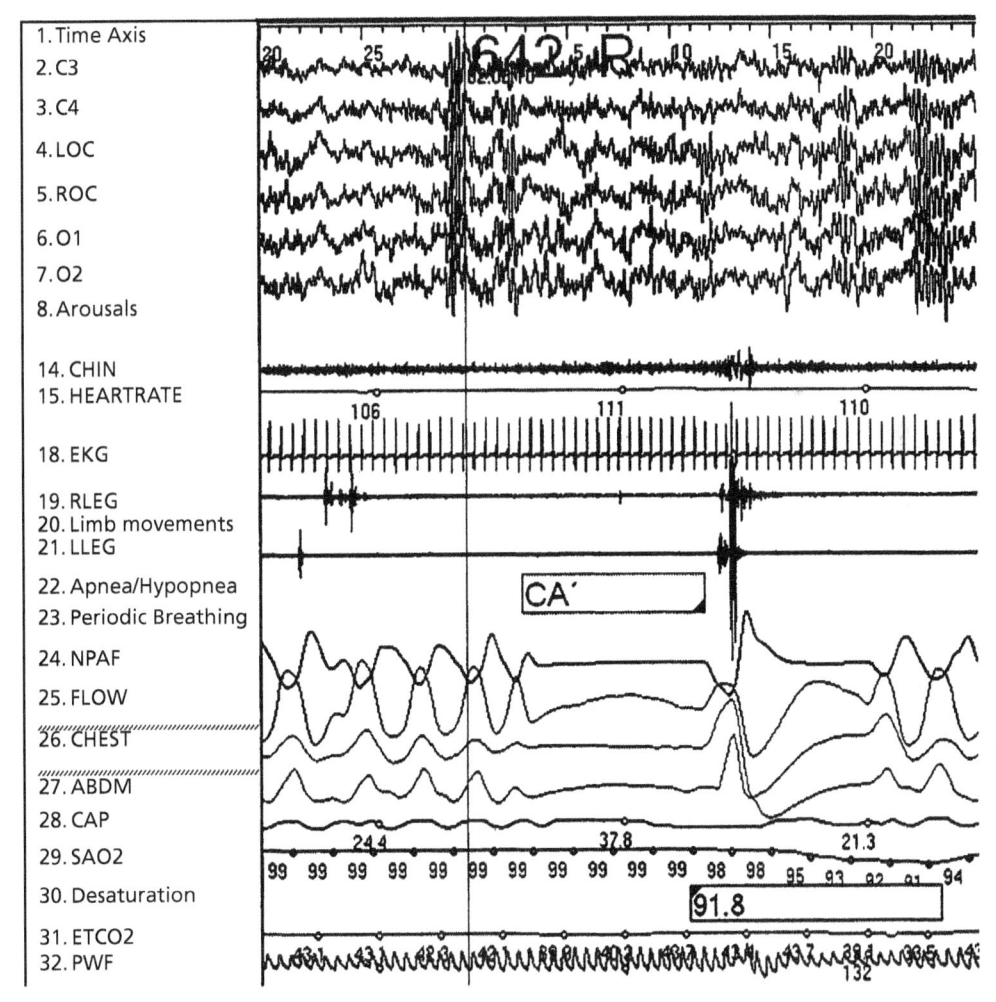

■ **FIGURE 6.3** This recording from an overnight polysomnogram shows a central apnea (CA). Note that there is a period of absent chest and abdominal movement (26. CHEST; 27. ABDM) with associated absence of airflow in multiple channels (nasal pressure transducer, NPAF; thermistor, FLOW, and end-tidal CO2 capnography, CAP).

sometimes associated with prematurity, improves with advancing postconceptual age. In some patients, central apnea is physiologically driven, such as during periods of sleep-wake transition or when sleeping at high altitudes. Whereas respiratory drive during wakefulness is under the control of cortical regions, respiratory drive during sleep is predominantly under brainstem control. Therefore, pathological brainstem processes, such as a Chiari I malformation, can be associated with central sleep apnea and central hypoventilation (marked by an increase in arterial carbon dioxide tension). Central hypoventilation in children may also occur secondary to hydrocephalus, hypoxic-ischemic encephalopathy, achondroplasia with stenosis of the foramen magnum, trauma, brainstem tumors, encephalitis, familial dysautonomia, and mitochondrial disorders (73). Rarely, central sleep apnea can occur in the setting of congenital central hypoventilation syndrome.

Whenever feasible, the cause of secondary hypoventilation should be treated (e.g., placement of a ventriculoperitoneal shunt for hydrocephalus). The mainstay of management for children without a treatable cause should be chronic ventilatory support. Although central apnea in preterm infants can improve with caffeine and other respiratory stimulants, pharmacotherapy has not been successful in other forms of central hypoventilation. Noninvasive ventilation (e.g., BLPAP) has been used successfully, but must be monitored carefully to ensure adequate ventilatory control. Tracheostomy is usually required in patients with congenital central hypoventilation syndrome, and diaphragmatic pacers may allow increased mobility for those who require ventilatory support while both awake and asleep (73).

Case Three

A 6-year-old boy presents with loud snoring, gasping in sleep, and pauses in breathing according to his parents' report. His academic performance in first grade has been below average. He is irritable at times but does not nap or appear sleepy. On examination, he breathes primarily through his mouth and has moderately hypertrophied palatine tonsils. If obstructive sleep apnea is suspected, what should be done next?

Discussion: An overnight polysomnogram should be performed to evaluate for the presence and severity of obstructive sleep apnea. The polysomnogram provides a quantitative assessment, including the number of obstructive respiratory events per hour (an apnea-hypopnea index) and parameters of respiratory gas exchange (e.g., the oxygen saturation nadir, and the mean and peak end-tidal CO_2 values). In childhood, most obstructive respiratory events occur in REM sleep (when breathing patterns are irregular and muscle tone is low); accordingly, oxygen desaturations typically also cluster in REM sleep. If the polysomnogram confirms obstructive sleep apnea, a referral to an ear, nose, throat (ENT) physician would be reasonable; the tonsils are large, and this boy's prominent mouth breathing suggests adenoid hypertrophy. In most cases, adenotonsillectomy will resolve the upper airway obstruction and may also improve daytime behavior, including school performance.

Seizures and Sleep

Seizures can occur during sleep as well as during wakefulness. Indeed, some patients have seizures more frequently, or even exclusively, during sleep. There are several seizure types in which events are prominent in sleep, including benign rolandic epilepsy, electrical status epilepticus of sleep, and nocturnal frontal lobe epilepsy. Benign rolandic epilepsy begins in childhood and typically resolves in adolescence; seizures occur in the evening hours, often in the wake-sleep transition period. The classic clinical presentation of benign rolandic epilepsy includes brief, partial, hemifacial motor seizures, with or without somatosensory symptoms (74), also often involving jerking of the ipsilateral the upper extremity; concurrent drooling and speech arrest are often seen, with preserved alertness (75). More rarely, patients may have secondarily generalized tonic-clonic seizures (74). The EEG demonstrates epileptiform activity (sharp waves, often followed by slow waves) in centrotemporal, midtemporal, frontocentral, centroparietal, or centro-occipital locations (74). With a typical presentation, anticonvulsant treatment is not always required.

Electrical status epilepticus of sleep is a dramatic finding: a normal EEG pattern during wakefulness changes to a generalized spike-wave pattern during sleep. The diffuse epileptiform activity is nearly persistent (e.g., often more than 85% of the NREM sleep record). Electrical status epilepticus of sleep may be associated with cognitive and language dysfunction, although a precise temporal relationship between the appearance or presence of the EEG abnormality and clinical features has not been established. In a given patient, electrical status epilepticus of sleep may wax and wane in severity but can be seen over years (76). No single therapy is recognized as effective, although there are reports of treatment attempted with intravenous immunoglobulin, prednisone, diazepam, and/or levitiracetam (76).

Autosomal dominant nocturnal frontal lobe epilepsy is a genetic epilepsy syndrome that manifests as abnormal activity during sleep. One subtype is paroxysmal arousals, in which patients have a brief (<20 second) stereotyped sequence of behavior (including eye opening, rising from the bed with abnormal limb posturing, and showing an expression of apparent fear or surprise). Nocturnal paroxysmal dystonia is marked by dystonic posturing of the limbs, trunk, or head; there may be associated bizarre or violent (ballistic) movements. The duration is often less than 2 minutes. Episodic nocturnal wandering is more rare; these events include paroxysmal ambulation during sleep, possibly accompanied by screaming or agitated behavior, and lasting 1 to 3 minutes (77,78). Nocturnal frontal lobe epilepsy has a mean age of onset of 10 to 12 years. For any of these frontal lobe epilepsy manifestations, it is difficult to capture ictal discharges by EEG, so an empiric trial with carbamazepine (which is especially effective) may be warranted if the events are clinically suspicious for seizures. Differentiating nocturnal frontal lobe epilepsy from arousal parasomnias (such as confusional arousals or agitated sleepwalking) can be challenging, but features supporting seizures include a slightly later onset of events (adolescence) with stability over time (i.e., persistence with advancing age), relatively short duration of events, stereotyped features particularly at onset, and the presence of dystonic posturing (79). Genetic studies in families have shown that autosomal dominant frontal lobe epilepsy is linked to mutations in nicotinic acetylcholine receptor subunits (*CHRNA4* and *CHRNB2*) (80).

The relationships between sleep and epilepsy extend beyond these associations with specific epilepsy syndromes. Interictal epileptiform discharges are increased by sleep and sleep deprivation. Seizure frequency can be exacerbated by chronic sleep deprivation, and case series have supported improved seizure control in patients following OSA treatment (81,82). The greatest frequency for focal discharges is in slow wave sleep, where neuronal synchrony is promoted. On the other hand, epileptiform discharges decrease dramatically during REM sleep (83). If a complex partial seizure or secondarily generalized seizure occurs during sleep, subsequent sleep is less efficient, with altered sleep architecture, including decreased REM sleep and, in some cases, less slow wave sleep. (84). Consequently, excessive daytime sleepiness in patients with epilepsy can result from seizure burden as well as anticonvulsant effects and any concurrent sleep disorders. Patients with tic disorder and Tourette syndrome also have decreased sleep efficiency, and similarly this disturbed sleep may affect daytime behavior (85,86).

From published data on anticonvulsants, phenytoin and valproic acid increase stage 1 sleep, whereas benzodiazepines decrease slow wave sleep. Phenobarbital, benzodiazepines, carbamazepine, and phenytoin all decrease REM sleep (83). Tiagabine increases sleep efficiency and slow wave sleep; similarly, gabapentin increases slow wave sleep. Felbamate actually appears to decrease daytime drowsiness, whereas many anticonvulsants typically increase sleepiness during the day. A small open-label study involving children and young adults with epilepsy and severe learning disabilities, who were given melatonin in doses ranging from 2 to 6 mg at night, showed no significant effect of melatonin on seizure frequency; 11 of 13 subjects slept better with melatonin (87).

Periodic Limb Movements in Sleep and Restless Legs Syndrome

Periodic limb movements in sleep (PLMS) was originally termed nocturnal myoclonus and occurs as rhythmical extensions of the big toe, with ankle dorsiflexion and knee/hip flexion; these movements cluster in episodes that may last minutes to hours. Arousals may result from intense movements. If numerous, these arousals or awakenings may result in nonrestorative sleep. PLMS may be associated with other sleep/wake complaints, including insomnia and daytime sleepiness; accordingly, the term periodic limb movement disorder may be applied. PLMS may occur in 6% of the general population, with increasing prevalence noted with advancing age. PLMS is felt to be much less common in childhood (88). PLMS is diagnosed through overnight polysomnography by scoring leg movements recorded through electromyogram leads at the anterior tibialis muscles (4). A periodic limb movement index greater than 5 in children is considered abnormal (42).

Restless legs syndrome (RLS) is associated with episodes of distressing paresthesias (described as "crawling" sensations, burning, tingling, itching, or stabbing) that occur mostly between the knees and ankles. There is no objective test for RLS, but rather the diagnosis is supported by the patient's or parent's report of the symptoms, including the quality, severity, and time of day when the symptoms appear (typically worse or only occurring in the evening or night) and the motor responses to these sensations (e.g., an urge to move, with partial or total relief of unpleasant sensations at least as long as the activity continues) (42). There is currently no standardized questionnaire developed for use with children, and it may be difficult for children to describe RLS sensations in their own words. Because several studies indicate an autosomal dominant inheritance for primary (idiopathic) RLS (75), physicians should ask about affected family members. In adults, secondary RLS has been associated with many neurological disorders (including polyneuropathies, myelopathies, and multiple sclerosis), anemia (including iron and folate deficiencies), uremia, diabetes, hypothyroidism, and medication use (especially tricyclic antidepressants and serotonin reuptake inhibitors). In children, there have been associations with low body iron stores (indicated by low serum ferritin values) and RLS/PLMS; improvement in symptoms has been noted following iron repletion (89).

Narcolepsy

Narcolepsy is a chronic disorder characterized by excessive sleepiness often presenting as repeated naps or lapses into sleep throughout the day. The "narcolepsy tetrad" includes (a) excessive daytime sleepiness, (b) cataplexy, (c) hypnogogic (occurring at sleep onset) or hypnopompic (occurring with awakening from sleep) hallucinations, and (d) sleep paralysis. Excessive daytime sleepiness, the hallmark of narcolepsy, may be the sole symptom present. Cataplexy, a sudden loss of bilateral muscle tone provoked by a strong emotion (often telling or hearing a joke), is pathognomonic for narcolepsy. On the other hand, sleep paralysis and hypnogogic/hypnopompic hallucinations are not specific for narcolepsy. Nocturnal sleep is also abnormal on polysomnography, with a short REM latency and increased fragmentation (arousals and awakenings).

An important development that furthered understanding of the pathophysiology of narcolepsy has been the discovery of the hypocretin (orexin) signaling system. In approximately 90% of patients with narcolepsy and cataplexy, low cerebrospinal fluid levels of hypocretin-1 have been documented. These low levels are thought to reflect loss, perhaps from an autoimmune mechanism, of hypocretin neurons in the posterior-lateral hypothalamus. While potentially useful, CSF hypocretin-1 testing is not yet readily available. Although almost all patients with cataplexy are positive for DQB1*0602, some 12% to 38% of the general population are also positive, resulting in low test specificity (42). HLA typing can be commercially performed.

The diagnosis of narcolepsy is typically made from the history and supported by overnight polysomnography followed by MSLT. On the MSLT, a short mean sleep latency and the presence of two or more naps that include REM sleep is considered abnormal (42). The differential diagnosis for narcolepsy includes insufficient sleep, obstructive sleep apnea, periodic limb movement disorder, RLS, idiopathic hypersomnolence, and other disorders with excessive consequent daytime sleepiness.

Treatment consists of appropriate sleep hygiene measures, short-acting stimulant or wake-promoting medications (e.g., methylphenidate, modafinil) for treatment of daytime sleepiness, and REM-suppressant medications (e.g., imipramine, venlafaxine) for cataplexy.

Case Four

A 17-year-old young man is excessively sleepy during the day, falling asleep in class, and taking afternoon naps regularly. There is no convincing history of cataplexy, but he does report rare episodes consistent with sleep paralysis and hypnogogic hallucinations. An overnight polysomnogram showed increased arousals, a high obstructive apnea-hypopnea index, and increased PLMS. The MSLT demonstrated an abnormally short mean sleep latency (7.5 minutes), with two REM sleep episodes. Does this patient have narcolepsy?

Discussion: This is a complicated presentation, and the determination of narcolepsy cannot be made until the obstructive sleep apnea is addressed. Excessive daytime sleepiness can be due to many causes, and certainly this patient's sleep apnea can produce pathological sleepiness by fragmentation of overnight sleep and can result in REM sleep during the MSLT. Thus, the abnormal MSLT results in this patient are not of themselves diagnostic of narcolepsy. A further consideration in this case is the elevated periodic limb movement index, which may be seen both in patients with obstructive sleep apnea and in patients with narcolepsy, as well as potentially occurring as an independent finding. Although sleep paralysis and hypnogogic hallucinations are part of the classic narcolepsy tetrad, they also occur in healthy individuals. To sort out these considerations, the patient's obstructive sleep apnea should be treated first, with a repeat polysomnogram and MSLT afterward. Resolution of sleep apnea may be associated with normal repeat sleep study results. On the other hand, a consistently abnormal MSLT with normal respiratory features on an overnight polysomnogram would lend support for excessive sleepiness in the setting of narcolepsy or idiopathic hypersomnolence.

Attention Deficit Hyperactivity Disorder and Sleep Disorders

Sleep disturbances in subjects with ADHD are frequently reported by their parents (90–96) as well as the children (97) and young adults (98) themselves, and include difficulties in falling asleep, snoring, nocturnal and early morning awakenings, restless sleep, enuresis, and daytime tiredness. Sleep diary data indicate increased bedtime resistance and challenging parent-child interactions at bedtime (99).

ATTENTION DEFICIT HYPERACTIVITY DISORDER AND OBJECTIVE SLEEP STUDIES

Actigraphy, an established and reliable method for naturalistic sleep-wake studies in children and adults (18,100–102), has shown varied results in ADHD studies from longer sleep duration (99), significant night-to-night variability in sleep structure (96,101), delayed sleep onset (96), higher rates of periodic limb movement disorder (96), to no changes (95).

Polysomnograms in children with ADHD also show varied results, including a reduced amount of REM sleep and longer latency to the first REM period (103–108); increased REM duration (109) and two recent studies (107,110) found no differences in sleep architecture between children with ADHD and children with reading disorders. Most of the polysomnographic studies investigating sleep in the ADHD population consist of small sample sizes, include various age ranges with no consideration given to pubertal status, lack control groups (108) or limited normative data, and do not consider psychosocial variables (socioeconomic status; sleep hygiene) (90,111). Some of the studies include medication-free periods prior to enrollment (103,105), whereas others do not address the potentially confounding medication issue at all.

A recent meta-analysis of existing controlled actigraphy and polysomnographic studies in nonmedicated ADHD children (101,107,109,112–116) did not find any significant differences in sleep onset latency and sleep architecture parameters. Two of those studies also measured daytime alertness and found shorter mean sleep latency in the ADHD group (107,116); however, the times were still within the normal time range (10 to 20 minutes). Higher levels of nocturnal movements were reported in three of these studies (109,110,113).

SLEEP-DISORDERED BREATHING AND ATTENTION DEFICIT HYPERACTIVITY DISORDER

Children with severe forms of sleep-disordered breathing, such as obstructive sleep apnea, are at risk of failure to thrive, hypertension, and heart failure (73). Children with milder forms such as habitual snoring may present with daytime sleepiness, behavioral problems, and learning difficulties (64,117–126). Parental reports of snoring, 63% in an ADHD cohort referred to a sleep clinic (96), is sevenfold that reported in the general population. Also, significant sleep-disordered breathing was found in 7% (96), more than twice the estimated prevalence in the general population.

Improvement in aggression, hyperactive behaviors, attention, and vigilance in children with moderate to severe obstructive airways has been reported after adenotonsillectomy (127). Similarly, case reports of two ADHD adults with obstructive sleep apnea treated with CPAP had significant improvement and no longer required treatment with methylphenidate (128). In a prospective, nonrandomized study of a cohort of 78 children (ages 5 to 13) scheduled for adenotonsillectomy, compared with 27 controls, Chervin et al. (129) found mild to moderate sleep apnea in 51% versus 4% of controls; 22% versus 7% also met criteria for ADHD. The frequency of ADHD was similar for those with and without sleep apnea. Fifty percent of the 22 children with ADHD no longer met criteria 1 year after the surgical procedure. This is significant, given that ADHD is generally persistent, with only a 20% remission rate reported in adolescents and 30% in young adults (130).

Several reports suggest that sleep-disordered breathing is a potential causal factor in ADHD and that its treatment may improve ADHD. Many of the studies, however, have methodological problems with assessment measures and study design. In a prospective study of 229 children (ages 2 to 13) who completed initial and 4-year follow-up surveys, 13% were found to have a new-onset hyperactivity, and these children also had received higher sleep-disordered breathing scores at baseline; unfortunately, the study design did not include a control group and used less than stringent criteria for determining hyperactivity (131). In addition, neurobehavioral deficits (attention, social, anxious/depressive) have been reported in a study of children with and without snoring that excluded children with ADHD (122). A higher prevalence of snoring but not obstructive sleep apnea has been reported in children with ADHD, and no sleep variable accounted for a significant proportion of neurobehavioral dysfunction (123). In that study, although both snorers and nonsnorers scored within the normal range for neurobehavioral deficits, the snorers had greater symptoms. In a separate study using actigraphy in children with ADHD without any sleep-disordered breathing (SDB) and controls, Gruber and Sadeh (114) found an association between sleep measures and impairment in complex neurobehavioral tasks in controls but not in the ADHD group. Rather, increased instability of sleep parameters was found in the ADHD group. Chervin and Archbold (132) studied 112 children referred for sleep-disordered breathing and found that children with or without sleep-disordered breathing on polysomnography had similar levels of hyperactivity. In a study of well-characterized ADHD children that excluded sleep-disordered breathing, RLS, and daytime sleepiness, overnight polysomnography showed longer REM sleep latency and decreased percentage of REM sleep but was otherwise normal (108). In summary, although sleep-disordered breathing may play a role in a few ADHD cases, it is unlikely to be a contributing factor in most cases.

ATTENTION DEFICIT HYPERACTIVITY DISORDER AND RESTLESS LEGS SYNDROME/PERIODIC LIMB MOVEMENT DISORDER

As reviewed by Cortese et al. (133), the prevalence of RLS symptoms in ADHD patients ages 2 to 18, ranged from 10.5% to 24% (134,135) and RLS from 11.5% to 44% (136,137). PLMS rates of 26% to 64% (96,136,138) have been reported in children with ADHD, with associated arousals and sleep fragmentation; several others have not replicated these high prevalence rates of PLMS in ADHD. In a health screening survey of 450 students ages 7–14 years using a modified sleep scale, children with a diagnosis of ADHD had significantly higher scores for periodic limb movement disorder but not for sleep-disordered breathing (139).

The prevalence of ADHD with RLS has been reported to be between 18% and 25% (140,141) in children and 26% in adults (142). The prevalence of ADHD in children with periodic limb movement disorder ranged from 44% (143) to 91% in a retrospective review of polysomnography, which found that 117 of 129 children with ADHD had documented PLMS (>5 per hour) and that 15 of 16 children had PLMS of greater than 25 per hour (144).

Dopaminergic dysfunction has been associated with both ADHD and RLS (145–147). In addition, iron deficiency has been reported in RLS (147) and ADHD (112). A potential relationship may exist because iron is an essential cofactor for tyrosine hydroxylase, the rate limiting enzyme in the synthesis of dopamine. Although ADHD did not respond to stimulants in a small group of children with combined RLS and ADHD, it improved significantly in 3 of 7 children after dopaminergic therapy (e.g., levodopa; pergolide) (148).

Taken together, the relationship between ADHD and sleep disorders is complex. Neurobehavioral studies in adult subjects have found that partial sleep deprivation does cause significant behavioral and cognitive dysfunction (149). The few studies investigating the influence of partial sleep deprivation on the functioning of children and adolescents found a relationship between shortened sleep and learning and behavior problems (150–154). Adolescents with irregular sleep schedules had more behavior problems and lower academic achievement than students with stable sleep schedules (11).

Thus, sleep disorders that decrease or fragment sleep, such as RLS and OSA, probably exacerbate daytime ADHD but are not causal. However, these sleep disorders probably do not cause ADHD. In a single study (142) that included a comparison group of insomnia patients, RLS patients had higher ADHD ratings than insomnia patients, suggesting increased risk independent of sleep deprivation. However, the mechanisms behind insomnia and sleep fragmentation may differ and are not necessarily comparable.

Attention deficit hyperactivity disorder is one of the most common neuropsychiatric disorders, with estimated prevalence rates of 5% to 10% in school-aged children (155), 4% in college students (156), and approximately 2.5% in adults (156,157). Given that RLS is estimated to occur in 5% to 10% of adults (158) and 1% to 2% in children (159), and that snoring is estimated to occur in 3% to 12% and OSA in 1% to 3% of children (160), it is also to be expected that these disorders would co-occur.

Excessive movement during sleep was included in the diagnostic criteria of ADHD in earlier versions of the *Diagnostic and Statistical Manual of Mental Disorders* (DSM) (161), as well as in some of the commonly used, early ADHD rating scales (162); however, the excessive movement criteria during sleep was omitted in later versions of the DSM (163) because it was not specific to the diagnosis. A more recent survey (164), which also takes into account comorbid conditions, attributes sleep problems to comorbidity and medications rather than necessarily to ADHD.

Case Five

T.T. is a 12-year-old boy who was diagnosed with ADHD at age 6. Parents have chosen not to use medication treatment and depend primarily on behavioral interventions and educational accommodations. Homework has always been a challenging time, and this past year T.T. is spending up to 3 to 4 hours per night attempting to complete homework under parental supervision. This is frequently pushing bedtime to 10 p.m. with subsequent daytime sleepiness. What management steps should be taken?

> **Discussion:** Homework is a challenging task for children with ADHD. As children move to the higher grades, homework demands increase, impinging on sleep time. Several management options could be considered. One is to consider medication treatment for the ADHD that would help the youngster complete class work and homework in less time. Another option is to request a homework-based accommodation from school that would limit homework time.

Attention Deficit Hyperactivity Disorder Medications and Sleep

Methylphenidate (Ritalin, Concerta) and amphetamine (Adderall) compounds are the first-line agents for the treatment of ADHD and sleep problems are often reported to worsen with treatment (90,165,166). In clinical trials of children and adolescents, insomnia was reported in 16% of subjects treated with Adderall XR during a 4-week trial (167), which was found to persist in 11% of subjects during a 24-month maintenance study (168). Insomnia was also reported in 29.5% of subjects treated with Concerta in a short term study (169) and in 14% during a 12-month maintenance study (170).

Results from objective studies are mixed. An actigraphy study in a cohort of ADHD children reported increased sleep onset latency, as well as decreased sleep efficiency and total sleep time, with methylphenidate treatment compared with placebo (171). Similar findings were reported in an adult ADHD sample in which decreased nocturnal awakenings were also found (172). Polysomnography and actigraphy data from a recent double-blind cross-over trial comparing methylphenidate (thrice daily) with atomoxetine in children also showed decreased night awakening with both medications and shorter sleep-onset latencies only with atomoxetine, a selective norepinephrine reuptake inhibitor also Food and Drug Administration (FDA) approved for ADHD (173).

Sleep efficiency may have an impact on medication response. In a recent study, children with ADHD were found to improve on vigilance performance measures with methylphenidate if their sleep efficiency, measured with actigraphs, was poor, but not if their sleep efficiency was good (174).

Clonidine in combination with stimulants has been found helpful in improving sleep in ADHD children (175); however, the safety of the combination is not well studied. Atomoxetine may be another option for some, but not for most ADHD children (176). Melatonin (3 to 6 mg) has also been reported to advance sleep onset and increase total sleep time; however, this has not been shown to have any effect on ADHD, cognitive performance, or quality of life (177,178).

Case Six

B.B., an 8-year-old with ADHD, has always been very energetic and tireless, and at bedtime he has difficulty in settling down. Once asleep, he stays asleep throughout the night but is the first one up in the morning. This past month, Concerta was started and subsequently sleep onset was delayed for about 30 minutes. His parents are surprised that during the day he is not tired. What role is the medication playing?

Discussion: For some children treated with Concerta (long-acting methylphenidate preparation) sleep onset can be delayed. An alternative to Concerta would include other methylphenidate compounds that have different delivery mechanisms (e.g., Ritalin LA, Metadate CD) that result in lower concentrations at the end of the day and have less impact on sleep onset.

Common Neuropsychiatric Disorders Presenting with Sleep Problems

In nonreferred, healthy school-aged children, actigraph recordings found an association between decreased sleep and teacher-reported symptoms of externalizing behaviors (aggression, attentional and social problems) (179). In neuropsychiatric studies of school-aged children, subjective sleep difficulties are frequently associated with internalizing disorders, such as depression, anxiety, and behavioral problems (180). The relationship is complex and bidirectional; that is, the behavior and emotional and behavioral problems can also cause sleep difficulties (150).

Depressed children and adolescents frequently report insomnia, hypersomnia, night time awakenings, daytime fatigue, circadian reversal, and poor sleep quality (181,182). Suicidality is more common in adolescents with reports of sleep problems (183). Inconsistent results have been reported in controlled studies using objective measures. Some polysomnography studies found no significant differences in sleep architecture between depressed and nondepressed children and adolescents (184–189), whereas others have reported longer sleep latency and shorter REM latency (181,190–194). Gender differences have also been noted; greater sleep disturbances, including shorter REM latency, decreased amount of slow-wave sleep, fewer minutes of slow wave sleep in the first NREM period, and more arousals, were seen in depressed boys, whereas depressed girls did not differ from healthy controls (195). In another study, decreased delta amplitude was reported in females (196).

In one study of bipolar disorder, for which decreased need for sleep is one of the diagnostic criteria (197), 40% of children with mania versus 6.2% with ADHD had decreased need for sleep (198,199). In a community sample of children with the behavioral profile of pediatric bipolar disorder, polysomnography results indicated poorer sleep efficiency, more awakenings after sleep onset, decreased REM sleep, and longer periods of slow-wave sleep than what was observed in controls (200). Rao et al. (201) also reported that adolescents who subsequently develop a bipolar course had significantly less REM sleep compared with those with a major depressive disorder.

In community settings, incremental increases in trait anxiety have been associated with nightmares in 5- to 11-year-olds (202). In 300 8-year-old twin pairs, bedtime resistance was the main sleep difficulty associated with anxiety symptoms, whereas difficulties in getting to sleep, night awakenings, early awakenings, and parasomnias were associated with symptoms of depression. In clinical samples, parental and child reports indicate significant sleep disturbances in children with generalized anxiety disorder or overanxious disorder (203–205). In a recent study, 88% of children and adolescents with anxiety disorders (generalized, separation, social) were found to have at least one sleep-related problem (e.g., major ones include insomnia, nightmares, reluctance/refusal to go to sleep alone), whereas 55% had three or more according to self and parental reports, which decreased after pharmacological treatment of anxiety using fluvoxamine (206). Longitudinal studies found that the presence of sleep problems at age 4 years predicted anxiety and depression in adolescence (207), and more than half of 5- to 9-year-olds with parental reports of sleep problems were found to develop an adult anxiety disorder (208).

Traumatic events (e.g., natural disasters, accidents, illnesses, painful experiences, physical and sexual abuse, witnessing a trauma) can result in acute stress reactions that can include emotional, behavioral, cognitive, and physiological symptoms. When these symptoms persist or recur in the absence of a real threat, they can lead to an acute stress disorder or posttraumatic stress disorder (PTSD) that can have additional symptoms of intrusive recollections, numbing, avoidance, and hyperarousal (197). Children may be more vulnerable than adults, given that the stress response has been reported to be less adaptive in children than adults (209). In addition, small children with PTSD have been reported to lack the normal inhibitory modulation of the startle response (210). As reviewed by Caffo and Belaise (211), comorbid conditions, such as mood, anxiety, sleep, and behavioral problems, can also occur after traumatic events. In addition, specific trauma such as head injury can also lead to ADHD (212) with its associated risk for sleep difficulties.

Problems with sleep onset, sleep duration, anxiety, and parasomnias are frequently reported in children with autism spectrum disorder (213), even in those with normal intelligence quotient (IQ) levels (214). Actigraphy studies also show longer time to fall asleep, more time awake during the night, lower sleep efficiency, and more extreme sleep times (215,216); however, children with reported sleeplessness did not differ from those without sleeplessness (216).

Polysomnography studies report inconsistent results. One study noted shorter sleep periods, total sleep time, and time in bed compared to controls (217). In contrast, neither other studies (218,219) nor spectral power analysis found differences from controls (219).

Sleep disorders and neuropsychiatric disorders, therefore, have bidirectional effects. Longitudinal study design that permits assessment of age-related sleep changes would be ideal in deciphering the bidirectional effects of sleep and neuropsychiatric disorders. In addition, given that children and adolescents frequently have more than one neuropsychiatric disorder [e.g., 28% of children with major depressive disorder also meet criteria for ADHD (195)], future studies need to take into account comorbidity. In one ADHD study that considered comorbid conditions, sleep problems were found to be associated with comorbidity and medications and not necessarily with ADHD (164).

Future Directions

Increasing the awareness of children, their parents, and health care providers about the causes and consequences of disordered sleep will help highlight appropriate choices for sleep hygiene and encourage evaluation when needed. Improving the sleep of a child offers benefits not only for the patient but also for the entire household. Some disorders, such as delayed sleep phase syndrome, are commonly encountered but difficult to treat; in many cases, standardized protocols could allow for a more critical review of treatment strategies. Another area for future development would be pharmacotherapy for pediatric sleep disturbances. Although multiple agents have been evaluated in adults for management of insomnia, RLS/PLMS, and narcolepsy, few pediatric drug trials have been performed or even planned. Specific pharmacokinetic and therapeutic efficacy data are certainly needed to bring pediatric sleep treatments up to par. Given the exciting advances in understanding narcolepsy as well as the support for family aggregation in many other pediatric sleep disorders, goals for the next decade should also include large studies to enhance assessment of genetic risk factors and to foster the discovery of potential novel treatment strategies for sleep disorders in children based on gene-environment interactions. Taken together, the future of pediatric sleep medicine looks very promising, and the greatest advances will be possible through an interdisciplinary approach to research and patient care.

Questions

1. The stage of sleep characterized by K-complexes and sleep spindles is
   A. stage 1.
   B. stage 2.
   C. stage 3.
   D. stage 4.
   E. REM sleep.

2. Management of arousal disorder parasomnias can include
   A. safety measures.
   B. minimizing sleep deprivation.
   C. reassuring parents.
   D. medications (rarely).
   E. all of the above.

3. A 4-year-old boy is found to have obstructive sleep apnea by overnight-polysomnography. What is the next step?
   A. Initiate CPAP therapy.
   B. Introduce a weight loss plan.
   C. Give supplemental oxygen at night.
   D. Refer to an ear, nose, and throat (ENT) surgeon for evaluation and possible adenotonsillectomy.
   E. No treatment is needed.

4. Which of the following is not typically associated with narcolepsy?
   A. hypnogogic hallucinations
   B. cataplexy
   C. episodic rage
   D. excessive daytime sleepiness
   E. sleep paralysis

5. Periodic limb movements in sleep
   A. are diagnosed by overnight polysomnography.
   B. never result in arousals.
   C. may be associated with RLS.
   D. A and C.
   E. A, B, and C.

6. Bedtime delaying tactics result in shorter total sleep time but not in diminished sleep quality.
   A. true
   B. false

7. Which of the following strategies has not been found effective in the management of behavioral insomnia?
   A. Bedtime is intentionally delayed until sleep cues become associated with positive experiences, followed by gradual return to an earlier time.
   B. Practice graduated extinction, which involves increasing the time interval between successive parental checks.
   C. Practice modified extinction, which involves having the parents remain in the child's room while ignoring behavior.
   D. Practice extinction that involves having parents respond to child's crying on an intermittent basis.

8. Delayed sleep phase syndrome is only due to cultural factors.
   A. true
   B. false

9. Nightmares are characterized by terrifying dreams and vivid recall of the dream and swift return to sleep.
   A. true
   B. false

10. Factors that can contribute to sleep apnea include the following:
    A. adenotonsillar hypertrophy.
    B. obesity.
    C. anxiety.
    D. A and B only.

Answers

1. B
2. E
3. D
4. C
5. D
6. A
7. D
8. B
9. B
10. D

REFERENCES

1. Rechtschaffen A, Kales A. *A manual of standardized terminology, techniques and scoring system for sleep stages of human sleep.* Bethesda, MD: National Institutes of Health; 1968. Publication no 204.1.
2. Marcus CL et al. Normal polysomnographic values for children and adolescents. *Am Rev Respir Dis.* 1992;146(5 Pt 1):1235–1239.
3. Standards and indications for cardiopulmonary sleep studies in children. American Thoracic Society. *Am J Respir Crit Care Med.* 1996;153:866–878.
4. Recording and scoring leg movements. The Atlas Task Force. *Sleep.* 1993;16:748–759.
5. Carskadon MA, et al. Guidelines for the multiple sleep latency test (MSLT): a standard measure of sleepiness. *Sleep.* 1986;9:519–524.
6. Sadeh A, Sharkey KM, Carskadon MA. Activity-based sleep-wake identification: an empirical test of methodological issues. *Sleep.* 1994;17:201–207.
7. Hering E, et al. Sleep patterns in autistic children. *J Autism Dev Disord.* 1999;29:143–147.
8. Allik H, Larsson JO, Smedje H. Sleep patterns of school-age children with Asperger syndrome or high-functioning autism. *J Autism Dev Disord.* 2006;36:585–595.
9. Chervin RD, et al. Pediatric sleep questionnaire (PSQ): validity and reliability of scales for sleep-disordered breathing, snoring, sleepiness, and behavioral problems. *Sleep Med.* 2000;1(1):21–32.
10. Owens JA, Spirito A, McGuinn M. The Children's Sleep Habits Questionnaire (CSHQ): psychometric properties of a survey instrument for school-aged children. *Sleep.* 2000;23:1043–1051.
11. Wolfson AR, Carskadon MA. Sleep schedules and daytime functioning in adolescents. *Child Dev.* 1998;69:875–887.
12. Iglowstein I, et al. Sleep duration from infancy to adolescence: reference values and generational trends. *Pediatrics.* 2003;111:302–307.
13. Schulz H, et al. REM latency: development in the first year of life. *Electroencephalogr Clin Neurophysiol.* 1983;56:316–322.
14. Montgomery-Downs HE, et al. Polysomnographic characteristics in normal preschool and early school-aged children. *Pediatrics.* 2006;117:741–753.
15. Mindell JA, et al. Behavioral treatment of bedtime problems and night wakings in infants and young children. *Sleep.* 2006;29:1263–1276.
16. Carey WB. Night waking and temperament in infancy. *J Pediatr.* 1974;84:756–758.
17. Owens-Stively J, et al. Child temperament, parenting discipline style, and daytime behavior in childhood sleep disorders. *J Dev Behav Pediatr.* 1997;18:314–321.
18. Sadeh A. Assessment of intervention for infant night waking: parental reports and activity-based home monitoring. *J Consult Clin Psychol.* 1994;62(1):63–68.
19. Goodlin-Jones BL, et al. Night waking, sleep-wake organization, and self-soothing in the first year of life. *J Dev Behav Pediatr.* 2001;22:226–233.
20. Baker S, Zee PC. Sleep wake cycle disorders. In: Kryger M, Roth T, Dement W, eds. *Principles and Practice of Sleep Medicine.* Philadelphia: WB Saunders; 2000:606–614.
21. Uchiyama M, et al. A polysomnographic study on patients with delayed sleep phase syndrome (DSPS). *Jpn J Psychiatry Neurol.* 1992;46(1):219–221.
22. Watanabe T, et al. Sleep and circadian rhythm disturbances in patients with delayed sleep phase syndrome. *Sleep.* 2003;26:657–661.
23. Wyatt JK, Stepanski EJ, Kirkby J. Circadian phase in delayed sleep phase syndrome: predictors and temporal stability across multiple assessments. *Sleep.* 2006;29:1075–1080.
24. Shibui K, Uchiyama M, Okawa M. Melatonin rhythms in delayed sleep phase syndrome. *J Biol Rhythms.* 1999;14(1):72–76.
25. Carskadon MA, Vieira C, Acebo C. Association between puberty and delayed phase preference. *Sleep.* 1993;16:258–262.
26. Archer SN, et al. A length polymorphism in the circadian clock gene Per3 is linked to delayed sleep phase syndrome and extreme diurnal preference. *Sleep.* 2003;26:413–415.
27. Iwase T, et al. Mutation screening of the human Clock gene in circadian rhythm sleep disorders. *Psychiatry Res.* 2002;109(2):121–128.
28. Hohjoh H, et al. Significant association of the arylalkylamine N-acetyltransferase (AA-NAT) gene with delayed sleep phase syndrome. *Neurogenetics.* 2003;4(3):151–153.
29. Hohjoh H, et al. Possible association of human leucocyte antigen DR1 with delayed sleep phase syndrome. *Psychiatry Clin Neurosci.* 1999;53:527–529.
30. Carskadon MA. Patterns of sleep and sleepiness in adolescents. *Pediatrician.* 1990;17(1):5–12.
31. Carskadon MA, et al. An approach to studying circadian rhythms of adolescent humans. *J Biol Rhythms.* 1997;12(3):278–289.
32. Carskadon MA, et al. Adolescent sleep patterns, circadian timing, and sleepiness at a transition to early school days. *Sleep.* 1998;21:871–881.
33. Pack AI, et al. Characteristics of crashes attributed to the driver having fallen asleep. *Accid Anal Prev.* 1995;27:769–775.
34. Czeisler CA, et al. Chronotherapy: resetting the circadian clocks of patients with delayed sleep phase insomnia. *Sleep.* 1981;4:1–21.
35. Oren DA, Wehr TA. Hypernyctohemeral syndrome after chronotherapy for delayed sleep phase syndrome. *N Engl J Med.* 1992;327:1762.

36. Rosenthal NE, et al. Phase-shifting effects of bright morning light as treatment for delayed sleep phase syndrome. *Sleep.* 1990;13:354–361.
37. Watanabe T, et al. Effects of phototherapy in patients with delayed sleep phase syndrome. *Psychiatry Clin Neurosci.* 1999;53:231–233.
38. Cole RJ, et al. Bright-light mask treatment of delayed sleep phase syndrome. *J Biol Rhythms.* 2002;17(1):89–101.
39. Mundey K, et al. Phase-dependent treatment of delayed sleep phase syndrome with melatonin. *Sleep.* 2005;28:1271–1278.
40. Broughton R. NREM arousal parasomnias. In: Kryger MH RT, Dement WC, ed. *Principles and Practice of Sleep Medicine.* 3rd ed. Philadelphia: WB Saunders; 2000:693–706.
41. Fisher C, et al. A psychophysiological study of nightmares and night terrors. I. Physiological aspects of the stage 4 night terror. *J Nerv Ment Dis.* 1973;157(2):75–98.
42. AASM. *International Classification of Sleep Disorders.* 2nd ed. *Diagnostic and Coding Manual.* Westchester, IL: American Academy of Sleep Medicine; 2005.
43. Mahowald MW, Bornemann MC, Schenck CH. Parasomnias. *Semin Neurol.* 2004;24:283–292.
44. Hublin C, et al. Prevalence and genetics of sleep-walking: a population-based twin study. *Neurology.* 1997;48:177–181.
45. Rosen GM, Ferber R, Mahowald MW. Evaluation of parasomnias in children. *Child Adolesc Clin North Am.* 1996;5:601–616.
46. Sheldon SH. Parasomnias in childhood. *Pediatr Clin North Am.* 2004;51:69–88, vi.
47. Mason TB 2nd, Pack AI. Sleep terrors in childhood. *J Pediatr.* 2005;147:388–392.
48. Mahowald M. Arousal and sleep-wake transition parasomnias. In: Lee-Chiong TL SM, Carskadon MA, ed. *Sleep Medicine.* Philadelphia: Hanley and Belfus; 2002:207–213.
49. Guilleminault C, et al. Sleepwalking and sleep terrors in prepubertal children: what triggers them? *Pediatrics.* 2003;111(1):e17–25.
50. Mahowald MW, et al. The role of a sleep disorder center in evaluating sleep violence. *Arch Neurol.* 1992;49:604–607.
51. Broughton R. NREM parasomnias. In: Kryger MH RT, Dement WC, ed. *Principles and Practice of Sleep Medicine.* Philadelphia: WB Saunders; 2000:693–706.
52. Hallstrom T. Night terror in adults through three generations. *Acta Psychiatr Scand.* 1972;48:350–352.
53. Kales A, et al. Hereditary factors in sleepwalking and night terrors. *Br J Psychiatry.* 1980;137:111–118.
54. Robinson A, Guilleminault C. Disorders of arousal. In: Chokroverty SHW, Walters AS, ed. *Sleep and Movement Disorders.* Philadelphia: Butterworth Heinemann; 2003:265–272.
55. Smedje H, Broman JE, Hetta J. Associations between disturbed sleep and behavioural difficulties in 635 children aged six to eight years: a study based on parents' perceptions. *Eur Child Adolesc Psychiatry.* 2001;10(1):1–9.
56. Smedje H, Broman JE, Hetta J. Short-term prospective study of sleep disturbances in 5-8-year-old children. *Acta Paediatr.* 2001;90:1456–1463.
57. Kazak AE, et al. Posttraumatic stress, family functioning, and social support in survivors of childhood leukemia and their mothers and fathers. *J Consult Clin Psychol.* 1997;65(1):120–129.
58. Green SM, Sherwin TS. Incidence and severity of recovery agitation after ketamine sedation in young adults. *Am J Emerg Med.* 2005;23(2):142–144.
59. Ipsiroglu OS, et al. Self-reported organic and nonorganic sleep problems in schoolchildren aged 11 to 15 years in Vienna. *J Adolesc Health.* 2002;31:436–442.
60. Brunetti L, et al. Prevalence of obstructive sleep apnea syndrome in a cohort of 1,207 children of southern Italy. *Chest.* 2001;120:1930–1935.
61. Hunt CE. Neurocognitive outcomes in sleep-disordered breathing. *J Pediatr.* 2004;145:430–432.
62. Clinical practice guideline: diagnosis and management of childhood obstructive sleep apnea syndrome. *Pediatrics.* 2002;109:704–712.
63. Kennedy JD, Waters KA. 8. Investigation and treatment of upper-airway obstruction: childhood sleep disorders I. *Med J Aust.* 2005;182:419–423.
64. Gottlieb DJ, et al. Sleep-disordered breathing symptoms are associated with poorer cognitive function in 5-year-old children. *J Pediatr.* 2004;145:458–464.
65. Marcus CL, et al. Upper airway dynamic responses in children with the obstructive sleep apnea syndrome. *Pediatr Res.* 2005;57:99–107.
66. Arens R, Marcus CL. Pathophysiology of upper airway obstruction: a developmental perspective. *Sleep.* 2004;27:997–1019.
67. Arens R, et al. Changes in upper airway size during tidal breathing in children with obstructive sleep apnea syndrome. *Am J Respir Crit Care Med.* 2005;171:1298–1304.
68. Redline S, et al. Studies in the genetics of obstructive sleep apnea. Familial aggregation of symptoms associated with sleep-related breathing disturbances. *Am Rev Respir Dis.* 1992;145(2 Pt 1):440–444.
69. Gislason T, et al. Familial predisposition and cosegregation analysis of adult obstructive sleep apnea and the sudden infant death syndrome. *Am J Respir Crit Care Med.* 2002;166:833–838.
70. Redline S, et al. The familial aggregation of obstructive sleep apnea. *Am J Respir Crit Care Med.* 1995;151(3 Pt 1):682–687.
71. Redline S, et al. Risk factors for sleep-disordered breathing in children. Associations with obesity,

race, and respiratory problems. *Am J Respir Crit Care Med.* 1999;159(5 Pt 1):1527–1532.
72. Ovchinsky A, et al. The familial aggregation of pediatric obstructive sleep apnea syndrome. *Arch Otolaryngol Head Neck Surg.* 2002;128:815–818.
73. Marcus CL. Sleep-disordered breathing in children. *Am J Respir Crit Care Med.* 2001;164:16–30.
74. Gobbi G, Boni A, Filippini M. The spectrum of idiopathic rolandic epilepsy syndromes and idiopathic occipital epilepsies: from the benign to the disabling. *Epilepsia.* 2006;47 (suppl 2):62–66.
75. Raizen DM, Mason TB, Pack AI. Genetic basis for sleep regulation and sleep disorders. *Semin Neurol.* 2006;26:467–483.
76. Van Hirtum-Das M, et al. Children with ESES: variability in the syndrome. *Epilepsy Res.* 2006;70(suppl 1):S248–258.
77. Provini F, Plazzi G, Lugaresi E. From nocturnal paroxysmal dystonia to nocturnal frontal lobe epilepsy. *Clin Neurophysiol.* 2000;111 (suppl 2):S2–8.
78. Provini F, et al. Nocturnal frontal lobe epilepsy. A clinical and polygraphic overview of 100 consecutive cases. *Brain.* 1999;122 (Pt 6):1017–1031.
79. Derry CP, Duncan JS, Berkovic SF. Paroxysmal motor disorders of sleep: the clinical spectrum and differentiation from epilepsy. *Epilepsia.* 2006;47:1775–1791.
80. Ryvlin P, Rheims S, Risse G. Nocturnal frontal lobe epilepsy. *Epilepsia.* 2006;47(suppl 2):83–86.
81. Malow BA. Sleep deprivation and epilepsy. *Epilepsy Curr.* 2004;4(5):193–195.
82. Malow BA, et al. Identification and treatment of obstructive sleep apnea in adults and children with epilepsy: a prospective pilot study. *Sleep Med.* 2003;4:509–515.
83. Bazil CW. Effects of antiepileptic drugs on sleep structure: are all drugs equal? *CNS Drugs.* 2003;17:719–728.
84. Bazil CW. Nocturnal seizures. *Semin Neurol.* 2004;24:293–300.
85. Kirov R, et al. Sleep patterns in children with attention-deficit/hyperactivity disorder, tic disorder, and comorbidity. *J Child Psychol Psychiatry.* 2007;48:561–570.
86. Kostanecka-Endress T, et al. Disturbed sleep in children with Tourette syndrome: a polysomnographic study. *J Psychosom Res.* 2003;55(1):23–29.
87. Jones C, Huyton M, Hindley D. Melatonin and epilepsy. *Arch Dis Child.* 2005;90:1203.
88. Mindell JA, Mason TBA. Sleep problems and disorders. In: Osborn LM, DeWitt TG, First LR, Zenel JA, eds. *Pediatrics.* Philadelphia: Elsevier Mosby; 2005:1608–1613.
89. Simakajornboon N, et al. Periodic limb movements in sleep and iron status in children. *Sleep.* 2003;26:735–738.
90. Corkum P, Tannock R, Moldofsky H. Sleep disturbances in children with attention-deficit/hyperactivity disorder. *J Am Acad Child Adolesc Psychiatry.* 1998;37:637–646.
91. Ball JD, et al. Sleep patterns among children with attention-deficit hyperactivity disorder: a reexamination of parent perceptions. *J Pediatr Psychol.* 1997;22:389–398.
92. Stein MA. Unravelling sleep problems in treated and untreated children with ADHD. *J Child Adolesc Psychopharmacol.* 1999;9(3):157–168.
93. Barkley RA, DuPaul GJ, McMurray MB. Comprehensive evaluation of attention deficit disorder with and without hyperactivity as defined by research criteria. *J Consult Clin Psychol.* 1990;58:775–789.
94. Kaplan BJ, et al. Sleep disturbance in preschool-aged hyperactive and nonhyperactive children. *Pediatrics.* 1987;80:839–844.
95. Wiggs L, Montgomery P, Stores G. Actigraphic and parent reports of sleep patterns and sleep disorders in children with subtypes of attention-deficit hyperactivity disorder. *Sleep.* 2005;28:1437–445.
96. Crabtree VM, Ivanenko A, Gozal D. Clinical and parental assessment of sleep in children with attention-deficit/hyperactivity disorder referred to a pediatric sleep medicine center. *Clin Pediatr (Phila).* 2003;42:807–813.
97. Owens JA, et al. Parental and self-report of sleep in children with attention-deficit/hyperactivity disorder. *Arch Pediatr Adolesc Med.* 2000;154:549–555.
98. Gau SS, et al. Association between sleep problems and symptoms of attention-deficit/hyperactivity disorder in young adults. *Sleep.* 2007;30:195–201.
99. Corkum P, et al. Actigraphy and parental ratings of sleep in children with attention-deficit/hyperactivity disorder (ADHD). *Sleep.* 2001;24:303–312.
100. Sadeh A, et al. Sleep and psychological characteristics of children on a psychiatric inpatient unit. *J Am Acad Child Adolesc Psychiatry.* 1995;34:813–819.
101. Gruber R, Sadeh A, Raviv A. Instability of sleep patterns in children with attention-deficit/hyperactivity disorder. *J Am Acad Child Adolesc Psychiatry.* 2000;39:495–501.
102. de Souza L, et al. Further validation of actigraphy for sleep studies. *Sleep.* 2003;26:81–85.
103. Nahas AD, Krynicki V. Effect of methylphenidate on sleep stages and ultradian rhythms in hyperactive children. *J Nerv Ment Dis.* 1977;164(1):66–69.
104. Haig JR, Schroeder CS, Schroeder SR. Effects of methylphenidate on hyperactive children's sleep. *Psychopharmacologia.* 1974;37(4):185–188.
105. Greenhill L, et al. Sleep architecture and REM sleep measures in prepubertal children with

attention deficit disorder with hyperactivity. *Sleep.* 1983;6:91–101.
106. Busby K, Firestone P, Pivik RT. Sleep patterns in hyperkinetic and normal children. *Sleep.* 1981;4:366–383.
107. Lecendreux M, et al. Sleep and alertness in children with ADHD. *J Child Psychol Psychiatry.* 2000;41:803–812.
108. Sangal RB, Owens JA, Sangal J. Patients with attention-deficit/hyperactivity disorder without observed apneic episodes in sleep or daytime sleepiness have normal sleep on polysomnography. *Sleep.* 2005;28:1143–1148.
109. Kirov R, et al. Is there a specific polysomnographic sleep pattern in children with attention deficit/hyperactivity disorder? *J Sleep Res.* 2004;13(1):87–93.
110. Konofal E, et al. High levels of nocturnal activity in children with attention-deficit hyperactivity disorder: a video analysis. *Psychiatry Clin Neurosci.* 2001;55(2):97–103.
111. Cortese S, et al. Sleep and alertness in children with attention-deficit/hyperactivity disorder: a systematic review of the literature. *Sleep.* 2006;29:504–511.
112. Konofal E, et al. Iron deficiency in children with attention-deficit/hyperactivity disorder. *Arch Pediatr Adolesc Med.* 2004;158:1113–1115.
113. Huang YS, et al. Sleep disorders in Taiwanese children with attention deficit/hyperactivity disorder. *J Sleep Res.* 2004;13:269–277.
114. Gruber R, Sadeh A. Sleep and neurobehavioral functioning in boys with attention-deficit/hyperactivity disorder and no reported breathing problems. *Sleep.* 2004;27:267–273.
115. Cooper J, et al. No evidence of sleep apnea in children with attention deficit hyperactivity disorder. *Clin Pediatr (Phila).* 2004;43:609–614.
116. Golan N, et al. Sleep disorders and daytime sleepiness in children with attention-deficit/hyperactive disorder. *Sleep.* 2004;27:261–266.
117. Ali NJ, Pitson DJ, Stradling JR. Snoring, sleep disturbance, and behaviour in 4–5 year olds. *Arch Dis Child.* 1993;68:360–366.
118. Ferreira AM, et al. Snoring in Portuguese primary school children. *Pediatrics.* 2000;106(5):E64.
119. Chervin RD, et al. Inattention, hyperactivity, and symptoms of sleep-disordered breathing. *Pediatrics.* 2002;109:449–456.
120. Gozal D. Sleep-disordered breathing and school performance in children. *Pediatrics.* 1998;102(3 Pt 1):616–620.
121. Urschitz MS, et al. Habitual snoring, intermittent hypoxia, and impaired behavior in primary school children. *Pediatrics.* 2004;114:1041–1048.
122. O'Brien LM, et al. Neurobehavioral implications of habitual snoring in children. *Pediatrics.* 2004;114:44–49.
123. O'Brien LM, et al. Sleep disturbances in children with attention deficit hyperactivity disorder. *Pediatr Res.* 2003;54:237–243.
124. Guilleminault C, et al. Children and nocturnal snoring: evaluation of the effects of sleep related respiratory resistive load and daytime functioning. *Eur J Pediatr.* 1982;139(3):165–171.
125. Blunden S, et al. Behavior and neurocognitive performance in children aged 5–10 years who snore compared to controls. *J Clin Exp Neuropsychol.* 2000;22:554–568.
126. Rosen CL, et al. Increased behavioral morbidity in school-aged children with sleep-disordered breathing. *Pediatrics.* 2004;114:1640–1648.
127. Ali NJ, Pitson D, Stradling JR. Sleep disordered breathing: effects of adenotonsillectomy on behaviour and psychological functioning. *Eur J Pediatr.* 1996;155(1):56–62.
128. Naseem S, Chaudhary B, Collop N. Attention deficit hyperactivity disorder in adults and obstructive sleep apnea. *Chest.* 2001;119:294–296.
129. Chervin RD, et al. Sleep-disordered breathing, behavior, and cognition in children before and after adenotonsillectomy. *Pediatrics.* 2006;117:e769–778.
130. Biederman J, et al. Young adult outcome of attention deficit hyperactivity disorder: a controlled 10-year follow-up study. *Psychol Med.* 2006;3:167–179.
131. Chervin RD, et al. Snoring predicts hyperactivity four years later. *Sleep.* 2005;28:885–890.
132. Chervin RD, Archbold KH. Hyperactivity and polysomnographic findings in children evaluated for sleep-disordered breathing. *Sleep.* 2001;24:313–320.
133. Cortese S, et al. Restless legs syndrome and attention-deficit/hyperactivity disorder: a review of the literature. *Sleep.* 2005;28:1007–1013.
134. Harnish M, et al. The relationship between sleep disorders and attention deficit hyperactivity disorder (ADHD): objective findings. *Sleep.* 2001;24:A14.
135. Chervin RD, et al. Conduct problems and symptoms of sleep disorders in children. *J Am Acad Child Adolesc Psychiatry.* 2003;42:201–208.
136. Picchietti DL, et al. Periodic limb movement disorder and restless legs syndrome in children with attention-deficit hyperactivity disorder. *J Child Neurol.* 1998;13:588–594.
137. Konofal E, et al. Restless legs syndrome and serum ferritin levels in ADHD children. *Sleep.* 2003;26:A136.
138. Picchietti DL, et al. Further studies on periodic limb movement disorder and restless legs syndrome in children with attention-deficit hyperactivity disorder. *Mov Disord.* 1999;14:1000–1007.
139. Gaultney JF, Terrell DF, Gingras JL. Parent-reported periodic limb movement, sleep disordered breathing, bedtime resistance behav-

iors, and ADHD. *Behav Sleep Med.* 2005;3(1):32–43.
140. Chervin RD, et al. Associations between symptoms of inattention, hyperactivity, restless legs, and periodic leg movements. *Sleep.* 2002;25:213–218.
141. Kotagal S, Silber MH. Childhood-onset restless legs syndrome. *Ann Neurol.* 2004;56:803–807.
142. Wagner ML, Walters AS, Fisher BC. Symptoms of attention-deficit/hyperactivity disorder in adults with restless legs syndrome. *Sleep.* 2004;27:1499–1504.
143. Crabtree VM, et al. Periodic limb movement disorder of sleep in children. *J Sleep Res.* 2003;12(1):73–81.
144. Picchietti DL, Walters AS. Moderate to severe periodic limb movement disorder in childhood and adolescence. *Sleep.* 1999;22:297–300.
145. Allen RP, et al. Restless legs syndrome: diagnostic criteria, special considerations, and epidemiology. A report from the restless legs syndrome diagnosis and epidemiology workshop at the National Institutes of Health. *Sleep Med.* 2003;4(2):101–119.
146. Trenkwalder C, et al. L-dopa therapy of uremic and idiopathic restless legs syndrome: a double-blind, crossover trial. *Sleep.* 1995;18:681–688.
147. Allen RP, et al. MRI measurement of brain iron in patients with restless legs syndrome. *Neurology.* 2001;56:263–265.
148. Walters AS, et al. Dopaminergic therapy in children with restless legs/periodic limb movements in sleep and ADHD. Dopaminergic Therapy Study Group. *Pediatr Neurol.* 2000;22:182–186.
149. Babkoff H, Caspy T, Mikulincer M. Subjective sleepiness ratings: the effects of sleep deprivation, circadian rhythmicity and cognitive performance. *Sleep.* 1991;14:534–539.
150. Dahl RE. The impact of inadequate sleep on children's daytime cognitive function. *Semin Pediatr Neurol.* 1996;3:44–50.
151. Kahn A, et al. Sleep problems in healthy preadolescents. *Pediatrics.* 1989;84:542–546.
152. Quine L. Sleep problems in children with mental handicap. *J Ment Defic Res.* 1991;35(Pt 4):269–290.
153. Randazzo AC, et al. Cognitive function following acute sleep restriction in children ages 10–14. *Sleep.* 1998;21:861–868.
154. Thorpy MJ, et al. Delayed sleep phase syndrome in adolescents. *J Adolesc Health Care.* 1988;9(1):22–27.
155. Scahill L, Schwab-Stone M. Epidemiology of ADHD in school-age children. *Child Adolesc Psychiatr Clin North Am.* 2000;9:541–555, vii.
156. Heiligenstein E, et al. Preliminary normative data on DSM-IV attention deficit hyperactivity disorder in college students. *J Am Coll Health.* 1998;46(4):185–188.
157. Kooij JJ, et al. Internal and external validity of attention-deficit/hyperactivity disorder in a population-based sample of adults. *Psychol Med.* 2005;35:817–827.
158. Phillips B, et al. Epidemiology of restless legs symptoms in adults. *Arch Intern Med.* 2000;160:2137–2141.
159. Erman MK. Selected sleep disorders: restless legs syndrome and periodic limb movement disorder, sleep apnea syndrome, and narcolepsy. *Psychiatr Clin North Am.* 2006;29:947–967; abstract viii–ix.
160. Katz E, Marcus CL. Diagnosis of obstructive sleep apnea syndrome in infants and children. In: Sheldon S, Feber R, Kryger M, eds. *Principles and Practice of Pediatric Sleep Medicine.* Philadelphia: Elsevier Saunders; 2005.
161. American Psychiatric Association. *Diagnostic and Statistical Manual of Mental Disorders (DSM-III).* Washington, DC: American Psychiatric Association; 1980.
162. Goyette CH, Conners CK, Ulrich RF. Normative data on revised Conners Parent and Teacher Rating Scales. *J Abnorm Child Psychol.* 1978;6(2):221–236.
163. Tahir E, et al. Association and linkage of DRD4 and DRD5 with attention deficit hyperactivity disorder (ADHD) in a sample of Turkish children. *Mol Psychiatry.* 2000;5:396–404.
164. Mick E, et al. Sleep disturbances associated with attention deficit hyperactivity disorder: the impact of psychiatric comorbidity and pharmacotherapy. *J Child Adolesc Psychopharmacol.* 2000;10:223–231.
165. Ring A, et al. Sleep disturbances in children with attention-deficit/hyperactivity disorder: a comparative study with healthy siblings. *J Learn Disabil.* 1998;31:572–578.
166. Efron D. Methylphenidate versus dextroamphetamine in ADHD. *J Am Acad Child Adolesc Psychiatry.* 1999;38:500.
167. Biederman J, et al. A randomized, double-blind, placebo-controlled, parallel-group study of SLI381 (Adderall XR) in children with attention-deficit/hyperactivity disorder. *Pediatrics.* 2002;110(2 Pt 1):258–266.
168. McGough JJ, et al. Long-term tolerability and effectiveness of once-daily mixed amphetamine salts (Adderall XR) in children with ADHD. *J Am Acad Child Adolesc Psychiatry.* 2005;44:530–538.
169. Wolraich ML, et al. Randomized, controlled trial of oros methylphenidate once a day in children with attention-deficit/hyperactivity disorder. *Pediatrics.* 2001;108:883–892.
170. Wilens T, et al. ADHD treatment with once-daily OROS methylphenidate: interim 12-month results from a long-term open-label study. *J Am Acad Child Adolesc Psychiatry.* 2003;42:424–433.
171. Schwartz G, et al. Actigraphic monitoring during sleep of children with ADHD on methylphenidate and placebo. *J Am Acad Child Adolesc Psychiatry.* 2004;43:1276–1282.

172. Boonstra AM, et al. Hyperactive night and day? Actigraphy studies in adult ADHD: a baseline comparison and the effect of methylphenidate. *Sleep.* 2007;30:433–442.
173. Sangal RB, et al. Effects of atomoxetine and methylphenidate on sleep in children with ADHD. *Sleep.* 2006;29:1573–1585.
174. Gruber R, et al. Performance on the continuous performance test in children with ADHD is associated with sleep effiiciency. *Sleep.* 2007;30:1003–1009.
175. Prince JB, et al. Clonidine for sleep disturbances associated with attention-deficit hyperactivity disorder: a systematic chart review of 62 cases. *J Am Acad Child Adolesc Psychiatry.* 1996;35:599–605.
176. Gibson AP, et al. Atomoxetine versus stimulants for treatment of attention deficit/hyperactivity disorder. *Ann Pharmacother.* 2006;40:1134–1142.
177. Weiss MD, et al. Sleep hygiene and melatonin treatment for children and adolescents with ADHD and initial insomnia. *J Am Acad Child Adolesc Psychiatry.* 2006;45:512–519.
178. Van der Heijden KB, et al. Effect of melatonin on sleep, behavior, and cognition in ADHD and chronic sleep-onset insomnia. *J Am Acad Child Adolesc Psychiatry.* 2007;46:233–241.
179. Aronen ET, et al. Sleep and psychiatric symptoms in school-age children. *J Am Acad Child Adolesc Psychiatry.* 2000;39:502–508.
180. Ivanenko A, Crabtree VM, Gozal D. Sleep in children with psychiatric disorders. *Pediatr Clin North Am.* 2004;51:51–68.
181. Dahl RE, et al. Sleep onset abnormalities in depressed adolescents. *Biol Psychiatry.* 1996;39:400–410.
182. Ryan ND, et al. The clinical picture of major depression in children and adolescents. *Arch Gen Psychiatry.* 1987;44:854–861.
183. Roberts RE, Roberts CR, Chen IG. Impact of insomnia on future functioning of adolescents. *J Psychosom Res.* 2002;53(1):561–569.
184. Bertocci MA, et al. Subjective sleep complaints in pediatric depression: a controlled study and comparison with EEG measures of sleep and waking. *J Am Acad Child Adolesc Psychiatry.* 2005;44:1158–1166.
185. Dahl RE, et al. EEG sleep in adolescents with major depression: the role of suicidality and inpatient status. *J Affect Disord.* 1990;19(1):63–75.
186. Dahl RE, et al. Electroencephalographic sleep measures in prepubertal depression. *Psychiatry Res.* 1991;38:201–214.
187. Kutcher S, et al. REM latency in endogenously depressed adolescents. *Br J Psychiatry.* 1992;161:399–402.
188. Puig-Antich J, et al. Sleep architecture and REM sleep measures in prepubertal children with major depression: a controlled study. *Arch Gen Psychiatry.* 1982;39:932–939.
189. Young W, et al. The sleep of childhood depressives: comparison with age-matched controls. *Biol Psychiatry.* 1982;17:1163–1168.
190. Emslie GJ, et al. Children with major depression show reduced rapid eye movement latencies. *Arch Gen Psychiatry.* 1990;47:119–124.
191. Goetz RR, et al. EEG sleep of young adults with major depression: a controlled study. *J Affect Disord.* 1991;22(1–2):91–100.
192. Emslie GJ, et al. Sleep EEG findings in depressed children and adolescents. *Am J Psychiatry.* 1987;144:668–670.
193. Emslie GJ, et al. Sleep EEG features of adolescents with major depression. *Biol Psychiatry.* 1994;36:573–581.
194. Lahmeyer HW, Poznanski EO, Bellur SN. EEG sleep in depressed adolescents. *Am J Psychiatry.* 1983;140:1150–1153.
195. Robert JJ, et al. Sex and age differences in sleep macroarchitecture in childhood and adolescent depression. *Sleep.* 2006;29:351–358.
196. Armitage R, et al. Delta sleep EEG in depressed adolescent females and healthy controls. *J Affect Disord.* 2001;63(1–3):139–148.
197. American Psychiatric Association. *Diagnostic and Statistical Manual of Mental Disorders.* 4th ed. DSM-IV-TR (Text Revision). 4th ed. Washington, DC: American Psychiatric Association; 2004.
198. Geller B, et al. Phenomenology of prepubertal and early adolescent bipolar disorder: examples of elated mood, grandiose behaviors, decreased need for sleep, racing thoughts and hypersexuality. *J Child Adolesc Psychopharmacol.* 2002;12(1):3–9.
199. Geller B, et al. DSM-IV mania symptoms in a prepubertal and early adolescent bipolar disorder phenotype compared to attention-deficit hyperactive and normal controls. *J Child Adolesc Psychopharmacol.* 2002;12(1):11–25.
200. Mehl RC, et al. Correlates of sleep and pediatric bipolar disorder. *Sleep.* 2006;29:193–197.
201. Rao U, et al. Heterogeneity in EEG sleep findings in adolescent depression: unipolar versus bipolar clinical course. *J Affect Disord.* 2002;70:273–280.
202. Mindell JA, Barrett KM. Nightmares and anxiety in elementary-aged children: is there a relationship. *Child Care Health Dev.* 2002;28:317–322.
203. Kendall PC, Pimentel SS. On the physiological symptom constellation in youth with generalized anxiety disorder (GAD). *J Anxiety Disord.* 2003;17:211–221.
204. Masi G, et al. Generalized anxiety disorder in referred children and adolescents. *J Am Acad Child Adolesc Psychiatry.* 2004;43:752–760.
205. Pina AA, et al. Diagnostic efficiency of symptoms in the diagnosis of DSM-IV: generalized anxiety disorder in youth. *J Child Psychol Psychiatry.* 2002;43:959–967.

206. Alfano CA, Ginsburg GS, Kingery JN. Sleep-related problems among children and adolescents with anxiety disorders. *J Am Acad Child Adolesc Psychiatry.* 2007;46:224–232.
207. Gregory AM, O'Connor TG. Sleep problems in childhood: a longitudinal study of developmental change and association with behavioral problems. *J Am Acad Child Adolesc Psychiatry.* 2002;41:964–971.
208. Gregory AM, et al. Prospective longitudinal associations between persistent sleep problems in childhood and anxiety and depression disorders in adulthood. *J Abnorm Child Psychol.* 2005;33:157–163.
209. Perry BD, Azad I. Posttraumatic stress disorders in children and adolescents. *Curr Opin Pediatr.* 1999;11:310–316.
210. Ornitz EM, Pynoos RS. Startle modulation in children with posttraumatic stress disorder. *Am J Psychiatry.* 1989;146:866–870.
211. Caffo E, Belaise C. Psychological aspects of traumatic injury in children and adolescents. *Child Adolesc Psychiatr Clin North Am.* 2003;12:493–535.
212. Stoddard FJ, Saxe G. Ten-year research review of physical injuries. *J Am Acad Child Adolesc Psychiatry.* 2001;40:1128–1145.
213. Richdale AL. Sleep problems in autism: prevalence, cause, and intervention. *Dev Med Child Neurol.* 1999;41(1):60–66.
214. Couturier JL, et al. Parental perception of sleep problems in children of normal intelligence with pervasive developmental disorders: prevalence, severity, and pattern. *J Am Acad Child Adolesc Psychiatry.* 2005;44:815–822.
215. Allik H, Larsson JO, Smedje H. Insomnia in school-age children with Asperger syndrome or high-functioning autism. *BMC Psychiatry.* 2006;6:18.
216. Wiggs L, Stores G. Sleep patterns and sleep disorders in children with autistic spectrum disorders: insights using parent report and actigraphy. *Dev Med Child Neurol.* 2004;46:372–380.
217. Elia M, et al. Sleep in subjects with autistic disorder: a neurophysiological and psychological study. *Brain Dev.* 2000;22(2):88–92.
218. Godbout R, et al. A laboratory study of sleep in Asperger's syndrome. *Neuroreport.* 2000;11(1):127–130.
219. Tani P, et al. Sleep in young adults with Asperger syndrome. *Neuropsychobiology.* 2004;50(2):147–152.

CHAPTER 7

Headaches in Children and Adolescents

A. DAVID ROTHNER AND DAVID W. DUNN

Headache, a frequently occurring disorder in children and adolescents, causes considerable discomfort and leads to time lost from school and work. It affects the family as well as afflicted children and adolescents. The majority of headaches in children and adolescents are not associated with structural or organic disease. In evaluating and treating headaches in children and adolescents, physicians must consider physical, psychological, and socioeconomic factors in determining the correct diagnosis and selecting optimal therapy. A thorough history coupled with complete general physical and neurological examinations, as well as the use of selected laboratory tests, will guide the clinician to the correct diagnosis. Treatment is most effective when both the specific headache type and its etiology are known (1).

Physicians caring for headache patients of any age understand that headache may be a symptom of a medical disorder, a primary headache disorder without a medical cause, or a psychiatric disorder. In particular, they recognize that headaches may be one component of a psychiatric disorder, may be associated with psychiatric disorders, may be precipitated by psychological difficulties, or may be unrelated to the patient's emotional problems. Mental health workers have special skills that may be beneficial in both the evaluation and the treatment of headache syndromes in children and adolescents (2).

This chapter reviews the common types of headache seen in children and adolescents and provides a systematic approach to diagnosis and treatment. It also discusses the psychiatric, psychosocial, lifestyle, and socioeconomic and family factors that play a role in the pathogenesis and treatment.

History

Hippocrates described migraine 25 centuries ago (3). Years later Galen coined the term *hemicrania* (3). William Henry Day, a British pediatrician in his book, *Essays on Diseases in Children,* recognized that nonorganic, nonvascular headaches were the most common type of headache in children. He stated, "Headaches in the young are for the most part due to bad arrangements in their lives" (4). A milestone in the study of pediatric headache occurred in 1962 when Bille (5) published his data on the frequency of headache in 9,000 school children. More recently, four textbooks and two practice parameters that focus on pediatric headache have been published (4,6–11).

Epidemiology

See references 12 and 13 for a discussion of epidemiology. In the Bille treatise, the entire school age population of Uppsala, Sweden, between the ages of 7 and 15 years of age was studied. It was noted that by 7 years of age 2.5 % of children had frequent tension headaches, 1.4% had migraine, and 35% had infrequent headaches of other varieties. By age 15, 15.5% had frequent tension headaches, 5.3% had migraine, and 54% had frequent headaches of other varieties (5). The frequency of migraines in prepubertal boys is higher than in prepubertal girls. At puberty the frequency of migraine is higher in girls. In adults, the frequency of all types of headaches, except cluster headache, is higher in women. The frequency of chronic migraine, mixed migraine, and tension headache is lowest in children younger than 7 years and increases between the ages of 7 and 12. In children 12 to 18 years of age, chronic headaches are more common than acute episodic migraine alone. The overall prevalence of headache increases quite strikingly in the period from preschool to adolescence. Overall, headache prevalence by 7 years of age is 37% to 51% and at ages 7 to 15 years, from 57% to 82%. The incidence of migraine with aura in boys is 6 per 1,000 and peaks at 5 to 6 years of age. The incidence of migraine without aura in boys is 10 per 1,000 and peaks at 10 to 11 years of age. The incidence of migraine with aura in girls is 14 per 1,000 and peaks at 12 to 13 years of age. The incidence of migraine without aura in girls is 18 per 1,000 and peaks at 14 to 17 years of age.

Epidemiological studies in adults show an association between migraine and anxiety disorders (14,15). Most studies have found a bidirectional relationship, with migraine predicting subsequent depression and depression predicting migraine. The relationship between anxiety disorders and migraine is also bidirectional.

In addition, childhood- or adolescent-onset headaches are associated with depression and anxiety (15). The weight of the evidence suggests that pediatric migraine is associated with depression and that the association is stronger in girls and adolescents. Similarly, the association between pediatric migraine and anxiety seems to be stronger for girls than boys. In boys, there is also some evidence of an association between headaches and disruptive behavior disorders. Although studies are fewer, there appears to be a relationship between chronic daily headaches and depression, anxiety disorders, and suicidal ideation (16).

Classification

The "Second Edition of the International Classification of Headache Disorders" (ICHD), published in 2004, bases its classification on the presumed abnormality, its origin, and its pathophysiology or symptom complex. The criteria are neither specific nor sensitive to the issues of headache in children and adolescents (17).

Authors have reviewed the initial classification and suggested modifications for the pediatric population (18). For example, the duration of headaches in children is shorter than in adults, and many young children have bilateral as opposed to unilateral headaches.

Headache can also be classified as primary or secondary. Primary headaches, such as migraine and cluster, have no underlying pathology; however, migraines frequently have a genetic basis. Secondary headaches are those due to an underlying pathological condition, such as a tumor, hemorrhage, hypertension, collagen vascular disorders, infection, hydrocephalus, trauma, or toxin.

In addition to the ICHD, it is helpful to classify headaches using the temporal pattern of the headache plotted against its severity (19). Four patterns can be identified:

1. Acute
2. Acute recurrent (migraine)
3. Chronic progressive (organic)
4. Chronic nonprogressive (Fig. 7.1), which includes tension-type headaches, chronic daily headaches, mixed migraine, tension headache, and chronic or transformed migraine

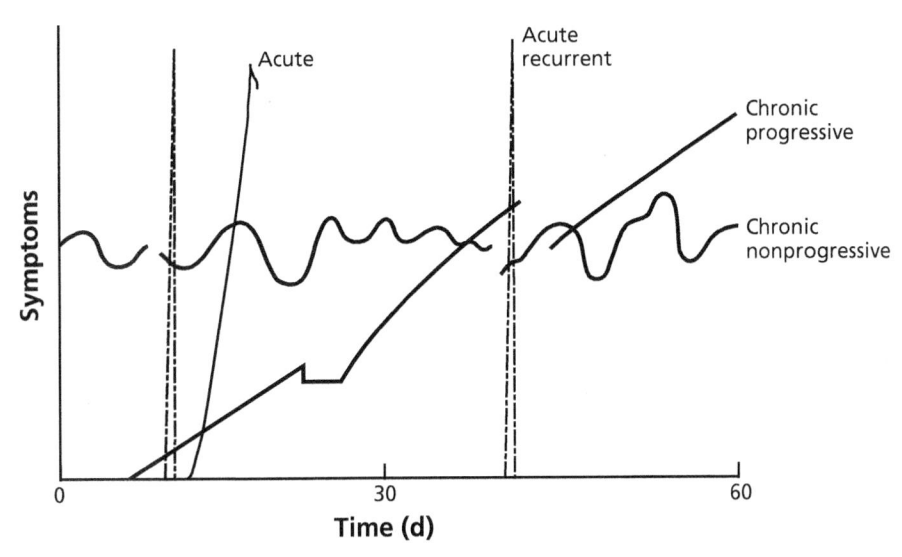

FIGURE 7.1 Types of headaches according to temporal patterns.

An acute headache is a single event with no history of a previous similar event. Most of these headaches are seen in the primary care setting. Many are associated with febrile illness or minor trauma. If the acute headache is associated with neurological symptoms or signs, an organic process should be suspected. The differential diagnosis of an acute headache, both generalized and localized, involves a wide variety of disorders (Table 7.1).

Acute headaches can also be seen in the setting of an emergency room. A summary of four studies indicates that the overwhelming majority of children and adolescents presenting to the emergency room with acute headache do not have serious neurological problems but rather migraine, tension-type headache, non–central nervous system (CNS) infection, or posttraumatic headache (Table 7.2) (20).

Acute recurrent headaches are usually migraines. If a similar headache has occurred and resolved several times, migraine is the most likely diagnosis. These headaches are painful but not life threatening. However, if the migraine is associated with neurological

TABLE 7.1 DIFFERENTIAL DIAGNOSIS OF ACUTE HEADACHE

Acute Generalized	Acute Localized
Systemic infection	Sinusitis
CNS infection	Otitis
Toxic: lead, cocaine	Ocular abnormality
Postseizure	Dental disease
Electrolyte imbalance	Trauma
Hypertension	Occipital neuralgia
Hypoglycemia	Temporomandibular joint dysfunction
Postlumbar puncture	
Trauma	
Embolic	
Vascular thrombosis	
Hemorrhage	
Collagen disease	
Exertional	

CNS, central nervous system.

TABLE 7.2 HEADACHE IN THE EMERGENCY WARD

Non–Life Threatening

Upper respiratory infections, migraines, tension type headache, minor trauma

Life Threatening—Serious

Brain tumor, shunt malfunction, intracranial hemorrhage, meningitis/aseptic meningitis, post seizure, subdural/epidural hemorrhage, toxins/substance abuse

---

symptoms or signs, other potentially life-threatening causes must be considered (Table 7.3).

As time passes, symptoms of increased intracranial pressure, progressive neurological disease, or focal or generalized neurological signs sometimes accompany the headache. As with acute recurrent headaches, if a progressive headache is associated with neurological symptoms or signs, potentially life-threatening causes must be considered (Table 7.4). Although most evolve over time, they may present precipitously.

Chronic nonprogressive headaches are also known as tension-type headaches, muscle contraction headaches, mixed headaches, chronic migraine, transformed migraine, or co-morbid headache. The episodic variety occurs fewer than 10 to 15 days per month and children with it are seldom seen in consultation. If, however, the headaches occur more than 10 to 15 days per month, interfere with normal school and family function, or are associated with medication overuse or excessive school absences, then the patient needs to be evaluated. These headaches are not associated with symptoms of increased intracranial pressure or progressive neurologic disease. They often combine features of tension type and migraine. Examinations of patients are normal both during the headache and between headaches. Laboratory studies are generally nonrevealing. These headaches, although not life-threatening, are among the most refractory to treatment. They are often associated with psychological factors, lifestyle issues, overuse of medications, excessive school absences, and low socioeconomic status.

These headaches are also often associated with other somatic complaints, such as recurrent abdominal pain, musculoskeletal pains, fatigue, and dizziness, and may be the early symptoms of anxiety or depression. Pain symptoms are part of the current *Diagnostic and Statistical Manual of Mental Disorders* (DSM) diagnostic criteria for separation anxiety disorder, pain disorder, generalized anxiety disorder, and somatization disorder. Although not part of the diagnostic criteria for a depressive episode, headaches and other somatic complaints are frequent presenting symptoms of mood disturbance in childhood.

Pathophysiology

Both extracranial and intracranial structures may be sensitive to pain (21,22). Pain from extracranial and intracranial structures from the front half of the skull are mediated via the

TABLE 7.3 ACUTE RECURRENT HEADACHE

Migraine
Tension type headache
Hypertension
Medications
Toxins
Postictal

TABLE 7.4 CHRONIC PROGRESSIVE HEADACHE

Tumor
Pseudotumor cerebri (IIH)
Chronic meningitis/brain abscess
Subdural hematoma
Hydrocephalus
Subacute shunt malfunction

IIH, idiopathic intracranial hypertension.

fifth cranial nerve. Pain from the occipital half of the skull is mediated via the upper cervical nerves. Inflammation, irritation, displacement, traction, dilation, and invasion of any of these pain sensitive structures will cause headache or head pain. However, the child's age, illness, fatigue, nutrition, psychological factors, ethnic factors, and previous experience with pain will modify the child's perception of headache and other pain. The severity of the pain should *not* be taken as an absolute indicator of the severity of the underlying process or even its organicity.

Biochemical, neurotransmitter, and regional cerebral blood flow studies have produced the trigeminal vascular hypothesis for the pathogenesis of migraine. This hypothesis considers migraine an inherited sensitivity of the trigeminal vascular system (21). Cortical, thalamic, or hypothalamic mechanisms initiate an attack in individuals who are genetically predisposed to be sensitive to internal or external stimuli. Impulses spread to the cranial vasculature and brainstem nuclei and produce a cascade of neurogenic inflammation and secondary vascular reactivity. Vascular peptides are released and activate endothelial cells, mast cells, and platelets, which then increase extracellular amines, peptides, and other metabolites that result in sterile inflammation and pain transmitted centrally via the trigeminal nerve.

Spreading depression begins in the visual cortex and propagates to the periphery at a speed of 3mm per minute. The human aura propagates in a similar fashion (22).

Improved understanding of the relationship of headaches to serotonin has resulted in both improved acute and chronic treatments. Serotonin receptors are implicated in constriction of cerebral blood vessels. The antimigraine agents dihydroxy-ergotamine and the triptans have potent activity at the 5HT1D and 5HT1B receptor sites. A number of potent 5HT1 antagonists, such as methysergide, cyproheptadine, amitriptyline, and verapamil, are effective in preventing migraine attacks. In addition, antiepileptic drugs (AEDs) that involve both calcium and sodium channels, such as sodium valproate, topiramate, and gabapentin, are useful in prevention.

The reasons for the association between headaches and psychopathology remain unclear, but there are suggestions that dysregulation of the serotonergic and gamma-aminobutyric acid (GABA)–ergic systems may be involved in migraine, depression, and anxiety. Neural pathways involving the periaqueductal gray have been implicated in pain regulation and receive input from limbic system pathways involved in emotion.

Genetics

Migraine is a familial disorder (23). Many patients with migraine (80%) have a first-degree relative with the disorder. In twins the pairwise concordance was highest for monozygotic twins and less for dizygotic twines. Migraine without aura is a multifactorial disorder with both genetic and environmental contributors. Migraine with aura has a stronger genetic pattern, often transmitted via the mother.

Hemiplegic migraine is often familial. It is a channelopathy resulting from a genetic mutation.

Evaluation

Evaluation of the child or adolescent with headaches is the key to appropriate treatment (10,24). A properly obtained history is necessary to differentiate the various headache types, their etiologies, and their comorbidity. Physicians should conduct a private interview with adolescents regarding physical abuse, sexual activity, sexual abuse, substance abuse, and other personal aspects of their medical, social, and academic history.

The history begins with details of pregnancy, labor, delivery, early childhood development, school function, previous medical problems, previous medications for headache, and the use of medication on a chronic basis for other disorders. Physicians should inquire about over-the-counter as well as prescription medicines. Both the patient and the parent should be questioned regarding anxiety, tension, nervousness, depression, inappropriate behavior, sleep schedules, and school function and absences. The family history should detail any family members with migraine, tension-type headaches, and psychological or psychiatric disorders. A second set of questions deals with the headache itself (Table 7.5).

The third set of questions should deal with symptoms, in addition to headache, of increased intracranial pressure or progressive neurological disease, including, ataxia, other balance problems, excessive lethargy, seizures or loss of consciousness, visual disturbances, focal or generalized weakness, vertigo or dizziness, personality change, loss of abilities, or change in school performance. Physicians should consider potentially ominous etiologies if children have had a change in a previous headache pattern, the severity of the headaches has increased dramatically, or the headache pain awakens them from sleep.

A general physical examination is necessary. If the child psychiatrist does not perform this general examination, the patient should be referred to a primary care physician. Careful attention should be paid to the vital signs, and any abnormality of blood pressure or temperature should be recorded. The skin must be closely examined for striae, rashes, and bruising

TABLE 7.5 INQUIRIES ABOUT HEADACHE

1. Do you have one type or two types of headaches?
2. How did the headache begin?
3. How long has the headache been present?
4. Are the headaches static, intermittent, or progressive?
5. How often does the headache occur?
6. Do the headaches occur at any special time or under special circumstances?
7. Are the headaches related to specific foods, medications, or activities?
8. Are there warning symptoms?
9. Where is the pain located?
10. What is the quality of the pain?
11. Are there associated symptoms?
12. How long does the headache last?
13. What do you do during the headache?
14. What makes the headache better?
15. What makes the headache worse?
16. Do symptoms continue between the headaches?
17. Are you being treated for any other problem?
18. Do you take any medication for any reason regularly or intermittently?
19. Does anyone else in your family have headaches?
20. What do you think is causing your headache?

or neurocutaneous abnormalities, such as café-au-lait spots. Looking for signs of sinusitis and temporal mandibular joint dysfunction, the physician should palpate and auscultate the skull, neck, and sinuses. In the overwhelming majority of patients with tension-type headaches and migraine, the general physical examination reveals no abnormality.

If the child psychiatrist does not perform a neurological examination, the patient should be referred to a pediatric neurologist. The pediatric neurologist must pay special attention to any signs of trauma or nuchal rigidity. The head circumference, optic fundi, eye movements, strength, reflexes, and coordination should be recorded. Children and adolescents with tension headaches and migraine should always have a normal neurological as well as a general physical examination.

Laboratory Studies

The choice of laboratory studies depends on the differential diagnosis. Routine laboratory tests are not helpful in patients with migraine or tension headaches. If, however, the patient is critically ill or the history or examinations suggest the presence of increased intracranial pressure or a progressive neurological disease, testing is necessary.

The electroencephalogram (EEG) is of limited value in the evaluation of headaches. Nonspecific abnormalities are found in normal children, and 9% of children with migraine will have benign focal epileptiform discharges without any evidence of epilepsy (25). If the patient has exhibited loss or alteration of consciousness or abnormal movements, an EEG may be useful. Evoked potentials have no proven value.

The diagnosis of structural CNS disorder has been made both rapid and accurate by the use of computed tomography (CT) and magnetic resonance imaging (MRI) (26). Both techniques are safe, rapid, and accurate in evaluating intracranial contents. They are useful in diagnosing congenital malformations, cranial infections, trauma, neoplasms, and degenerative, neurocutaneous, and vascular disorders. In acute situations, they may be life-saving. Although MRI incurs greater costs, takes longer, and may require sedation, it may demonstrate lesions not visible on the CT scan, including sinus pathology and disorders of white matter and of the craniocervical junction. In the majority of patients with migraine or tension headaches who have no symptoms of progressive neurological dysfunction or increased intracranial pressure and normal neurological examinations, imaging is not required. Imaging in these patients is normal or shows "unrelated" abnormalities.

Psychological Interview and Projective Testing

Questionnaires and psychological tests are useful in individuals with chronic, recurrent, or disabling headaches who are unresponsive to initial treatment (7,27,28). When academic problems coexist, educational testing including intelligence quotient (IQ) and achievement tests may be indicated. Personality testing may be helpful.

Patients with headache frequently exhibit a variety of behavioral symptoms. Lifestyle factors, psychological factors, and learned behavioral patterns often maintain symptoms. Experience and research support the value of headache diaries, structured interviews, self-report measures, and objective psychological testing. Evaluations should assess the pain, the child, and the child's environment. Close attention should be paid to parent-child interaction. Many parents consciously or unconsciously are "enablers" and promote the continuation of the headache. Physicians should emphasize that the headache is genuine and the goal of assessment is to investigate factors that might be causing, worsening, or maintaining the problem.

Specific Headache Syndromes

ACUTE GENERALIZED HEADACHE

Kandt and Levin (29) published a study of 37 children seen in the pediatrician's office for headache: 30% had an infection, such as pharyngitis or otitis. Patients with a family history of migraine are more likely to have headache. Sleep disorders are more common in headache patients.

If an acute headache is associated with neurological symptoms or signs, an organic disorder must be suspected and referral to a pediatric neurologist is indicated. The etiologies of headaches in children and adolescents presenting to the emergency room with headache have been reviewed previously (Table 7.2). Nonserious problems are usually related to respiratory infections, minor trauma, stress, and migraine. (Serious medical conditions represent 3% to 17% of these patients.) Neurological problems include aseptic meningitis, hydrocephalus, postseizure headaches, tumors, pseudotumor cerebri, and CNS infections.

ACUTE RECURRENT MIGRAINE

Migraine is an acute recurrent headache characterized by episodic periodic and paroxysmal attacks of pain, separated by pain-free intervals (30,31). Notably, migraines do not occur daily. Symptoms associated with acute migraine include pallor, irritability, anorexia, abdominal pain, nausea, vomiting, photophobia, phonophobia, and a desire to sleep.

Young children have bifrontal or bilateral headaches that occur more frequently in the afternoon or after school. As children become teenagers, headaches are more frequently unilateral, vomiting is less frequent, and the peak time of occurrence shifts to the morning.

Typical migraines in children and adolescents do not occur daily. Children tend to have one to four attacks per month. The headaches are shorter in duration in children than adults. They usually are relieved by sleep and analgesics. In teenagers, the number of attacks per month increases. The duration of the attacks increases, and the attacks seem more difficult to control. In later adolescence, migraine may be noted to be superimposed on more frequent, almost daily headaches. This syndrome has been referred to as chronic migraine, transformed migraine, comorbid headaches, or mixed headaches.

Several articles have suggested that stress precipitates migraine. Authors have stated that patients with migraine are frequently "different" in terms of their personalities; however, this suggestion has not been well documented. Symptoms of anxiety and depression may precipitate migraine, may be associated with migraine, or may result from migraine.

Migraine has been proposed as a marker for depression in children and adolescents, but most children and adolescents with migraine are unlikely to show clinically significant levels of depression. Patients, however, who have chronic daily headaches or chronic migraine may have depression and or anxiety. Clinical interviews may reveal elevated rates of dysthymia, adjustment disorders, and depressed mood among adolescents with migraine but usually not major depression. It appears that children and adolescents with migraine have more depressive symptoms when compared with peers without headache. A recent study by Bigal et al. (32) showed that in adolescents who have a family history of migraines, the family's economic status has little or no effect; however, in adolescents without a family history of migraines, the family's economic status is associated with a greater prevalence of headache.

There is some reason to believe that the level of anxiety in individuals with recurrent pediatric headache may increase both as they mature and as they have more and more headaches. Children and adolescents with anxiety are likely to experience more frequent and severe headaches. Headache severity increases as anxiety levels increase.

Migraine with aura

Migraine with aura occurs in 15% to 30% of patients with migraine. A visual aura, including brightly colored lights, moving lights, scotomata, and fortification spectra, precedes the headache by 15 to 30 minutes. It often ceases when the actual headache pain begins. Somatic disturbances, such as dysphasia, dysesthesias, hemiplegia, and speech disturbance, may also occur but are transient. Patients describe the headache's location as contralateral to the aura, and the pain as severe and throbbing. The headache is followed by anorexia, abdominal pain, nausea, and vomiting. Children suffering a migraine appear pale, avoid light and noise, and seek sleep because it frequently relieves their pain.

Migraine without aura

Migraine without aura, known as common migraine, is the most prevalent form of migraine in children and adolescents. Although no visual aura occurs, children with these migraines often have autonomic aura, which includes pallor, irritability, lethargy, and personality change. A headache that follows the autonomic aura is usually bifrontal or bitemporal in younger children but unilateral in adolescents. It is throbbing and frequently accompanied by anorexia and nausea. Vomiting occurs frequently in younger children. Sleep often relieves all the symptoms. Episodes usually last approximately 2 hours and occur one to four times per month. However, there is a wide variability in the frequency, severity, and duration of attacks.

COMPLEX MIGRAINE

Paroxysmal headache and transient neurological abnormalities characterize complex migraine (33). The neurological deficits are secondary to both neuronal and vascular factors. Most attacks resolve spontaneously without permanent sequelae. It is important, however, to differentiate complex migraine from more serious intracranial conditions, such as tumor, arteriovenous malformation (AVM), vascular occlusion, or stroke. MRI with MR angiography (MRA) of the cervical and intracranial vessels may differentiate migraine from such conditions. Hypercoagulability may also play a role. Collagen vascular and metabolic diseases are found less frequently. If the child psychiatrist elicits a history of migraine associated with neurological abnormalities, albeit transient, referral to a pediatric neurologist is indicated.

HEMIPLEGIC MIGRAINE

Hemiplegic migraine is the association of recurrent hemiparesis, which usually resolves within 24 hours, and headache that may precede, accompany, or follow the hemiparesis. The differential diagnosis of this disorder includes thromboembolism, AVM, Moya Moya syndrome, metabolic disorders, collagen vascular disease, tumor, and hypercoagulable disorders. Oral contraceptives, hyperlipidemia, and smoking, as well as family history of stroke, may increase the frequency of neurological complications. Even mild head trauma may precipitate hemiplegic migraine. Because three genes have been associated with hemiplegic migraine, if there is a family history of similar disorder, genetic testing is advisable (23).

OPHTHALMOPLEGIC MIGRAINE

Ophthalmoplegic migraine, now termed neuritis of the third nerve, is the association of a complete or incomplete third nerve palsy with an ipsilateral headache. As with other migraine disorders, the headache may precede, accompany, or follow the neurological deficit. In this disorder, the pain is orbital or retro-orbital and the examination reveals a unilateral dilated pupil and lateral deviation of that eye. In addition, the patient may have ptosis and diplopia. MRI with contrast demonstrates hyperintensity of the third nerve that resolves after the syndrome has cleared. It is important to differentiate this disorder from an aneurysm causing headache and a third cranial nerve palsy.

BASILAR ARTERY MIGRAINE

This form of migraine, also called Bickerstaff disease, is identified by recurrent attacks of occipital headache in conjunction with neurological symptoms referable to the cerebellum and brainstem. The symptoms may be unilateral or bilateral. Children with this migraine variant may present with visual symptoms, sensory symptoms, dizziness, vertigo, nausea and vomiting, ataxia, dysarthria, monoparesis, hemiparesis, or quadriparesis. On rare occasions, they lose consciousness. Symptoms usually clear within 24 hours. The differential diagnosis includes epilepsy, vascular disease, and demyelinating disease. EEG, MRI, and MRA may be required to exclude a structural lesion in the cerebellum and brainstem.

CONFUSIONAL MIGRAINE

This disorder, which simulates a toxic encephalopathy, most commonly occurs in adolescents. In it, headache is associated with or followed by confusion and a receptive or expressive aphasia. Attacks clear within 6 to 12 hours. The differential diagnosis of this disorder includes minor head trauma, viral infections, and drug abuse. The evaluation may consist of toxicology screening, electroencephalography, MRI, and a lumbar puncture. Data concerning efficacy of preventive measures in any of these syndromes are not available.

MIGRAINE VARIANTS

Even when headache is not necessarily prominent, migraine variants imply episodic, recurrent, transient neurological events in a known migraine patient, in a patient who will later develop migraine, or in one who has a family history of migraine.

PAROXYSMAL VERTIGO

This syndrome occurs in children between 2 and 6 years of age. The episodes are sudden and brief and consist of an inability to maintain equilibrium. There is no loss of consciousness. Nystagmus may be present. Symptoms last a few minutes. These patients may develop the more common forms of migraine in later years.

PAROXYSMAL TORTICOLLIS

This is a rare disorder that comprises recurrent episodes, lasting from hours to days, of head-tilt with headache, nausea, and vomiting in infants and young children. Many of these children also develop the more common forms of migraine in life in later years.

CYCLICAL VOMITING

This disorder is a periodic syndrome and consists of recurrent episodes of unexplained abdominal pain, nausea, and vomiting. Headache may not be present. The episodes occur periodically, such as once a month, and last 24 hours. The episodes frequently begin late at night or early in the morning. The children vomit multiple times per hour. Daily stomachaches are not cyclical vomiting. Structural gastrointestinal abnormalities and metabolic causes must be excluded. The recurrent episodes may be prevented by prophylactic migraine therapy. Despite this therapy, many continue to have these episodes. Many patients require intravenous (IV) fluids each time. It often remits at puberty. The more common forms of migraine may follow.

ALICE IN WONDERLAND SYNDROME

This rare disorder consists of bizarre visual hallucinations and spatial distortions occasionally associated with migraine. Children describe micropsia, macropsia, and disorders of perception. They rarely seem frightened and often relate the experience with detailed descriptions. Some investigators consider these visual symptoms to be part of a migraine aura. The symptoms may be time-locked to a migraine attack and do not persist. In fact, many patients have no associated headache. Between attacks, patients are free of psychiatric symptoms. This syndrome has been reported with infectious mononucleosis, complex partial seizures, occipital epilepsy, and drug ingestions as well as in psychiatric disorders.

RETINAL MIGRAINE

Patients exhibiting monocular scotomas, blindness, or hemianopia, without headache, are referred to as having *migraine sine hemicrania*. This disorder appears to be more common in girls during adolescence.

EPILEPSY AND MIGRAINE

Epilepsy and migraine are both common disorders and may coexist in a single patient (34,35). The association of episodic headache, nausea and vomiting, and an abnormal EEG has been erroneously termed "epilepsy equivalent." Such episodes are most often actually migraine with an abnormal EEG. Epileptiform EEGs occur in up to 9% of migraine patients, even if they do not have epilepsy. If a patient has altered consciousness or convulsive movements, the diagnosis of epilepsy should be considered. In such cases, prolonged video-EEG monitoring may be necessary.

Management of Migraine

The best approach to the child or adolescent with migraine is based on the patient's age, the frequency and severity of attacks, the presence of an aura, the child's reliability, and the child's attitude toward medication (30,36,37). Physicians must also consider the child's comorbidities, such as anxiety, depression, epilepsy, sleep disorders, obesity, hypertension, and eating disorders. Once physicians assure the patient and parents that there are no serious underlying problems, headaches often become less frequent and less distressing. Physicians often suggest both acute and preventative lifestyle changes, nonpharmacological management, and pharmacological treatments.

LIFESTYLE

Lifestyle issues that must be explored include sleep disorders, eating and dietary issues, school function, school attendance, family issues, and bullying. It is often surprising that modifying existing behaviors can significantly improve headaches. Education of the parents and the child regarding headaches, their causes, and treatments is beneficial.

Many adolescents are sleep deprived and follow erratic schedules. Physicians should identify problems with the patient's falling asleep, snoring, parasomnias, and nocturnal awakenings. Especially because sleep deprivation and schedules are crucial, the physician should impose a 6-week trial of a standard bedtime and arousal time. Dietary habits are also important. Good nutrition should be discussed. Breakfast should not be missed. Foods containing vasoactive substances—alcohol, caffeine, chocolate, aged cheese with tyramine, luncheon meats with nitrates, and foods containing monosodium glutamate (MSG)—should be avoided for a period of 6 to 8 weeks as a therapeutic trial.

Another problem is that adolescents often self-medicate. Abuse of over-the-counter medications promotes rebound headache. Combination medications containing aspirin, caffeine, barbiturates, and narcotics should be avoided.

If the patient's school absences are excessive, further evaluation is indicated. School avoidance may indicate anxiety or a more problematical psychiatric issue.

PHARMACOLOGICAL THERAPY

Pharmacological therapy (11,38,39) can be divided into two stages: (a) suppression of the acute attack and its symptoms of pain, nausea, and vomiting and (b) prophylaxis or prevention of future attacks (Table 7.6).

Suppression of acute symptoms includes pain medications, such as acetaminophen or nonsteroidal anti-inflammatory drugs (NSAIDs), singly or in combination. Physicians should avoid prescribing narcotics and barbiturates. Antiemetics may relieve nausea and vomiting and may allow the patient to take additional medicine by mouth. The sublingual forms, although costly, can be effective and carry few side effects. Promoting sleep with mild sedatives is helpful because sleep often aborts migraines.

Abortive medications include ergotamines, (Midrin, a combination medication that includes isometheptene and acetaminophen), NSAIDs, acetaminophen, and the triptans. There are five "regular" triptans and two long-acting triptans. It should be noted that even though all of these medications are used in adolescents, the Food and Drug Administration (FDA) has specifically approved none for the treatment of migraine patients age 17 or younger.

The authors' preference is to begin with an antiemetic if nausea is severe or vomiting is present. An antiemetic is followed by diphenhydramine, 1 mg per kilogram, and ibuprofen, 10 mg per kilogram. The patient should then go to a dark, quiet room and apply a cold com-

TABLE 7.6 MIGRAINE: SYMPTOMATIC TREATMENT

Medication	Dosage	Comment
Analgesics		
Acetaminophen[a]	10–15 mg/kg/dose q4–6h	Available as suppository
Ibuprofen[a]	4–10 mg/kg/dose q6–8h	No suppository available
Antiemetics		
Trimethobenzamide	15–20 mg/kg/day divided q6h	100-mg/200-mg suppository
Prochlorperazine[b]	0.4 mg/kg/day divided q6–8h	2.5-, 5-, and 25-mg suppository Extrapyramidal reactions

[a]May be used together.

[b]Use with caution.

TABLE 7.7 MIGRAINE: SYMPTOMATIC ABORTIVE[a,b]

Medication	Dosage	Comment
Midrin/Duradrin[a]	2 caps at onset/1 qh × 3	>50 kg = maximum of 5 caps
	1 cap at onset/1 qh × 2	35–50 kg = maximum of 3 caps
Ergot	2 mg sublingual	>50 kg
	May repeat × 1 in 1 h	
Sumatriptan	0.06–0.1 mg/kg subcutaneously	See protocol
	Oral 25 mg	35–50 kg
	Oral 50 mg = 100 mg	>50 kg
	Nasal 5 mg	35–50 kg
Zolmitriptan	Nasal 20 mg	>50 kg
DHE Nasal Spray[a]	2.5–5.0 mg	>50 kg
	As directed	>50 kg

[a]Not approved for children younger than 18 years.

[b]See package insert regarding side effects.

press. If 2 hours later the patient is not improved, the diphenhydramine can be repeated and acetaminophen at 15 mg per kilogram could be added. If after two or three such attacks this regimen is found to be inadequate, consideration can be given to the addition of a triptan (Table 7.7). The parents are informed that the drug is not FDA approved.

The smallest dose of a triptan should be used in conjunction with diphenhydramine and ibuprofen. If 2 hours later the patient is no better, one can add acetaminophen and repeat the triptan. If after several attacks this is insufficient and there are no side effects, the next higher dose of triptan can be carefully considered.

Prophylactic medications should be considered in children or adolescents who have frequent migraines in whom symptomatic or abortive medications are not effective. In particular, they should be considered in children and adolescents who are missing excessive days at school or work or who have frequent or prolonged attacks. These medications should be used for 3 to 6 months and then be slowly tapered. If a specific agent does not work after 6 to 8 weeks, another medication should be substituted.

If the patient has comorbid anxiety or depression, the choice of prophylactic medication should allow for both disorders to be treated with a single medication.

Medications used in preventing migraine include antihistamines, ß-blockers, tricyclic antidepressants, calcium channel blockers, and AEDs. As with abortive migraine drugs, it should be noted that none of these medications have been specifically approved by the FDA for the prevention of migraine in children or adolescents. It should also be noted that if propranolol is being used for migraine prophylaxis, it might aggravate or cause depression. Cyproheptadine may cause somnolence and weight gain. The calcium channel blockers may cause constipation. NSAIDs used as a prophylactic on a daily basis may cause rebound headache or gastric distress. Amitriptyline has been associated with drowsiness, weight gain and prolongation of the QTc interval. Many physicians do an electrocardiogram (ECG) prior to the initiation of that medication (Table 7.8).

NONPHARMACOLOGICAL THERAPY

Nonpharmacological therapy focuses on the elimination of trigger factors, a regular diet, normal sleep patterns, discontinuation of inappropriate and over-used analgesics, stress relief, and use of counseling, relaxation therapy, biofeedback, and yoga (40).

Eliminating foods containing vasoactive substances, as mentioned previously, should be eliminated. Medications that may precipitate or aggravate migraine include vasodilators, bronchodilators, oral contraceptives, and stimulants.

TABLE 7.8 MIGRAINE: PROPHYLACTIC TREATMENT

Drug	Dosage	Side Effects
Cyproheptadine	0.25 mg/kg/day ⅓ in a.m.—⅔ hs	Sedation, appetite stimulation
Propranolol	0.6–1.5 mg/kg/day, divide 2 doses	Cardiac, vivid dreams, depression
Amitriptyline	0.1–2 mg/kg/day hs	Cardiac, sedation
Verapamil	4–8 mg/kg/day; divide 3 doses	Cardiac, constipation
Valproate	10–30 mg/kg/day; divide 2 or 3 doses	Hepatic and pancreatic dysfunction, anorexia or weight gain
Topiramate	25 mg/day to start	Impaired concentration, decreased appetite

Biofeedback has been specifically useful in children and adolescents with migraine, particularly those wishing to avoid using medication. Both muscle relaxation training using electromyogram (EMG) feedback and thermal regulation using hand warming have been successful. When family stress is a contributing factor, family counseling has been useful. When academic failure complicates the situation, remediation and evaluation of learning issues may be helpful.

ALTERNATIVE MEDICINES

Alternative and complementary medications are widely used by the general public but somewhat less so in children (41). Although data supporting their use are sparse, judicious use of these medicines may be helpful in the overall management of the patient.

The most commonly used supplements are riboflavin, magnesium, and coenzyme Q 10. Magnesium oxide is commonly given bid or tid, up to 9 mg/kg/24 hours. Riboflavin (vitamin B_2) is given twice a day up to 400 µg per 24 hours. Coenzyme Q 10 is given three times a day from 100 to 300 mg per day.

Herbals most commonly used include feverfew and butterbur. The strength of preparations varies, and caution should be used when prescribing these substances. Data are limited.

PROGNOSIS

Bille conducted a 40-year follow-up of school children with migraine: 23% were migraine free before 25 years of age. Boys were significantly more often improved than girls. He suggested that 30% of patients will go into remission permanently, 30% will continue having migraine on a regular basis, and 40% will have migraine for a while, go into remission, and then re-experience migraine. Others have suggested that migraine or vascular headaches during childhood evolve into a daily headache syndrome in adults (42). This is called "transformed migraine." This process is exacerbated by overuse of medication, obesity, and psychological factors, such as depression or anxiety.

Chronic Progressive Headaches

If a patient presents with headache that worsens in frequency and severity over time, especially if that headache is associated with symptoms of increased intracranial pressure or an abnormal neurological examination, a pathological intracranial process should be suspected (43). Consultation is necessary.

Pseudotumor cerebri, also known as idiopathic intracranial hypertension (IIH), causes an intermittent or constant headache (44). Pulsatile tinnitus may be present. Papilledema is almost invariably present at the time of the presentation. Markedly increased intracranial pressure causes a sixth nerve palsy. The retinal blind spot enlarges and visual fields constrict. The syndrome is common in both children and adolescents, but in adolescents it is more common in females. Children have no coexisting obesity, but adolescents often have obesity and menstrual irregularity. Potential precipitants include withdrawal of steroid therapy, hypervitaminosis A, and the use of minocycline or outdated tetracycline for the treatment of acne. MRI and neuro-ophthalmology consultation should be obtained. The former is normal, but the latter usually shows an enlarged blind spot and constricted visual fields as well as papilledema. A lumbar puncture should then be performed. The opening pressure is usually elevated above 250 mm of water. Treatment includes repeated lumbar punctures, diuretics, and steroids. Weight loss in an obese patient is invaluable. The patient needs to be monitored closely by an ophthalmologist for changes in visual fields and visual acuity. If the vision is progressively impaired, consideration has to be given to lumbar peritoneal shunting or optic nerve sheath decompression. Patients with this disorder should be referred to a pediatric neurologist for ongoing management.

Chronic Nonprogressive Headaches

Chronic nonprogressive headaches are common in adolescents (45,46). The terminology used for this disorder is variable and changing. Many patients with intermittent migraine, as they use more and more medication, develop transformed migraine. Physicians use various terms for chronic nonprogressive headache, including transformed migraine, chronic migraine, and comorbid headaches. In general, the term "chronic daily headache" refers to a combination of both migraine and tension-type headaches occurring daily.

Bille reported that there were three times more chronic tension-type headaches than migraine by 15 years of age. Chronic daily headache may occur in 1% of adolescents and 4% of adults. It is the most difficult headache type to treat. The clinical features of chronic daily headaches in children are similar to those noted in adults. The headaches are described as frontal and pressure-like or band-like. There is associated tenderness in the occipital and cervical regions. The pain may be present for a portion of the day or the entire day. The pain may be only "moderate" when compared with the severe pain associated with acute migraine. Many adolescents with chronic daily headache continue their activities. Intermittent migraines coexist 5 to 10 days per month. A few patients are bothered by light and noise and mild nausea. Some excessively use over-the-counter medications. Others have stopped taking such medications, as they were not helpful. Many adolescents identify fatigue from erratic sleep and stressful situations at school, at home, or with peers as aggravating factors. The headache impairs their concentration, causes irritability and anxiety, and creates academic difficulties. These headaches rarely awaken patients from sleep, but patients may have problems falling and staying asleep. Food does not seem to play an important role, as it does in migraine. Exercise does not usually exacerbate the headache. Rest may temporarily relieve the headaches. Many of these patients are honor students, and self-imposed stress may play a role. More girls than boys have this disorder. About 15% to 20% have excessive school absences. A minority is home tutored. Most of the patients and their families need help in recognizing lifestyle factors as a major contributor to the headaches. Psychological evaluation and counseling may aid them in recognizing issues that play a role in their headaches.

Inadvertently, many parents actually perpetuate and exacerbate their children's chronic daily headaches by providing secondary gain in the form of attention and relief from responsibilities and household chores.

In contrast to migraines, chronic daily headaches are usually not preceded by an aura and many are bilateral. This pain is frequently described in a vague, nonspecific manner. Associated symptoms may include blurred vision, fatigue, dizziness, and syncope. Except for the headache, patients have no symptoms of increased intracranial pressure or progressive neurological disease. Most have no underlying medical condition. A minority has coexisting chronic fatigue, fibromyalgia, or recurrent abdominal pain. By definition, laboratory studies and neuroimaging are negative.

If the patient has had daily or constant headache for longer than 8 weeks, no symptoms of increased pressure, and a normal general physical and neurological examination, an organic source is unlikely. A psychiatric evaluation is generally appropriate.

Patients with chronic daily headache frequently show a variety of associated psychological and behavioral symptoms (47). Both the psychological factors and learned behavioral patterns are often related to the maintenance of their headache symptom. Although the methodology used for evaluation differs, experience and research support the use of direct and indirect measures, including headache diaries, structured self-report measures, and objective psychological testing. Evaluation should evaluate three core areas: (a) the pain itself, including antecedents, precipitants, and responses; (b) effect on the patient, including global psychological and social function; and (c) the patient's environment, including physical, family, school, and social factors.

Both covert and overt depression, as well as anxiety, occur in patients with chronic daily headaches. The controlled studies indicate significantly more depressive symptoms in these patients compared with headache-free controls, although the strict criteria for depression may not be met. In addition, more anxiety is reported. Stress is variable from individual to individual. What one person considers stressful may seem trivial to another. An individual subjective interpretation of an event may determine how stressful it is and whether intervention would be effective. Factors considered precipitants in children and adolescents with chronic daily headaches include a genetic predisposition, major negative life changes, or life events, including divorce, moving, and death of a close friend or relative. Achievement motivation and fear of failure as well as somatic preoccupation also play important roles. It should be noted that many headache patients are above-average students who, despite doing very well in school or at extracurricular activities, or both, are not attending school. Some headache patients have had previous somatic complaints, including recurrent abdominal pain, limb pain, and fibromyalgia-like symptoms. Pain models in their family may be present.

At the Cleveland Clinic, the psychological evaluation includes standardized testing and a structured interview with the child and at least one parent. Typically, the patient and parents are seen together for a brief overview of the evaluation process and for a general review of the problem and current family situation. The parents are then interviewed separately, as is the patient. The purpose of psychological testing is discussed along with the framework used to understand headache. After the introduction, the parents are interviewed while the patient completes some standardized testing. The patient is then interviewed privately, and the parents may complete standardized forms. Frequently conclusions and recommendations for treatments are discussed with the parents and the patient at the time of the initial visit.

Mental health professionals can be helpful in the treatment of children and adolescents with headaches. Relaxation, self-hypnosis, and coping are efficacious in the long-term treatment of recurrent pediatric headache. Biofeedback may also help in some patients. Potential problems may be the lack of availability of behavioral therapies and limited insurance coverage of behavioral therapies. More research is needed to compare efficacy and combinations of pharmacological and behavioral therapies.

Physicians should consider cognitive behavioral and family therapies for children or adolescents with intractable headaches and psychopathology. Treatment of depression and anxiety may reduce reactivity to stress and thus decrease the frequency and severity of headaches and improve the child's or adolescent's quality of life. Serotonin reuptake inhibitors are first-line agents for treatment of depression and anxiety in children and adolescents. There has been a warning from the FDA that combining selective serotonin reuptake inhibitors (SSRIs) with triptans, agents used in the treatment of acute migraine attacks, might precipitate a serotonin syndrome. However, the data for this recommendation are limited and the risk appears to be small. Tricyclic antidepressants have been used successfully for the preventive therapy of migraine and may have a role in the treatment of anxiety, although there is no evidence of their effectiveness in childhood depression. Cyproheptadine, although possibly efficacious in the prevention of migraine, has been associated with the emergence of depressive symptoms.

Even if overt depression is not present, tricyclic antidepressants, specifically amitriptyline, may be quite useful when combined with psychological interventions. If either overt depression or anxiety is present, specific medications are often useful.

Because many adolescents are sensitive to the side effects of tricyclics, the authors begin amitriptyline with a 5-mg dose, one-half of a 10-mg tablet, at bedtime. Every 2 weeks, the dose is increased by 5 mg until a dose of 20 to 30 mg, which is about 0.5 mg per kilogram, is achieved. The patient is seen in follow-up 6 to 8 weeks after the initial visit. Often the combination of lifestyle changes and low-dose amitriptyline therapy is successful. If, however, significant depression coexists, a child psychiatry consultation is needed. Amitriptyline may cause sedation, dry mouth, postural hypotension, and weight gain. If the dosage is built up slowly and a low dose is ultimately used, these problems can be minimized. An ECG to rule out prolonged QT_C prior to initiating the medication is recommended. Levels are occasionally checked in order to prove compliance.

Daily use of NSAIDs, acetaminophen, analgesics, or caffeine-containing compounds should be avoided. These medications may perpetuate the headache pain. Patients with sensitive or tender muscles may benefit from physical therapy and daily exercise. Trigger-point injections, although not well studied in adolescence, may occasionally be indicated.

The outcome of these therapies in the long-term prognosis in these patients has not been well studied. Because stress, anxiety, and depression seem to participate in the development and maintenance of headache, headache specialists usually recommend the combination of psychological medical intervention and lifestyle changes using a conservative model. Patients must attend school regularly, or they will not get better. At all costs, they should avoid school absences and medication overuse. They also must have 8 hours of sleep at night.

Summary

Chronic headache—at least in some of its syndromes—affects many children and adolescents. A thorough history, physical examination, and neurological evaluation with charting of the temporal pattern of the headache and evaluation of psychosocial factors will usually reveal the correct diagnosis. Laboratory testing in most instances is unnecessary. Psychological factors, important in all headache syndromes, should be evaluated in each and every case. A comprehensive approach to the patient's problem, including medical and psychological factors, will usually result in improvement.

Questions

1. Which of the following statements regarding migraine in children and adolescents is true?
   A. Migraine is more common in prepubertal girls than boys.
   B. Depression and anxiety are comorbid with migraine.
   C. In 50% of children, migraine is associated with an aura.
   D. Migraine is associated with an abnormal EEG.

2. What proportion of children and adolescents with migraine has a family history of migraine?
   A. 20%
   B. 40%
   C. 60%
   D. 80%

3. With which of the following conditions does chronic progressive headache occur?
   A. brain tumor
   B. migraine
   C. hypertension
   D. epilepsy

4. Which of the following statements regarding chronic, nonprogressive headaches is true?
   A. They usually involve a daily combination of tension and migraine type headache.
   B. They are exacerbated by overuse of medications for migraine.
   C. They can impair concentration and interfere with sleep.
   D. All of the above are true.

5. Triggers for migraine include all but which of the following?
   A. Chinese food with MSG
   B. chocolate
   C. bananas
   D. hot dogs

6. In Bille's landmark 40-year follow-up study of school children with migraine, what proportion had permanent remission by adulthood?
   A. 5%
   B. 30%
   C. 60%
   D. 90%

Answers

1. **B.** In children and adolescents, as in adults, depression and anxiety are comorbid with migraine. Migraine is more common in young women than young men. Far fewer than 50% of children with migraine have an aura before a migraine attack.

2. **D**
3. **A**
4. **D**
5. **C**
6. **B**

REFERENCES

1. Rothner AD, Winner P. Headaches in children and adolescents. In: Silberstein S, Lipton R, Dalessio D, eds. *Headache and Other Head Pain*. New York: Oxford; 2001:539–561.
2. Powers SW, Gilman DK, Hershey AD. Suggestions for a psychosocial approach to treating children and adolescents who present with headache. *Headache*. 2006;46(suppl 3):S149–S150.
3. Isler H. Retrospect: the history of thought about migraine from Aretaeus to 1920. In: Blau JN, ed. *Migraine*. London: Chapman and Hall; 1987:659–674.
4. Day WH. *Essays on Diseases of Children*. London: J & A Churchill; 1873.
5. Bille BS. Migraine in school children. *Acta Paediatr Scand*. 1962;51(suppl 136):1.

6. Winner P, Rothner AD, eds. *Headache in Children and Adolescents.* Hamilton and London: BC Decker; 2001.
7. McGrath PA, Hillier LM, eds. *The Child with Headache: Diagnosis and Treatment.* Seattle: IASP Press; 2001.
8. Abu-Arafeh I. *Childhood Headache.* London: Mac Keith Press; 2002.
9. Guidetti V, et al. *Headache and Migraine in Childhood and Adolescence.* London: Martin Dunitz, Ltd; 2002.
10. Lewis DW, et al. Practice parameter: evaluation of children and adolescents with recurrent headaches: report of the Quality Standards Subcommittee of the American Academy of Neurology and the Practice Committee of the Child Neurology Society. *Neurology.* 2002;63:2215–2224.
11. Lewis D, et al. Practice parameter: pharmacological treatment of migraine headache in children and adolescents: report of the American Academy of Neurology Quality Standards Subcommittee and the Practice Committee of the Child Neurology Society. *Neurology.* 2004;59:490–498.
12. Lipton RB. Classification and epidemiology of headaches in children. *Curr Opin Neurol.* 1997;10:231–236.
13. Juang KD, et al. Comorbidity of depressive and anxiety disorders in chronic daily headache and its subtypes. *Headache.* 2000;40:818–823.
14. White KS, Farrell AD. Anxiety and psychosocial stress as predictors of headache and abdominal pain in urban early adolescents. *J Pediatr Psychol.* 2006;31:582–596.
15. Anttila P, et al. Psychiatric symptoms in children with primary headache. *J Am Acad Child Adolesc Psychiatry.* 2004;43:412–419.
16. Wang SJ, et al. Psychiatric comorbidity and suicide risk in adolescents with chronic daily headache. *Neurology.* 2007;68:1468–1473.
17. The International Classification of Headache Disorders, ed 2. Headache Classification Subcommittee of the International Headache Society. *Cephalalgia.* 2004;(suppl 1):1–160.
18. Seshia S, et al. International Headache Society Criteria and childhood headache. *Dev Med Child Neurol.* 1994;36:419–428.
19. Rothner AD. Headaches in children: a review. *Headache.* 1979;19:156.
20. Lewis DW, Queshi FA. Acute headache in the pediatric emergency department. *Headache.* 2000;40:200–203.
21. Goadsby PJ. Migraine pathophysiology. In: Winner P, Rothner AD, editors. *Headache in Children and Adolescents.* Hamilton, ON: BC Decker; 2001:47–59.
22. Moskowitz MA. Basic mechanisms in vascular headache. *Neurol Clin.* 1990;8:801–815.
23. Montagna P. Molecular genetics of migraine headaches: a review. *Cephalalgia.* 2000;20:3–14.
24. Rothner AD, ed. Evaluation of headache. In: *Headache in Children and Adolescents.* Hamilton and London: BC Decker; 2001.
25. Kinast M, et al. Benign focal epileptiform discharges in childhood migraine (BFEDC). *Neurology.* 1982;32:1309.
26. Schwedt TJ, Guo Y, Rothner AD. "Benign" imaging abnormalities in children and adolescents with headache. *Headache.* 2006;46:387–398.
27. Maizels M, Smitherman TA, Penzien DB. A review of screening tools for psychiatric comorbidity in headache patients. *Headache.* 2006;46(suppl 3):S98–S109.
28. Just U, et al. Emotional and behavioral problems in children and adolescents with primary headache. *Cephalalgia.* 2003;23:206–213.
29. Kandt R, Levine R. Headache and acute illness in children. *J Child Neurol.* 1987;2:22.
30. Wasiewksi WW, Rothner AD. Pediatric migraine headache diagnosis, evaluation, and management. *Neurologist.* 1999;5:122–134.
31. Winner P, Lewis D. Clinical features of migraine. In: Guidetti V, Russell G, Sillanpaa M, eds. *Headache and Migraine in Childhood and Adolescence.* London: Martin Dunitz, Ltd; 2002.
32. Bigal ME, et al. Migraine in adolescents: Association with socioeconomic status and family history. *Neurology.* 2007;69:16–25.
33. Rothner AD. Complicated migraine and migraine variants. *Curr Pain Headache Rep.* 2002;4:233–239.
34. Andermann E, Andermann F. Migraine-epilepsy relationships: epidemiological and genetic aspects. In: Andermann FA, Lugaresi E, eds. *Migraine and Epilepsy.* Boston: Butterworth; 1987:281–291.
35. Bigal ME, et al. Epilepsy and migraine. *Epilepsy Behav.* 2003;4(suppl 2):S13–24.
36. Lewis D, Winner P. Migraine, migraine variants, and other primary headache syndromes. In: *Headache in Children and Adolescents.* Hamilton and London: BC Decker; 2001.
37. Rothner AD. Primary care management of headache in children and adolescents. *Headache Manage.* 2002;24(2).
38. Levin DS. Drug therapies for childhood headache. In: McGrath P, Hillier L, eds. *The Child with Headache: Diagnosis and Treatment.* Seattle: ISAP Press; 2001.
39. Winner P, Linder SL, Wasiewski WW. Pharmacologic treatment of headache. In: *Headache in Children and Adolescents.* Hamilton and London: BC Decker; 2001.
40. McGrath P, Stewart D, Koster A. Nondrug therapies for childhood headache. In: McGrath P, Hillier L, eds. *The Child with Headache: Diagnosis and Treatment.* Seattle: ISAP Press; 2001.
41. Holroyd KA, Mauskop A. Complementary and alternative treatments. *Neurology.* 2003;60(suppl 2):S58–62.

42. Monastero R, et al. Prognosis of migraine headaches in adolescents: a 10-year follow-up study. *Neurology.* 2006;67:1353–1356.
43. Cohen BH. Headaches as a symptom of neurological disease. *Semin Pediatr Neurol.* 1995;2:144–151.
44. Gordon K. Pediatric pseudotumor cerebri: descriptive epidemiology. *Can J Neurol Sci.* 1997;24:219–221.
45. Rothner AD. Miscellaneous headache syndromes in children and adolescents. *Semin Pediatr Neurol.* 1995;2:159–164.
46. Powers SW, Gilman DK, Hershey AD. Headache and psychological functioning in children and adolescents. *Headache.* 2006;46:1404–1415.
47. Trautmann E, Lackschewitz H, Kroner-Herwig B. A review. Psychological treatment of recurrent headache in children and adolescents—a meta-analysis. *Cephalalgia.* 2006;26:1411–1426.

CHAPTER 8

Pediatric Brain Tumors

DAVID L. KAYE, PATRICIA K. DUFFNER,
AND MICHAEL E. COHEN

Background

Intracranial tumors are the second most common malignancy in childhood (exceeded only by leukemia) and are the leading cause of cancer-related deaths in this age group. In 1992, when the first edition of this book was published, the incidence of malignant brain tumors in children younger than 15 years (Third National Cancer Survey) was 2.4 per 100,000 (1). In the period 1990 to 1994 the Central Brain Tumor Registry of the United States (CBTRUS) reported an incidence of brain tumors in children 0 to 19 years as 3.77 per 100,000, and most recently, the incidence in the same age group had risen to 4.3 per 100,000 (2). CBTRUS reported that in 2005 the number of newly diagnosed nonmalignant and malignant brain tumors in children 0 to 19 in the United States was 2,590. This overall increase in reported cases has been reflected in individual tumor types, including a rise in the incidence of ependymomas in children younger than 2 years and in astroglial tumors in children younger than 4 years (3). Part of the increase in the reported incidence may reflect enhanced neuroimaging of benign tumors, which might previously have been misdiagnosed on computed tomography (CT) scan as encephalomalacia. The possible role of environmental factors in the increasing incidence of brain tumors is being explored.

Although the incidence of brain tumors may be rising, the survival of children with certain types of brain tumors is also increasing. Today children with average-risk medulloblastomas have an 80% progression-free survival, those with high-risk medulloblastomas have progression-free survivals of 60% to 80%, and children with cerebral low-grade gliomas have 80% progression-free survivals (4). In general, children have significantly better survivals than adults. Five-year survival of children 0 to 19 years reported by the SEER (Surveillance Epidemiology and End Results) registries was 64.8%, compared with 10.7% for patients 55 to 64 years of age (2).

Brain tumors occur more commonly in children 0 to 4 years, in whom the incidence is 5.0 per 100,000, compared with children in the 10- to 14-year and 15- to 19-year age groups, in whom the incidence is 3.9 per 100,000. There is also a difference according to gender, as brain tumors are more common in boys than in girls (4.5 vs. 4.0 per 100,000), and they are also more common in white children than black children (4.5 vs. 2.9 per 100,000) (2).

The current World Health Organization classification of brain tumors is based on site, histologic type, and degree of malignancy. One fourth of all brain tumors in children are benign, a much lower percentage than in adults. Gliomas, the most common histological grouping in children, refer to any neoplasm deriving from interstitial tissue cells of the nervous system and include such diverse tumors as astrocytomas, oligodendrogliomas, ependymomas, and glioblastoma multiforme among others. Medulloblastomas are the next most common histopathological grouping. Among children 0 to 14 years of age, the most common histopathological groupings are pilocytic astrocytomas (21%) and embryonal tumors, including medulloblastomas (17%). In contrast among the 15- to 19-year group, pilocytic astrocytomas represent 15% of tumors, whereas embryonal tumors, including medulloblastomas, represent only 6%. The most common sites for brain tumors in children 0 to 19 years are the brainstem and cerebellum (31%), followed by the cerebral hemispheres (25.6%) (2).

The survivals of children with certain types of brain tumors have steadily increased over the past 20 years. The most striking increase has been in children with standard-risk medulloblastomas whose current survivals are approximately 80% (5). These improved survivals, however, are by no means found in all children. Children with diffuse intrinsic pontine gliomas still face almost certain death within 2 years. Most of the improved survivals are due to advances in surgery, anesthesia, radiation techniques, and the advent of chemotherapy. As a result, there are now an increasing number of long-term survivors who are at risk for sequelae including cognitive decline, endocrinopathies, second tumors, leukoencephalopathy, and vasculopathy. Most centers therefore use a multidisciplinary team approach toward these children. Members of the team include neurologists, oncologists, neurosurgeons, radiation therapists, psychiatrists, psychologists, endocrinologists, pediatricians, and social workers.

Signs and Symptoms

NONLOCALIZING SYMPTOMS

The signs and symptoms of brain tumors reflect the location and nature of the tumor, the age and development of the child, the neurological system with which the tumor interferes, and the presence or absence of increased intracranial pressure. A number of symptoms associated with brain tumors are considered nonlocalizing. For example, signs of increased intracranial pressure may result from obstruction of cerebrospinal fluid (CSF) pathways or a mass growing within a fixed volume. Symptoms of increased intracranial pressure may be delayed, however, due to the ability of the young child to expand the skull. Young children may therefore present with a biphasic pattern of illness, in which temporary relief of symptoms accompanies sutural diastasis, rather than with the relentless progression of symptoms present in older children.

The nonlocalizing symptoms of increased intracranial pressure include headache, vomiting, diplopia, and personality change. Headache is a particularly important symptom. Although most children with headaches do not have an intracranial mass lesion, certain warning signs should alert the examiner to this possibility (6–10) (Table 8.1).

TABLE 8.1. HIGH-RISK HEADACHE WARNING SIGNS

- Headaches that wake the child from sleep or occur first thing in the morning
- Persistently focal headaches
- Headaches of less than 6 months' duration
- Headaches associated with nausea and vomiting (especially in the absence of a family history of migraine)
- Headaches that increase with Valsalva maneuvers
- Headaches that are associated with confusion, disorientation, or abnormal neurological findings

In general, most children whose headaches are due to brain tumors typically develop other neurological symptoms or have findings on neurological examination particularly involving the extraocular movements or fundi by 8 weeks following onset of symptoms, and most assuredly within 4 to 6 months (11). Chronic headaches of long duration are rarely associated with intracranial neoplasms.

Nausea and vomiting, also important nonlocalizing symptoms of intracranial mass lesions, may reflect either increased intracranial pressure or direct irritation of the vomiting center in the floor of the fourth ventricle. In general, vomiting occurs in the morning and then improves as the day progresses. As noted earlier, headaches associated with vomiting are of concern if there is no family history of migraine. Persistent or recurrent vomiting should suggest intracranial pathology and merits a neurodiagnostic evaluation.

Recent personality change occurs commonly with brain tumors and may be associated with tumors in a variety of locations, not just the supratentorial region. Lethargy, irritability, and apathy are typically present. The tendency of a child to withdraw, become indifferent to playmates, or refuse to participate in play or school activities may indicate depression, but these symptoms are also seen in the context of organic disease. A deterioration in academic functioning is also commonly observed. Although these symptoms are frequently observed at presentation, they are usually seen along with other neurological signs and symptoms. An emotional, behavioral, or school-related symptom is the first symptom noted in a small percentage (up to 10%) of children with brain tumors (8). It is the extremely rare child who presents solely with these symptoms and no other neurological sign or symptom. In addition to the frequent personality changes noted previously, children with brain tumors may present with specific psychiatric disorders. A wide range of psychiatric disorders has been reported in the medical literature in association with central nervous system (CNS) tumors. These include changes in mentation, delirium, and agitation, which may be nonspecific and reflect intracranial pressure. Other cases mimicking obsessive-compulsive disorder (12), psychosis, mania, depression, and/or anorexia nervosa (13) have also been reported in children; schizophrenia, panic, and other anxiety disorders have also been reported in adults. Anorexia, bulimia, somnolence, failure to thrive, sexual precocity, or symptoms of an autonomic nature also raise the suspicion of disease of the hypothalamic-pituitary axis. The caveat resulting from these observations is that in the assessment of a new-onset acute or subacute psychiatric illness in a child, a careful history and neurological examination are essential in excluding an organic etiology.

NONLOCALIZING SIGNS

Nonlocalizing signs of increased intracranial pressure include papilledema, sixth nerve palsy, and increasing head circumference. Papilledema should always suggest increased intracranial pressure. Early signs of papilledema are an increase in the blind spot and/or loss of color vision in the presence of normal visual acuity. In contrast, visual loss and optic atrophy may indicate long-standing increased intracranial pressure.

Sixth nerve palsy, causing an inability to abduct the affected eye, is associated with diplopia. It is considered a nonlocalizing sign, as it can develop due to compression of the nerve against bony prominences resulting from diffuse increased intracranial pressure.

Although this chapter does not focus on infants and very young children, it is still important to recognize that in young children skulls will expand to accommodate a mass lesion, and as such, attention should be paid not just to the absolute head circumference but to the changing of percentiles as well.

LOCALIZING SIGNS AND SYMPTOMS

Cerebral hemispheres

The most common tumors in this location are astrocytomas, anaplastic astrocytomas, glioblastoma multiforme, primitive neuroectodermal tumors, ependymomas, oligodendrogliomas, and meningiomas. Supratentorial tumors tend to present later, with increased intracranial pressure, than those arising in the posterior fossa. This is because with cerebral hemisphere tumors, signs of pressure reflect tumor bulk rather than obstruction of CSF pathways.

Headaches are a very common presenting symptom in patients with tumors of the cerebral hemispheres. At times a focal headache can be highly correlated with tumor location, but diffuse headaches, due to increased intracranial pressure, are more common.

Because certain supratentorial tumors, such as oligodendrogliomas and desmoplastic neuroepithelial tumors, are extremely epileptogenic in nature, seizures are frequently the presenting symptom. Those tumors located in the sensorimotor region tend to be particularly epileptogenic. Most seizures are either partial seizures with simple or complex symptomatology, with or without secondary generalization. Seizures tend to be a good prognostic sign, as they occur more commonly with low-grade rather than high-grade tumors. Although most children with seizures do not have mass lesions, tumor should be suspected in those patients with long-standing seizure disorders who undergo changes in school performance or behavior, change in type or frequency of seizure, an alteration on neurological examination, or development of a slow-wave dysrhythmia on electroencephalogram (14).

Other signs and symptoms of supratentorial mass lesions include motor, sensory, and hemianopic defects. Because most brain tumors are compressive rather than destructive, motor abnormalities can be subtle and may reveal only a pronator drift, decreased arm swing, or slight dragging of the leg as opposed to the dense hemiparesis arising from a cerebrovascular accident.

Midline tumors

Midline tumors include optic pathway tumors, hypothalamic tumors, thalamic tumors, craniopharyngiomas, pineal tumors, and ventricular tumors. Optic pathway tumors and hypothalamic tumors are typically juvenile pilocytic astrocytomas. They are commonly associated with abnormalities of the visual axis and endocrinopathies. Visual loss may reflect either direct involvement of the optic nerves or chiasm or may be due to optic atrophy arising from chronic increased intracranial pressure. The presence of nystagmus in a young child, often associated with a chiasmatic mass, may erroneously be attributed to congenital nystagmus or spasmus nutans (15). Visual field abnormalities may be a sign of a craniopharyngioma, chiasmatic tumor, or a lesion compressing the optic tracts or radiations.

Endocrine dysfunction may include weight loss or weight gain. Weight loss is typical of infants with the diencephalic syndrome due to a tumor in the hypothalamus (16), whereas older children may experience an increase in weight due to damage to the satiety center in the hypothalamus. Other endocrinopathies include diabetes insipidus, growth failure, and hypothyroidism.

Precocious puberty is another endocrinopathy that should raise the suspicion of CNS disease. Children with certain pineal tumors have excessive androgen effects. Therefore minimal testicular enlargement will be found in the presence of a large penis; axillary, inguinal, and facial hair; and increase in both bone age and longitudinal growth. In contrast, males with precocious puberty secondary to hypothalamic lesions tend to have large testes with other signs of sexual precocity.

Children with pineal region tumors may present with Parinaud syndrome (failure of upward gaze, pupils that react better to accommodation than direct light, lid retraction, and convergence or retraction nystagmus). In addition, these children may have hydrocephalus, ataxia, pyramidal signs, and obtundation.

Children with craniopharyngiomas may present with signs and symptoms of increased intracranial pressure, endocrinopathies, and visual field defects (17).

Posterior fossa tumors

The posterior fossa is the most frequent location of tumors in childhood. Cerebellar astrocytomas, medulloblastomas, ependymomas, and brainstem gliomas are the most common posterior fossa tumors that develop in childhood. Children with tumors in the cerebellum typically present with disorders of coordination. Tumors in the midline tend to be associated with truncal ataxia, whereas tumors in the cerebellar hemispheres are more likely associated with appendicular ataxia. Scanning speech, hypotonia, pendular reflexes, and skew deviation of the eyes are less common. Patients with tumors of the cerebellum typically present with signs and symptoms of increased intracranial pressure due to obstruction of the fourth ventricle or aqueduct of Sylvius. In children, cerebellar astrocytomas tend to be diagnosed later than medulloblastomas, which are more malignant.

Children with tumors in the pons have the typical triad of cranial neuropathies, cerebellar signs, and long tract signs. Because of the tumor's location on the ventral aspect of the pons, increased intracranial pressure occurs either late or not at all. Tumors in the midbrain, in contrast, are typically associated with increased intracranial pressure due to obstruction of the aqueduct of Sylvius, whereas medullary and cervicomedullary tumors are associated with bulbar signs, spasticity, and ataxia.

Ependymomas of the fourth ventricle tend to occur in very young children. They present with signs and symptoms of increased intracranial pressure as well as cranial neuropathies arising from compression or invasion of the floor of the fourth ventricle. Truncal ataxia is also common.

Neurological Evaluation

All children presenting with histories suggestive of intracranial structural disease require a complete examination by a neurologist, including comprehensive history, physical examination, and neuroimaging studies. Although CT scans provide a good screening test for children with headaches but no warning signs on examination, magnetic resonance imaging (MRI) is the procedure of choice when a brain tumor is suspected (18).

The evaluation of a child with a brain tumor consists of MRI of the brain with and without gadolinium and, in those tumors that seed the CSF, MRI of the neuraxis. In addition, examination of the CSF for abnormal cytology as well as tumor markers (in the case of pineal region tumors) completes the initial workup in most cases (19). Because medulloblastomas can occasionally metastasize to the bone marrow and bones, bone marrow aspiration and radionuclide bone scans are performed at baseline.

MR angiography can also be helpful in identifying vascular lesions, thus eliminating the need in most cases for more invasive angiography. MR spectroscopy has been used to identify tumor, determine response to therapy, and distinguish tumor from necrosis (20).

Surveillance neuroimaging of the neuraxis in children with tumors that have the potential to seed the CSF (e.g., medulloblastomas) is typically recommended on national cancer group studies. Although it is unclear how much early identification affects survival of those children who have already received radiation therapy, most investigators believe that early identification of metastatic disease is indicated (21).

Medical-Surgical Treatment

Surgery is the first approach to the treatment of almost all brain tumors. The only exceptions are the optic pathway tumor, especially in children with neurofibromatosis, some tectal tumors, and the diffuse intrinsic pontine glioma. In all other cases, surgery permits pathological confirmation of the tumor, relief of pressure, opening of CSF pathways, and removal of tumor, allowing adjuvant treatment to be more effective. In the past 10 years it has become abundantly clear that a gross total removal of tumor is associated with significantly better survivals for children with medulloblastomas and ependymomas. In some tumors such as cerebellar astrocytomas, meningiomas, choroid plexus papillomas, and optic gliomas (in those children with complete visual loss), a complete resection is associated with a cure without need for further therapy. With the advent of the operating microscope, CT- and MRI-guided surgery, microdissection, and the laser, tumors that previously were considered too dangerous to approach due to their location can be safely biopsied and either removed or at least subtotally resected.

Radiation remains the standard therapy for brain tumors in older children and adolescents. Because of concerns about the long-term effects of radiation, however, a number of modifications have been instituted. For example, children with average-risk medulloblastoma—that is, treated with gross total resection, age older than 3 years, and no metastases—are now treated with reduced-dose radiation to the neuraxis (2400 cGy vs. 3600 cGy) coupled with chemotherapy. This approach has led to no decline in survivals. Indeed, although there are no studies in which standard-dose radiation is compared with reduced neuraxis radiation plus adjuvant chemotherapy, survivals approach 80% (5).

Another change in radiation treatment involves the volume of radiation. Three-dimensional (3-D) conformal radiation to the tumor bed is now standard for children with ependymomas and infants with medulloblastomas. Hyperfractionation, in which radiation is delivered twice daily in smaller doses, has also been used in several brain tumor trials. All of these changes reflect the concerns of the neuro-oncology community regarding the delayed neurocognitive toxicity of radiation. Recently, several studies have incorporated radiation sensitizers such as carboplatin (22).

Chemotherapy is given in an adjuvant fashion on most of the national cancer cooperative group studies today. For some tumors, such as glioblastoma multiforme and primitive neuroectodermal tumors, chemotherapy is given along with full-dose radiation. In children with average-risk medulloblastomas, the use of adjuvant chemotherapy has allowed a reduction in the dose of radiation delivered to the neuraxis. In the case of germinomas, the volume of radiation can be significantly reduced if adjuvant chemotherapy is administered. The most commonly used agents for high-grade tumors are cyclophosphamide, cisplatin, etoposide, vincristine, and the nitrosoureas (BCNU or CCNU). In addition to being given in an adjuvant role, chemotherapy is now the primary therapy for young children with low-grade tumors, that is, optic pathway and hypothalamic tumors. The most common chemotherapeutic agents for this group are carboplatinum, vincristine, etoposide, vinblastine and temozolomide. For many of these children, chemotherapy has permitted a delay of radiation therapy and, in some cases, has completely eliminated the need for it. Chemotherapy not only is given as the primary postoperative therapy for low-grade tumors but has become an important primary treatment for infants and young children with malignant brain tumors (23). In these studies, radiation therapy has been delayed, eliminated completely, or limited to small volume (conformal radiation) to the tumor bed. Most recently, very high dose chemotherapy with either bone marrow transplantation or peripheral stem cell support has become a focus of investigators.

Long-term Outcome

Children's lives are impacted by brain tumors in multiple domains. Over time, disruptions occur in neurological, endocrinological, neurocognitive, psychosocial, and psychiatric functioning. Second primary malignancies may occur. Indeed, studies of health-related quality of life indicate that the vast majority of survivors of pediatric brain tumors have deficits in multiple domains of functioning. Of all child cancer survivors, pediatric brain tumor survivors have some of the poorest outcomes (24–27).

NEUROLOGICAL STATUS

Survivors of pediatric brain tumors frequently have at least one neurological sequela in the years following recovery (25,26,28,29). Ataxia, hemiparesis and hemiplegia, epilepsy, slowed speech, and visual impairments are the most common difficulties. A number of studies suggest that many of these children experience significant pain. Perhaps up to one fourth have multiple neurological disabilities.

ENDOCRINOPATHY

Endocrinopathies are another important late effect of radiation therapy and chemotherapy. The most common is growth hormone deficiency. Approximately 80% of children who receive craniospinal radiation therapy will develop growth failure. The resulting growth hormone deficiency is primarily due to radiation damage to the ventromedian nucleus of the hypothalamus (growth hormone releasing factor). Growth failure is also related to radiation damage to the vertebral bodies, especially when young children receive neuraxis radiation (30). Other contributing factors to growth failure include untreated hypothyroidism, poor nutrition, and precocious puberty. No data support the concept that treatment with growth hormone will lead to early tumor relapse (31,32). Although growth hormone treatment is not as effective as in children with idiopathic growth hormone deficiency, it should be instituted promptly or children irradiated for brain tumors will not reach their appropriate adult height. Treatment to delay fusion of the epiphyses in those children who develop precocious puberty will also increase adult height.

Another important endocrinopathy that develops as a result of radiation therapy is hypothyroidism. Approximately 30% of children who have received craniospinal radiation will develop primary hypothyroidism as a result of radiation to the thyroid gland. Adding chemotherapy may increase the incidence to 60%. A smaller number of children will develop secondary or tertiary hypothyroidism. Complications of hypothyroidism include lethargy, poor school performance, and growth failure.

Patients treated for brain tumors may also develop gonadal dysfunction. Boys treated with cyclophosphamide may develop oligospermia or even azospermia. Girls may develop ovarian dysfunction from spinal radiation.

ONCOGENESIS

Radiation therapy and chemotherapy are known to predispose to second malignancies. Radiation to the brain, even in low doses, has been associated with the development of meningiomas and gliomas. Second primary tumors tend to be biologically aggressive and are often poorly responsive to treatment. They usually occur within the radiation port with a latency of 5 to 25 years. Gliomas tend to occur earlier (median of 9 years from original diagnosis) compared with meningiomas (17 years). Children who are irradiated before 5 years of age are at the greatest risk for developing gliomas (33). In addition to intracranial tumors and intraspinal tumors, radiation to the neuraxis is associated with the development of thyroid carcinoma (34). Chemotherapy, particularly the alkylating agents and the topoisomerase inhibitors, has been associated with the development of leukemia and myelodysplastic syndrome. As more chemotherapy is used in children with brain tumors, the incidence of second malignancies has risen (35).

NEUROCOGNITIVE DEFICITS

As the survivals of children with certain types of brain tumors have increased, attention has been increasingly directed toward the assessment of long-term survivors who may suffer from the adverse effects of CNS therapy. Most of the early research focused on the effects of cranial irradiation on cognition. More recently the role of chemotherapy in cognitive decline has also been a source of study.

Beginning in the 1980s, several investigators reported that children who had received cranial irradiation as treatment for their brain tumors were experiencing cognitive difficulties. Moreover, the cognitive decline became progressively worse over at least a decade (36,37). Subsequently, investigators identified several risk factors for this iatrogenic dementia including perioperative morbidity, especially the posterior fossa syndrome, supratentorial location of tumor, young age at time of radiation, large-volume radiation, and high-dose radiation. Those children who developed radiation vasculopathy or leukoencephalopathy were at especially high risk. Another risk factor contributing to cognitive decline includes seizures and the consequent anticonvulsant therapies these children receive.

Until recently, most chemotherapy was considered to have acute adverse effects but no delayed neurotoxicity. The exception was thought to be methotrexate, which has been associated with causing a decline in intelligence quotient (IQ) and the development of white matter changes on MRI in both children with leukemia and those with brain tumors, even in the absence of treatment with cranial irradiation (38,39). A recent study by Dietrich et al. (40), however, has demonstrated that other chemotherapeutic agents, in dosages comparable to those given in the clinical arena, are toxic to neural progenitor cells and oligodendrocytes. The agents that investigators studied included BCNU and cisplatin, both agents frequently used in the treatment of children with brain tumors. As most treatment regimens employ both radiation therapy and chemotherapy, it is difficult to determine the role of each in cognitive decline. Because the primary concern has been with cranial irradiation, attempts have been made to reduce the dose of radiation to the neuraxis from 3600 to 2400 cGy for children with average-risk medulloblastoma. Unfortunately, this reduction in radiation dose was associated with an increased risk of early relapse, early isolated neuraxis relapse, and both lower 5-year event-free survivals and overall survivals than those seen with standard radiation (41,42). A subsequent trial added chemotherapy (CCNU, CDDP, and vincristine) to the regimen of reduced neuraxis radiation, with resulting excellent survivals (43). However, there was still a 15- to 20-point decline in IQ for most patients (44). Future studies plan to reduce the dose of radiation to the neuraxis even further to 1800 cGy, without taking into consideration the possible role that chemotherapy may be playing in the cognitive decline.

Although the cause of treatment-induced dementia is not clear, there appears to be an association between cognitive decline and white matter loss (45). Mulhern et al. (46) studied children treated with radiation, with and without chemotherapy, using quantitative MRI and were able to correlate white matter loss with cognitive deficits. The white matter loss was attributed to damage to oligodendrocytes and endothelial cells. Whether treatment with chemotherapy alone would have produced the same findings is not yet known, although Noble's work suggests that it seems likely.

The specific neuropsychological deficits identified in brain tumor patients vary widely, but the greatest reported difficulties are in attention, memory (especially short-term and visuospatial memory, less so for long-term verbal memory), visuospatial organization, processing speed, and executive functioning (47–49). Some have suggested that mathematics is a particular problem, but this finding is not universal. There is a growing acceptance that the decline in IQ scores that occurs in very young children who have been irradiated for brain tumors is not due to loss of knowledge but rather a delay in acquiring new information in an age-appropriate fashion (50–52).

In summary, pediatric brain tumor survivors generally experience cognitive decline. The degree of cognitive decline is variable, with some (especially those diagnosed in adolescence) showing little effect and others showing catastrophic declines. An average child loses 10 to 20 overall IQ points, with deficits mostly in the areas of attention, memory, processing speed, visuospatial organization, and executive functioning. Many factors contribute to this decline, including, foremost, early CNS irradiation but also including other factors related to the tumor, surgery and its complications, exposure to chemotherapy, seizures, and anticonvulsant therapies.

PSYCHOSOCIAL FUNCTIONING

Pediatric brain tumor (PBT) survivors have substantial difficulties at school and with peer relationships. Primarily as a result of cognitive changes already reviewed, as well as school absences for illness and treatment, PBT survivors generally require special education accommodations, services, and supports (29,53). They often have academic difficulties and educational testing has documented delays in reading, math, spelling, and writing scores. Chronic absences are not unusual and complicate academic achievement further. Despite these academic difficulties, these children do not present behavioral problems in the school setting. The vast majority of PBT survivors qualify for academic supports under Individuals with Disabilities Education Act (IDEA), and an individualized education plan (IEP) should be in place for these children and adolescents. In the long term, PBT survivors less frequently graduate from college and have limitations in their employability and work histories (53–55). Often they are not able to work in full-time competitive employment (56–60). Aside from academic and vocational concerns, peer relationships often change. Survivors are often described as more passive and withdrawn, leading more frequently to social isolation and being "left out" (61–64). Being bullied is sometimes noted but is not apparently widespread. Often friendship patterns change during the school years as established friendships drop off. As children reach adolescence and beyond, new friendships often emerge and a social niche is more easily found. Nevertheless, the elementary and middle school years can be socially painful. As survivors reach adulthood, they live independently and marry less frequently than their age mates (56–59,65).

PSYCHIATRIC STATUS

Although many studies have assessed the mental health of survivors, the vast majority have used general mental health parent- or self-report screening checklists, such as the Child Behavior Checklist as the sole measurement. These studies generally document that, compared with a control population, survivors in the immediate, short term, and longer term have higher rates of mental health or emotional problems, although these rates vary widely (25% to 92%) (66). Typically, internalizing problems are found, with anxiety, depression, withdrawal, and passivity noted most commonly. It is unusual in these studies to note suicidal ideation or behavior in survivors, but recent studies have suggested there may be an increased rate of both suicidality and completed suicide in adult survivors of childhood cancer (67,68). No studies have investigated these issues specifically in PBT survivors. Externalizing problems also appear to be unusual. From a narrower psychiatric perspective, no studies have used diagnostic interviews or standardized instruments to assess for psychiatric disorder in large samples of PBT patients. As a result, little is known about rates or types of specific disorders. In a related study Ross et al. (69) reviewed the records of all 3,710 Danish pediatric cancer patients who had survived at least 3 years to ascertain rates of psychiatric hospitalization. Of the total cohort, 978 were PBT survivors. Using national registry data, they followed up all cases for a mean of 15 years or until death. Although there was no increase in rates of psychiatric hospitalization for the cohort as a whole, the brain tumor survivors had more than a twofold increase in the rates of hospitalization (nearly 9% had been hospitalized). Discharge diagnoses suggested elevated rates of schizophrenia and psychotic disorders, although exposure to radiation therapy did not increase the risk of hospitalization. No other studies have investigated or confirmed these findings.

Psychosocial and Neuropsychiatric Treatments

As the number of survivors has increased there is a need for the development of treatments to address the psychosocial and neuropsychiatric difficulties of PBT survivors. Multiple treatment approaches have been described in the literature, primarily within the past 5 years. These treatment approaches have targeted the emotional stressors associated with having a life-threatening illness, the social difficulties, and the neurocognitive deficits of survivors. Psychosocial interventions have been developed to address the emotional stressors and the social difficulties, whereas cognitive retraining efforts and psychotropic medications have been used to have an impact on neurocognitive deficits.

PSYCHOSOCIAL APPROACHES TO TREATMENT

Although few investigators have developed psychosocial approaches specifically for PBT survivors, a number have done so for childhood cancer survivors in general. Most of these approaches have targeted both families and the child survivor. A recent meta-analysis (70) suggests that current psychosocial interventions are modestly effective in diminishing distress and improving adjustment for parents, although few effects have been noted for the child survivors. A promising approach has considered childhood cancer through the lens of post-traumatic stress disorder (PTSD). Stuber et al. (71) suggested that although a full PTSD syndrome is not typical, many children and parents respond to cancer as a repeated trauma and report posttraumatic symptoms. Kazak et al. (72) has referred to this as pediatric medical traumatic stress (PMTS) and has developed a model treatment approach for children and their families. This approach posits three phases of medical traumatic stress (73). The first phase (phase I) includes the stress associated with the early symptoms and diagnosis of cancer. The National Child Traumatic Stress Network has created a set of materials for health care providers aimed at phase I and the prevention of PMTS. (These resources can be accessed online at http://www.nctsnet.org/nccts/nav.do?pid=typ_mt_ptlkt.) Phase II includes the ongoing stress associated with the sequelae of the cancer and its treatment. Phase III refers to the later and longer term stressors that occur after the initial shock and acute threat have subsided. Approaches to phase II and III include family-based psychoeducational and cognitive-behavioral interventions. Initial data support the effectiveness of this approach (74,75) for both parents and adolescent survivors.

The social skills deficits of PBT survivors are another potentially fruitful area for intervention. Although these are frequently noted in the literature, few approaches have been described to assist PBT survivors. Notably, social deficits are not typically found in children with chronic illness in general and cancer in particular (76,77). The social skills deficits of PBT survivors are likely related to compromise of the CNS and neurocognitive changes. Barakat et al. (78) developed a specific social skills training group for PBT survivors and piloted a study that showed encouraging results for improving social skills.

School and vocational difficulties have been identified in PBT survivors, but no psychosocial interventions have been described in the literature. This would be another rich area for future research.

NEUROCOGNITIVE APPROACHES TO TREATMENT

Neurocognitive approaches include both cognitive remediation and psychopharmacology. Cognitive remediation is an intervention approach that stems from work with children who have suffered traumatic brain injury (79,80). Butler and Copeland (81) have described an innovative program that integrates brain injury rehabilitation (i.e. cognitive remediation), cognitive-behavioral, and educational psychology approaches to PBT and other cancer survivors with cognitive deficits. Pilot data have demonstrated improved attentional processes, and a larger clinical trial is currently under way.

Although infrequent, studies of psychopharmacological treatment in PBT survivors have also been done. These studies have investigated the use of methylphenidate (MPH) to enhance the attentional deficits common in PBT survivors. Meyers et al. (82) did a small open-label study using MPH in adult brain tumor survivors that showed significant improvements in a wide array of cognitive functions. Thompson et al. (83) conducted a randomized double-blind placebo controlled trial to test the immediate response of childhood cancer survivors (more than 70% were PBT survivors) to MPH. They found that measures of attention were significantly improved at 90 minutes on a continuous performance test. In a larger, 3-week crossover extension of this study, Mulhern et al. (84) confirmed significant clinical improvement at home and school with MPH. Statistical "effect sizes" were in the 0.4 to 0.7 range (mild to moderate range of efficacy). Low-dose MPH [0.3 mg/kg immediate release (IR) or 10 mg twice daily maximum] was as effective as moderate-dose MPH (0.6 mg/kg or 20 mg twice daily maximum). Generally, MPH was well tolerated, with 5% experiencing severe adverse effects. Almost all of these were in the higher dose MPH group. Consistent with other studies of patients with brain damage or mental retardation, it would thus appear that MPH is less effective in this population than when used in typical children and that lower doses should generally be used. There are no studies of the use of psychotropic medications [e.g., atypical antipsychotics, selective serotonin reuptake inhibitors (SSRIs), mood stabilizers] in this population. In adults, there is a small, 24 week Phase II trial of donepezil that showed positive effects on cognitive functioning, mood, and general quality of life (85).

Conclusion

Brain tumors are the second most common cancer and the most common solid malignancy in the pediatric population. Because of improved treatments, survival rates have improved greatly in the past 30 years. As a consequence, the population of long-term survivors has grown substantially. Comprehensive monitoring and treatment by a multidisciplinary team are required by survivors, who often have long-term psychological, cognitive, and academic difficulties, as well as endocrinological, sensory, and neurological complications. Promising treatments to address the psychosocial needs of these patients and their families are being developed but are still in their infancy. The psychiatric needs of this population are not yet well defined, although they appear to be common. Psychopharmacological approaches are beginning to be utilized and investigated. Child and adolescent psychiatrists can contribute much to the multidisciplinary teams needed to care for these patients.

Case One

Two years prior to neurological evaluation, M.T. (a 15-year-old girl) had been diagnosed as having anorexia nervosa. At the time of initial presentation, her neurological examination had been normal. Because of persistent somatic complaints, she was hospitalized for re-evaluation. She complained primarily of occipital headaches. She also noted difficulty in swallowing, which was attributed to "globus hystericus," and dizziness and unsteady gait, which were considered a form of astasia-abasia. She was alert but emaciated. On examination she had nystagmus, chronic papilledema, and decreased visual acuity. She also had marked truncal ataxia. Neuroimaging revealed a large cystic mass with fourth ventricular outflow obstruction. At surgery a cystic cerebellar astrocytoma was completely removed. She is free of tumor 15 years later.

Discussion: This adolescent originally presented with weight loss and anorexia. Neurological examination and a radionuclide brain scan were normal. Over time, her myriad physical complaints were attributed to psychosomatic disease. In reality, the occipital headache and neck pain were due to irritation of the cervical roots secondary to incipient tonsillar herniation, the "globus hystericus" was due to bulbar dysfunction, and her "astasia-abasia" was secondary to the cerebellar mass lesion. Once her initial psychiatric diagnosis of anorexia nervosa was made, she unfortunately never received another detailed neurological examination, which would have readily revealed the cerebellar and brainstem signs.

In addition to the weight loss due to nausea and vomiting, which occurs in children with posterior fossa tumors (secondary to either increased intracranial pressure or direct irritation of the medullary vomiting center), disorders of eating may also occur in patients with tumors in the hypothalamus and pituitary gland. For example, infants with pilocytic astrocytomas of the hypothalamus may present with the diencephalic syndrome, in which they are emaciated but hyperalert and retain normal longitudinal growth. In contrast, some children with tumors in the hypothalamic-pituitary axis may experience excessive weight gain, especially when the satiety center is damaged due to tumor infiltration. This is always a concern in those children with acute lymphoblastic leukemia who develop hyperphagia. Differentiating the weight gain due to infiltration of the satiety center by leukemic cells from that due to steroids can be challenging and requires cytologic examination of the CSF. Damage to the satiety center also occurs following surgery for craniopharyngiomas The resulting hyperphagia can be extremely debilitating.

Case Two

R.D., a 13-year-old girl, presented at 6 years of age with generalized tonic-clonic seizures. She had a normal neurological examination and normal electroencephalogram (EEG) and MRI. She was a good student, and there were no interpersonal conflicts in the home. Seizures were well controlled with carbamazepine until age 13 years, when she had a gradual personality change over several months. She began acting out sexually, her academic achievement declined markedly, and she was in severe conflict with her parents. Simultaneously, her seizures increased in frequency and changed in description. Seizures that had been generalized tonic-clonic were now characterized as staring followed by picking at her clothing and uttering nonsense syllables. The neurological examination remained normal. She had been diagnosed as having an adolescent adjustment disorder, but a repeat EEG revealed a slow wave focus in the left temporal lobe and neuroimaging demonstrated a calcified mass in the left temporal lobe. She underwent a total resection of an oligodendroglioma. She has remained seizure-free without medication, cognitively normal, and without behavioral difficulties for 10 years.

Discussion: This patient had a 7-year history of seizures that had changed in character from generalized tonic clonic to partial complex. In addition, she had a change in personality and school performance. Her original EEG, which had been normal, later revealed a slow wave focus suggesting structural disease. At surgery an oligodendroglia was found. Although many of her personality traits were compatible with an adolescent adjustment reaction, there were enough warning signs to suggest an organic cause for her psychological dysfunction. As noted earlier in this chapter, although brain tumors are an uncommon cause of seizures in children, any child with a long-standing history of a seizure disorder who develops a change in personality, change in seizure type or control, decline in school performance, change in neurological examination, or change in EEG pattern warrants an investigation for an occult neoplasm. (14)

Case Three

S.B. presented at 10 years of age with a 3-month history of intermittent frontal headaches occurring throughout the day. In the 3 weeks prior to evaluation, the patient complained of nausea and nonprojectile vomiting. He was previously a good student, but his grades had recently declined. There had been family turmoil with an alcohol-dependent father and a sister who had conduct disorder symptoms. Examination revealed a slight boy whose height and weight were in the 5th percentile. Visual acuity was 20/100 in the left eye but 20/20 in the right, with evidence of a right hemianopsia. Neuroimaging revealed a calcified mass obstructing the foramen of Monro with secondary dilatation of the ventricles. A diagnosis of craniopharyngioma was suspected and confirmed after surgery. The postoperative course was uneventful except for the development of diabetes insipidus, which was readily controlled with vasopressin. Over the next 1½ years the patient developed excessive weight gain, became morbidly obese, and stopped socializing with his friends. Whereas previously he had been active in sports, following surgery he became withdrawn and poorly motivated, and was no longer interested in peers. Five years after surgery he remained obese, had dropped out of school, and generally appeared amotivational.

Discussion: This patient had a rather characteristic course for patients with craniopharyngioma. He initially presented with growth retardation, headache, vomiting, and visual compromise. The headache and vomiting resulted from increased intracranial pressure secondary to ventricular obstruction. The growth retardation was a direct effect of the craniopharyngioma, involving either hypothalamic or pituitary structures. Visual loss was secondary to impingement of the mass on the left optic nerve and tract. Despite total surgical removal of the tumor, the patient developed diabetes insipidus and required replacement therapy with antidiuretic hormone (ADH). Excessive eating secondary to organic disease responds in a limited way to behavioral therapy techniques. Abulia may occur for years and eventually resolve. In patients with craniopharyngiomas, psychiatric manifestations occur as a result of the treatment. Cure rates for this tumor following treatment are 80% to 90%. Unfortunately, morbidity (i.e., endocrinopathies, visual loss, and personality change) approaches 80%. (17)

Case Four

L.B. was adopted at birth and had struggled academically in school beginning in kindergarten. He was classified by the Committee for Special Education (CSE) and received resource room assistance and speech therapy from first grade on. He was described as a very social child at that time. In second grade his parents separated and he adjusted adequately. His development remained otherwise unremarkable until the sixth grade. At that time his academic functioning deteriorated, which was thought to be due to increased academic expectations in middle school. However, at the beginning of seventh grade he had a generalized tonic-clonic seizure. In the subsequent evaluation he was discovered to have a left temporal lobe oligodendroglioma. He was treated with surgery and chemotherapy but no radiation therapy. The tumor stabilized but did not decrease in size. L.B. was initially treated successfully for his seizures with phenytoin. Subsequently, he struggled even more academically, requiring special classroom placements. He became more passive and socially more withdrawn. His speech became slower. At 13 years, he developed additional seizure-like phenomena that eventually were diagnosed as stress-related episodes. By 14 years, he had dysthymia and sought psychiatric treatment. He preferred psychotherapy and was not treated with medications at that time. He improved modestly and was functioning better at school and with peers. He continued in this state until he had the acute onset of mutism, difficulties in caring for himself, and psychotic symptoms (including paranoia and auditory hallucinations). He was admitted to the hospital, where he was noted to be disoriented. A presumptive diagnosis of status epilepticus was made, but EEG monitoring was negative. Repeat MRI revealed that his tumor was smaller than shown on the last study; his neurological examination was otherwise unremarkable and showed no signs of an acute neurological event. He was started on low-dose risperidone and he seemed to improve somewhat. An underlying organic cause for his mental status change was exhaustively investigated, yet nothing came up positive. After 3 weeks he was marginally improved, and lorazepam was initiated with a working diagnosis of catatonia. He improved markedly within 24 hours and was discharged to home after 4 more days. He remained on the risperidone and lorazepam for the next month and he continued to improve markedly. He was weaned slowly off the lorazepam and risperidone and he continued to recover. Three months later he was back to baseline.

Discussion: Although more dramatic than most, this case captures the complexity of many children with PBTs. His case involved a premorbid speech and learning disability, an unknown psychiatric genetic background, family disruption, a seizure disorder (and treatment with anticonvulsants), and a left temporal brain tumor. The etiology for his recent acute deterioration was never found, but fortunately he recovered. Given his history it was assumed that his symptoms were related to his neurological condition yet the negative medical workup and EEG, as well as the improved MRI, did not support this diagnosis. Empirical treatment and supportive measures, including close contact with the family throughout the ordeal, led to a positive outcome.

Questions

1. Which of the following headache symptoms is *not* considered to be high risk for an underlying intracranial mass lesion?
   A. focal headache
   B. headaches that occur in the morning
   C. headaches that increase with Valsalva maneuvers
   D. headaches of more than 6 months duration
   E. headaches with vomiting and negative family history

2. Which of the following is considered an early sign associated with papilledema?
   A. increase in blind spot
   B. loss of vision
   C. seizures
   D. lethargy

3. Which of the following tumors is most often associated with seizures?
   A. glioblastoma multiforme
   B. desmoplastic neuroepithelial tumor
   C. diffuse intrinsic pontine glioma
   D. craniopharyngioma

4. Which of the following tumors is associated with Parinaud syndrome?
   A. optic glioma
   B. cerebellar astrocytoma
   C. diffuse intrinsic pontine glioma
   D. pineoblastoma

5. Which of the following tumors cannot be cured with a gross total resection?
   A. cerebellar astrocytoma
   B. intraorbital optic glioma
   C. choroid plexus papilloma
   D. medulloblastoma

6. In pediatric brain tumor patients, which of the following factors is most correlated with later neurocognitive deficit?
   A. development of hydrocephalus
   B. chemotherapy exposure
   C. radiotherapy exposure
   D. type of tumor
   E. location of tumor

7. Which of the following psychiatric conditions is most correlated with PBTs?
   A. suicidality
   B. psychosis
   C. anxiety and depression
   D. conduct disorder

8. Which of the following psychotropic medications has evidence to support their use in children with brain tumors?
   A. Adderall
   B. risperidone
   C. fluoxetine
   D. methylphenidate

Answers

1. D
2. A
3. B
4. D
5. D
6. C
7. C
8. D

REFERENCES

1. Young JL, Miller RW. Incidence of malignant tumors in US children. *J Pediatr.* 1975;86:254–258.
2. CBTRUS (2005). Statistical Report: Primary Brain Tumors in the United States, 1998–2002. Central Brain Tumor Registry of the United States, Hinsdale, IL.
3. Gurney JG, et al. Trends in cancer incidence among children in the US. *Cancer.* 1996;78: 532–541.
4. Robertson PL. Advances in the treatment of pediatric brain tumors. *J Am Soc Exp Neurother.* 2006;3:276–391.

5. Packer RJ, Gajjar A, Vezina G, Rorke-Adams L. Phase III study of craniospinal radiation therapy followed by adjuvant chemotherapy for newly diagnosed average-risk medulloblastoma. *J Clin Oncol.* 2006;24:4202–4208.
6. Abu-Arafeh, Macleod S. Serious neurological disorders in children with chronic headache. *Arch Dis Child.* 2005;90:937–940.
7. Boiardi A. Headache in brain tumors: a symptom to reappraise critically. *Neurol Sci.* 2004;25:S143–147.
8. Wilne SH, et al. The presenting features of brain tumours: a review of 200 cases. *Arch Dis Child.* 2006;91:502–506.
9. Mehta V, et al. Latency between symptom onset and diagnosis of pediatric brain tumors: an Eastern Canadian geographic study. *Neurosurgery.* 2005;51:365–372.
10. Medina LS, et al. Children with headache: clinical predictors of surgical space-occupying lesions and the role of neuroimaging. *Radiology.* 1997;202:819–824.
11. Honig P, Chaney E. Children with brain tumor headaches. *Am J Dis Child.* 1982;136:121–124.
12. Caplan R, et al. Middle Childhood onset of interictal psychosis. *J Am Acad Child Adolesc Psychiatry.* 1991;30:893–896.
13. Chipkevitch E. Brain tumors and anorexia nervosa syndrome. *Brain Dev.* 1994;16:175179.
14. Page LK, Lombroso CT, Matson DD. Childhood epilepsy with late detection of cerebral glioma. *J Neurosurg.* 1969;31:253–261.
15. Kelly TW. Optic glioma presenting as spasmus nutans. *Pediatrics.* 1970;45:295–296.
16. Russell A. A diencephalic syndrome of emaciation in infancy and childhood. *Arch Dis Child.* 1951;26:274
17. Karavitaki N, et al. Craniopharyngiomas. *Endocr Rev.* 2006;27:371–397.
18. Medina LS, Kuntz KM, Pomeroy S. Children with headache suspected of having a brain tumor: a cost effective analysis of diagnostic strategies. *Pediatrics.* 2001;108:255–263.
19. Allen JC. Controversies in the management of intracranial germ cell tumors. *Neurol Clin.* 1991;9:441–452.
20. Tzika AA, et al. Spectroscopic and magnetic resonance imaging predictors of progression in pediatric brain tumors. *Cancer.* 2004;100:1246–1256.
21. Minn AY, et al. Surveillance neuroimaging to detect relapse in childhood brain tumors: a Pediatric Oncology Group study. *J Clin Oncol.* 2001;19:4135–4140.
22. Allen J, et al. A phase I/II study of carboplatin combined with hyperfractionated radiotherapy for brainstem gliomas. *Cancer.* 1999;86:1064–1069.
23. Duffner PK, et al. Postoperative chemotherapy and delayed radiation in children less than 3 years of age with malignant brain tumors. *N Engl J Med.* 1993;328:1725–1731.
24. Fuemmeler BF, Elkin TD, Mullins LL. Survivors of childhood brain tumors: behavioral, emotional, and social adjustment. *Clin Psychol Rev.* 2002;22:547–585.
25. Hudson MM, et al. Health status of adult long-term survivors of childhood cancer: a report from the childhood cancer survivor study. *JAMA.* 2003;290:1583–1592.
26. Oeffinger KC, et al. Childhood Cancer Survivor Study. Chronic health conditions in adult survivors of childhood cancer. *N Engl J Med.* 2006;355:1572–1582.
27. Speechley KN, et al. Health-related quality of life among child and adolescent survivors of childhood cancer. *J Clin Oncol.* 2006;24:2536–2543.
28. Packer RJ, et al. Long-term neurologic and neurosensory sequelae in adult survivors of a childhood brain tumor: childhood cancer survivor study. *J Clin Oncol.* 2003;21:3255–3261.
29. Upton P, Eiser C. School experiences after treatment for a brain tumour. *Child Care Health Dev.* 2006;32(1):9–17.
30. Shalet SM, et al. Effect of spinal irradiation on growth. *Arch Dis Child.* 1987;62:461–464.
31. Packer RJ, et al. Growth Hormone replacement therapy in children with medulloblastoma: use and effect on tumor control. *J Clin Oncol.* 2001;19:480–487.
32. Clayton PE, et al. Does growth hormone cause relapse of brain tumors? *Lancet.* 1987;1:711–717.
33. Neglia JP, et al. New primary neoplasms of the central nervous system in survivors of childhood cancer: a report from the Childhood Cancer Survivor Study [see comment]. *J Natl Cancer Inst.* 2006;98:1528–1537.
34. Roggli VL, Estrada R, Fechner RE. Thyroid neoplasia following irradiation for medulloblastoma. *Cancer.* 1979;43:2232–2238.
35. Duffner PK, et al. Second malignancies in young children following treatment wit POG 8633: prolonged postoperative chemotherapy and delayed RT for children <3 years of age with malignant brain tumors. *Ann Neurol.* 1998;44:313–316.
36. Hoppe-Hirsch E, et al. Medulloblastoma in childhood: progressive intellectual deterioration. *Childs Nerv Syst.* 1990;6:60–65.
37. Duffner PK. Long-term effects of radiation therapy on cognitive and endocrine function in children with leukemia and brain tumors. *Neurologist.* 2004;10:293–310.
38. Riva D, et al. Intrathecal methotrexate affects cognitive function in children with medulloblastoma. *Neurology.* 2002;59:48–53.
39. Mahoney DH Jr, et al. Acute neurotoxicity in children with B-precursor acute lymphoid leukemia: an association with intermediate-dose intravenous methotrexate and intrathecal triple therapy: a Pediatric Oncology Group Study. *J Clin Oncol.* 1998;16:1712–1722.

40. Dietrich J, et al. CNS progenitor cells and oligodendrocytes are targets of chemotherapeutic agents in vitro and in vivo. *J Biol.* 2006;5:22–22.23.
41. Deutsch M, et al. Results of a prospective randomized trial comparing standard dose neuraxis radiation with reduced neuraxis radiation in patients with low stage medulloblastoma. *Pediatr Neurosurg.* 1996;24:167–177.
42. Thomas PR, et al. Low-stage medulloblastoma: final analysis of trial comparing standard-dose with reduced-dose neuraxis irradiation. *J Clin Oncol.* 2000;18:3004–3011.
43. Packer RJ, et al. Treatment of children with medulloblastoma with reduced dose craniospinal radiation and adjuvant chemotherapy: a Children's Cancer Group study. *J Clin Oncol.* 1999;17:2127–2136.
44. Ris MD, et al. Intellectual outcome after reduced dose radiation therapy plus adjuvant chemotherapy for medulloblastoma: a Children's Cancer Group Study. *J Clin Oncol.* 2001;19:3470–3476.
45. Reddick WE, et al. Developmental model relating white matter volume to neurocognitive deficits in pediatric brain tumor survivors. *Cancer.* 2003;97:2512–2519.
46. Mulhern RK, et al. Neurocognitive deficits in medulloblastoma survivors and white matter loss. *Ann Neurol.* 1999;46:834–841.
47. Anderson VA, et al. Cognitive and academic outcome following cranial irradiation and chemotherapy in children: a longitudinal study. *Br J Cancer.* 2000;82:255–262.
48. Butler RW, Haser JK. Neurocognitive effects of treatment for childhood cancer. *Mental Retardation Dev Disabilities Res Rev.* 2006;12:184–191.
49. Mulhern RK, Butler RW. Neurocognitive sequelae of childhood cancers and their treatment. *Pediatr Rehab.* 2004;7(1):1–14; discussion 15–16.
50. Mabbott DJ, et al. Serial evaluation of academic and behavioral outcome after treatment with cranial radiation in childhood. *J Clin Oncol.* 2005;23:2256–2263.
51. Palmer SL, et al. Patterns of intellectual development among survivors of pediatric medulloblastoma: a longitudinal analysis. *J Clin Oncol.* 2001;19:2302–2308.
52. Reimers TS, Mortensen EL, Schmiegelow K. Memory deficits in long-term survivors of childhood brain tumors may primarily reflect general cognitive dysfunctions [Journal Article. Research Support, Non-U.S. Gov't]. *Pediatr Blood Cancer.* 2007;48:205–212.
53. Mitby PA, et al. Childhood Cancer Survivor Study Steering Committee. Utilization of special education services and educational attainment among long-term survivors of childhood cancer: a report from the Childhood Cancer Survivor Study. *Cancer.* 2003;97:1115–1126.
54. Hays DM, et al. Educational, occupational, and insurance status of childhood cancer survivors in their fourth and fifth decades of life. *J Clin Oncol.* 1992;10:1397–1406.
55. Kelaghan J, et al. Educational achievement of long-term survivors of childhood and adolescent cancer. *Med Pediatr Oncol.* 1998;16:320–326.
56. Mostow EN, et al. Quality of life in long-term survivors of CNS tumors of childhood and adolescence. *J Clin Oncol.* 1991;9:592–599.
57. Langeveld NE, et al. Educational achievement, employment and living situation in long-term young adult survivors of childhood cancer in the Netherlands. *Psycho-oncology.* 2003;12:213–225.
58. Lannering B, et al. Long-term sequelae after pediatric brain tumors: their effect on disability and quality of life. *Med Pediatr Oncol.* 1990;18:304–310.
59. Ness KK, et al. Limitations on physical performance and daily activities among long-term survivors of childhood cancer. *Ann Intern Med.* 2005;143:639–647.
60. Syndikus I, et al. Long-term follow-up of young children with brain tumors after irradiation. *Int J Radiat Oncol Biol Phys.* 1994;30:781–787.
61. Carpentieri SC, et al. Psychosocial and behavioral functioning among pediatric brain tumor survivors. *J Neuro-Oncol.* 2003;63:279–287.
62. Nassau JH, Drotar D. Social competence among children with central nervous system-related chronic health conditions: review. *J Pediatr Psychol.* 1997;22:771–793.
63. Noll RB, et al. Social, emotional, and behavioral functioning of children with cancer. *Pediatrics.* 1999;103:71–78.
64. Vannatta K, et al. A controlled study of peer relationships of children surviving brain tumors: teacher, peer, and self ratings. *J Pediatr Psychol.* 1998;23:279–287.
65. Rauck AM, et al. Marriage in the survivors of childhood cancer: a preliminary description from the childhood cancer survivor study. *Med Pediatr Oncol.* 1999;33:60–63.
66. Zebrack BJ, et al. Psychological outcomes in long-term survivors of childhood brain cancer: a report from the childhood cancer survivor study. *J Clin Oncol.* 2004;22:999–1006.
67. Recklitis CJ, Lockwood RA, Rothwell MA, et al. Suicidal ideation and attempts in adult survivors of childhood cancer. *J Clin Oncol* 2006;24(24):3852–7.
68. Howard RA, Inskip PD, Travis LB. Suicide after childhood cancer. *J Clin Oncol.* 2007;25:731; author reply 733–734.
69. Ross L, et al. Psychiatric hospitalizations among survivors of cancer in childhood or adolescence. *N Engl J Med.* 2003;349:650–657.
70. Pai A, et al. A meta-analysis of the effects of psychological interventions in pediatric oncology on outcomes of psychological distress and adjustment. *J Pediatr Psychol.* [Special Section on Families, Youth and HIV: First Generation Intervention Studies] 2006;31:978–988.

71. Stuber ML, et al. Is posttraumatic stress a viable model for understanding responses to childhood cancer? *Child Adolesc Psychiatric Clin North Am.* 1998;7:169–182.
72. Kazak AE, et al. An integrative model of pediatric medical traumatic stress. *J Pediatr Psychol.* 2006; 31:343–355.
73. Stuber ML, et al. The medical traumatic stress toolkit. *CNS Spectrums.* 2006;11(2):137–142.
74. Kazak AE, et al. Treatment of posttraumatic stress symptoms in adolescent survivors of childhood cancer and their families: a randomized clinical trial. *J Fam Psychol.* 2004;18:493–504.
75. Kazak AE. Evidence-based interventions for survivors of childhood cancer and their families. *J Pediatr Psychol.* 2005;30(1):29–39.
76. Noll RB, et al. Social, emotional, and behavioral functioning of children with cancer. *Pediatrics.* 1999;103:71–78.
77. Gerhardt CA, et al. Social and romantic outcomes in emerging adulthood among survivors of childhood cancer. *J Adolesc Health.* 2007;40(5): 462.e9–15.
78. Barakat LP, et al. Evaluation of a social-skills training group intervention with children treated for brain tumors: a pilot study. *J Pediatr Psychol.* 2003;28:299–307.
79. Anderson DM, et al. Medical and neurocognitive late effects among survivors of childhood central nervous system tumors. *Cancer.* 2001;92: 2709–2719.
80. Butler RW, Mulhern RK. Neurocognitive interventions for children and adolescents surviving cancer. *J Pediatr Psychol.* 2005;30(1):65–78.
81. Butler R, Copeland DR. Attentional processes and their remediation in children treated for cancer: a literature review and the development of a therapeutic approach. *J Int Neuropsychol Soc.* 2002;8:115–124.
82. Meyers CA, et al. Methylphenidate therapy improves cognition mood, and function of brain tumor patients. *J Clin Oncol.* 1998;16:2522–2527.
83. Thompson SJ, et al. Immediate neurocognitive effects of methylphenidate on learning-impaired survivors of childhood cancer. *J Clin Oncol.* 2001;19:1802–1808.
84. Mulhern RK, et al. Short-term efficacy of methylphenidate: a randomized, double-blind, placebo-controlled trial among survivors of childhood cancer. *J Clin Oncol.* 2004;22:4795–4803.
85. Shaw EG, et al. Phase II study of donepezil in irradiated brain tumor patients: effect on cognitive function, mood, and quality of life. *J Clin Oncol.* 2006;24:1415–1420.

CHAPTER 9

Functional Neuroimaging in Pediatric Populations

DANIEL J. SIMMONDS AND STEWART H. MOSTOFSKY

The advent of functional magnetic resonance imaging (fMRI) has allowed us to see the living brain "at work." fMRI studies in children have been an important step in understanding neural circuits involved in motor, sensory, cognitive, and behavioral functions that are key to normal development, as well as differences in those functions associated with pediatric clinical populations. This chapter is divided into three sections. First, it presents the general principles of fMRI, as well as its advantages over different neuroimaging techniques and its limitations, including specific caveats of the application of fMRI to pediatric populations. Second, it focuses on the specific applications of fMRI to attention deficit hyperactivity disorder (ADHD) as an example of a population extensively studied using fMRI, discussing behavioral findings in ADHD and how fMRI findings in the disorder complement understanding of its clinical profile. Finally, the chapter concludes with how the strategies for using fMRI to study ADHD can be extended to other clinical populations and how these data will inform the neural bases both of clinical disorders and of typical development.

Functional Magnetic Resonance Imaging

Magnetic resonance imaging uses a series of radio frequency (RF) pulses in combination with time-varying magnetic fields in order to image biological tissue. Inside the MRI scanner, hydrogen atoms within a person's body align with the static magnetic field. Electromagnetic RF pulses delivered by the scanner excite the hydrogen nuclei and disrupt their alignment with the magnetic field. After excitation, the nuclei undergo both longitudinal relaxation, in which the nuclei realign with the static magnetic field, that is, the net magnetization recovers along the longitudinal (parallel) axis, and transverse relaxation, in which the net magnetization in the transverse (perpendicular) plane decreases as the nuclei lose their phase coherence. The longitudinal relaxation process is called T1 recovery and is what contributes to anatomical T1-weighted images, whereas the transverse relaxation process leads to T2 decay, which contributes to anatomical T2-weighted images, and T2* decay. The latter is especially relevant to fMRI, as it forms the basis of blood-oxygenation-level dependent (BOLD) imaging (1).

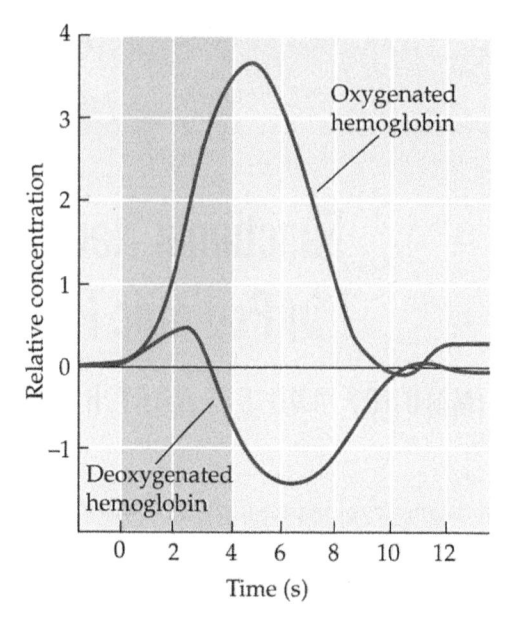

■ **FIGURE 9.1** Illustration depicting the "hemodynamic response," which is characterized by changes in oxygenated and deoxygenated hemoglobin that follow neuronal activity, called the "hemodynamic response." The concentration of deoxygenated hemoglobin rapidly increases, peaking at approximately 2 seconds, then declines, reaching its lowest value at approximately 6 seconds, and then increases again, returning to baseline at about 10 seconds. The concentration of oxygenated hemoglobin rises sharply after neuronal activity, peaking at about 5 to 6 seconds, then declines, reaching baseline at about 10 seconds. (From Huettel SA, Song AW, McCarthy G. *Functional Magnetic Resonance Imaging*. Sunderland, MA: Sinauer Associates; 2004; with permission.)

MECHANISMS OF THE BLOOD-OXYGENATION-LEVEL–DEPENDENT RESPONSE

The basis for the BOLD contrast is the sensitivity of $T2^*$-weighted images to local amounts of deoxygenated hemoglobin, which disrupt the static magnetic field in the scanner due to its strong paramagnetic properties. Deoxygenated hemoglobin changes in accordance with the metabolic demands of neurons; increases in neuronal activity result in an increase in metabolic demands, necessitating the delivery of oxygen to the active neurons. Hence, neuronal activity is reflected by a delayed increase in oxygenated hemoglobin and a decrease in deoxygenated hemoglobin. This "hemodynamic response," which is equivalent to the BOLD contrast, generally peaks about 4 to 6 seconds after neuronal activity (Fig. 9.1) (2). By taking a number of BOLD-sensitive images over time, localized changes in deoxyhemoglobin concentration corresponding to a priori task-dependent models can be measured. For fMRI, these images are usually acquired using echo-planar imaging (EPI), which is sensitive to the BOLD contrast and allows the brain to be rapidly imaged in slices (3).

TASK DESIGN IN FUNCTIONAL MAGNETIC RESONANCE IMAGING

Given that the brain is never "at rest" and local metabolic demands are constantly changing, traditional fMRI studies typically rely on contrasting activation during the experimental task with a baseline condition, such as a rest period or a different task. This technique is called "cognitive subtraction," whereby it is inferred that differences in the BOLD contrast, or "activation," between the two conditions are due to cognitive processes present in the experimental condition but not in the baseline condition.

Early fMRI studies used a block design approach adapted from positron emission tomography (PET) studies, whereby individuals perform a task for a period of time, and activation is averaged across the whole block. Due to fMRI's superior temporal resolution in comparison to PET, many investigators quickly moved to event-related designs, whereby activation due to a single event can be modeled. Early event-related fMRI studies used periodic designs in which events were separated by more than 15 seconds in order to allow the hemodynamic response to relax, so that the BOLD signal did not saturate with rapidly repeated events (4); however, these designs were inefficient and inconsistent with the psychodynamic properties of tasks used to examine behavior outside the scanner. More recently, designs began to incorporate "jittering," in which events occur at irregular intervals, allowing for interevent intervals as low as 500 ms (5).

Recently, newer methods of analysis have emerged, such as functional connectivity, which permit analysis of functional brain activation in the absence of an experimental task. Such studies of "resting-state" brain activity are further discussed later in this chapter.

ADVANTAGES OF FUNCTIONAL MAGNETIC RESONANCE IMAGING

There are several advantages to using fMRI rather than other functional neuroimaging techniques. Perhaps the most convincing is that fMRI is noninvasive, unlike PET and single-photon emission computed tomography (SPECT), which require injection of radioactive contrast agents. Its noninvasive nature makes fMRI better suited for longitudinal studies and pediatric studies (6).

Another advantage of fMRI is its balance of spatial resolution and temporal resolution. Typical fMRI studies have a spatial resolution on the scale of 2 to 4 mm, allowing detection of BOLD contrast changes (activation) in relatively small brain structures, such as the amygdala. On the temporal scale, whole-brain image volumes in fMRI are typically taken every 2 to 3 seconds, which is a high enough resolution to sample the hemodynamic response to single events. In contrast, PET has a temporal resolution ranging from 90 seconds for ^{15}O to 30 to 40 minutes for ^{18}F, due to its low signal-to-noise ratio (2). The temporal constraints of PET limit its use to studies with block designs, in contrast with the rapid event-related capabilities of fMRI.

LIMITATIONS OF FUNCTIONAL MAGNETIC RESONANCE IMAGING

Although fMRI has the best spatial resolution of the current human neuroimaging techniques and is capable of imaging brain function on a millimeter scale, it is unable to capture activity on a submillimeter scale, as manifested in individual neurons, axons, and synapses. In addition, the temporal resolution of fMRI, on the scale of seconds, cannot detect electrophysiological changes, which are on the scale of milliseconds; this is possible in humans only by using techniques such as electroencephalography (EEG), which has poor spatial resolution, and magnetoencephalography (MEG), which can detect activity only from neurons that are oriented perpendicular to the scalp.

An important consideration in fMRI is that the changes in signal are on the scale of 1% to 3%, depending on the strength of the scanner. To achieve enough power to detect a signal, a large number of trials must be averaged, which results in longer tasks and longer time spent in the scanner. This also means that sample sizes must be adequate to achieve enough power on a group level.

Another limitation in fMRI, particularly with EPI, is the presence of magnetic susceptibility artifacts that occur at air-tissue interfaces, most notably in the orbitofrontal cortex, adjacent to the nasal sinuses. The artifacts are due to magnetic field inhomogeneities, causing signal loss and compromised images of these regions. However, recently developed scanning techniques show promise for minimizing these artifacts (7,8). Other scanner artifacts include those caused by metals with ferromagnetic material entering the scanner. Although some metal, such as dental fillings, do not induce artifact, implants with ferromagnetic material may preclude individuals from being scanned.

Head motion during scanning, which tends to occur more in children, is another factor that compromises image quality. Given the fine spatial resolution of fMRI, even slight movements can cause the same brain region to be measured at different locations in space and alter the images. The need to restrict movement limits the use of tasks requiring verbal responses because oral movements are likely to result in changes in head position. Various software packages that can correct for motion artifacts are available (9); however, if the motion is correlated with the task (e.g., face imitation task in which subjects are required to mimic facial movements seen on a screen), it may be difficult to correct for motion without removing effects of interest. Approaches for minimizing motion in pediatric populations are discussed in the following section.

CAVEATS OF PEDIATRIC FUNCTIONAL MAGNETIC RESONANCE IMAGING

Using fMRI in pediatric populations poses unique methodological challenges. As mentioned in the previous section, one major limitation of fMRI is its susceptibility to even small amounts of motion, necessitating the subject to remain very still during scanning. This can be difficult for children, especially those with clinical diagnoses such as ADHD. To reduce motion during scanning, several methods of restraint are available, including bite bars, forehead and chin straps, and pillow/foam padding; however, many of these restraints will be unappealing to children. As such, minimizing these restraints will enhance tolerability.

Claustrophobia is another common challenge, given the relatively narrow and small space within the scanner. The head coil that is necessary for scanning can further compound this feeling. In addition, the scanner emits loud noises, which can be distressing to children who are sensitive to such stimuli, such as those with autism. All of these factors underlie the importance of having children participate in a "mock scan," which simulates the environment and noises of the actual scanner. First, the mock scanner gives children a chance to acclimate to the scanner environment, which can help to reduce anxiety associated with entering the actual scanner for testing (10). Second, behavior management approaches, involving feedback with use of reinforcers, can be used to train children to lie still over the course of the mock scan, which subsequently helps to reduce motion during the actual scan (11). Finally, the mock scanner gives children the opportunity to ask questions before, rather than during, the time when the actual scanning takes place.

Another critical issue for pediatric fMRI is distractibility and boredom. Children frequently tend toward self-entertainment such as humming and singing, especially in boring or tedious environments, and hence need periodic reminders of which behaviors are unacceptable in the scanner, although training in the mock scanner may help alleviate this. One of the most common causes of these unacceptable behaviors is using a task that is developmentally inappropriate, that is, one that is either too difficult or too easy. Suitable tasks are those in which the instructions are explained simply and clearly so that the child understands and can comply, cognitive demands are commensurate with the child's level, and duration is minimized in order to avoid the risk of the child's not cooperating late in the session.

There are aspects of fMRI image processing for which special considerations exist with regard to the study of children. As each individual's brain is unique, both in size and in morphology, all individual brains need to undergo "spatial normalization" to a common template to facilitate comparisons. Most fMRI studies utilize a standardized adult template;

using such a template may be problematical in pediatric studies, though, given that brain size and morphology change over the course of development. In typically developing children, this issue can be addressed by using a standardized pediatric template (12). However, in pediatric clinical populations in which distinct morphological differences exist, such as ADHD, the use of a template based only on typically developing children may create difficulties, leading to group activation differences that are due to better anatomical normalization in the typically developing group rather than actual differences in brain function. In these situations, creating a customized template based on the control and affected sample is preferable as it would allow equal representation of both groups in the template. An alternative or complementary approach, especially important in populations with noted reductions in brain volume, is covarying functional activation with local amounts of gray matter to determine whether differences in activation are due to functional abnormalities or differences in neuronal mass/registration error (13).

Functional Magnetic Resonance Imaging Studies of Attention Deficit Hyperactivity Disorder

The biological substrates of ADHD are still uncertain, despite the fact that the disorder affects about 5% of school-aged children and frequently persists into adulthood (14). Understanding the neural basis of ADHD is critical to improving accurate diagnosis and helping to guide treatment. Recent studies have focused on three sets of neural findings in ADHD: abnormalities in response inhibition and resting state and neural effects of pharmacotherapy.

RESPONSE INHIBITION IN ATTENTION DEFICIT HYPERACTIVITY DISORDER

The clinical features in ADHD, including hyperactivity and impulsivity, and findings from neuropsychological studies (15–17) have contributed to leading hypotheses that ADHD is associated with impairments in executive control functions. There has been a particular emphasis on response inhibition (18), which refers to an inability to suppress behaviors that are inappropriate in a given context, and this has been the most examined domain in fMRI studies of ADHD. In the experimental setting, the most widely used tasks to assess response inhibition are the Go/No-go task and the Stop Signal task. In both of these tasks, a series of cued simple motor responses ("Go" trials requiring a button push) are accompanied by occasional "Stop" or "No-go" cues requiring suppression of this motor response. Impaired response inhibition, as measured by elevated commission error rates relative to typically developing children, is consistently observed in ADHD (15–17). Group differences in other behavioral measures have also been reported in ADHD. Specifically, children with ADHD show greater reaction times and reaction time variability during Go trials relative to typically developing children, suggesting that deficits in motor/behavioral control do not solely manifest as impaired response inhibition (17,19,20).

fMRI studies of response inhibition in "normal" adult populations have emphasized the involvement of circuits between the striatum and prefrontal regions, including the medial frontal wall, inferior frontal cortex and dorsolateral prefrontal cortex (21,22); however, localization of prefrontal activation is inconsistent across studies. These inconsistencies may be task dependent. One study examined healthy adults performing two versions of the Go/No-go task: a simple Go/No-go task with well-ingrained stimulus-response associations (green = Go, red = No-go) and a counting Go/No-go task in which the stimulus-response associations changed after each stimulus (green = Go, red = Go if preceded by an even number of green stimuli, No-go if preceded by an odd number of green stimuli). The latter task requires constant manipulation of stimulus-response associations in working memory. Prefrontal activation in the simple task was localized to the rostral portion of the superior medial wall (pre-SMA), whereas greater activation in the counting task was present in right lateral prefrontal and inferior parietal regions as well as the pre-SMA, suggesting that these regions are recruited under conditions of increased working memory load (Fig. 9.2) (23). A similar systematic approach is warranted for examining differences in activation associated with response inhibition in both typically developing children and children with ADHD.

Current pediatric fMRI studies of response inhibition in ADHD are outlined in Table 9.1 (24–36). Most of the studies show differences in striatal and frontal regions; however, similar to what is seen in adults, frontal differences vary across studies and may be task dependent. Several of the tasks use novel stimuli, such as cartoon characters (27,33), objects (e.g., airplanes) (25,26,30), multiple letters (24,28,29,34), and arrows (31,32,35), which may have increased the need to maintain recently learned rules in working memory and necessitated recruitment of regions involved in working memory. In addition, tasks involving multiple stimuli tend to involve the anterior cingulate cortex, which has a well-established role in error detection.

Given the apparently task-dependent variation of findings across studies, a methodological approach in which task design is systematically varied, similar to the approach discussed above in adults, would be a useful strategy to elucidate the neural mechanisms underlying impaired response inhibition in ADHD. As a first step, it would be advantageous to focus on the components solely involved in inhibition of relatively simple responses, thus focusing on response inhibition in this specific domain and minimizing involvement of more complicated neural systems necessary for regulation of cognition and behavior. This was recently accomplished in a group of 25 children with ADHD and 25 typically developing controls using the simple Go/No-go task described above (green = Go, red = No-go) (36). Findings revealed no between-group differences associated with the habitual Go trials; however, the children with ADHD showed decreased frontal No-go activation in the pre-SMA (Fig. 9.3). The findings suggest that abnormalities in circuits important for motor response selection contribute to deficits in response inhibition in children with ADHD and lend support to the growing awareness of ADHD-associated anomalies in medial frontal regions important for control of voluntary actions.

Findings of increased reaction time variability associated with Go responses provide further evidence for abnormalities in regions important for motor response preparation and control in children with ADHD (17,19,20). Further, this variability positively correlates with response inhibition performance, such that greater variability is associated with increased commission errors (19,37,38), suggesting that common neural circuits may underlie both ADHD-associated impairments in both response preparation and response inhibition. This idea is supported by fMRI data on response variability during performance of a Go/No-go task by 30 typically developing children (37) that showed that less variability (better performance) during Go trials was associated with No-go activation in the pre-SMA.

These findings suggest that dysfunction within the pre-SMA may be central to impaired response inhibition in ADHD; this hypothesis is supported by anatomical findings of decreased cortical thickness in ADHD localized to the pre-SMA (39). However, findings from other fMRI studies, revealing activation differences in various prefrontal regions, suggest that abnormalities may not be localized to the pre-SMA (Table 9.1). Further, although some anatomical findings highlight pre-SMA abnormalities in ADHD, others suggest more diffuse volumetric differences (40,41). An alternative explanation would be that ADHD is associated with broad abnormalities across frontal circuits; these abnormalities may contribute to impaired response inhibition in more complex contexts involving control of cognitive and

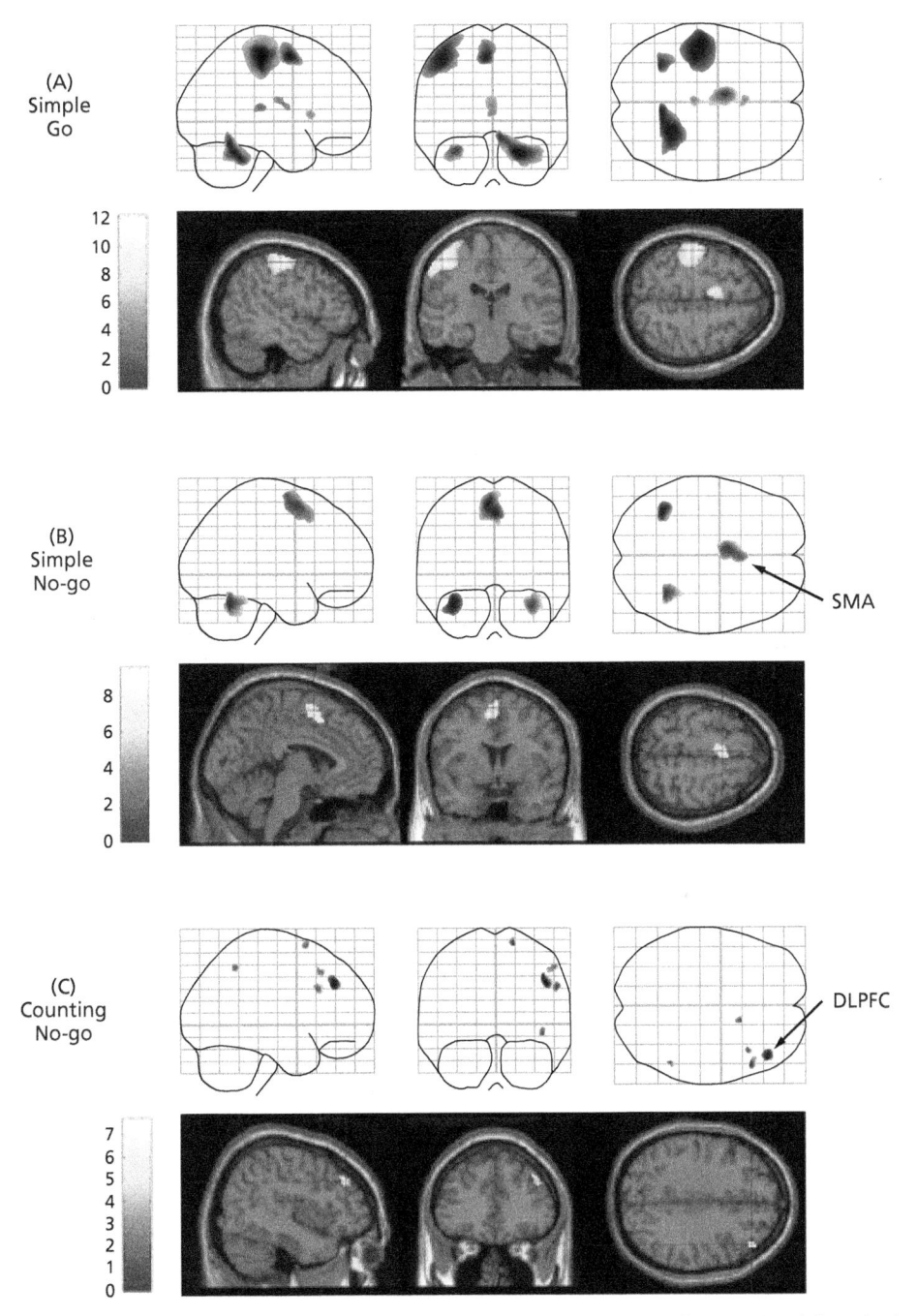

FIGURE 9.2 Glass-brain and sectional maps from reference 23 depicting the fMRI results of the "simple" and "counting" Go/No-go tasks. The simple task used well-ingrained stimulus-response associations (green = Go, red = No-go), whereas in the counting task, red was either Go if preceded by an even number of greens or No-go if preceded by an odd number of greens. For the simple task **(A)**, No-go activation in the frontal lobe was localized to the pre-SMA. In the counting task **(B)**, activation was also seen in the right dorsolateral prefrontal cortex, which was significantly greater than that seen in the simple task **(C)**. (From Mostofsky SH, Simmonds DJ. Response inhibition and response selection: two sides of the same coin. *J Cogn Neurosci*. In press. with permission).

TABLE 9.1 fMRI STUDIES OF RESPONSE INHIBITION IN CHILDREN WITH ADHD

Year	Author	Participants (ADHD/TD)	Age Range	Task	Stimuli	Design	Contrasts	ADHD Activation Differences
1998	Vaidya et al. (24)	10/6	8–13	Go/No-go[a]	Letters	Block	Go/No-go—Go only	1. ↓ striatum 2. ↑ striatum, ↑ frontal
1999	Rubia et al. (25)	7/9	12–18	Stop-Signal	Objects (e.g., airplanes)	Block	Stop/Go—Go only	↓ right mesial frontal, right IFG, left caudate
2001	Rubia et al. (26)	7/9	12–18	Stop-Signal	Objects (e.g., airplanes)	Block	Stop/Go—Go only	↓ right mesial frontal, right IFG, left caudate
2003	Durston et al. (27)	7/7	6–10	Go/No-go	Cartoon characters	Event-related	No-go—Go	↓ left caudate, ↑ right SFG, right MFG, right IPL, right STG, PCG, precuneus, occipital
2004	Tamm et al. (28)	14/12	14–18	Go/No-go	Letters	Event-related	No-go—Oddball Go	↓ medial frontal wall, ↑ temporal
2004	Schulz et al. (29)	10/9	15–19	Go/No-go	Letters	Event-related	No-go—Go	↓ right PG, right ITG, left hippocampus, right occipital, bilateral cerebellum, ↑ bilateral MFG, bilateral IFG, left medial frontal wall, bilateral IPL, right precuneus
2005	Booth et al. (30)	12/12	9–11	Go/No-go	Multiple colored shapes	Block	Go/No-go—Go only	↓ medial frontal wall, bilateral MFG, right IFG, bilateral PG, bilateral caudate, left GP, right amygdala, cuneus, occipital, thalamus
2005	Rubia et al. (31)	16/21	9–17	Stop-Signal	Arrows	Event-related	Successful Stop—Unsuccessful Stop	SS – US: ↓ right orbital/PG, right STG
2005	Vaidya et al. (32)	10/10	NRS[c]	Go/No-go[b]	Arrows and letters	Event-related	Unsuccessful Stop—Go No-go—"Neutral" Go	US – Go: ↓ PCG, precuneus No significant differences
2006	Durston et al. (33)	11/11	8–19	Go/No-go	Cartoon characters	Event-related	No-go—Go	↓ left IFG, left ACG, left premotor, right MFG, left IPL
2006	Pliszka et al. (34)	17/15	9–15	Stop-Signal	Letters	Event-related	Successful Stop—Go Unsuccessful Stop—Go	SS – Go: ↑ ACG US – Go: ↓ ACG
2006	Smith et al. (35)	17/18	NRS[d]	Go/No-go	Arrows	Event-related	No-go—Oddball Go	↓ left mesial frontal
2007	Suskauer et al. (36)	25/25	8–12	Go/No-go	Green and red spaceships	Event-related	No-go—baseline	↓ pre-SMA, right TPJ, right cerebellum, bilateral occipital

ADHD, attention deficit hyperactivity disorder; TD, typically developing; IFG, inferior frontal gyrus; SFG, superior frontal gyrus; MFG, middle frontal gyrus; IPL, inferior parietal lobule; STG, superior temporal gyrus; PCG, posterior cingulate gyrus; PG, precentral gyrus; ITG, inferior temporal gyrus; GP, globus pallidus; ACG, anterior cingulate gyrus; pre-SMA, presupplementary motor area; TPJ, temporoparietal junction.

[a] Used two different Go/No-go tasks (a) Stimulus controlled: both Go/No-go and Go only blocks contained an equal number of stimuli and (b) response controlled: Go/No-go blocks contained half as many stimuli, but an equal number of motor responses.

[b] Combined a Go/No-go task with a modified Eriksen Flanker task, in which distractor stimuli are presented that may be congruent or incongruent with the target stimulus; No-go trials occurred when the distractor stimuli were "X."

[c] No range specified: ADHD: 8.8 ± 0.9; TD: 9.2 ± 1.3.

[d] No range specified: ADHD: 14.1 ± 2.0; TD: 12.8 ± 2.0.

(A) Within-group contrasts for Go related activation

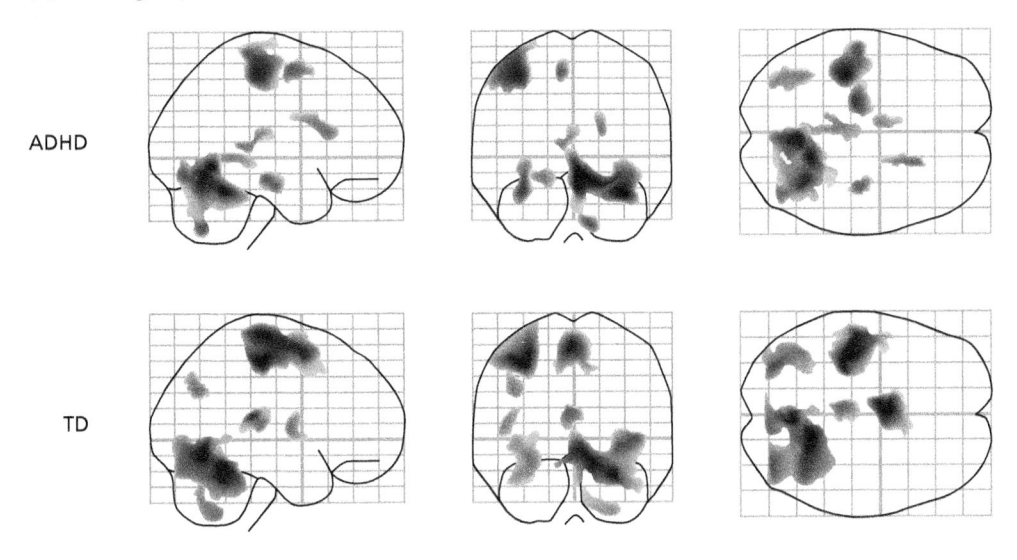

ADHD

TD

(B) Within-group contrasts for No-go related activation

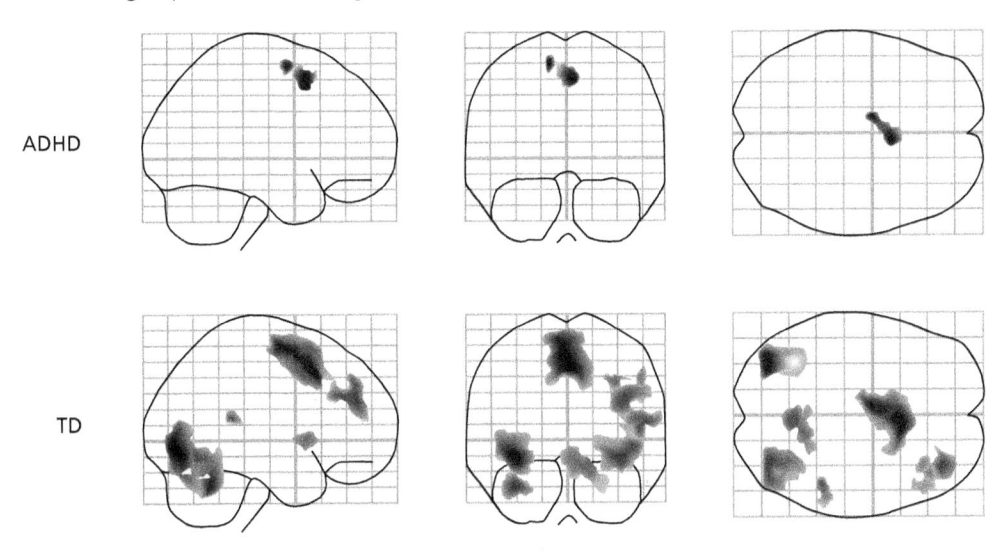

ADHD

TD

■ **FIGURE 9.3** Transparent brain maps showing effects for **(A)** Go and **(B)** No-go events. Neurological convention is used (right side of image = right hemisphere). **A:** For Go events, there were no significant group differences; both groups showed activation in the left primary sensorimotor cortex, left supplementary motor area, bilateral cerebellum and bilateral occipital lobes. **B:** For No-go events, children with ADHD showed less general activation than their typically developing (TD) peers; both groups showed activation in the pre-SMA, but this activation was significantly greater in the TD group than in the ADHD group. (From Suskauer SJ, et al. fMRI evidence for abnormalities in response selection in ADHD: differences in activation associated with response inhibition but not habitual motor response. *J Cogn Neurosci.* In press. with permission.)

socio-emotional function, which may explain the variation in prefrontal activation differences across studies. Following a systematic approach, these competing hypotheses could be tested by using a design previously applied to adults (23) and extrapolating to children with ADHD and typically developing controls, in order to examine whether broader frontal differences are seen under conditions of increased cognitive demands.

Although response inhibition has been emphasized as a core deficit in ADHD, it is not the only domain of executive function that is impaired in ADHD. Behavioral deficits have been noted with a moderate effect size across all executive function domains, including planning, vigilance, set shifting, and working memory (42). Despite this, few fMRI studies have examined these domains in children with ADHD. One recent study compared children with ADHD and typically developing controls on a mental rotation task testing spatial working memory; although no differences in task performance were found, children with ADHD had decreased activation in striatal and inferior parietal regions relative to their typically developing peers (43). Another study from the same group found poorer performance on the mental rotation task as well as decreased activation in prefrontal, inferior parietal, and striatal regions in children with ADHD (44). These regional differences are similar to those seen in fMRI studies of response inhibition, reinforcing notions of abnormalities of circuits between the striatum and other regions (frontal, parietal) in ADHD.

ATTENTION DEFICIT HYPERACTIVITY DISORDER AND THE RESTING STATE

Moving beyond traditional analyses, such as those contrasting tasks versus baseline in block and event-related designs, some investigators have started to examine functional activation in the absence of an a priori task–dependent design. This can be accomplished using functional connectivity analyses that compare the time courses of functional activation between remote brain regions. These types of analyses are important for ADHD as well as other neuropsychiatric disorders because they do not require performance of tasks, which may be difficult for clinical groups, and they also have the potential to show functional differences that are not experimentally driven.

As it is apparent that impairments in ADHD are not limited to (nor explained by) a single experimental domain, it is possible that ADHD is not associated with specific motor or cognitive deficits, but rather differences in the tonic resting state that may be attributed to differences in arousal (45). This is also reflected in the consistent finding of increased reaction time variability seen in ADHD (17,19,46), which is thought to be reflective of deficient ability to regulate one's tonic state, or "state regulation." A number of fMRI studies have investigated the resting state in ADHD; a few are described later.

T2 relaxometry is a measure of steady-state blood flow that has been applied to children with ADHD. One study using this technique found increased T2 relaxation times in the striatum, which correlated with behavioral measures of ADHD; methylphenidate normalized T2 relaxation times in the striatum for hyperactive children with ADHD, but not for normoactive children with ADHD (47). Similar findings were seen in the cerebellar vermis (48), a region of the cerebellum connected with the striatum.

Differences in resting state activity can also be assessed by examining differences in functional connectivity, which measures similarity of the time course of BOLD signal change between distinct brain regions. Using a variation on functional connectivity called "regional homogeneity," in which functional connectivity is calculated between the voxels within a single region rather than between regions, investigators found that children with ADHD showed decreased regional homogeneity in fronto-striatal-cerebellar circuits (49). Another series of studies has examined low-frequency fluctuations in BOLD signal; one study found decreased low-frequency fluctuations in prefrontal and cerebellar regions (50), and another found increased low-frequency connectivity in ADHD between the anterior cingulate cortex and striatal-cerebellar circuits, which was hypothesized to result from an abnormality in autonomic control functions (51). A number of other methods for calculating functional connectivity have come into common use in the neuroimaging community but have not yet been employed to study ADHD; certainly, more investigations are warranted.

EXAMINATION OF TREATMENT EFFECTS IN ATTENTION DEFICIT HYPERACTIVITY DISORDER

Several lines of evidence suggest that an imbalance in the dopaminergic system may contribute to ADHD (46,52). Dopamine receptors are highly concentrated in the striatum and the frontal cortex, regions implicated as being abnormal in ADHD. Moreover, evidence from genetic studies implicates genes involved in dopaminergic regulation in ADHD, most notably loci for the dopamine postsynaptic D4 receptor (DRD4) and the DAT transporter system (DAT1) (52,53). These factors likely explain why stimulant medications such as methylphenidate, which affect dopamine receptors, are generally effective medications for the treatment of ADHD (46).

Very few fMRI studies to date have examined treatment effects in ADHD. With respect to stimulant medication, an early fMRI study evaluated the effects of methylphenidate in children with ADHD during performance of Go/No-go tasks (24). Methylphenidate improved response inhibition performance and increased activation in both the prefrontal cortex and the striatum in children with ADHD, suggesting that fronto-striatal regions function abnormally in ADHD and that methylphenidate may normalize activity in these regions. Methylphenidate was also shown to normalize striatal activity during attention tasks (54), and this common finding across different task types strongly suggests that methylphenidate normalizes dopaminergic activity in the striatum.

Summary and Applications to Other Pediatric Populations

Functional MRI is a powerful tool that can help to elucidate the neural basis of normal and abnormal cognitive and psychiatric development in children. Considerable pediatric fMRI research is emerging across a wide range of psychiatric disorders, including autism, dyslexia, conduct disorder, Tourette syndrome, anxiety disorder, bipolar and other mood disorders, and eating disorders (55). As two brief examples of this, fMRI has been used to examine differences in the function of the amygdala, in depression and anxiety; in autism fMRI has been used to detect differences in activation of the fusiform gyrus and limbic system in response to viewing emotive faces and to detect differences during motor imitation within the "mirror neuron" system, which encompasses the frontal operculum, inferior parietal lobe, and superior temporal sulcus. This chapter focused exclusively on ADHD as it is one of the most extensively studied psychiatric disorders, and furthermore, it centered primarily on one behavioral aspect of ADHD, namely, response inhibition, rather than other aspects, such as working memory, which require further research. It also addressed the tonic resting state and studies of treatment effects in ADHD. fMRI findings revealed that fronto-striatal circuits may be abnormal in ADHD, consistent with research from other domains, including genetics and anatomical neuroimaging. However, one important area that has been lacking in fMRI studies of ADHD is examination of age-related changes in the disorder related to development. As a future direction, it is important for fMRI studies to examine, in either a longitudinal or cross-sectional fashion, these development effects and how they may factor into presentation of the disorder, potentially revealing critical points for intervention.

Although ADHD is a relatively narrow topic, the chapter was intended to highlight key fMRI concepts that can be applied to research on all disorders; this includes fMRI methods, designs and limitations, interplay between behavioral and brain findings, comparisons of adult and child data, and discussion of whether adult hypotheses and methods can and should be extrapolated to children. Several prominent lines of investigation—genetic, metabolic, neuroanatomical, animal model, and neuroimaging—are critical to understanding the neurobiological basis of disorders. As fMRI is a relatively new technology, it does not yet have any established clinical use in psychiatric disorders, although it is used frequently in presurgical mapping of motor and language areas in cases of epilepsy. However, functional neuroimaging, and fMRI in particular, can make important contributions by providing insight into how the typically developing brain functions and the brain basis of altered development of cognitive, behavioral, and motor functions that define these pediatric disorders. The identified differences in brain function can serve as endophenotypes for correlation with genetic variations and as markers in investigations of candidate therapies; in doing so, they can help establish an improved framework for understanding the genetic and neurochemical basis of these disorders as well as for improving medical and behavioral management of the children who have them.

Questions

1. What are some of the differences between fMRI and other neuroimaging methods?
   A. fMRI has superior temporal resolution to EEG.
   B. fMRI has superior spatial resolution to EEG.
   C. fMRI has poorer spatial resolution than EEG.
   D. fMRI requires the injection of radioactive tracers.

2. What is the scanner measuring during BOLD fMRI?
   A. density of neurons in different areas of the brain
   B. electrical activity of neurons
   C. total amounts of oxygenated and deoxygenated hemoglobin
   D. changes in the concentrations of oxygenated and deoxygenated hemoglobin

3. What are some limitations of fMRI?
   A. It is sensitive to small motion artifacts.
   B. Susceptibility artifacts present near air-tissue interfaces make it more difficult to examine these regions.
   C. The presence of ferromagnetic materials inside an individual may preclude them from being scanned.
   D. All of the above.

4. In what ways could other technologies and lines of study be combined usefully with fMRI and what types of questions could these combinations address?
   A. combining fMRI and EEG to capitalize on the spatial resolution of fMRI and the temporal resolution of EEG
   B. combining fMRI and genetics to understand how brain function differs based on genotype
   C. combining fMRI and psychopharmacological treatment to understand how brain function is affected by treatment
   D. all of the above

5. Picture a task in which children look at pictures of faces every 2 seconds, and have to judge what gender the face is. What type of analysis would be most suitable for this study?
   A. block analysis
   B. event-related analysis
   C. resting-state functional connectivity analysis
   D. all equally appropriate

6. Picture a task in which children with autism and typically developing children are instructed to tap their right hand rapidly for 30 seconds, then their left hand rapidly for 30 seconds, then rest for 30 seconds, with the sequence repeating several times. The results show that for the contrast of "right hand tap minus rest," typically developing children show greater activation in a certain region of the cerebellum than children with autism. What can you say conclusively about the findings?

   A. Typically developing children have greater cerebellar activity during tapping than do children with autism.
   B. Typically developing children have less cerebellar activity during rest than do children with autism.
   C. Both A and B are conclusive.
   D. Neither A nor B is conclusive.

Answers

1. **B**
2. **D**
3. **D**
4. **D**
5. **B**
6. **D**

Acknowledgments

We would like to thank Dr. Roma Vasa and Dr. Stacy Suskauer for their helpful comments in improving the chapter.

REFERENCES

1. Ogawa S, et al. Brain magnetic resonance imaging with contrast dependent on blood oxygenation. *Proc Natl Acad Sci USA.* 1990;87:9868–9872.
2. Huettel SA, Song AW, McCarthy G. *Functional Magnetic Resonance Imaging.* Sunderland, MA: Sinauer Associates; 2004.
3. Wilke M, et al. Functional magnetic resonance imaging in pediatrics. *Neuropediatrics.* 2003;34:225–233.
4. Bandettini PA, Cox RW. Event-related fMRI contrast when using constant interstimulus interval: theory and experiment. *Magn Reson Med.* 2000;43:540–548.
5. Dale AM. Optimal experimental design for event-related fMRI. *Hum Brain Mapp.* 1999;8(2–3):109–114.
6. Byars AW, et al. Practical aspects of conducting large-scale functional magnetic resonance imaging studies in children. *J Child Neurol.* 2002;17:885–890.
7. Deichmann R, et al. Optimized EPI for fMRI studies of the orbitofrontal cortex. *Neuroimage.* 2003;19(2 Pt 1):430–441.
8. Glover GH, Law CS. Spiral-in/out BOLD fMRI for increased SNR and reduced susceptibility artifacts. *Magn Reson Med.* 2001;46:515–522.
9. Oakes TR, et al. Comparison of fMRI motion correction software tools. *Neuroimage.* 2005;28:529–543.
10. Casey BJ, et al. Activation of prefrontal cortex in children during a nonspatial working memory task with functional MRI. *Neuroimage.* 1995;2:221–229.
11. Slifer KJ, et al. Behavior analysis of motion control for pediatric neuroimaging. *J Appl Behav Anal.* 1993;26:469–470.
12. Wilke M, Schmithorst VJ, Holland SK. Assessment of spatial normalization of whole-brain magnetic resonance images in children. *Hum Brain Mapp.* 2002;17(1):48–60.
13. Oakes TR, et al. Integrating VBM into the general linear model with voxelwise anatomical covariates. *Neuroimage.* 2007;34:500–508.
14. Biederman J. Attention-deficit/hyperactivity disorder: a life-span perspective. *J Clin Psychiatry.* 1998;59(suppl 7):4–16.
15. Willcutt EG, et al. Neuropsychological analyses of comorbidity between reading disability and attention deficit hyperactivity disorder: in search of the common deficit. *Dev Neuropsychol.* 2005;27(1):35–78.
16. Geurts HM, et al. How specific are executive functioning deficits in attention deficit hyperactivity disorder and autism? *J Child Psychol Psychiatry.* 2004;45:836–854.
17. Wodka EL, et al. Evidence that response inhibition is a primary deficit in ADHD. *J Clin Exp Neuropsychol.* 2007;29:345–356.
18. Barkley RA. Behavioral inhibition, sustained attention, and executive functions: constructing a unifying theory of ADHD. *Psychol Bull.* 1997;121(1):65–94.
19. Klein C, et al. Intra-subject variability in attention-deficit hyperactivity disorder. *Biol Psychiatry.* 2006;60:1088–1097.
20. Lijffijt M, et al. A meta-analytic review of stopping performance in attention-deficit/

hyperactivity disorder: deficient inhibitory motor control? *J Abnorm Psychol.* 2005;114:216–222.
21. Aron AR, Poldrack RA. The cognitive neuroscience of response inhibition: relevance for genetic research in attention-deficit/hyperactivity disorder. *Biol Psychiatry.* 2005;57:1285–1292.
22. Mostofsky SH, Simmonds DJ. Response inhibition and response selection: two sides of the same coin. *J Cogn Neurosci.* 2008;20:751–761.
23. Mostofsky SH, et al. fMRI evidence that the neural basis of response inhibition is task-dependent. *Brain Res Cogn Brain Res.* 2003;17:419–430.
24. Vaidya CJ, et al. Selective effects of methylphenidate in attention deficit hyperactivity disorder: a functional magnetic resonance study. *Proc Natl Acad Sci USA.* 1998;95:14494–14499.
25. Rubia K, et al. Hypofrontality in attention deficit hyperactivity disorder during higher-order motor control: a study with functional MRI. *Am J Psychiatry.* 1999;156:891–896.
26. Rubia K, T et al. Neuropsychological analyses of impulsiveness in childhood hyperactivity. *Br J Psychiatry.* 2001;179:138–143.
27. Durston S, et al. Differential patterns of striatal activation in young children with and without ADHD. *Biol Psychiatry.* 2003;53:871–878.
28. Tamm L, et al. Event-related FMRI evidence of frontotemporal involvement in aberrant response inhibition and task switching in attention-deficit/hyperactivity disorder. *J Am Acad Child Adolesc Psychiatry.* 2004;43:1430–1440.
29. Schulz KP, et al. Response inhibition in adolescents diagnosed with attention deficit hyperactivity disorder during childhood: an event-related FMRI study. *Am J Psychiatry.* 2004;161:1650–1657.
30. Booth JR, et al. Larger deficits in brain networks for response inhibition than for visual selective attention in attention deficit hyperactivity disorder (ADHD). *J Child Psychol Psychiatry.* 2005;46:94–111.
31. Rubia K, et al. Abnormal brain activation during inhibition and error detection in medication-naive adolescents with ADHD. *Am J Psychiatry.* 2005;162:1067–1075.
32. Vaidya CJ, et al. Altered neural substrates of cognitive control in childhood ADHD: evidence from functional magnetic resonance imaging. *Am J Psychiatry.* 2005;162:1605–1613.
33. Durston S, et al. Activation in ventral prefrontal cortex is sensitive to genetic vulnerability for attention-deficit hyperactivity disorder. *Biol Psychiatry.* 2006;60:1062–1070.
34. Pliszka SR, et al. Neuroimaging of inhibitory control areas in children with attention deficit hyperactivity disorder who were treatment naive or in long-term treatment. *Am J Psychiatry.* 2006;163:1052–1060.
35. Smith AB, et al. Task-specific hypoactivation in prefrontal and temporoparietal brain regions during motor inhibition and task switching in medication-naive children and adolescents with attention deficit hyperactivity disorder. *Am J Psychiatry.* 2006;163:1044–1051.
36. Suskauer SJ, et al. fMRI evidence for abnormalities in response selection in ADHD: differences in activation associated with response inhibition but not habitual motor response. *J Cogn Neurosci.* In press.
37. Simmonds DJ, et al. Functional brain correlates of response time variability in children. *Neuropsychologia.* 2007;45:2147–2157.
38. Verte S, et al. The relationship of working memory, inhibition, and response variability in child psychopathology. *J Neurosci Methods.* 2006;151(1):5–14.
39. Shaw P, et al. Longitudinal mapping of cortical thickness and clinical outcome in children and adolescents with attention-deficit/hyperactivity disorder. *Arch Gen Psychiatry.* 2006;63:540–549.
40. Mostofsky SH, et al. Smaller prefrontal and premotor volumes in boys with attention-deficit/hyperactivity disorder. *Biol Psychiatry.* 2002;52:785–794.
41. Castellanos FX, et al. Developmental trajectories of brain volume abnormalities in children and adolescents with attention-deficit/hyperactivity disorder. *JAMA.* 2002;288:1740–1748.
42. Willcutt EG, et al. Validity of the executive function theory of attention-deficit/hyperactivity disorder: a meta-analytic review. *Biol Psychiatry.* 2005;57:1336–1346.
43. Vance A, et al. Right parietal dysfunction in children with attention deficit hyperactivity disorder, combined type: a functional MRI study. *Mol Psychiatry.* 2007;12:826–832.
44. Silk T, et al. Fronto-parietal activation in attention-deficit hyperactivity disorder, combined type: functional magnetic resonance imaging study. *Br J Psychiatry.* 2005;187:282–283.
45. Sergeant J. The cognitive-energetic model: an empirical approach to attention-deficit hyperactivity disorder. *Neurosci Biobehav Rev.* 2000;24(1):7–12.
46. Castellanos FX, Tannock R. Neuroscience of attention-deficit/hyperactivity disorder: the search for endophenotypes. *Nat Rev Neurosci.* 2002;3:617–628.
47. Teicher MH, et al. Functional deficits in basal ganglia of children with attention-deficit/hyperactivity disorder shown with functional magnetic resonance imaging relaxometry. *Nat Med.* 2000;6:470–473.
48. Anderson CM, et al. Effects of methylphenidate on functional magnetic resonance relaxometry of the cerebellar vermis in boys with ADHD. *Am J Psychiatry.* 2002;159:1322–1328.
49. Cao Q, et al. Abnormal neural activity in children with attention deficit hyperactivity disorder: a resting-state functional magnetic resonance imaging study. *Neuroreport.* 2006;17:1033–1036.

50. Zang YF, et al. Altered baseline brain activity in children with ADHD revealed by resting-state functional MRI. *Brain Dev.* 2007;29(2): 83–91.
51. Tian L, et al. Altered resting-state functional connectivity patterns of anterior cingulate cortex in adolescents with attention deficit hyperactivity disorder. *Neurosci Lett.* 2006;400(1–2): 39–43.
52. Swanson JM, et al. Etiologic subtypes of attention-deficit/hyperactivity disorder: brain imaging, molecular genetic and environmental factors and the dopamine hypothesis. *Neuropsychol Rev.* 2007;17(1):39–59.
53. Bobb AJ, et al. Molecular genetic studies of ADHD: 1991 to 2004. *Am J Med Genet B Neuropsychiatr Genet.* 2005;132(1):109–125.
54. Shafritz KM, et al. The effects of methylphenidate on neural systems of attention in attention deficit hyperactivity disorder. *Am J Psychiatry.* 2004;161:1990–1997.
55. Seyffert M, Castellanos FX. Functional MRI in pediatric neurobehavioral disorders. *Int Rev Neurobiol.* 2005;67:239–284.

CHAPTER 10

Neurofibromatosis Type 1 and Tuberous Sclerosis Complex

KALEB H. YOHAY AND MARTHA B. DENCKLA

Neurofibromatosis type 1 (NF1) and tuberous sclerosis complex (TSC) are autosomal dominant genetic conditions that affect multiple organ systems. Although both are tumor syndromes, the pathology related to both disorders extends far beyond the development of tumors. A significant amount of the morbidity associated with these two disorders results from their effects on cognition, behavior, and attention.

Neurofibromatosis Type 1

Neurofibromatosis type 1, also known as von Recklinghausen disease, is a common genetic disorder that affects multiple organ systems. It is inherited in autosomal dominant fashion and has an incidence of about 1 in 3,000 (1). Penetrance is 100% although there is wide variation in phenotype severity (2). Mosaicism may also occur. The NF1 gene is located on chromosome 17q11.2 and encodes for a protein called neurofibromin (3). Neurofibromin belongs to a family of proteins called GTPase activating proteins (GAP), which downregulate the proto-oncogene p21-RAS.

The diagnosis of NF1 is based on the presence of clinical features (Table 10.1). NF1 is usually diagnosed in infancy or early childhood. Essentially all patients with NF1 meet the criteria by young adulthood, with more than 95% meeting clinical criteria by age 8. About half of children with sporadic NF1 will meet the diagnostic criteria by age 1 (4). Genetic testing for NF1 is available but is of limited utility in the clinical setting and is generally reserved only for equivocal cases. Mutation analysis is not helpful in predicting phenotype or prognosis, with the exception of cases in which the entire gene is deleted, which may predict more severe disease (5).

Clinical Features

CAFÉ-AU-LAIT MACULES AND FRECKLING

Café-au-lait macules (CALs) are the most consistent manifestation of NF1 and are typically the first diagnostic criteria met by patients with NF1. These hyperpigmented macules are often present at birth and generally appear within the first year of life (4). They may increase in both size and number with age, although later in adulthood may fade.

TABLE 10.1 CLINICAL DIAGNOSTIC CRITERIA FOR NEUROFIBROMATOSIS 1 (NF1)

NF1 is present in a person who has two or more of the following signs:
Six or more café-au-lait macules >5 mm in greatest diameter in prepubertal individuals or >15 mm in greatest diameter after puberty
Two or more neurofibromas of any type or one or more plexiform neurofibromas
Freckling in the axial or inguinal region
A tumor of the optic pathway
Two or more Lisch nodules
A distinctive osseous lesion, such as sphenoid wing dysplasia, or thinning of the cortex of the long bones (with or without pseudarthrosis)
A first-degree relative with NF1 by the above criteria

Adapted from Neurofibromatosis. Conference statement, National Institutes of Health Consensus Development Conference. *Arch Neurol.* 1988; 45:575–578; with permission.

CALs are common in the normal population, with approximately 25% of the general population having one to three CALs. Greater than 95% of all patients with NF1 have CALs. CALs are generally oval with relatively smooth borders (Fig. 10.1). They usually range in size between 1 and 4 cm. Larger, more irregularly shaped CALs can be seen in NF1 but may also be indicative of other disorders associated with the presence of CALs such as McCune-Albright syndrome.

Axillary or inguinal freckling is also a diagnostic criterion for NF1. Freckling in NF1 is distinct in that it appears in non–sun-exposed areas such as the armpits, the groin area, or other intertriginous areas (Fig. 10.2). The freckling generally appears during childhood. Older patients with NF1 may develop more diffuse hyperpigmentation and freckling.

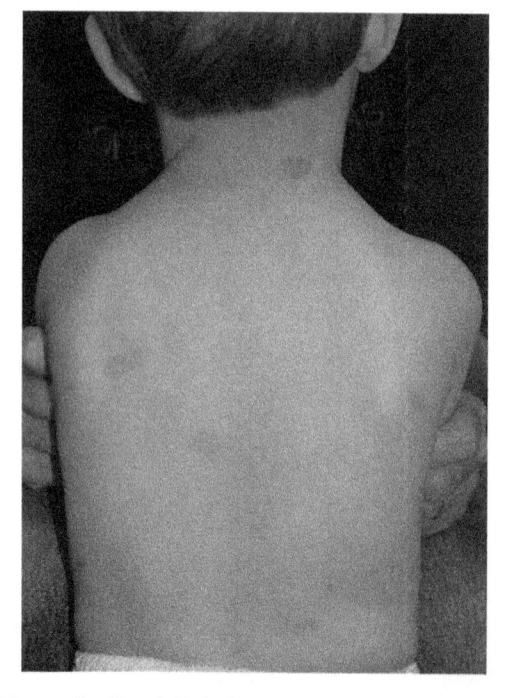

■ **FIGURE 10.1** Café-au-lait macules (CALs). Typical appearance of CALs in a 4-year-old boy with NF1. They are typically ovoid and smooth bordered.

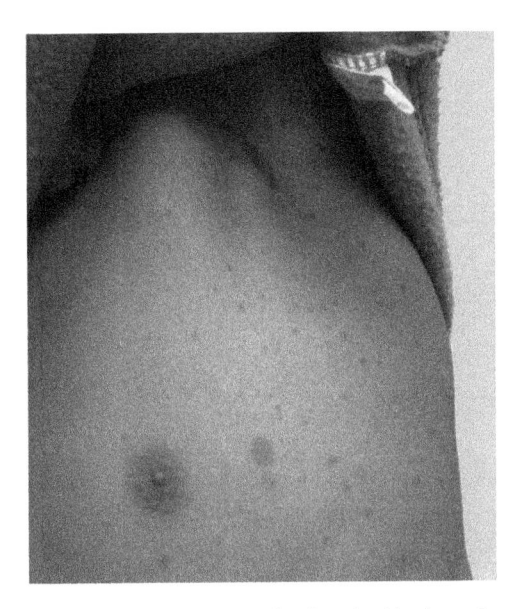

■ FIGURE 10.2 Axillary freckling. Typical appearance of axillary freckles in an 8-year-old girl with NF1.

NEUROFIBROMAS

Neurofibromas are the defining characteristic of NF1. Neurofibromas can be divided into several subtypes: cutaneous neurofibromas, subcutaneous neurofibromas, nodular plexiform neurofibromas, and diffuse plexiform neurofibromas. All types are composed of the mix of Schwann cells, fibroblasts, and mast cells (6). Cutaneous neurofibromas are soft, fleshy tumors that arise from the peripheral nerve sheath at the skin's surface (Fig. 10.3). They generally appear during late childhood or young adulthood (4). They can vary in color, size, and density. Some are sessile, whereas others are pedunculated. They are not premalignant but are often cosmetically significant and may cause itching or, less commonly, pain. Subcutaneous neurofibromas are generally firm, often tender nodules that arise along the course of the peripheral nerve below the surface of the skin. They also generally appear during adolescence or young adulthood. Like cutaneous neurofibromas, these are not considered to be premalignant but may become cosmetically significant or

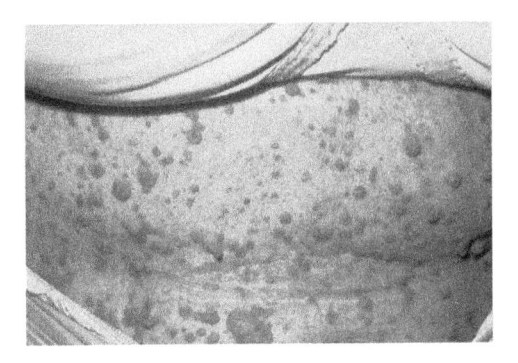

■ FIGURE 10.3 Cutaneous neurofibromas. Cutaneous neurofibromas are soft, fleshy benign growths arising from intracutaneous nerves. They can be sessile or pedunculated and can vary markedly in color, size and density. (From Goodheart HP, MD. *Goodheart's Photoguide of Common Skin Disorders*. 2nd ed. Philadelphia: Lippincott Williams & Wilkins; 2003; with permission.)

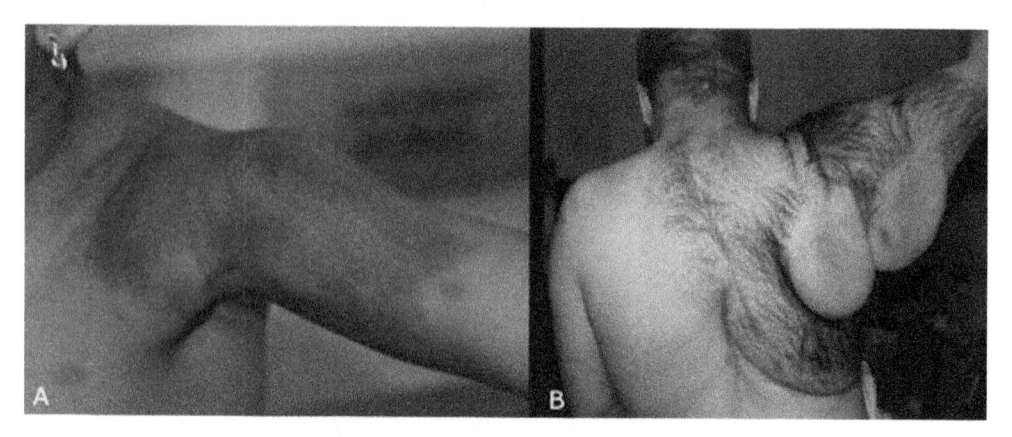

FIGURE 10.4 A: Plexiform neurofibroma in the shoulder of a 4-year-old girl with neurofibromatosis type 1 (NF1). Underlying the area of rough, hyperpigmented skin is a palpable, heterogeneous, mobile, painless mass. **B:** Plexiform neurofibroma in a 38-year-old man with NF1.

cause discomfort. Nodular plexiform neurofibromas arise along the proximal nerve roots and, because of their proximity to the spinal cord, can cause cord compression as well as vertebral erosion and scoliosis. Diffuse plexiform neurofibromas often involve multiple nerve fascicles or long lengths of nerve fibers. These are thought to be congenital and their origin may not be apparent initially (Fig. 10.4). Plexiform neurofibromas can be particularly problematical, in that they can become quite large, causing disfigurement or functional impairment or impingement on vital organs or structures.

Currently, no effective medical treatments for neurofibromas are available. Cutaneous neurofibromas may be removed with traditional plastic surgical techniques or by laser ablation. However, removal of cutaneous neurofibromas is generally reserved for those that cause discomfort or are cosmetically significant. Plexiform neurofibromas are particularly difficult to treat because they are generally large, irregular, and highly vascular and often involve numerous nerves. As a result, complete resection is generally not achievable and surgery is reserved for situations in which there is significant functional impairment, severe discomfort, or disfigurement. Furthermore, their growth patterns are variable, which makes treatment choices more difficult. These masses may stay quiescent throughout life, causing little or no morbidity, or may go through periods of rapid growth. They also have the potential for malignant transformation to a malignant peripheral nerve sheath tumor (MPNST). The lifetime risk of malignant transformation is probably between 5% and 13% (7,8).

CENTRAL NERVOUS SYSTEM TUMORS

Optic pathway gliomas (OPGs) are the most common central nervous system (CNS) tumor in patients with NF1. OPGs occur in up to 15% of patients with NF1 and generally develop during the first decade of life (9,10). These tumors are histologically low-grade astrocytomas arising anywhere along the optic pathway (Fig. 10.5). Most optic pathway gliomas are asymptomatic; however in the one third that are symptomatic, patients typically present with vision loss or proptosis or both. They may also present with signs of early onset of puberty if the tumor originates near the optic chiasm. Most patients with NF1 and optic pathway gliomas are managed conservatively with serial neuroimaging and ophthalmologic evaluation. For patients with progressive symptomatic disease, treatment with chemotherapy and, less commonly, surgery or radiation may be considered.

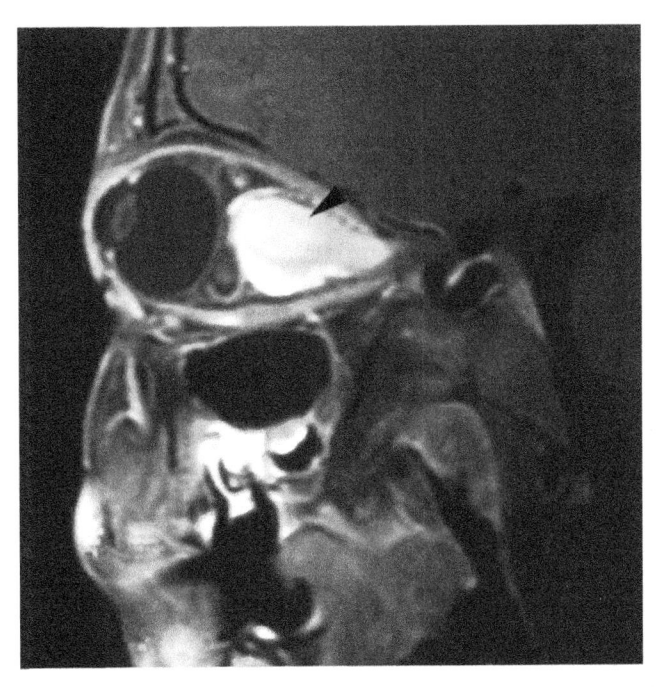

■ **FIGURE 10.5** Optic pathway glioma in a 5-year-old boy with neurofibromatosis type 1 (NF1). This sagittal magnetic resonance imaging (MRI) of the orbits demonstrates an avidly enhancing mass (*arrowhead*) within the optic nerve displacing the globe forward.

Patients with NF1 have an elevated risk for the development of brainstem gliomas. Unlike brainstem gliomas in the non-NF1 population, they are typically slow growing and asymptomatic and may not require treatment (11,12). There may also be an increased risk of development of other intracranial tumors, including low- and high-grade astrocytomas, medulloblastomas, meningiomas, ependymomas, and malignant schwannomas of the cranial nerves (13,14).

NON–CENTRAL NERVOUS SYSTEM MALIGNANCY

The most common malignancies seen in patients with NF1 are MPNSTs. These tumors are very aggressive, often fatal sarcomas. The lifetime risk of the development of a MPNST is between 5% and 13% (7,8). Typically, malignant transformation of the plexiform neurofibroma is heralded by rapid, asymmetrical growth of a known plexiform neurofibroma and new onset of significant pain. Imaging with magnetic resonance imaging (MRI) or positron emission tomography (PET) may be helpful in diagnosing MPNSTs. Treatment is difficult and generally requires a combination of surgical resection and chemotherapy.

Patients with NF1 are at low but increased risk of development of several other non–CNS malignancies, including juvenile chronic myelogenous leukemia, pheochromocytoma, and rhabdomyosarcoma.

OCULAR MANIFESTATIONS

The most common eye finding in patients with NF1 is the presence of Lisch nodules. These are small, pigmented, raised hamartomas present on the iris. These are best visualized using a slit lamp examination but may be seen through direct visualization. Lisch nodules generally cause no apparent symptoms. Congenital glaucoma is occasionally seen in NF1.

SKELETAL MANIFESTATIONS

Patients with NF1 are at increased risk for development of several bony lesions, including sphenoid wing dysplasia, pseudarthrosis, vertebral dysplasias, and scoliosis. Sphenoid wing dysplasia is a congenital abnormality of the sphenoid bone of the skull. This may be a disfiguring complication and may occur with or without the presence of an associated plexiform neurofibroma. It may result in intrusion of the temporal lobe into the orbit, causing a pulsatile proptosis. Pseudarthrosis, or false joint, may result from thinning of the long bone cortex, most commonly of the tibia, followed by pathological fracture and poor bone regrowth and healing. Pseudarthroses most typically manifest prior to the age of 2 years. Scoliosis occurs in more than 10% of patients with NF1. It may be a result of deformation of the vertebral bodies by nodular plexiform neurofibromas in the vertebral foramina or from dysplasia of the vertebral bodies.

CARDIOVASCULAR ABNORMALITIES

Patients with NF1 are also at increased risk of congenital and acquired cardiovascular abnormalities. These include vasculopathy, hypertension, and a wide range of congenital heart defects. Symptomatic vasculopathy is relatively uncommon but may result in stenosis, inclusion, aneurysm formation, or fistula formation. The most common symptomatic lesions are renal artery stenosis, leading to hypertension or stenosis of the internal carotid arteries, or middle cerebral artery stenosis, resulting in stroke, brain hypoperfusion, or seizures.

Hypertension may be seen in children with NF1 most commonly as a result of renal artery stenosis. Adult patients with NF1 may develop hypertension as a result of the development of pheochromocytoma, primary hypertension, or, less commonly, renal artery stenosis.

OTHER CENTRAL NERVOUS SYSTEM MANIFESTATIONS

Seizures are a relatively uncommon manifestation of NF1 with a prevalence of approximately 4%. They may be focal or generalized and may begin at any age. Macrocephaly occurs in approximately one half of children with NF1. Most commonly, macrocephaly is due to increased brain volume. Less commonly, it is due to hydrocephalus from aqueductal stenosis.

Unidentified bright objects (UBOs) are characteristic lesions in the brain seen on MRI in patients with NF1 (Fig. 10.6). These lesions most likely represent areas of myelin vacuolization and are not thought to be malignant or premalignant. They have no mass effect or contest enhancement on neuroimaging. They are generally not associated with focal neurological deficits; however, it has been suggested that the location or number of UBOs may be correlated with the degree of cognitive and behavioral dysfunction.

COGNITIVE AND BEHAVIORAL MANIFESTATIONS

Behavioral and cognitive manifestations are common in NF1 and represent a major source of morbidity. Intellectual development, learning disabilities, psychosocial impairments, attention problems, and emotional difficulties have all been associated with NF1.

Overall, intelligence appears to be somewhat affected in the NF1 population. The incidence of mental retardation in patients with neurofibromatosis is quite low with approximately 4% to 8% of patients having intelligence quotients (IQs) less than 70 (15). However, numerous studies have repeatedly shown that although patients with NF1 have IQs within the normal range, there is a downward shift in IQ of between 5 and 10 points when compared with unaffected siblings (16–18). There does not seem to be a consistent pattern in differences between the verbal IQ and performance IQ (19–23).

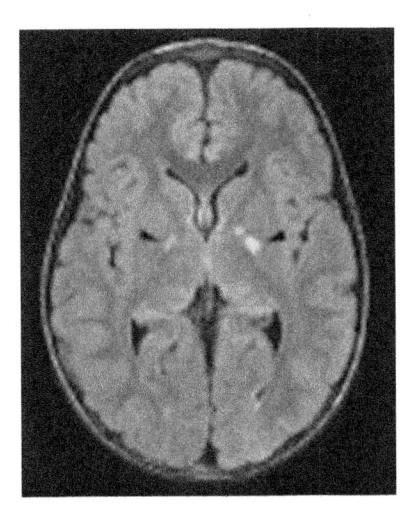

■ FIGURE 10.6 Unidentified bright objects (UBOs) in a patient with neurofibromatosis type 1 (NF1). This axial magnetic resonance imaging (MRI) [FLuid Attenuated Inversion Recovery (FLAIR) sequence] shows T2 bright lesions in the internal capsule bilaterally (*black arrowheads*). These do not enhance and cause no mass effect, typical of UBOs.

LEARNING DISABILITIES AND COGNITIVE PHENOTYPE

The prevalence of learning disabilities in children with NF1 is clearly increased with rates reported between 20% and 65% (24–30), compared with approximately 10% in the general population (30a). Specific patterns of learning disability have long been postulated, in particular that the cognitive phenotype of NF1 is primarily characterized by the presence of nonverbal learning disabilities. Over two decades ago Eliason (30b) demonstrated a high incidence of visual perceptual disability in children with NF1 (56%). Studies comparing children with NF1 to their unaffected siblings have demonstrated a leftward shift of the IQ and increased incidence of subtle neurological signs and visuospatial dysfunction (31–33). In particular, the Judgment of Line Orientation test, a measure of visuospatial function, is consistently abnormal in children with NF1 and learning disabilities (34). Other studies have demonstrated poor performance on tests of spatial memory (35) and visual motor integration (36). However, other work suggests that children with NF1 and learning disabilities demonstrate a broad range of cognitive deficits, such that the concept of a cognitive phenotype may not be useful. More recent studies have demonstrated that verbal learning disabilities may be as common as nonverbal learning disabilities (37–42) and may include impairments in phonological awareness, expressive and receptive vocabulary, verbal reasoning, and academic achievement in reading and writing (38). Furthermore, deficits in attention and organizational skills have also been demonstrated (43–45).

Attention deficit hyperactivity disorder (ADHD) also occurs with increased frequency in the NF1 population. In one study of children with NF1, 42% met criteria for ADHD, compared with 13% of their unaffected siblings (46). In another study of 81 children with neurofibromatosis, 38% met criteria for ADHD compared with 12% in their unaffected siblings. Furthermore, 46% of children with NF1 and a specific or global learning delay met criteria for ADHD (47). Children with NF1 and ADHD appear to respond to treatment with stimulants similarly to children having ADHD without NF1 (48).

Research examining the relationship between NF1 and other psychiatric disturbances such as anxiety and depression is quite limited, although some preliminary results suggest an association (49).

The underlying pathogenic mechanisms for the cognitive and behavioral aspects of NF1 are not well understood. In addition to its role as a tumor suppressor, neurofibromin may also play a role in embryonic CNS development (50,51). Dysfunction of neurofibromin may therefore result in underlying brain structural abnormalities and cognitive dysfunction; however, neuropathological data to support or refute this are scarce (52). Neuroimaging has provided the best tool for identifying structural and cognitive correlates. Some studies have suggested an association with UBOs and cognitive deficits. UBOs occur in 60% to 70% of children younger than 16 years with NF1, although they often disappear later in adulthood (53,54). The relationship between UBOs and cognition is complex. The presence of UBOs during childhood has been shown to be a predictor of cognitive dysfunction during adulthood (55). The number of locations UBOs occupy may correlate more with cognitive function than the total number or volume of UBOs (56). Location of the UBOs may also be important. One study demonstrated that thalamic lesions were associated with poorer cognitive function (57). Interestingly, magnetic resonance spectroscopy reveals abnormalities in the thalami of patients with NF1. These abnormalities are most pronounced in patients with UBOs in the thalami but were observed to be also present to a lesser extent in patients without UBOs in the thalami (58). This certainly suggests that UBOs may be only a small visible part of the underlying brain pathology present in NF1. Megalencephaly, which may be the result of both gray and white matter volumes (59), has also been suggested to possibly correlate with some aspects of cognitive dysfunction (60).

Tuberous Sclerosis Complex

Tuberous sclerosis complex is a relatively common genetic disorder that affects multiple organ systems and is primarily characterized by the development of benign neoplasms of the brain, skin, and kidneys. It may be inherited in autosomal dominant fashion (30%) or arise by spontaneous mutation (70%). Two genes are associated with TSC: TSC1 located on chromosome 9q34 and TSC2 located on chromosome 16p33.3. TSC1 encodes for a protein called hamartin, and TSC2 encodes for a protein called tuberin. These two proteins interact to form a complex that has been shown to be important in several intracellular signaling pathways. TSC has an incidence of about 1 in 6,000 (61) and has wide phenotypic variability. Recent studies have demonstrated that patients with mutations in TSC1 may have a milder phenotype than those with mutations in TSC2. (62,63). The diagnosis of TSC is generally made on the basis of clinical criteria (Table 10.2). Genetic testing is available, but poor sensitivity limits its clinical utility.

Clinical Features

CUTANEOUS MANIFESTATIONS

Skin lesions are very common in TSC and are often the presenting manifestation leading to diagnosis. With the exception of hypomelanotic macules, skin lesions are the result of hamartomatous growth. Hypomelanotic macules, also known as ash leaf lesions, are one of the most consistent features of TSC, occurring in up to 97% of patients (64) (Fig. 10.7). These are often present at birth and may become more numerous with age. They can occur anywhere on the body but tend to be most prominent on the trunk and buttocks. Hypomelanotic macules are not specific to TSC.

Facial angiofibromas are seen in up to three fourths of patients with TSC (64). These pink or reddish papular lesions involve the cheeks and nasolabial folds, sparing the up-

TABLE 10.2 CLINICAL DIAGNOSTIC CRITERIA FOR TUBEROUS SCLEROSIS COMPLEX (TSC)

Major Criteria	Minor Criteria
Facial angiofibromas or forehead plaque	Multiple pits in dental enamel
Nontraumatic ungual or periungual fibroma	Hamartomatous rectal polyps[c]
Hypomelanotic macules (three or more)	Bone cysts[d]
Shagreen patch (connective tissue nevus)	Cerebral white matter radial migration lines[a,d]
Multiple retinal nodular hamartomas	Gingival fibromas
Cortical tuber[a]	Nonrenal hamartoma[c]
Subependymal nodule	Retinal achromic patch
Subependymal giant-cell astrocytoma	"Confetti" skin lesions
Cardiac rhabdomyoma, single or multiple	Multiple renal cysts[c]
Lymphangiomyomatosis[b]	
Renal angiomyolipoma[b]	

Definite TSC: either two major features or one major feature plus two minor features; probable TSC: one major plus one minor feature; possible TSC: either one major feature or two or more minor features.
[a]When cerebral cortical dysplasia and cerebral white matter migration tracts occur together, they should be counted as one rather than two features of tuberous sclerosis.
[b]When both lymphangiomyomatosis and renal angiomyolipomas are present, other features of tuberous sclerosis should be present before a definite diagnosis is assigned.
[c]Histologic confirmation is suggested.
[d]Radiographic confirmation is sufficient.
Adapted from Roach ES, Gomez MR, Northrup H. Tuberous sclerosis complex consensus conference: revised clinical diagnostic criteria. *J Child Neurol.* 1998;13:624; with permission.

per lip, typically in a malar distribution (Fig. 10.8). They generally begin to appear during the preschool years and become more prominent with age. Forehead fibrous plaques are similar lesions seen in about 20% of patients with TSC. These are slightly elevated brownish or flesh-colored plaques made up of coalesced nodules. Shagreen patches are irregular areas of raised roughened skin often described as having an orange peel–like

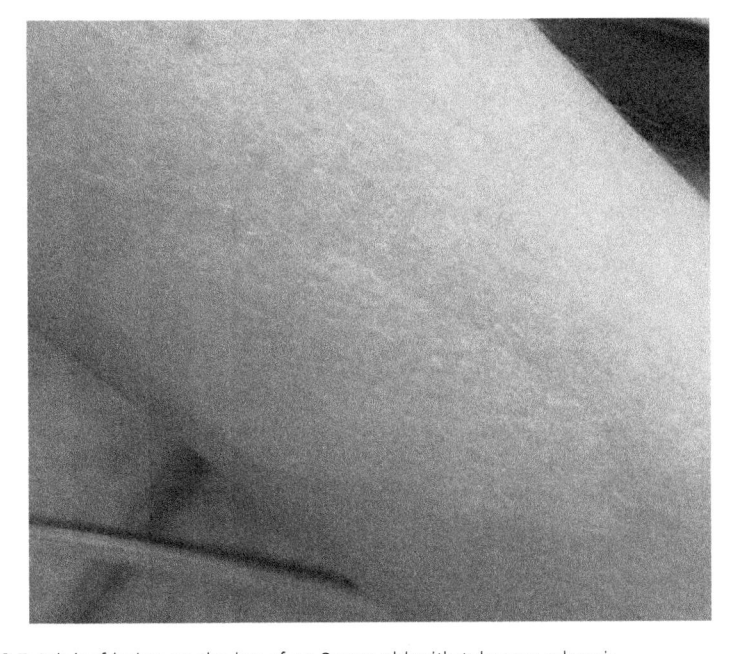

■ **FIGURE 10.7** Ash leaf lesion on the leg of an 8-year-old with tuberous sclerosis.

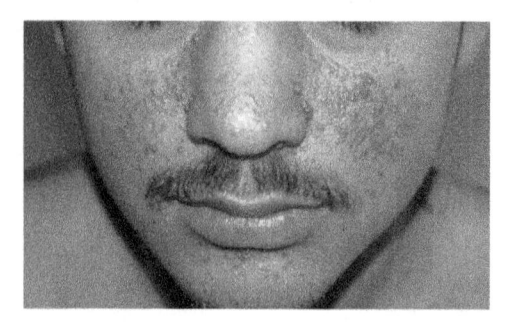

■ **FIGURE 10.8** Angiofibroma in a patient with tuberous sclerosis. Note the prominence in the malar regions and similarity in appearance to acne. (From Goodheart HP, MD. *Goodheart's Photoguide of Common Skin Disorders.* 2nd ed. Philadelphia: Lippincott Williams & Wilkins; 2003; with permission.)

texture (Fig. 10.9). They are seen in approximately one half of patients with TSC and generally manifest around the time of puberty (64). They tend to be most commonly located in the lumbosacral region but can appear elsewhere. Periungual or subungual fibromas are pink or flesh-colored nodules that grow in the fingernail or toenail beds in patients with TSC (Fig. 10.10).

CARDIAC MANIFESTATIONS

The most common cardiac manifestation of TSC is cardiac rhabdomyoma. These lesions may be seen in more than half of patients with TSC, although most cause no significant medical problems and regress spontaneously with age (65). When symptomatic, cardiac rhabdomyomas may present with heart failure, arrhythmia, or murmurs.

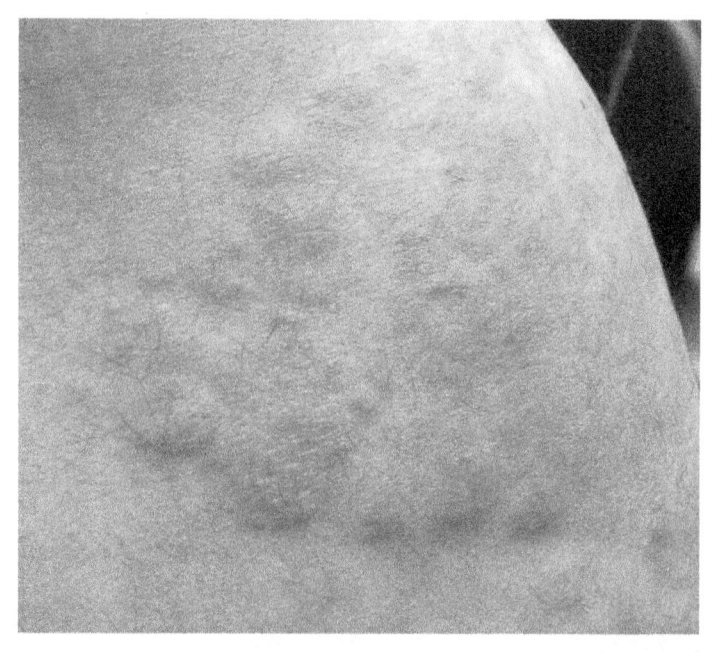

■ **FIGURE 10.9** Shagreen patch on the flank of a 12-year-old with tuberous sclerosis. The skin is raised and somewhat rough.

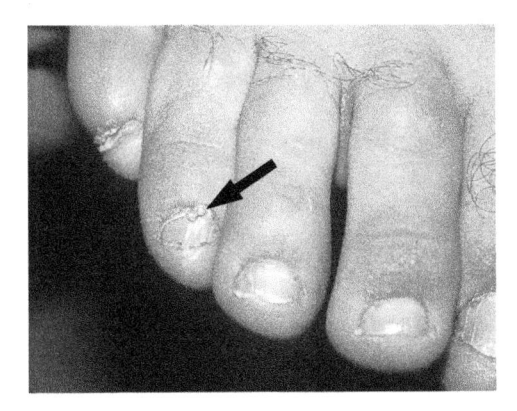

FIGURE 10.10 Periungual fibromas in a patient with tuberous sclerosis. (From Goodheart HP, MD. *Goodheart's Photoguide of Common Skin Disorders*. 2nd ed. Philadelphia: Lippincott Williams & Wilkins; 2003; with permission.)

RENAL MANIFESTATIONS

The most common renal complication of TSC is the growth of angiomyolipomas. These are benign tumors composed of immature smooth muscle cells, fat cells, and abnormal blood vessels. They are typically multiple and involve both kidneys at time of diagnosis. They occur in more than three fourths of patients with TSC, although most remain asymptomatic (66–68). When symptomatic, angiomyolipomas typically present with either renal failure or hypertension on the basis of encroachment on normal kidney tissue or hemorrhage due to aneurysm formation. Hemorrhage can be a life-threatening complication and is most commonly seen with angiomyolipomas more than 3 cm in diameter (68). Angiomyolipomas greater than 3 to 4 cm are often treated with embolization. Renal cysts are also common in TSC and, like angiomyolipomas, typically affect both kidneys. Renal cysts are more likely to present with hypertension and renal insufficiency or failure and are unlikely to present with hemorrhage. A relationship between TSC and renal carcinoma has been postulated but not yet clearly established (69,70).

OPHTHALMOLOGICAL MANIFESTATIONS

Several retinal abnormalities can be seen in patients with TSC; however, they are usually asymptomatic and only rarely cause any functional vision loss. Retinal hamartomas are seen in approximately half of patients with TSC. Punched-out areas of retinal depigmentation may also be seen. In addition, patients with TSC may develop angiofibromas of the eyelid, strabismus, or colobomas.

PULMONARY MANIFESTATIONS

Lymphangioleiomyomatosis (LAM) is a condition characterized by proliferation of atypical smooth muscle–like cells in the lungs and diffuse, progressive cystic destruction of lung tissue. It occurs almost exclusively in young adult women. It typically presents with dyspnea, hemoptysis, chest pain, chylothorax, and/or pneumothorax. It occurs in approximately one third of women with TSC (71–73). LAM is a chronic, sometimes progressive illness with a 10-year survival rate of about 90% (74).

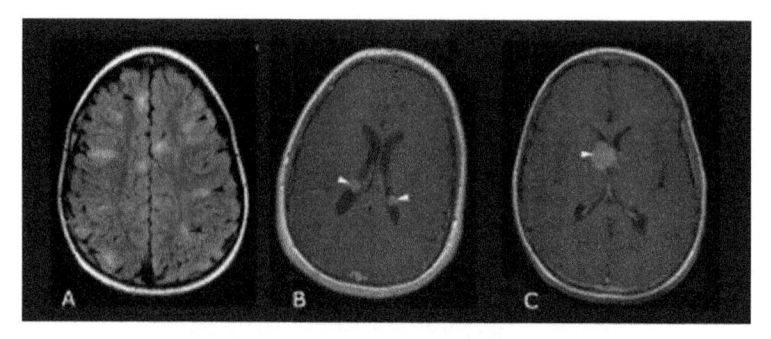

■ **FIGURE 10.11** Intracranial manifestations of tuberous sclerous. **A:** This axial FLAIR magnetic resonance imaging (MRI) demonstrates numerous bright lesions involving the cortex and subcortical white matter consistent with tubers *(closed arrows)*. **B:** This axial T1 MRI with contrast demonstrates enhancing nodules *(open arrows)* along the subependymal lining of the lateral ventricles, typical of subependymal nodules seen in most patients with tuberous sclerosis complex (TSC). **C:** This axial T1 MRI with contrast demonstrates an enhancing mass *(open arrows)* originating near the foramen of Monro, typical of a subependymal giant-cell astrocytoma (SEGA).

CENTRAL NERVOUS SYSTEM MANIFESTATIONS

Neurological complications of TSC are common and are one of the most prominent sources of morbidity and mortality in patients with TSC.

INTRACRANIAL MANIFESTATIONS

Cortical tubers are seen in as many as 95% of patients with TSC (75). Tubers (Fig. 10.11A) are composed of disorganized neurons and dysmorphic giant astrocytes. The border zone between gray and white matter becomes indistinct, and the normal six-layered lamination pattern of neurons in the cortex is lost. The number of cortical tubers has been shown to be correlated with the severity of seizures and cerebral dysfunction (76).

Lesions in the white matter are also commonly seen in TSC. These lesions represent areas of demyelination, dysmyelination, hypomyelination, or heterotopic neurons or glia along paths of cortical migration (75,77).

Subependymal nodules (SENs) are seen in most patients with TSC (62,75,78). SENs are hamartomatous lesions composed of dysplastic astrocytes and auroral cells located in the subependymal region (Fig. 10.11B). They appear as small lumps along the walls of the lateral ventricles that calcify with age. They often cluster around the foramen of Monro.

Subependymal giant-cell astrocytomas (SEGAs) are low-grade glioneuronal tumors that are seen in approximately 8% to 18% of patients with TSC (62,75,79). They typically originate near the foramen of Monro and, as a result, often cause obstructive hydrocephalus and may require surgical resection (Fig. 10.11C).

Seizures and epilepsy are very common in patients with TSC, with reported incidences ranging between 75% and 96% (62,80–82). Seizures most typically begin during infancy and early childhood, with incidence decreasing with increasing age. Seizures can be either generalized or partial in onset. Infantile spasms are seen in approximately one third of patients with TSC (62).

COGNITIVE AND BEHAVIORAL MANIFESTATIONS

Behavioral and cognitive impairments are common in TSC, with approximately one half of patients showing some degree of intellectual impairment and 60% diagnosed with behavioral problems such as autism, pervasive developmental disorder (PDD), obsessive compulsive disorder (OCD), or ADHD.

Intelligence can be normal or severely impaired in TSC. The TSC population appears to have a bimodal distribution of IQ. Approximately 70% of patients with TSC fall into a normal distribution, with mean scores 12 points below those of unaffected siblings, whereas about 30% of patients cluster around IQs in the profoundly impaired range (IQs less than 20) (83). Even those with normal IQs may have academic problems or learning disabilities. Learning disabilities in TSC have not been systematically studied; however, the incidence of learning disabilities in patients with IQs greater than 70 has been reported to be as high as 60% (62).

There is a broad range of estimates of the incidence of autism and PDD in patients with TSC; however, the incidence of classic autism is probably around 25%, with approximately 40% to 50% meeting diagnostic criteria for autism or PDD (83,84). Autism and PDD are more prevalent in patients with TSC and global intellectual impairment than in those with normal intelligence. Approximately half of patients with TSC meet the diagnostic criteria for ADHD (83).

Other psychiatric diagnoses may be associated with TSC, although few systematic data are available. The rates of anxiety, depressive disorders, OCD, and psychosis may be increased (83). A recent report suggests that up to 45% of adults with TSC demonstrate a high degree of psychological distress, particularly anxiety and depression (85).

Case One

M.J. is a 13-year-old boy with no significant past medical history. He attends eighth grade and is an honors student. One month prior to presentation he began complaining to his mother about episodes of mild substernal chest pain. Over the following weeks the pain increased in both severity and frequency. He was taken to his primary care physician, who performed an electrocardiogram (ECG) in the office, which was normal. Because of continued discomfort he was referred to a pediatric cardiologist. While at the cardiologist's office it was noted that his blood pressure was 200/120 mm Hg. He was admitted to the hospital. An echocardiogram was performed, which was normal. A renal ultrasound demonstrated a mass in the left kidney. Subsequently, a computed tomography (CT) of the abdomen was performed, which demonstrated a large heterogeneous mass in the left kidney. Serum catecholamine levels were normal, ruling out a pheochromocytoma.

On examination, M.J. is a well-developed and well-nourished young man in no apparent distress. He is alert and oriented but makes poor eye contact. He is exceedingly shy and very reticent. He answers questions with short, clipped responses. His affect is flat. His general physical examination is notable for four hypopigmented macules located on his left forearm, left upper back, right lower back, and right abdomen. In addition, he has an area of roughened, orange peel–like skin located over the left lower back consistent with a shagreen patch. His neurological examination demonstrates no focal abnormalities.

Based on these findings a clinical diagnosis of tuberous sclerosis was made. An MRI scan of the brain was obtained to evaluate for the presence of CNS manifestations. The MRI scan demonstrated multiple cortical and subcortical lesions consistent with tubers as well as multiple nonenhancing nodules along the subependymal wall. A 6-mm-diameter enhancing mass was also located near the left foramen of Monro, consistent with a small SEGA. There was no evidence of hydrocephalus.

M.J. subsequently underwent a resection of the left kidney. Essentially, the entire left kidney had been replaced by tumor, and no viable tissue remained. Pathological evaluation of the specimen revealed an angiomyolipoma. His blood pressure initially required treatment with nifedipine and labetalol, but he was able to be weaned successfully postoperatively.

M.J. is currently being monitored with serial brain MRI scans, to check for progression of the presumed SEGA. His right kidney is currently free of evidence of any cystic disease or angiomyolipomas, but he is being monitored with yearly renal ultrasound. After a recent psychiatric evaluation, M.J. was diagnosed with social anxiety disorder for which he is being treated with fluoxetine.

Case Two

P.C. is a 14-year-old girl with a long-standing history of NF1. She was noted to have numerous CALs, but the diagnosis of NF1 was not made until she was 8 years old when axillary and inguinal freckling and several cutaneous neurofibromas were noted. Subsequent ophthalmological evaluation revealed numerous Lisch nodules. She has a history of learning disabilities, for which she gets special help in school. She has been diagnosed with attention deficit disorder, which has responded well to treatment with stimulants. An MRI scan of the brain was obtained at age 9 because of new onset of headaches. The MRI of the brain revealed numerous UBOs in the deep cerebellar gray matter, brainstem, and internal capsule. Her headaches responded to treatment with naproxen sodium. At age 10, P.C. noticed a new nodule beneath the occipital scalp. It was mobile and nontender; however it bothered her whenever she brushed her hair. Over the past several years the nodule has grown slowly. In the past 2 months the nodule has increased rapidly in its rate of growth and has become intermittently painful.

On examination P.C. is alert, conversational, oriented, and in no apparent distress. Examination of her scalp reveals a large mass measuring approximately 10 × 8 cm that is protruding from the occipital region just to the left of midline. The skin overlying the mass has a paucity of hair and is rough in texture. The mass is heterogeneous in consistency with some portions being soft while others are rock hard. It is moderately tender to palpation. Skin examination reveals numerous CALs scattered across her limbs and torso, freckling in the axillary and inguinal regions, and several 2- to 6-mm cutaneous neurofibromas, some sessile, some pedunculated, scattered across her torso and arms. She has mild scoliosis. Neurological examination demonstrates no focal abnormalities.

Because of the rapid increase in growth of the presumed plexiform neurofibroma of her occipital scalp, along with a new onset of pain, P.C. underwent MRI and PET scans. The MRI demonstrated heterogeneity and cystic changes within the mass as well as avid enhancement. There was no bony erosion or intracranial encroachment. The PET scan demonstrated increased glucose uptake within the mass, which was concerning for possible malignancy.

P.C. underwent a gross total resection of the scalp mass. Pathological evaluation demonstrated the mass to be an MPNST with a very high mitotic index. P.C. is currently undergoing radiation therapy.

Case Three

G.B. is a 4-year-old girl with a past medical history notable for short stature. G.B. is one of triplets. She was born at 32 weeks of gestation and weighed 4 lb. 2 oz. She has always been at or below the 2nd percentile for height, 25th percentile for weight, and 95th percentile for head circumference. Her two brothers are of normal stature. Developmentally, she has achieved motor milestones appropriately, although she has always reached those milestones 1 or 2 months after her brothers. She continues to be somewhat clumsy. She receives early intervention for mild language delay and articulation problems.

Because of her short stature, G.B. underwent evaluation by a pediatric endocrinologist. Growth hormone levels were found to be low normal. In preparation for initiation of growth hormone therapy, an MRI scan of the brain was ordered. The MRI scan demonstrated an expansile nonenhancing mass in the medulla. In addition, there are numerous T2 bright lesions particularly in the deep white matter of the cerebellum and in the basal ganglia.

G.B. has had no recent headaches, complaints of visual changes, new weakness or clumsiness, sensory symptoms, behavioral changes, respiratory problems, chewing or swallowing problems, change in weight or appetite, developmental regression, or gait abnormalities.

She has a long-standing history of numerous brown birthmarks, all of which are quite faint. There is no known history of cutaneous nodules; however, she has had a prominence of the dorsum of the left foot since infancy, which has always been attributed to asymmetrical distribution of body fat.

On examination, G.P. is alert and playful. Some of her speech is at times difficult to understand due to some mild articulation deficits. Her head circumference is approximately 95th percentile for age. She has numerous (more than six greater than 0.5 cm) CALs scattered across her torso and limbs. There is one small CAL on her forehead but no axillary or inguinal freckles, and no Lisch nodules. A soft, fleshy, nontender mass is present on the dorsum of her left foot. The skin overlying the mass is normal. Her neurological examination is notable for diffuse moderate hypotonia.

Based on her clinical findings of numerous CALs and a mass consistent with a plexiform neurofibroma of the left foot, the diagnosis of NF1 was made. She also has the associated features of relative macrocephaly, UBOs, and an asymptomatic mass in the medulla, consistent with a low-grade astrocytoma. Given the typically benign natural history of low-grade brainstem tumors in children with neurofibromatosis, the decision was made to monitor the mass with serial MRI scans. No other intervention is planned unless the mass progresses and becomes symptomatic, in which case surgery would be considered.

Questions

1. The presence of six or more CALs in a child
   A. is necessary for the diagnosis of NF1.
   B. is common in tuberous sclerosis.
   C. may be normal.
   D. merits careful monitoring due to the risk of malignant transformation.
   E. none of the above.

2. With regard to pain in patients with NF1:
   A. Pain is commonly associated with cutaneous neurofibromas.
   B. Pain may be an indicator of malignant transformation of a plexiform neurofibroma.
   C. Pain may be an indicator of malignant transformation of a cutaneous neurofibroma.
   D. Headache may be a sign of the presence of UBOs.
   E. None of the above.

3. Epilepsy is commonly seen in patients with
   A. neurofibromatosis 1.
   B. neurofibromatosis 2.
   C. tuberous sclerosis.

D. all of the above.
E. none of the above.

4. A 6-year-old girl presents with eight CALs ranging in size from 1 to 5 cm and freckling in the axillary region. Her parents are healthy and have no stigmata of neurofibromatosis. The parents are considering having a second child. In counseling the parents about the risk of NF1 in the second child, you tell them

   A. that the risk of having a second child with NF1 is uncertain, as the diagnosis in the first child is not certain.
   B. that NF1 is an autosomal dominant condition and therefore their risk of having a second child with NF1 is 50%.
   C. that NF1 is an autosomal recessive condition and therefore their risk of having a second child with NF1 is 25%.
   D. that their risk of having a second child with NF1 is essentially the same as the risk in the general population (approximately 1 in 3,000).
   E. that they should not have any more children.

5. With regard to renal complications in patients with NF1 and TSC:

   A. Hypertension in a child with NF1 is often due to the development of a pheochromocytoma.
   B. Hypertension in a child with TSC is usually due to renal artery stenosis.
   C. Hypertension in children with TSC may result from the development of angiomyolipomas or renal cysts.
   D. The renal cysts seen in TSC are at high risk for hemorrhage.
   E. Renal angiomyolipomas in children with TSC are always symptomatic.

6. An 8-month-old infant presents with generalized epilepsy. On examination she has three hypomelanotic macules and a raised area of roughened skin consistent with a shagreen patch. Family history for TSC is negative. Genetic testing is performed and is negative for mutations in the TSC1 and TSC 2 genes. The diagnosis of tuberous sclerosis is

   A. ruled out by the negative genetic test.
   B. questionable, due to the negative genetic test.
   C. very likely, on the basis of clinical manifestations.
   D. definite, on the basis of clinical manifestations.
   E. impossible to make at this age in the absence of a family history of tuberous sclerosis.

7. Regarding the cognitive and behavioral manifestations of NF1 and TSC:

   A. Autism and pervasive developmental delay are commonly seen in both NF1 and TSC.
   B. Intelligence is severely impaired in the majority of patients with NF1 and TSC.
   C. Even in patients with normal intelligence, learning disabilities are seen in the majority of children with NF1 or TSC.
   D. ADHD is uncommon in NF1 or TSC.

Answers

1. C. CALs are common in the general population. They are the most commonly met diagnostic criteria of an NF1 but are not necessary for the diagnosis. They may be seen occasionally in tuberous sclerosis. They are not premalignant.

2. B. New onset of pain in a plexiform neurofibroma may be the first indication of malignancy. Cutaneous neurofibromas may itch, but it is uncommon for them to be painful. Cutaneous neurofibromas do not undergo malignant transformation. The headaches are common in NF1 but are not associated with UBOs.

3. C. Seizures are very common in TSC, occurring in the vast majority of patients. Seizures are uncommon in NF1 and NF2.

4. D. Because the parents show no signs or symptoms of neurofibromatosis, it is most likely that this patient represents a sporadic mutation. As such, the parents are not carriers and the risk for future offspring is that of the general population. The only exception to this rule is in the rare instance that the parents have gonadal mosaicism, in which case there is some increased risk. NF1 is an autosomal dominant condition, and each child that the patient has in the future carries a 50% risk of inheriting the mutated gene.

5. C. Angiomyolipomas and renal cysts both occur in patients with tuberous sclerosis and can cause impaired renal function and hypertension. The most common cause of hypertension in children with NF1 is renal artery stenosis. Pheochromocytoma is more commonly a cause of hypertension in adult patients with NF1. Angiomyolipomas carry a high risk of hemorrhage, whereas renal cysts do not. Renal angiomyolipomas and renal cysts are often asymptomatic in children with tuberous sclerosis.

6. D. The diagnosis of tuberous sclerosis is made on the basis of clinical findings. This patient has two major features (three or more hypomelanotic macules and a shagreen patch) and therefore meets criteria for definite TSC. The genetic tests for TSC carry a fairly high false-negative rate, so a negative result does not rule out TSC. A positive family history is not necessary for the diagnosis of tuberous sclerosis.

7. C. Learning disabilities are very common in patients with NF1 and TSC, even in patients who are of normal intelligence. Autism and PDD are commonly seen in tuberous sclerosis and only occasionally in NF1. Attention deficit disorder is prevalent in both disorders.

REFERENCES

1. Littler M, Morton NE. Segregation analysis of peripheral neurofibromatosis (NF1). *J Med Genet.* 1990;27:307–310.
2. Riccardi VM, Lewis RA. Penetrance of von Recklinghausen neurofibromatosis: a distinction between predecessors and descendants. *Am J Hum Genet.* 1988;42:284–289.
3. Basu TN, et al. Aberrant regulation of ras proteins in malignant tumour cells from type 1 neurofibromatosis patients. *Nature.* 1992;356:713–715.
4. DeBella K, Szudek J, Friedman JM. Use of the national institutes of health criteria for diagnosis of neurofibromatosis 1 in children. *Pediatrics.* 2000;105(3 Pt 1):608–614.
5. Cnossen MH, et al. Deletions spanning the neurofibromatosis type 1 gene: implications for genotype-phenotype correlations in neurofibromatosis type 1? *Hum Mutat.* 1997;9:458–464.
6. Lott IT, Richardson EP Jr. Neuropathological findings and the biology of neurofibromatosis. *Adv Neurol.* 1981;29:23–32.
7. Ducatman BS, et al. Malignant peripheral nerve sheath tumors. A clinicopathologic study of 120 cases. *Cancer.* 1986;57:2006–2021.
8. Evans DG, et al. Malignant peripheral nerve sheath tumours in neurofibromatosis 1. *J Med Genet.* 2002;39:311–314.
9. Listernick R, et al. Natural history of optic pathway tumors in children with neurofibromatosis type 1: a longitudinal study. *J Pediatr.* 1994;125:63–66.
10. Listernick R, et al. Optic gliomas in children with neurofibromatosis type 1. *J Pediatr.* 1989;114:788–792.
11. Molloy PT, et al. Brainstem tumors in patients with neurofibromatosis type 1: a distinct clinical entity. *Neurology.* 1995;45:1897–1902.
12. Pollack IF, Shultz B, Mulvihill JJ. The management of brainstem gliomas in patients with neurofibromatosis 1. *Neurology.* 1996;46:1652–1660.
13. Cohen BH, Rothner AD. Incidence, types, and management of cancer in patients with neurofibromatosis. *Oncology (Williston Park).* 1989;3(9):23–30.
14. Korf BR. Malignancy in neurofibromatosis type 1. *Oncologist.* 2000;5:477–485.
15. North KN, et al. Cognitive function and academic performance in neurofibromatosis. 1: consensus statement from the NF1 Cognitive Disorders Task Force. *Neurology.* 1997;48:1121–1127.
16. North K, et al. Cognitive function and academic performance in children with neurofibromatosis type 1. *Dev Med Child Neurol.* 1995;37:427–436.
17. Eldridge R, et al. Neurofibromatosis type 1 (Recklinghausen's disease). Neurologic and cognitive assessment with sibling controls. *Am J Dis Child.* 1989;143:833–837.
18. North KN, et al. Cognitive function and academic performance in neurofibromatosis. 1: consensus statement from the NF1 Cognitive Disorders Task Force. *Neurology.* 1997;48:1121–1127.

19. Hofman KJ, et al. Neurofibromatosis type 1: the cognitive phenotype. *J Pediatr.* 1994;124(4):S1–S8.
20. Moore BD III, et al. Neuropsychological profile of children with neurofibromatosis, brain tumor, or both. *J Child Neurol.* 1994;9:368–377.
21. Eldridge R, et al. Neurofibromatosis type 1 (Recklinghausen's disease). Neurologic and cognitive assessment with sibling controls. *Am J Dis Child.* 1989;143:833–837.
22. Wadsby M, Lindehammar H, Eeg-Olofsson O. Neurofibromatosis in childhood: neuropsychological aspects. *Neurofibromatosis.* 1989;2(5–6):251–260.
23. North KN, et al. Cognitive function and academic performance in neurofibromatosis. 1: consensus statement from the NF1 Cognitive Disorders Task Force. *Neurology.* 1997;48:1121–1127.
24. Legius E, et al. Neurofibromatosis type 1 in childhood: a study of the neuropsychological profile in 45 children. *Genet Couns.* 1994;5(1):51–60.
25. Moore BD III, et al. Neuropsychological profile of children with neurofibromatosis, brain tumor, or both. *J Child Neurol.* 1994;9:368–377.
26. North K, et al. Specific learning disability in children with neurofibromatosis type 1: significance of MRI abnormalities. *Neurology.* 1994;44:878–883.
27. North K, et al. Cognitive function and academic performance in children with neurofibromatosis type 1. *Dev Med Child Neurol.* 1995;37:427–436.
28. Stine SB, Adams WV. Learning problems in neurofibromatosis patients. *Clin Orthop Relat Res.* 1989;(245):43–48.
29. Kayl AE, Moore BD III. Behavioral phenotype of neurofibromatosis, type 1. *Ment Retard Dev Disabil Res Rev.* 2000; 6(2):117–124.
30. Hyman SL, Arthur SE, North KN. Learning disabilities in children with neurofibromatosis type 1: subtypes, cognitive profile, and attention-deficit-hyperactivity disorder. *Dev Med Child Neurol.* 2006;48:973–977.
30a. Altarac M, Saroha E. Lifetime prevalence of learning disability among US children. *Pediatrics.* 2007; 119 Suppl 1:S77–S83.
30b. Eliason MJ. Neurofibromatosis: implications for learning and behavior. *J. Dev Behav Pediatr.* 1986; 7(3):175–179.
31. Eldridge R, et al. Neurofibromatosis type 1 (Recklinghausen's disease). Neurologic and cognitive assessment with sibling controls. *Am J Dis Child.* 1989;143:833–837.
32. Hofman KJ, et al. Neurofibromatosis type 1: the cognitive phenotype. *J Pediatr.* 1994;124(4):S1–S8.
33. Schrimsher GW, et al. Visual-spatial performance deficits in children with neurofibromatosis type-1. *Am J Med Genet A.* 2003;120:326–330.
34. North KN, et al. Cognitive function and academic performance in neurofibromatosis. 1: consensus statement from the NF1 Cognitive Disorders Task Force. *Neurology.* 1997;48:1121–1127.
35. Varnhagen CK, et al. Neurofibromatosis and psychological processes. *J Dev Behav Pediatr.* 1988;9:257–265.
36. North K. Neurofibromatosis type 1: review of the first 200 patients in an Australian clinic. *J Child Neurol.* 1993;8:395–402.
37. Hofman KJ, et al. Neurofibromatosis type 1: the cognitive phenotype. *J Pediatr.* 1994;124(4):S1–S8.
38. Mazzocco MM, et al. Language and reading deficits associated with neurofibromatosis type 1: evidence for a not-so-nonverbal learning disability. *Dev Neuropsychol.* 1995;11:503–522.
39. North K, et al. Specific learning disability in children with neurofibromatosis type 1: significance of MRI abnormalities. *Neurology.* 1994;44:878–883.
40. North K, et al. Cognitive function and academic performance in children with neurofibromatosis type 1. *Dev Med Child Neurol.* 1995;37:427–436.
41. Legius E, et al. Neurofibromatosis type 1 in childhood: a study of the neuropsychological profile in 45 children. *Genet Couns.* 1994;5(1):51–60.
42. Hofman KJ, et al. Neurofibromatosis type 1: the cognitive phenotype. *J Pediatr.* 1994;124(4):S1–S8.
43. North K, et al. Cognitive function and academic performance in children with neurofibromatosis type 1. *Dev Med Child Neurol.* 1995;37:427–436.
44. Ferner RE, Hughes RA, Weinman J. Intellectual impairment in neurofibromatosis 1. *J Neurol Sci.* 1996;138(1–2):125–133.
45. Hofman KJ, et al. Neurofibromatosis type 1: the cognitive phenotype. *J Pediatr.* 1994;124(4):S1–S8.
46. Koth CW, Cutting LE, Denckla MB. The association of neurofibromatosis type 1 and attention deficit hyperactivity disorder. *Child Neuropsychol.* 2000;6(3):185–194.
47. Hyman SL, Arthur SE, North KN. Learning disabilities in children with neurofibromatosis type 1: subtypes, cognitive profile, and attention-deficit-hyperactivity disorder. *Dev Med Child Neurol.* 2006;48:973–977.
48. Mautner VF, et al. Treatment of ADHD in neurofibromatosis type 1. *Dev Med Child Neurol.* 2002;44(3):164–170.
49. Johnson H, et al. Psychological disturbance and sleep disorders in children with neurofibromatosis type 1. *Dev Med Child Neurol.* 2005;47:237–242.
50. Daston MM, Ratner N. Neurofibromin, a predominantly neuronal GTPase activating protein in the adult, is ubiquitously expressed during development. *Dev Dyn.* 1992;195(3):216–226.

51. Daston MM, et al. The protein product of the neurofibromatosis type 1 gene is expressed at highest abundance in neurons, Schwann cells, and oligodendrocytes. *Neuron.* 1992;8(3):415–428.
52. North KN, et al. Cognitive function and academic performance in neurofibromatosis. 1: consensus statement from the NF1 Cognitive Disorders Task Force. *Neurology.* 1997;48:1121–1127.
53. Itoh T, et al. Neurofibromatosis type 1: the evolution of deep gray and white matter MR abnormalities. *AJNR Am J Neuroradiol.* 1994;15:1513–1519.
54. North KN, et al. Cognitive function and academic performance in neurofibromatosis. 1: consensus statement from the NF1 Cognitive Disorders Task Force. *Neurology.* 1997;48: 1121–1127.
55. Hyman SL, et al. Natural history of cognitive deficits and their relationship to MRI T2-hyperintensities in NF1. *Neurology.* 2003;60:1139–1145.
56. Denckla MB, et al. Relationship between T2-weighted hyperintensities (unidentified bright objects) and lower IQs in children with neurofibromatosis-1. *Am J Med Genet.* 1996;67(1):98–102.
57. Goh WH, et al. T2-weighted hyperintensities (unidentified bright objects) in children with neurofibromatosis 1: their impact on cognitive function. *J Child Neurol.* 2004;19:853–858.
58. Wang PY, et al. Thalamic involvement in neurofibromatosis type 1: evaluation with proton magnetic resonance spectroscopic imaging. *Ann Neurol.* 2000;47:477–484.
59. Greenwood RS, et al. Brain morphometry, T2-weighted hyperintensities, and IQ in children with neurofibromatosis type 1. *Arch Neurol.* 2005;62:1904–1908.
60. Cutting LE, et al. Relationship of cognitive functioning, whole brain volumes, and T2-weighted hyperintensities in neurofibromatosis-1. *J Child Neurol.* 2000;15(3):157–160.
61. Osborne JP, Fryer A, Webb D. Epidemiology of tuberous sclerosis. *Ann N Y Acad Sci.* 1991;615:125–127.
62. Au KS, et al. Genotype/phenotype correlation in 325 individuals referred for a diagnosis of tuberous sclerosis complex in the United States. *Genet Med.* 2007;9(2):88–100.
63. Dabora SL, et al. Mutational analysis in a cohort of 224 tuberous sclerosis patients indicates increased severity of TSC2, compared with TSC1, disease in multiple organs. *Am J Hum Genet.* 2001;68(1):64–80.
64. Jozwiak S, et al. Skin lesions in children with tuberous sclerosis complex: their prevalence, natural course, and diagnostic significance. *Int J Dermatol.* 1998;37:911–917.
65. Jozwiak S, et al. Clinical and genotype studies of cardiac tumors in 154 patients with tuberous sclerosis complex. *Pediatrics.* 2006;118(4):e1146–e1151.
66. Ewalt DH, et al. Renal lesion growth in children with tuberous sclerosis complex. *J Urol.* 1998;160(1):141–145.
67. Casper KA, et al. Tuberous sclerosis complex: renal imaging findings. *Radiology.* 2002;225:451–456.
68. O'Callaghan FJ, et al. An epidemiological study of renal pathology in tuberous sclerosis complex. *BJU Int.* 2004;94:853–857.
69. Selle B, et al. Population-based study of renal cell carcinoma in children in Germany, 1980–2005: more frequently localized tumors and underlying disorders compared with adult counterparts. *Cancer.* 2006;107:2906–2914.
70. Tello R, et al. Meta analysis of the relationship between tuberous sclerosis complex and renal cell carcinoma. *Eur J Radiol.* 1998;27(2):131–138.
71. Costello LC, Hartman TE, Ryu JH. High frequency of pulmonary lymphangioleiomyomatosis in women with tuberous sclerosis complex. *Mayo Clin Proc.* 2000;75:591–594.
72. Moss J, et al. Prevalence and clinical characteristics of lymphangioleiomyomatosis (LAM) in patients with tuberous sclerosis complex. *Am J Respir Crit Care Med.* 2001;164:669–671.
73. Franz DN, et al. Mutational and radiographic analysis of pulmonary disease consistent with lymphangioleiomyomatosis and micronodular pneumocyte hyperplasia in women with tuberous sclerosis. *Am J Respir Crit Care Med.* 2001;164:661–668.
74. Johnson SR, et al. Survival and disease progression in UK patients with lymphangioleiomyomatosis. *Thorax.* 2004;59:800–803.
75. Braffman BH, et al. MR imaging of tuberous sclerosis: pathogenesis of this phakomatosis, use of gadopentetate dimeglumine, and literature review. *Radiology.* 1992;183:227–238.
76. Goodman M, et al. Cortical tuber count: a biomarker indicating neurologic severity of tuberous sclerosis complex. *J Child Neurol.* 1997;12(2):85–90.
77. Iwasaki S, et al. MR and CT of tuberous sclerosis: linear abnormalities in the cerebral white matter. *AJNR Am J Neuroradiol.* 1990;11: 1029–1034.
78. Inoue Y, et al. CT and MR imaging of cerebral tuberous sclerosis. *Brain Dev.* 1998;20:209–221.
79. Goh S, Butler W, Thiele EA. Subependymal giant cell tumors in tuberous sclerosis complex. *Neurology.* 2004;63:1457–1461.
80. Webb DW, Fryer AE, Osborne JP. Morbidity associated with tuberous sclerosis: a population study. *Dev Med Child Neurol.* 1996;38(2):146–155.
81. Jozwiak S, et al. Usefulness of diagnostic criteria of tuberous sclerosis complex in pediatric patients. *J Child Neurol.* 2000;15:652–659.
82. Sparagana SP, et al. Seizure remission and antiepileptic drug discontinuation in children

with tuberous sclerosis complex. *Arch Neurol.* 2003;60:1286–1289.
83. Prather P, de Vries PJ. Behavioral and cognitive aspects of tuberous sclerosis complex. *J Child Neurol.* 2004;19:666–674.
84. Smalley SL. Autism and tuberous sclerosis. *J Autism Dev Disord.* 1998;28:407–414.
85. Pulsifer MB, Winterkorn EB, Thiele EA. Psychological profile of adults with tuberous sclerosis complex. *Epilepsy Behav.* 2007;10: 402–406.

CHAPTER 11

Static Encephalopathies and Common CNS Anomalies

ELISABETH GUTHRIE

Introduction

Static encephalopathy is a general term that refers to nonprogressive dysfunction of the brain. Static encephalopathy may be acquired *in utero*, perinatally, or postnatally. Faulty maturation of the central nervous system (CNS), prematurity, and perinatal events, as well as vascular, infectious, or traumatic insults to the CNS throughout life can all result in nonprogressive disruption of the normally functioning brain. The clinical presentation of static encephalopathy depends on the nature, timing, cerebral location, and degree of the neurological insult.

Because childhood and adolescence represent particularly dynamic periods of brain development, static deficits may change in clinical presentation and significance over time. For example, an impairment compromising visuomotor function (hand–eye coordination) may not be evident in infancy or even the preschool period. The same impairment will create significant difficulties for the school-aged child, when academic and extracurricular demands rely more heavily on fine motor coordination. Likewise, a child with a neurocognitive profile consistent with an impairment of language pragmatics or semantics, which facilitate the more nuanced aspects of communication, will encounter greater difficulties during later childhood and adolescence, as the social complexities of communication increase. The insult or injury to the brain has not changed or progressed, but the developmental context of the deficit has evolved. Some clinicians refer to these phenomena as "growing into a deficit."

Many types of static encephalopathy are described in other chapters of this book, most notably in the chapter on intellectual disabilities. Therefore the static encephalopathy this chapter describes is limited primarily to cerebral palsy, as well as some congenital lesions involving the CNS, that a child and adolescent psychiatrist is likely to encounter in practice over time.

Certain infectious and metabolic processes involving the CNS may have an indolent course and transiently resemble static encephalopathy; however, these processes are arrested, not static, and as such are not covered here.

Cerebral Palsy

Cerebral palsy is caused by a nonprogressive insult to the developing brain that results in abnormalities of muscular movement, posture, and tone. The diagnosis of cerebral palsy in no

TABLE 11.1. GESTATIONAL AGE AND CEREBRAL PALSY

Gestational Age	Prevalence of CP per 1,000 Live Births
<28 wk	76.6
28–31 wk	40.4
32–36 wk	6.7

Adapted from Keogh J, Badawi N. The origins of cerebral palsy. *Curr Opin Neurol* 2006;19:129–134, with permission.

way infers a particular disease process or etiology, but, rather, describes a disorder of motor function that is nonprogressive, acquired in early infancy, and results in lifelong disability.

Cerebral palsy is the most common motor disability of childhood, with an overall prevalence of approximately 2 per 1,000 (1). The highest prevalence of cerebral palsy is among extremely low-birth-weight/extremely low-gestational-age infants (ELBW/ELGA) (Tables 11.1 and 11.2). As in many developmental disorders, male children are more commonly affected than are female children, although the reasons for this remain uncertain (2).

Despite the decline in the incidence of cerebral palsy among prematurely born infants, the prevalence of cerebral palsy has increased slightly over time (3,4). This modest increase in prevalence is attributed to the increased survival of premature infants, improved interventions for cerebral palsy over the life span that result in increased longevity, and a relatively stable rate of cerebral palsy among term births (5).

As many authors point out, it is important to underscore the fact that, despite the clear vulnerability of extremely premature low-birth-weight infants to cerebral palsy, in the vast majority of these infants, cerebral palsy does not develop (6,7).

Medical opinion regarding the etiology of cerebral palsy has changed significantly over the past two decades. Prior to the mid 1980s, the major cause of cerebral palsy was thought to be intrapartum asphyxia, with resultant hypoxic and ischemic injury to the neonatal brain. Research findings and epidemiological studies have disputed this line of causality as overly restrictive and inaccurate and point to a cascade of antenatal abnormalities and events that negatively affect placental functioning, immune mechanisms, and, ultimately, the fetal central nervous system as a more plausible mechanism resulting in the development of cerebral palsy. Many researchers conceptualize distinct differences between preterm and term infants in whom cerebral palsy develops. Gestational age and low birth weight have been studied most rigorously, but additional factors in the premature infant that compound the risk for cerebral palsy include intrauterine growth retardation (IUGR), failure to administer multiple doses of antenatal steroids during prolonged premature labor, and postnatal complications in the neonatal nursery, including respiratory distress, infection, intraventricular hemorrhage, and subsequent neonatal course (8,9).

Extreme prematurity, IUGR, and pre- and postnatal complications increase the likelihood of periventricular leukomalacia (PVL). Periventricular leukomalacia represents injury to deep cerebral white matter and is the most common pathologic correlate of cerebral

TABLE 11.2. BIRTHWEIGHT AND CEREBRAL PALSY

Birthweight	Prevalence of CP per 1,000 Live Births
<1,000 g	82
1,000–1,499 g	54
1,500–2,500 g	6.7

Adapted from Keogh J, Badawi N. The origins of cerebral palsy. *Curr Opin Neurol* 2006;19:129–134, with permission.

palsy. Free radicals and cytokines that are released after periods of hypoxic-ischemic stress injure the vulnerable periventricular brain tissue. Because the extremely premature infant's brain appears to be more susceptible to injury, it sustains damage to the periventricular white matter more frequently than the brain in near-term infants (10–12). Younger fetuses are also more susceptible to intrauterine infection, as evidenced by the elevated positive amniotic fluid cultures and cytokines in women who go into labor before 34 weeks' gestation, even in low-risk pregnancies (13). Intrauterine infection also places the infant at increased risk for PVL.

Cerebral palsy is classified according to muscle-tone characteristics (spastic, dyskinetic, ataxic, atonic) and location of motor impairment (diplegia, hemiplegia, quadriplegia). In spasticity, a consistent increase in muscle tone results in tonic muscle contraction and, over time, contractures. Dyskinesia refers to abnormal, involuntary changes in muscle tone that result in two types of movements: choreiform movements are rapid and jerky and result from sudden tonic/atonic changes in tone, whereas athetosis is a twisting, writhing motion that results from slower changes in muscle tone. A third type of cerebral palsy, ataxic, refers to abnormalities of balance and position that affect voluntary movement. (6,14). Finally, atonic, or hyptonic, cerebral palsy refers to persistent, diffuse absent or low muscle tone (14).

Spastic cerebral palsy is the most common form of cerebral palsy and represents damage to the pyramidal tracts. Spastic cerebral palsy is further classified by localization; spasticity affecting the lower extremities is referred to as diplegia; spasticity affecting ipsilateral upper and lower extremities is referred to as hemiplegia; and spasticity involving all four extremities is spastic quadriplegia (Fig. 11.1).

Spastic diplegic cerebral palsy is most commonly associated with prematurity and represents a clinical consequence of periventricular leukomalacia (1,7). As the affected child matures, the tonic contraction of large pelvic girdle and thigh muscle groups result in internal rotation and often displacement of the hip. Contraction of the thigh and

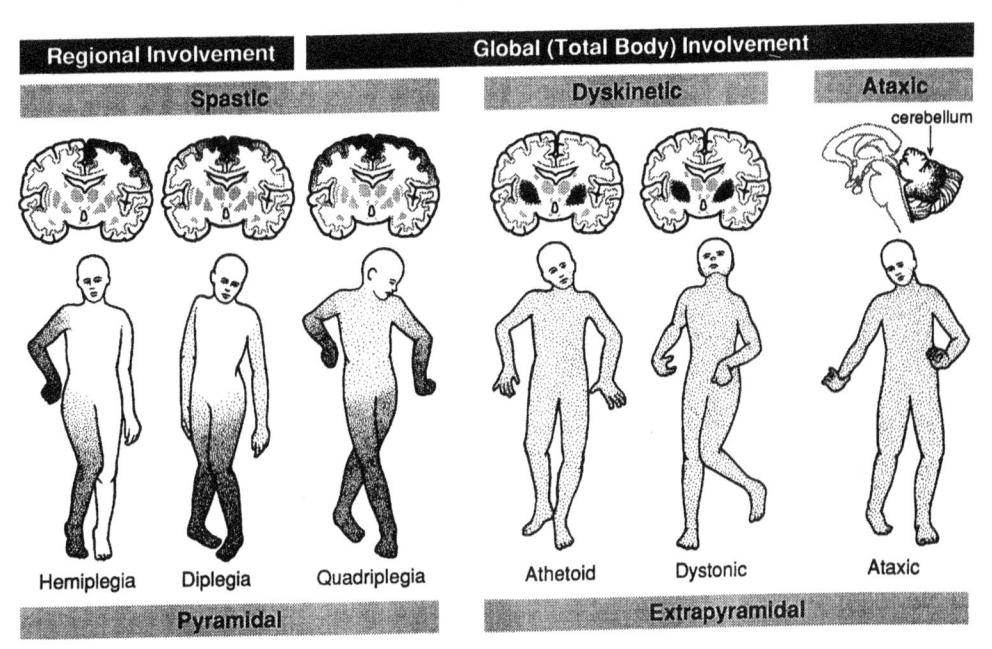

■ FIGURE 11.1. Different regions of the brain are affected in various forms of cerebral palsy. The darker the shading, the more severe the involvement. (Reprinted with permission from Pellegrino L. Cerebral palsy. In: Batshaw M, ed. *Children with disabilities*. Baltimore: Brookes Publishing, 2002:446.)

Scissoring **Toe Walking**

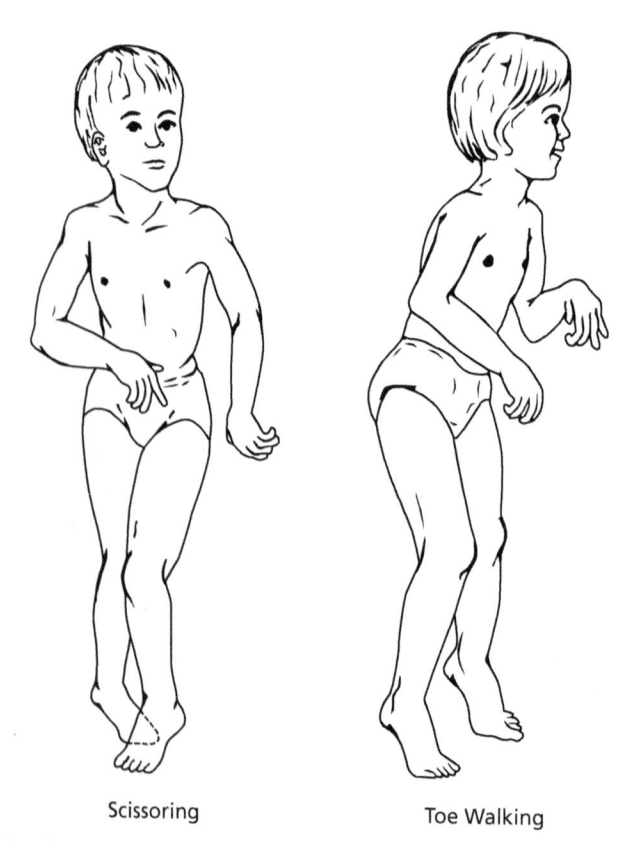

■ **FIGURE 11.2.** Scissoring results from increased tone in the muscles that control adduction and internal rotation of the hip. Toe-walking is due to an equinus position of the feet and increased extensor tone in the legs. (Reprinted with permission from Pellegrino L. Cerebral palsy. In: Batshaw M, ed. *Children with disabilities*. Baltimore: Brookes Publishing, 2002:451.)

calf muscles results in flexed knees that cross the midline and tight, shortened heel cords. The resultant gait is referred to as scissoring, and the shortened heel cords result in toe walking (Fig. 11.2).

Spastic hemiplegic cerebral palsy refers to ipsilateral upper- and lower-extremity involvement, with the upper extremity usually more affected than the lower. Spastic hemiplegia is often the result of a localized vascular injury, like stroke, and, as such, is the type of spastic cerebral palsy more commonly found in term infants (1,15). Because motor function is controlled by contralateral motor neurons, a spastic left-sided hemiplegia represents a right-sided cortical injury and vice versa. A youngster with hemiplegic cerebral palsy will have a flexed upper extremity and an ipsilateral rotated lower extremity with flexion at the knee and some heel-cord shortening. The gait does not appear scissored because both lower extremities are not involved; however, the involved leg often has the appearance of being dragged as compared with the unaffected side (6).

Dyskinetic cerebral palsies involve the entire body and represent injuries to deeper, extrapyramidal brain structures. In the past, kernicterus secondary to perinatal hyperbilirubinemia was the major cause of athetoid cerebral palsy. Today, dyskinetic cerebral palsy is generally the result of abnormalities of fetal brain development or severe perinatal hypoxia and ischemia in the term infant.

Atonic, or hypotonic, cerebral palsy refers to diffuse, persistent abnormalities of absent or low muscle tone despite preserved, or even exaggerated, deep tendon reflexes. By definition, the low tone is not secondary to peripheral nerve or muscle abnormalities. The central origins of atonic cerebral palsy are unknown (14).

Clinically, it is often difficult to detect cerebral palsy during the first year of life. Infants with cerebral palsy may be unable to coordinate oropharyngeal tasks, resulting in poor feeding and failure to thrive. Youngsters who have intermittent opisthonic posturing may roll over prematurely (before 2 to 3 months), and hemiplegic spasticity may lead to premature declaration of handedness (before 2 years of life), with the affected child favoring the unaffected upper extremity. A persistence of primitive reflexes and failure to meet motor milestones, especially ambulation, should alert the pediatrician to possible cerebral palsy. Some studies support developmental markers, including head control by 9 months, sitting independently by 20 months, and crawling by 30 months, to predict future ambulation. Failure to meet these developmental milestones, by 20 months for head control, 36 months for sitting, and 61 months for crawling, carries a poor prognosis for walking (16). Observations support a direct correlation between the duration of hypotonia and severity of cerebral palsy, such that those children with longer periods of hypotonia have more impairing cerebral palsy (14).

Timing in the development and the nature of the brain injury are critical factors in functional outcome. Usually, the more circumscribed the lesion responsible for cerebral palsy, the less devastating the long-term sequelae. For example, a vascular event (a stroke) in a term infant may result in hemiplegia without other sequelae. This is attributed to the observation that the infant's brain is more adaptable and able to compensate for localized injury.

The types of deficits and challenges that confront the child with cerebral palsy depend very much on the specific type of cerebral palsy and associated impairments. Between 40% and 50% of youngsters with cerebral palsy meet criteria for an additional diagnosis of mental retardation (8,17). More than half of the youngsters with spastic cerebral palsy demonstrate cognitive and adaptive capabilities within the normal range. However, an estimated 70% of children with dyskinetic cerebral palsy have subnormal intelligence (6,14). In approximately 40% to 50% of individuals with cerebral palsy, seizures (epilepsy) develop during childhood; 35% have a seizure disorder, and 16% to 20% have severe visual impairments (8,18). In 23% of premature infants with cerebral palsy, hydrocephalus develops, contrasted with 5% of term children with cerebral palsy, a discrepancy explained by the mechanism of CNS injury (8,19).

Rates of psychiatric disorders in youngsters with cerebral palsy are described as higher than expected (20). Problems with dependency, hyperactivity, and oppositional behavior are commonly reported by parents (21). Bipolar disorder has also been reported in older teens with cerebral palsy, although, because the cases are limited to two, the significance of this finding is unclear (22). Issues of autonomy and independence in adolescence are complicated by cerebral palsy. Because more severe cerebral palsy is frequently associated with additional cognitive and sensory impairments, it is unclear how much each of these variables may contribute to the elevated rates of psychopathology. In addition, most prevalence studies of psychiatric symptoms among individuals with cerebral palsy have relied on children attending clinics at larger academic institutions. This population of youngsters with cerebral palsy may reflect a higher number of more severely affected individuals, resulting in selection bias (21). In one study of children with hemiplegia that relied primarily on parent and teacher reports and, to a lesser degree, on individual assessments, 25% of the children were found to have an "emotional" disorder, 24% had a disorder of conduct, and another 26% had some form of hyperactivity (22). On 4-year follow-up, the externalizing behaviors persisted, with hyperactivity being most predictive of continued psychiatric problems (23).

Speech and language difficulties, which are known to be associated with increased psychiatric symptoms, are common problems for children with spastic and, to a lesser degree, dyskinetic cerebral palsy. Oropharyngeal musculature is often affected in cerebral palsy. As described earlier, when this occurs in infancy, feeding and growth difficulties commonly ensue. As an infant develops, the same musculature is recruited for speech, and other motor groups are used for nonverbal communication. Studies of speech and communication in children with cerebral palsy have described them as passive communicators who have more restricted repertoires for language communication than do their nonimpaired peers. Youngsters with cerebral palsy are less inclined to initiate conversation, answer open-ended questions, or exchange turns in a discourse with a familiar person. Not surprisingly, speech intelligibility is directly linked to these communication impairments (24). It is important that the psychiatrist be aware of these communicative constraints when working with the individual with cerebral palsy.

The task of the interdisciplinary team is not solely to treat the deficits, but also to delineate the individual's strengths and anticipate developmental challenges, to maximize function and growth. Motor impairment is managed primarily through physical therapy, pharmacological treatments (both oral and parenteral), orthopedic surgery, and, less commonly, neurosurgical intervention.

The mainstay of rehabilitation for individuals with cerebral palsy is physical therapy and movement (25,26). Maintaining and improving range of motion through active and passive exercise is critical for optimal motor function. Proper positioning, bracing, and splinting minimize malalignment and maximize functionality. Range-of-motion exercises that focus on stretching spastic muscles are often painful, as a spastic muscle will increase resistance to motion as the velocity of that motion increases. Youngsters, therefore, will often become reluctant and apprehensive regarding physical therapy, and it requires great skill on the part of the physical therapist, parents, and adjunct team members to maintain a therapeutic alliance.

Medications such as baclofen, dantrolene, and benzodiazepines may help to reduce increased muscle tone, although their efficacy remains somewhat controversial (27). Baclofen and benzodiazepines are often accompanied by significant drowsiness and fatigue. Less-common adverse effects include confusion, depression, disinhibition (benzodiazepines), and hallucinations (baclofen). Dantrolene is a calcium channel blocker and works directly on striated muscle. A common side effect of dantrolene also is sedation. The potential cognitive blunting of these adverse effects may impede academic success or compound preexisting learning problems.

Carbidopa-levodopa (Sinemet) and trihexyphenidyl (Artane) are often prescribed in the management of extrapyramidal dyskinesias. Trihexyphenidyl is an anticholinergic medication and, as such, may produce side effects that include agitation, nervousness, delusions, blurred vision, and tachycardia, among others. Carbidopa-levodopa is a dopamine agonist that can precipitate or exacerbate mood disorders and psychosis, along with other adverse physical effects.

Parenteral therapies in the form of nerve blocks and botulinum toxin avoid the untoward CNS side effects of sedation and lethargy. In nerve blocks, compounds that denature muscle are injected directly into motor nerves. When these same agents are injected more distally, at the junction of the motor nerve and striated muscle, the injection is referred to as a motor point block. Nerve blocks carry a risk of sensory nerve impairment. More recently, injectable botulinum toxin has become a routine part of treatment for dynamic contractures. Botulinum injections provide temporary and reversible inhibition of spasticity that generally lasts between 4 and 6 months. It is not clear whether repeated use of botulinum toxin produces significant functional improvement (28). As these invasive procedures are quite painful, and discomfort can persist for days afterward, repeated administration may call for cognitive and behavioral techniques to manage pain and anticipatory anxiety.

Individuals with spastic diplegia are at risk to develop hip dislocation over time. Adductor tenotomy before the hip-joint migration percentage (amount the hip articulation has deviated from proper alignment) reaches 50 degrees has been noted to reduce the trend toward lateral hip displacement (29). Some orthopedists recommend this surgery as a prophylactic intervention that should be done in ambulatory youngsters before 4 years of age for optimal results (30).

Additional treatments for cerebral palsy include neurosurgical interventions. Selective posterior rhizotomy is a neurosurgical intervention for spastic cerebral palsy that was introduced in the United States in the 1980s. The technique severs the dorsal nerve roots to muscle groups that are severely affected by spasticity, resulting in significantly reduced tone in the respective musculature. Rhizotomy must be followed up with a course of physical therapy geared at increasing range of motion, endurance, and relearning selected muscle use. A decrease in reported pain and observed anticipatory anxiety after rhizotomy has been associated with improved physical therapy compliance (31), although one study found rhizotomy ineffective (32).

An intrathecal baclofen infusion pump is a treatment option for intractable spasticity. This treatment places a catheter and pump subfascially in the thoracic spine. The device has proven to be effective in treating refractory spasticity (33). Primary complications include local inflammation and infection, which necessitate pump revision (34).

Hyperbaric oxygen has been studied and found to be ineffective in reversing or ameliorating motor impairments secondary to cerebral palsy (35,36).

Functional outcome and prognosis for the individual with cerebral palsy vary with severity and associated impairments. Intellectual functioning is a strong predictor of mortality and longevity. Even individuals with intelligence in the normal range have difficulty maintaining gainful employment because of their motor impairments (37).

Agenesis of the Corpus Callosum

The corpus callosum is the largest interhemispheric commissure in the human brain; however, its precise function remains somewhat elusive. *In utero*, corpus callosum development proceeds from the anterior to the posterior regions. Formation of the corpus callosum is a complex embryonic process involving multiple interdependent steps including midline patterning, the formation of the cerebral hemispheres, and neuronal and axonal migration across the midline to contralateral targets. Myelination of the corpus callosum begins posteriorly and proceeds anteriorly, beginning at approximately 3 months of life (38). Almost half of the fibers of the corpus callosum are not myelinated, suggesting that its role is not only the rapid transfer of information between cerebral hemispheres but also inhibition of such transfer (39). Excitatory transmission and inhibition of signaling facilitates integration of motor, sensory, and cognitive brain function. Some research supports the theory that the corpus callosum is necessary for acquiring skills but not necessary for maintaining these skills once learned.

Abnormalities in formation of the corpus callosum vary from complete agenesis (i.e., total absence) to hypogenesis (also referred to as partial agenesis) to hypoplasia, in which case the corpus callosum volume is less than that in age- and sex-matched norms.

Estimates on the prevalence of abnormalities of the corpus callosum vary and are complicated by selection bias. Most recent literature estimates that partial or complete agenesis of the corpus callosum occurs in approximately 1 in 4,000 individuals and has been found in 2.3% to 5% of radiographic studies performed on persons with developmental disability (40–42).

Agenesis of the corpus callosum has been described in two forms; in one form, the anomaly is limited primarily to the corpus callosum, with only minimal involvement of adjacent or phylogenetically similar structures; in the other, additional abnormalities of cell proliferation and migration are present. Individuals who have the more-circumscribed condition often have normal intelligence (43). Individuals with corpus callosum agenesis associated with additional abnormalities often have significant degrees of intellectual impairment and seizures.

Abnormalities of the corpus callosum have been found in association with numerous genetic syndromes (including Aicardi, Andermann, Apert, and Dandy-Walker syndromes), metabolic disorders (including Zellweger and Menkes), as well as autism and schizophrenia (44). In autism, evidence for intracortical underconnectivity that correlates with a reduction in corpus callosum size has been described (45). Clinically, these youngsters may appear as clearly dysmorphic, as in congenital syndromes, with midline defects such as cleft palate or extreme hypertelorism and macrocephaly, but as frequently may appear phenotypically unremarkable. Studies of neuropsychological profiles of individuals with partial or complete agenesis of the corpus callosum have found differences between verbal and performance IQ scores, although no consistent pattern has been described. (43). Language processing, as assessed by dichotic listening, may be more strongly lateralized in individuals with agenesis of the corpus callosum as compared with normal controls (46). Disturbances of higher language functioning, primarily language syntax and pragmatics, as well as prosody and humor, have been identified as deficits among individuals with agenesis of the corpus callosum. (47,48). Such deficits in communication are intriguing, as they may represent a neuroanatomical correlate for a pattern of social deficits described in youngsters who have difficulty understanding nonliteral language and emotional cues inherent in social communication.

Neural Tube Defects

Neural tube defects are the result of failure of fusion of the cranium or vertebral column or both that may be accompanied by herniation of the brain or spinal cord or both. Neural induction is a complex process whereby embryonic ectodermal tissue is influenced, and induced, by surrounding tissue to differentiate and mature into structures of the nervous system. (49). Neurulation, or the formation of the neural tube, of the fetal CNS occurs within the first 6 weeks of gestation (12,50). The complex genetic and environmental mechanisms that control this process are not fully understood, but they clearly play an important role in etiology. The prevalence of neural tube defects varies a great deal between populations and countries. The risk for having a child with a neural tube defect increases with advanced maternal age, lower socioeconomic status, and prenatal exposure to certain medications. In addition, because neural tube defects can be detected between 16 and 18 weeks *in utero* with an α-fetoprotein screen and subsequent ultrasonography, individuals who would not consider termination of a pregnancy that is complicated by a neural tube malformation have higher rates than the remainder of the population (51,52). The prevalence in the United States is estimated at 0.06% (6 per 10,000).

Neural tube malformations exist on a spectrum of severity. The most severe deformity, anencephaly, represents a failure of induction in brain development that results in spontaneous abortions or perinatal death. Encephalocele is the next most impairing deformity and results from a malformation of the brain and the skull during neural tube closure. Encephalocele describes the condition in which a portion of the brain protrudes outside the cranium. Anterior encephaloceles are generally less clinically impairing than posterior ones, but most children with encephaloceles have some degree of mental retardation (53).

Spina bifida refers to a failure of vertebral fusion. Spina bifida accounts for the majority of neural tube defects and, as such, is the type of spinal cord malformation a child psychiatrist is most likely to encounter in clinical practice. It is estimated that up to 10% of the population has the most benign form of neural tube anomaly, spina bifida occulta, in which a separation of vertebral arches is asymptomatic because no spinal cord involvement exists (50). Spina bifida lesions that involve the sac surrounding the spine, or meninges, or spinal cord or both are first seen with clinical symptoms that correspond to the location and nature of the malformation. Meningocele refers to an aperture in the spinal vertebrae that contains protruding meninges, but the spinal cord itself is not entrapped or involved. Myelomeningocele describes a malformation in which the meninges and spinal cord protrude, resulting in sensory loss and motor paralysis distally, and account for the majority of spina bifida lesions (54). Folic acid is now used prenatally to help prevent spina bifida (Fig. 11.3).

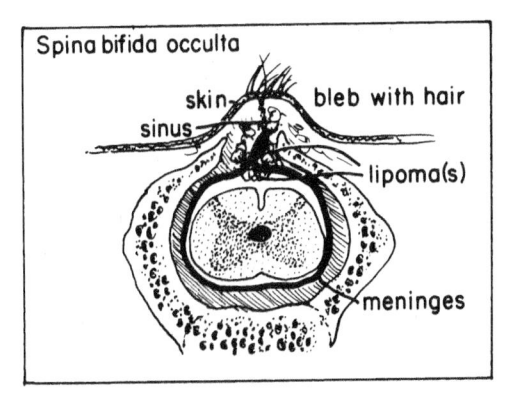

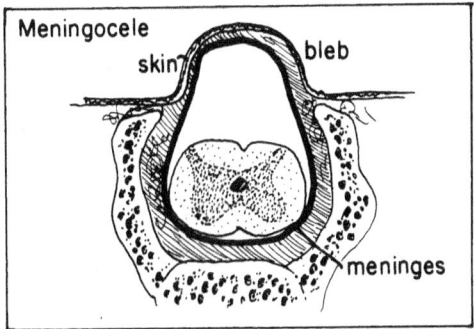

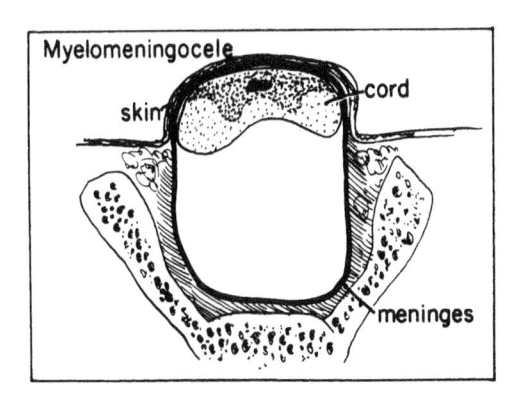

■ **FIGURE 11.3.** Illustrations of three common spinal neural tube defects of increasing severity. (Reprinted with permission from Pellock JM, Myer EC. Static encephalopathy and related disorders. In: Kaufman DM, Solomon GE, Pfeffer CR, eds. *Child and adolescent neurology for psychiatrists*. Baltimore: Williams & Wilkins, 1992:202.)

Thoracic level and high lumbar (L1 to L2) myelomeningoceles result in paralysis of the lower extremities and loss of sensation from the lower abdomen downward. Lower lesions result in varying degrees of paralysis and sensory loss, which is usually greater on the posterior surface of the lower extremities than on the anterior surfaces. Anal and genital sensation is lost.

In addition to the distal loss of function and sensation from the abnormal spinal cord, most children with myelomeningocele have abnormalities of brain development from faulty migration, including cortical heterotopias and dysplasias, abnormal gyrification, and malformations of the cerebellum and of the brainstem. A higher level of spinal lesion is a marker for more severe anomalies of brain development, which in turn are associated with poorer neurobehavioral outcomes. Higher myelomeningocele lesions may be associated with reductions in cerebrum and cerebellum volumes, lower scores on IQ testing, fewer academic skills, and less-adaptive behavior (55). Sleep apnea is common among children with myelomeningocele and important to recognize, as it compounds disturbances of behavior and cognition (56).

Specific neuropsychological profiles for youngsters with meningomyelocele have focused on problems with semantic and pragmatic language in addition to relative deficiencies in visuoperceptual and motor integration. Again, these problems are almost always related to faulty maturation and associated CNS anomalies, as is described in further detail later under the topic of hydrocephalus.

Social isolation is common among youngsters with meningomyelocele, due, initially, to their restricted activity and bladder incontinence and, later, by their higher cognitive-language deficits. Inability to participate in developmentally appropriate activities in the classroom, in sports, and in social gatherings, predisposes these patients to depression. Some research suggests that girls are at greater risk than boys for depressed mood, low self-esteem, and self-blame (57). The perceived amount of family support a child with meningomyelocele receives may ameliorate the depressive symptoms. Mood disturbance, neuropsychological difficulties, and poor academic achievement present a challenge to the family and physician.

Despite these challenges, the prognosis for myelomeningocele has improved greatly over the past 50 years. Survival into adulthood has increased by a factor of 8.5 (58). Approximately half of all adult survivors can ambulate short distances and have maintained urinary and bowel continence (59). The majority of youngsters with myelomeningocele have borderline IQ scores, followed by approximately 35% who score below 50 on FS IQ and require assistance with adaptive functioning (60).

Myelomeningocele in the lumbar and thoracic regions is almost always associated with a downward displacement of the brainstem and cerebellum called Arnold-Chiari malformations. Approximately 80% of children with myelomeningocele have hydrocephalus. Complications of Arnold–Chiari malformations and hydrocephalus are frequently associated with worse outcomes; however, these youngsters, who are usually born at term or mildly preterm, fare better than infants who acquire hydrocephalus secondary to prematurity (61).

Arnold-Chiari Malformation

Arnold–Chiari malformation results from anomalous development of skeletal and hindbrain structures, such that the cerebellum herniates, to varying degrees, through the foramen magnum. Type I Arnold–Chiari malformation describes a condition in which the medulla is displaced caudally into the cervical spinal column, and the most inferior cerebellum herniates through the foramen magnum. Type I is often asymptomatic until adolescence or young adulthood, when symptoms from medullary compromise may appear with recurrent apneic attacks, occipital headache, and neck pain, or signs of cervical compression (61). Compression of the hindbrain may result in subclinical syringomyelia and resultant scoliosis; rare reports exist of scoliosis in children with Chiari type I malformation without syringomyelia (62). Rarely, Chiari type I malformation results in aqueductal stenosis and resultant hydrocephalus (50,60).

In contrast, Chiari type II malformation is commonly diagnosed in childhood. The type II malformation consists of any of the anomalies present in type I in association with noncommunicating hydrocephalus. In type II, the elongation of the medulla is more pronounced, and the pons is often involved. Because the medulla and cerebellum are displaced into the spinal column, the cervical spinal roots are likewise shifted inferiorly and must travel upward to exit from their respective foramens. These additional structural changes may result in further compromise of cervical spine (61–63).

Dandy–Walker Malformation

Dandy–Walker is thought to be a defect of neural tube closure and is characterized by partial or complete agenesis of the cerebellar vermis and cystic dilatation of the fourth ventricle that shifts caudally to displace the cerebellar hemispheres. The incidence of Dandy–Walker is 1 per 25,000 to 30,000 births (50,60). Because the fourth ventricle cyst enlarges in infancy, hydrocephalus is not initially present but develops in most affected children by age 3 months of life. Associated anomalies include agenesis of the corpus callosum, aqueductal stenosis, and abnormalities of cortical migration, as well as midline defects of the palate, cardiovascular system, and cystic kidneys (63). Intellectual capability and motor function may vary; in one review of 19 cases, approximately 40% performed within normal range academically, and approximately 15% had severe mental retardation and spasticity (64,65).

Hydrocephalus

Hydrocephalus is a condition in which CSF production exceeds absorption. CSF is secreted by the choroid plexus and absorbed primarily by the arachnoid villi. In theory, any condition that increases CSF production or decreases CSF absorption can result in hydrocephalus. However, overproduction of CSF is an extremely rare clinical occurrence, and hydrocephalus is generally the result of impaired absorption of CSF.

The age at onset, degree, and etiology of hydrocephalus all affect the signs, symptoms, and morbidity of the condition. Because of the supple nature of the cranium in infancy, head circumference will enlarge to accommodate the increase in intracranial pressure secondary to hydrocephalus in the younger child. Fibrous closure of the sutures occurs by about 6 months of life, and ossification of the basal skull is complete by age 8 (60). After age 12, sutures are permanently fused, and the cranial vault is a closed system. Therefore hydrocephalus that arises in infancy will appear with macrocephaly and attenuated signs of increased intracranial pressure, whereas hydrocephalus that emerges later in childhood will result in increased pressure but not increased head circumference.

Hydrocephalus may be communicating or noncommunicating. In communicating hydrocephalus, the blocked absorption occurs outside of the ventricular system; in noncommunicating, a blockage exists within the ventricular system, obstructing the flow of CSF. A variety of clinical conditions predispose to the development of hydrocephalus.

TABLE 11.3. CAUSES OF COMMUNICATING AND NONCOMMUNICATING HYDROCEPHALUS

Causes of hydrocephalus:
   Increased CSF production
   Decreased CSF absorption
Causes of noncommunicating hydrocephalus:
   Foramen of Monro obstruction
   Third ventricle obstruction
   Aqueductal stenosis
     Congenital
     Infection
     External compression
   IV ventricle: posterior fossa tumor
   Obstruction to Luschka and Magendie foramina
     Infection
Causes of communicating hydrocephalus:
   Congenital abnormalities
     Arnold-Chiari malformation
   Infections
     Pus and adhesions, especially base of brain
Meningitis
   Subarachnoid hemorrhage
   Tumor
   Sinus thrombosis or obstruction of venous return

Reprinted with permission from Pellock JM, Myer EC. Static encephalopathy and related disorders. In: Kaufman DM, Solomon GE, Pfeffer CR, eds. *Child and adolescent neurology for psychiatrists.* Baltimore: Williams & Wilkins, 1992:199.

Hydrocephalus secondary to intraventricular hemorrhage (IVH) in very preterm infants is found in approximately 14 per 1,000 births, or 15% of infants with IVH (66,67). Communicating hydrocephalus may result from CNS complications of very premature births that compromise CSF absorption; IVH accounts for 90% of hydrocephalus in this population. Congenital malformations may give rise to hydrocephalus; as described earlier, approximately 90% of Arnold–Chiari type II malformations are complicated by hydrocephalus. Any space-occupying lesion of the central nervous system that obstructs the outflow of CSF may result in noncommunicating hydrocephalus (Table 11.3).

As stated earlier, infants born very prematurely in whom hydrocephalus develops secondary to IVH have worse outcomes with regard to cerebral palsy, seizures, and mental retardation, than infants born with hydrocephalus associated with myelomeningocele (67,68).

Obstructions that are transient, such as the posterior fossa cyst in Dandy–Walker malformation, can result in intermittent noncommunicating hydrocephalus. Intermittent noncommunicating hydrocephalus usually results in a less severe and more variable clinical picture, with episodic signs and symptoms that may be difficult to assess unless a child is seen repeatedly over time. Hydrocephalus that reaches a physiologic equilibrium or stasis is referred to as "arrested hydrocephalus" and is generally associated with less neurocognitive morbidity (69,70).

Shunt placement is indicated in cases of progressive hydrocephalus (71,72). Infants who are operated on later than a month after diagnosis have poorer outcomes with regard to cognitive and language function than do those children with hydrocephalus who undergo shunting within a month of diagnosis (73). The treatment of increased ICP secondary to hydrocephalus is surgical placement of a shunt. Ventriculoperitoneal shunts are the first choice, but occasionally a shunt will be placed from the ventricles into the atria of the heart (ventriculoatrial). In the latter case, the child should receive prophylactic antibiotics to prevent endocarditis, as would any patient with a cardiac prosthesis (74).

Normal-pressure hydrocephalus in children and adolescents is poorly understood but does exist. It may occur as the sequelae of neonatal IVH or later-life vascular, infectious, or traumatic events that result in communicating hydrocephalus with partial obstruction of arachnoid CSF resorption. The result is an indolent and mild form of progressive hydrocephalus with normal CSF pressure but a marked pulse-pressure gradient that results in gradual ventricular enlargement and progressive damage of brain tissue, especially the white matter.

The clinical presentation for hydrocephalus in the first 2 years of life includes macrocephaly, thinning of the cranium, and impairment in upward gaze (sundowning). Persistence of primitive reflexes and increased spasticity in the lower extremities should alert the pediatrician to possible increased intracranial pressure. Feeding difficulties and speech difficulties secondary to dysfunction of the lower brainstem due to pressure effects may be present. In the older child, complaints may occur of headache, vision changes, endocrine changes (precocious puberty or abnormal growth curves), and cognitive slowing and deterioration, as well as behavior changes, gait abnormalities, and incontinence (75).

Neuropsychological profiles of youngsters with hydrocephalus in general have a pronounced discrepancy between verbal and performance functions, with visuoperceptual and visuomotor impairments that affect learning (70,76). Children with hydrocephalus also have deficiencies in both receptive and expressive language. Despite rapid word decoding, children with hydrocephalus have poor reading comprehension that has been attributed to deficiencies in inference and integration of discourse (77,78). Additional research has revealed that children with myelomeningocele with normal IQs perform poorly on oral-discourse tasks that rely on similar skills of inference and integration. Some researchers suggest that these deficiencies of discourse interpretation and production may result from faulty cross-modal (i.e., corpus callosal) processing (77,79).

Shunt obstruction is the most common complication after shunt placement, followed by shunt infection. Symptoms of either complication can be insidious, and vigilant clinical assessment is required to assess any change in mental status. Shunt infections occur in approximately 10% of procedures (80,81). The morbidity associated with shunt infections, especially recurrent infection, is significant and includes new onset of seizure disorders and neurocognitive decline (82).

The Role of the Psychiatrist

A variety of clinical conditions that result in static encephalopathy have been described in this chapter. They are diverse with regard to etiology, presentation, and natural history. The role of the psychiatrist entrusted with the care of a child and the family with static encephalopathy, regardless of etiology, should follow some general tenets.

First, problems with speech and communication are common and must be considered and assessed. Language and speech impairments should be identified and augmented forms of communications put in place early in the evaluation process.

Whereas the advanced clinician may draw on prior experience with similar clinical situations, each child and illness is unique and should be approached anew. The psychiatrist is in an excellent position to discover not only what physiological and psychological limitations a child has but also how those limits are experienced by the child and the family. Thus a thorough evaluation, including psychological and preferably neuropsychological testing, is a critical component to a comprehensive evaluation. Collateral information from parents, siblings, and teachers, as well as physical, occupational, and speech therapists, is the key to revealing not only a child's struggles and deficits, but successes and areas of strength.

Participating as a member of a multidisciplinary team in the overall management of a child with static encephalopathy is critical in ensuring up-to-date communication and coordination of services.

As compliance with treatment regimens is paramount for good outcomes, the psychiatrist should help maximize the child's participation in rehabilitation with cognitive behavioral techniques geared at decreasing anticipatory anxiety, making pharmacological interventions (in collaboration with the pediatrician or neurologist) geared at pain reduction, and consultation with individual therapists to advance their working alliance with the child and family.

The psychiatrist is in the privileged position of anticipating problems a child will encounter during maturation. Educating parents about the changing physical, cognitive, social, and emotional aspects of development through early childhood, the school-age years, adolescence, and young adulthood may help them anticipate obstacles as their child "grows into a deficit." Facilitating difficult conversations that recognize differences between the affected child and siblings or peers is another task the psychiatrist should be prepared to provide. In doing so, the effective therapist helps minimize the negative impact of parental or patient denial while maintaining a reasonable positive outlook that is optimistic without being naive.

Learning problems of some sort are always present among youngsters with static encephalopathy, and their early recognition and intervention are paramount to a child's future academic success. Identification of learning problems and the institution of an appropriate individualized educational plan is challenging for families who have never interfaced with specialized education. Even youngsters with cerebral palsy who have above-average scores on cognitive/IQ testing usually encounter difficulties in the school system and warrant specialized educational services.

Beyond the identification of learning disabilities and other health impairments affecting school performance, youngsters with static encephalopathy are at greater risk for psychiatric diagnoses. The psychiatrist must remain vigilant for internalizing symptoms of anxiety and depression, and problems with separation, individuation, behavior, and psychosis. Careful assessment across multiple situations and at different times will be necessary to diagnose psychiatric illness accurately in a child with static encephalopathy. Specific psychiatric disorders, when present, should be treated with evidenced-based treatments when possible. Youngsters who meet criteria for a diagnosis of attention-deficit hyperactivity disorder should receive psychopharmacologic intervention, as well as parent education and possibly behavioral therapy, in addition to an individualized educational plan. Children and adolescents with mild to moderate depression should receive cognitive, behavioral, and interpersonal therapy. For refractory or moderate to severe depression, adjunct psychopharmacologic intervention should be considered. Caution is necessary when considering the use of a psychotropic, and this is especially true if the child or adolescent is taking other medications.

Last, all treatment recommendations not only should correspond to an accurate diagnosis but also must be appropriate to the mental, physical, and psychological capabilities of the child and the family.

Questions

1. Static encephalopathy may result from:
   A. Teratogenic exposure *in utero*
   B. Perinatal vascular events
   C. CNS infection
   D. Traumatic brain injury
   E. All of the above

2. Cerebral palsy is classified by:
   A. Location and severity
   B. Muscle type and functional outcome

C. Location and functional outcome
D. Muscle type and location
E. All of the above

3. Which of the following statements are correct?
   A. Youngsters with cerebral palsy have some degree of cognitive impairment.
   B. Eighty percent of all children with dyskinetic cerebral palsy have a seizure disorder.
   C. Fewer than half of all children with spastic cerebral palsy have cognitive and adaptive capabilities within the normal range.
   D. The types of deficits that confront the child with cerebral palsy are a function of the specific type of cerebral palsy and associated impairments in that child.
   E. All of these statements are true.

4. Myelomeningocele:
   A. Is a malformation in which the meninges and spinal cord protrude
   B. May be prevented with prenatal folate administration
   C. Is a malformation that results in sensory loss and motor paralysis distal to the lesion
   D. Is a condition that accounts for the majority of spina bifida lesions
   E. All of the above

5. Signs of increased intracranial pressure include all but one of the following:
   A. Impaired upward gaze
   B. Microcephaly
   C. Apnea
   D. Poor feeding
   E. Speech difficulties

6. Studies have shown that youngsters with agenesis of the corpus callosum have:
   A. Lower rates of anxiety disorders
   B. Increased suicidal ideation
   C. Increased learning disorders
   D. Increased depression
   E. None of the above

Answers

1. E
2. D
3. D
4. E
5. B
6. C

REFERENCES

1. Keogh J, Badawi N. The origins of cerebral palsy. *Curr Opin Neurol.* 2006;19:129–134.
2. Johnston MV, Hagberg H. Sex and the pathogenesis of cerebral palsy. *Dev Med Child Neurol.* 2007; 49:74–78.
3. Paneth N, Hong T, Korzeniewski S. The descriptive epidemiology of cerebral palsy. *Clin Perinatol.* 2006;33:251–267.
4. Himmelmann K, Hagberg G, Beckung E, et al. The changing panorama of cerebral palsy in Sweden, IX: prevalence and origin in the birth year period. *Acta Paediatr.* 2005;94:287–294.
5. Doyle LW, Anderson PJ. Improved neurosensory outcomes at 8 years of age of extremely low birth weight children born in Victoria over three distinct eras. *Arch Dis Child Fetal Neonatal Ed.* 2005; 90:F484–F488.
6. Pellegrino L. Cerebral palsy. In: Batshaw ML, ed. *Children with disabilities.* 5th ed. Baltimore: Paul H. Brookes, 2002:443–466.
7. Grether J, Nelson K, Emery E. Prenatal and perinatal factors and cerebral palsy in very low birth weight infants. *J Pediatr.* 1996;128: 407–414.
8. Liptak GS, Accardo PJ. Health and social outcomes of children with cerebral palsy. *J Pediatr.* 2004;145(2 suppl 1):S36–S41.
9. French NP, Hagan R, Evans SF, et al. Repeated antenatal corticosteroids: effects on cerebral palsy and childhood behavior. *Am J Obstet Gynecol.* 2004;190:588–595.
10. Kinney HC. The near-term (late preterm) human brain and risk for periventricular leukomalacia: a review. *Semin Perinatol.* 2006;30:81–88.
11. Filkerth R. Periventricular leukomalacia: overview and recent findings. *Pediatr Dev Pathol.* 2006;9:3–13.
12. Graham EM, Olcroft CJ, Rai KK, et al. Neonatal cerebral white matter injury in preterm infants is associated with culture-positive infections and

12. only rarely with metabolic acidosis. *Am J Obstet Gynecol.* 2004;191:1305–1310.
13. Hagberg H, Mallard C, Jacobsson B. Role of cytokines in preterm labour and brain injury. *Br J Obstet Gynecol.* 2005;112:16–18.
14. Menkes JH, Sarnat HB. Perinatal asphyxia and trauma. In: Menkes JH, Sarnat HB, eds. *Child neurology.* 6th ed. Philadelphia: Lippincott Williams & Wilkins, 2000:401–466.
15. Kirton A, deVeber G. Cerebral palsy secondary to perinatal ischemic stroke. *Clin Perinatol.* 2006;33: 367–386.
16. dePaz AC, Burnett SM, Braga LW. Walking prognosis in cerebral palsy: a 22-year retrospective analysis. *Dev Med Child Neurol.* 1994;36:130–134.
17. Beckung E, Hagberg G. Neuroimpairments, activity limitations, and participation restrictions in children with cerebral palsy. *Dev Med Child Neurol.* 2002;44:309–316.
18. Delgado M, Schulman J, Nanes M, et al. Discontinuation of antiepileptic drug treatment after two seizure-free years in children with cerebral palsy. *Pediatrics.* 1996;97:192–197.
19. Hagberg B, Hagberg G, Olow I, et al. The changing pattern of cerebral palsy in Sweden, VII: prevalence and origin in the birth-year period 1987–1990. *Acta Paediatr.* 1996;85:954–960.
20. Goodman R, Scott S. Brain disorders. In: Goodman R, Scott S, eds. *Child psychiatry.* Oxford: Blackwell Scientific, 1997:182–186.
21. McDermott S, Coker A, Mani S, et al. Population-based analysis of behavior problems in children with cerebral palsy. *J Pediatr Psychol.* 1997;21: 447–463.
22. Goodman R, Graham P. Psychiatric problems in children with hemiplegia: cross-sectional epidemiological survey. *Br Med J.* 1996;312:1065–1069.
23. Goodman R. The longitudinal stability of psychiatric problems in children with hemiplegia. *J Child Psychol Psychiatry.* 1998;39:347–354.
24. Pennington L, Goldbart J, Marshall J. Interaction training for conversational partners of children with cerebral palsy: a systemic review. *Int J Lang Commun Disord.* 2004;39:151–170.
25. O'Neil ME, Fragala-Pinkham MA, Westcott SL, et al. Physical-therapy clinical-management recommendations for children with cerebral palsy: spastic diplegia: achieving functional-mobility outcomes. *Pediatr Phys Ther.* 2006;18:49–72.
26. Damiano D. Activity, activity, activity: rethinking our physical therapy approach to cerebral palsy. *Phys Ther.* 2006;86:1534–1540.
27. Montane E, Vallano A, Laporte JR. Oral antispastic drugs in nonprogressive neurologic diseases: a systematic review. *Neurology.* 2004;63:1357–1363.
28. Singhi P, Ray M. Botulinum toxin in children with cerebral palsy. *Indian J Pediatr.* 2004;71: 1087–1091.
29. Terjesen T, Lie GD, Hyldmo AA, Knaus A. Adductor tenotomy in spastic cerebral palsy. *Acta Orthop.* 2005;76:128–137.
30. Pap K, Kiss S, Vizkelety T, Szoke G. Open adductor tenotomy in the prevention of hip subluxation in cerebral palsy. *Int Orthop.* 2005;29:18–20.
31. Miller AC, Johann-Murphy M, Pitten Cate IN. Pain, anxiety, and cooperativeneess in children with cerebral palsy after rhizotomy: changes throughout rehabilitation. *J Pediatr Psychol.* 1997;22:689–705.
32. McLaughlin JF, Bjornson KF, Astley SJ, et al. Selective dorsal rhizotomy: efficacy and safety in an investigator-masked randomized clinical trial. *Dev Med Child Neurol.* 1998;40:239–247.
33. Albright A, Awaad Y, Muhonen M, et al. Performance and complications associated with the synchromed 10-ml infusion pump for intrathecal baclofen administration in children. *J Neurosurg.* 2004;101(1 suppl):64–68.
34. Vender JR, Hester S, Waller JL, et al. Identification and management of intrathecal baclofen pump complications: a comparison of pediatric and adult patients. *J Neurosurg.* 2006;104(1 suppl):9–15.
35. Hardy P, Collet JP, Goldberg J, et al. Neuropsychological effects of hyperbaric oxygen therapy in cerebral palsy. *Dev Med Child Neurol.* 2002;44: 436–446.
36. Collet JP, Vaqrasse M, Marois P, et al. Hyperbaric oxygen for children with cerebral palsy: a randomized multicentre trial. *Lancet.* 2001;357:582–586.
37. Murphy K, Molnar G, Lankasky K. Medical and functional status of adults with cerebral palsy. *Dev Med Child Neurol.* 1995;37:1075–1084.
38. Barkovich AJ, Kjos B. Normal postnatal development of the corpus callosum as demonstrated by MR imaging. *AJNR Am J Neuroradiol.* 1988;9: 487–491.
39. Devinsky O, Laff R. Callosal lesions and behavior: history and modern concepts. *Epilepsy Behav.* 2003;4:607–617.
40. Bodensteiner J, Schaefer GB, Breeding L, Cowan L. Hypoplasia of the corpus callosum: a study of 445 consecutive MRI scans. *J Child Neurol.* 1994;9: 47–49.
41. Wang L, Huang C, Yeh T. Major brain lesions detected on sonographic screening of apparently normal term neonates. *Neuroradiology.* 2004;46: 368–373.
42. Jeret JS, Serur D, Wiesniewski K, Fisch C. Frequency of agenesis of the corpus callosum in the developmentally disabled population as determined by computerized tomography. *Pediatr Neurosci.* 1986;12:101–103.
43. Chiarello C. A house divided? Cognitive functioning with callosal agenesis. *Brain Lang.* 1980; 11:128–158.
44. Paul LK, Brown WS, Adolphs R, et al. Agenesis of the corpus callosum: genetic, developmental, and functional aspects of connectivity. *Nat Rev Neurosci.* 2007;8:287–299.
45. Just M, Cherkassky VL, et al. Functional and anatomical cortical underconnectivity in autism: evidence from an fMRI study of an executive-

46. Lassonde M, Bryden MP, Demers P. The corpus callosum and cerebral speech lateralization. *Brain Language*. 1990;38:195–206.
47. Sanders RJ. Sentence comprehension following agenesis of the corpus callosum. *Brain Language*. 1989;37:59–72.
48. Paul LK, Van Lancker-Sidtis D, Schieffer B, et al. Communicative deficits in agenesis of the corpus callosum: nonliteral language and affective prosody. *Brain Language*. 2003;85:313–324.
49. Sarnat HB, Menkes JH. Neuroembryology, genetic programming, and malformations of the nervous system, part 1: the new neuroembryology. In: Menkes JH, Sarnat HB, eds. *Child neurology*. 6th ed. Philadelphia: Lippincott Williams & Wilkins, 2000:227–305.
50. Liptak GS. Neural tube defects. In: Batshaw ML, ed. *Children with disabilities*. 5th ed. Baltimore: Paul H. Brookes, 2002:443–466.
51. Forrester MB, Merz RD. Prenatal diagnosis and elective termination of neural tube defects in Hawaii, 1986–1997. *Fetal Diagn Ther*. 2000;15:146–151.
52. Hendricks KA, Simpson JS, Larsen RD. Neural tube defects along the Texas–Mexican border, 1993–1995. *Am J Epidemiol*. 1999;149:1119–1127.
53. Padmanabhan R. Etiology, pathogenesis, and prevention of neural tube defects. *Congenit Anom*. 2006;46:55–67.
54. Pellock M. Static encephalopathy and related disorders. In: Kaufman DM, Solomon G, Pfeffer C, eds. *Child and adolescent neurology for psychiatrists*. Baltimore: Williams & Wilkins, 1992.
55. Fletcher J, Copeland K, Frederick J, et al. Spinal-lesion level in spina bifida: a source of neural and cognitive heterogeneity. *J Neurosurg*. 2005;102 (3 suppl):268–279.
56. Kirk V, Morielli A, Brouillette R. Sleep-disordered breathing in children with myelomeningocele: the missed diagnosis. *Dev Med Child Neurol*. 1999; 41:40–43.
57. Appleton P, Ellis NC, Minchom PE, et al. Depressive symptoms and self-concept in young people with spina bifida. *J Pediatr Psychol*. 1997;22:707–722.
58. Hunt GM, Poulton A. Open spina bifida: a complete cohort reviewed 25 years after closure. *Dev Med Child Neurol*. 1995;37:19–29.
59. Hunt GM. Non-selective intervention in newborn babies with open spina bifida: the outcome 30 years on for the complete cohort. *Eur J Pediatr Surg*. 1999;9:5–8.
60. Menkes J, Sarnat H. Malformations of the central nervous system. In: Menkes JH, Sarnat HB, eds. *Child neurology*. 6th ed. Philadelphia: Lippincott Williams & Wilkins, 2000:305–400.
61. Riveira C, Pascual J. Is Chiari type I malformation a reason for chronic daily headache. *Curr Pain Headache Rep*. 2007;11:53–55.
62. Tubbs RS, Doyle S, Conkin M, et al. Scoliosis in a child with Chiari I malformation and the absence of syringomyelia: case report and review of the literature. *Childs Nerv Syst*. 2006;22:1351–1354.
63. Stevenson KL. Chiari type II malformation: past, present, and future. *Neurosurg Focus* 2004;16:1–7.
64. Maria BL, Zinreich SJ, Carson BC, et al. Dandy Walker syndrome revisited. *Pediatr Neurosci*. 1987;13:45–51.
65. Tal Y, Freigang B, Dunn HG, et al. Dandy Walker Syndrome: analysis of 21 cases. *Dev Med Child Neurol* 1980;22:189–201.
66. Fernell E, Hagberg G. Infantile hydrocephalus: declining prevalence in preterm infants. *Acta Paediatr*. 1998;7:392–396.
67. Persson EK, Hagberg G, Uvebrant P. Hydrocephalus prevalence and outcome in a population-based cohort of children born 1989–1998. *Acta Paediatr*. 2005;94:726–732.
68. Cherian S, Whitelaw A, Thoresen M, et al. The pathogenesis of neonatal post-hemorrhagic hydrocephalus. *Brain Pathol*. 2004;14:305–311.
69. McLone DG, Partington MD. Arrest and compensation of hydrocephalus. *Neurosurg Clin North Am*. 1993;4:621–624.
70. Erickson K, Baron IS, Fantie BD. Neuropsychological functioning in early hydrocephalus. *Child Neuropsychol*. 2001;7:199–229.
71. Hanlo PW, Gooskens RJ, van Schooneveld M, et al. The effect of intracranial pressure on myelination and the relationship with neurodevelopmental in infantile hydrocephalus. *Dev Med Child Neurol*. 1998;39:286–291.
72. Fernell E, Hagberg B, Hagberg G, et al. Epidemiology of infantile hydrocephalus in Sweden: a clinical follow-up study in children born at term. *Neuropediatrics*. 1988;19:135–142.
73. Heinsbergen I, Rotteveel J, Roeleveld N, Grotenhuis A. Outcome in shunted hydrocephalic children. *Eur J Paediatr Neurol*. 2002;6:99–107.
74. Chiafery M. Care and management of the child with hydrocephalus. *Pediatr Nurs*. 2006;32:222–225.
75. Sarnat HB, Menkes JH. Neuroembryology, genetic programming, and malformations of the central nervous system, part 2: malformations of the central nervous system. In: Menkes JH, Sarnat HB, eds. *Child neurology*. 6th ed. Philadelphia: Lippincott Williams & Wilkins, 2000:305–400.
76. Fletcher JM, Francis DJ, Thompson NM, et al. Verbal and nonverbal skill discrepancies in hydrocephalic children. *J Clin Exp Neuropsychol*. 1992;14:593–609.
77. Dennis M, Jacennik B. The content of narrative discourse in children and adolescents after early-onset hydrocephalus and in normally developing age peers. *Brain Lang*. 1994;46:129–165.
78. Vachha B, Adams R. Language differences in young children with myelomeningocele and shunted hydrocephalus. *Pediatr Neurosurg*. 2003;39:184–189.

79. Barnes M, Faulkner H, Dennis M. Poor reading comprehension despite fast word decoding in children with hydrocephalus. *Brain Lang.* 2001;76:35–44.
80. Kulkarni AV, Drake JM, Lamberti-Pasculi M. Cerebral fluid shunt infection: a prospective study of risk factors. *J Neurosurg.* 2001;94:195–201.
81. Casey AT, Kimmings EJ, Kleinlugtebeld AD, et al. The long-term outlook for hydrocephalus in childhood: a 10-year cohort study of 155 patients. *Pediatr Neurosurg.* 1997;27:2:63–70.
82. Duhaime AC. Evaluation and management of shunt infections in children with hydrocephalus. *Clin Pediatr.* 2006;45:705–713.

CHAPTER 12

Intellectual Disability/Mental Retardation

MARIS D. ROSENBERG AND SUSAN VIG

Definition and Terminology

2002 AAMR DEFINITION OF MENTAL RETARDATION

The following definition of mental retardation was endorsed in 2002 by the American Association on Mental Retardation: "Mental retardation is a disability characterized by significant limitations both in intellectual functioning and in adaptive behavior as expressed in conceptual, social, and practical adaptive skills. This disability originates before age 18." (1). Implementation of the definition emphasizes the need to identify strengths, as well as limitations, of people with intellectual disability, and to develop profiles of supports that will optimize their functioning. The 2002 definition specifies that intellectual limitation is documented by an IQ approximately 2 standard deviations below the mean of a standardized intelligence test. Limitations in adaptive behavior (activities of daily living) are documented by the score on a test of adaptive behavior, based on information provided by a third party (parent, caregiver, or teacher).

CURRENT TERMINOLOGY

The term *mental retardation* is gradually being replaced by other terminology. In Great Britain, the terms "intellectual disability," "learning disability," and "learning difficulty" have long been preferred. Use of the term "learning disability" to represent intellectual and adaptive limitations has created confusion in the United States, where learning disabilities refer to academic deficits that are not consistent with intellectual potential.

In 2007, the American Association on Mental Retardation, a 130-year-old association representing disability professionals worldwide, changed its name to American Association on Intellectual and Developmental Disabilities. This change suggested that, in the United States and worldwide, the term "intellectual disability" might eventually replace the previous term "mental retardation."

The term "developmental delay" is often used to characterize intellectual disability in young children. Most experts agree that it should be used to describe children younger than 3 years. Some experts have suggested that mental retardation should not be diagnosed in children younger than 5 years. In many educational settings, "developmental delay" is used for children up to 8 years of age.

In the following discussion, the term "intellectual disability" (ID) will be used instead of "mental retardation," except where doing so would obscure meaning. Consistent with international usage, the term "children" includes adolescents.

Diagnostic Guidelines

In clinical settings, guidelines provided by the *Diagnostic and Statistical Manual of Mental Disorders*, Fourth Edition, Revised (2) are used to establish a formal diagnosis of ID (termed "mental retardation" in the diagnostic manual). This diagnosis is based on intellectual limitations (an IQ below 70 to 75) and deficits in adaptive behavior. Classification levels, based on IQ ranges, are mild (IQ of 50 to 55 to approximately 70), moderate (IQ 35 to 40 to 50 to 55), severe (IQ 20 to 25 to 35 to 40), and profound (IQ less than 20 to 25). The guidelines apply to children as well as adults, but do not specify the age at which this diagnosis may be made.

Prevalence

Prevalence estimates depend on how ID is defined. The prevalence of ID is generally thought to be approximately 2 1/2% of the population (3). Increasing the IQ cutoff to 75 increases prevalence and means that more people will be eligible for publicly funded entitlements and services. According to Sattler (4), 85% of people with ID have mild ID, 10% have moderate, 3.5% have severe, and 1.5% have profound ID. More males than females have ID. Durkin and Stein reported male-to-female ratios of 1.1 to 1.8:1 for mild ID and 1.1 to 1.4:1 for severe ID (5). Gillberg and Soderstrom (6) reported a male-to-female ratio of 1.3:1, based on population studies, hypothesizing that this gender difference might be attributable to X-linked genetic mechanisms.

Within the United States educational system, reluctance to use the label "mental retardation" has affected prevalence estimates. As Baroff (7) pointed out, school systems may avoid using the term mental retardation for children with mild ID and associated academic deficits. Baroff reported that between 1977 and 1997, a 38% decline occurred in students classified as "mentally retarded" and an increase of 202% of students classified as "learning disabled" (7).

Etiology

Determination of the cause of ID has important implications for the patient and family. For the patient, an accurate diagnosis can provide the care provider with information about medical problems that may occur in the patient's future, thus ultimately improving prognosis. For the family, the importance of identifying the cause of ID is threefold. First, parents often believe that their child's problems were directly caused by things the parent did or did not do during or before the pregnancy, and establishing a biologic etiology can allay that guilt. Next, establishing a diagnosis can provide the family with a greater sense of control, when armed with the knowledge of cause, treatment options, and prognosis. Finally, establishing a diagnosis can provide the parents, siblings and extended family with a realistic assessment of risk of recurrence of the condition in future progeny. For all of these reasons, vigorous attempts should be made to identify the cause of ID in the individual patient.

In many patients, no specific etiology will ever be identified. According to Srour et al. (8), the diagnostic yield in patients with global developmental delay is approximately 40%. Factors associated with the ability to identify an underlying cause included female gender, abnormal pre/perinatal history, absence of autistic features, presence of microcephaly, abnormal neurologic examination, and dysmorphic features. No association was found between the severity of the delay and the identification of underlying etiology. Van Karnebeek et al. (9) and Battaglia and Carey (10), however, reported that an etiologic diagnosis could be made in more than 50% of children with varying levels of ID based on history and examination alone, or history and physical findings with confirmatory laboratory studies. Serial evaluations over a period of several years have been suggested, in that clinical and behavior phenotypes can modify over time (11), and as new diagnostic techniques become available (12).

Recent advances in the area of genetics and genomics have made the determination of etiology increasingly possible. New technology has allowed the diagnosis of chromosomal anomalies associated with cognitive disabilities to be made with greater precision; molecular genetic techniques have broadened the scope of our understanding of mechanisms such as in mitochondrial inheritance, imprinting, uniparental disomy, and trinucleotide repeat disorders. Genomics, the study of the functions and interactions of all genes in the genome, has led to the understanding that complex disorders such as mental retardation are due to the interaction of genes, epigenetic (those that modify the expression of a gene) factors, and environmental factors. All this has rendered the genetic evaluation central to the assessment of an individual with cognitive delay. The reader is referred to several excellent reviews of current technology (13–15).

The Clinical Assessment

Despite the rapid expansion of knowledge in genomic medicine, the medical assessment of the child initially seen with ID, geared toward determining an etiology, is currently initiated in the clinical setting, not in the laboratory. Three recent statements by the American College of Medical Genetics (11), American Academy of Neurology and Child Neurology Society (16), and American Academy of Pediatrics Committee on Genetics (12) discussed the approach to the evaluation of children with ID and share many common elements. Each emphasizes the need for a careful history beginning with pregnancy, including exposure to teratogens, and perinatal course. Family history should include a pedigree of three generations or more, detailing the presence of developmental disorders (with careful attention to distribution e.g., suggestion of X-linked inheritance), congenital malformations, psychiatric illness, and frequent miscarriages/stillbirths/early childhood deaths. Physical and neurologic examinations focus on growth parameters, dysmorphic features (documenting minor anomalies with detailed measurements, skin changes with Wood's lamp), and neuromuscular and behavioral features that suggest a specific syndrome.

Genetic Testing

Chromosomal anomalies have been detected in individuals with ID with a frequency ranging between 9% and 36% by using high resolution (>650 bands) karyotyping (12). Van Karnebeek et al. (9) reported such abnormalities to be present in all levels of ID and in both genders, with a median frequency of 1 in 10, with a higher number of anomalies (more than six) significantly increasing the likelihood of a chromosomal anomaly (9). Shevell et al. (16) reported the range of chromosomal anomalies to be between 2.3% and 11.6% and suggested ". . . cytogenetic testing is indicated in the evaluation of the child with developmental delay even in the absence of clinical features or dysmorphic features suggestive of a syndrome."

Fluorescence in situ hybridization (FISH) techniques, by using fluorescently labeled cDNA probes, have been used to increase the yield of genetic testing for the cause of ID. FISH can be used to confirm a clinical suspicion of a microdeletion syndrome, many of which have specific behavioral phenotypes, such as Williams (del 7p), Prader–Willi/

Angelman syndrome (del 15p), catch 22 syndrome (del 22q), and Smith–Magenis syndrome (del 17p). In addition, rearrangements leading to deletions of the functional end of the chromosome (subtelomeric region) are thought to be responsible for a significant number of structural chromosomal abnormalities not previously detected with routine karyotype analysis. (17). Biesecker et al. (18) found a 6% rate of subtelomere abnormalities detected by FISH in a variety of subjects evaluated for ID, growth retardation, major and minor anomalies, and familial versus sporadic occurrence. DeVries et al. (19) proposed a five-item checklist designed to increase the yield of subtelomeric studies. The presence of three or more features (family history of ID, prenatal-onset growth retardation, postnatal poor growth/overgrowth, two or more facial dysmorphic features, or one or more nonfacial dysmorphic features and/or congenital abnormalities) would allow the exclusion of 20% of cases without missing a subtelomeric abnormality.

Molecular genetic testing for fragile X syndrome has been recommended for children with undiagnosed ID, particularly in the presence of a family history or physical features suggestive of this diagnosis (11,12,16). Fragile X syndrome is the most common inherited form of ID occurring in 1 of 4,000 males and 1 of 8,000 females. The prevalence of the fragile X mutation is reported to vary with severity of retardation, ranging from 1% in borderline IQ or mild ID to 4.1% in more-severe degrees of MR (9). De Vries et al. (19) proposed a seven-item clinical checklist that increased the molecular diagnostic yield to 7.6%. Features include a family history of ID, long jaw or high forehead, large or protuberant ears or both, hyperextensible joints, soft and velvety palmar skin with redundancy on the dorsum of the hands, testicular enlargement, and behaviors of initial shyness and lack of eye contact followed by friendliness and verbosity. Molecular testing also is suggested to confirm diagnoses in syndromes in which the gene has been identified, such as in Rett syndrome, or in cases in which an atypical presentation of a known syndrome is suspected.

Not yet widely clinically available, the newest diagnostic technology, molecular karyotyping using microarray comparative genomic hybridization, allows the detection of abnormal copy numbers of DNA sequences throughout the entire human genome. This approach can reveal causative chromosomal microdeletions or duplications or both in 10% to 20% of patients with unexplained MR and congenital malformations (14). Nucleic acid probes are deposited on microarray platforms, which, when hybridized to test DNA, detect sequence variations known as single-nucleotide polymorphisms (SNPs). Microarrays have been developed to analyze hundreds of thousands of SNPs that compose an individual's genome. The challenge lies in determining those copy-number alterations that cause disease versus those that are unique to the individual but have no clinical consequence. CGH will not replace routine chromosomal analysis, in that chromosomal rearrangements such as inversions or translocations, as well as low-level mosaicism may be missed by this technology (14).

Neuroimaging

CT and MRI studies are not considered mandatory in the evaluation of children with ID. Moeschler et al. (12), in their review of the literature, reported abnormal findings in approximately 30% of patients with ID. However, such findings led to an etiologic or syndrome diagnosis in only up to 3.9% of patients. Diagnostic yield was higher with an abnormal neurological examination. Shevell et al. (16) thus recommend neuroimaging (MRI preferable to CT) in cases with abnormal neurological examination (focal motor findings or microcephaly). Curry et al. (11) also do not recommend routine neuroimaging in the normocephalic patient without clinical neurological signs.

Metabolic Testing

Routine metabolic screening, in the absence of suggestive clinical history or abnormal laboratory findings, is reported to have a diagnostic yield of less than 1% (9,11,12,16). Targeted metabolic studies are suggested with specific clinical or laboratory findings such as growth failure, recurrent unexplained illness, neurologic findings, specific dysmorphic features, or laboratory abnormalities (lactic acidosis, hyperammonemia).

Figure 12.1details the diagnostic algorithm published by the AAP Committee on Genetics based on the approach suggested by van Karnebeek et al. (9).

Characteristics of Children with ID

PRESENTATION

The presentation of intellectual disability in children varies by level of severity; in general, the more severe the level, the earlier the age at presentation, controlling for environmental factors. Failure to achieve expected motor milestones in the first year of life generally corresponds to levels of moderate retardation and below; a thorough medical workup for causal factors is indicated. Mild mental retardation is typically manifest by a delay in attainment of language milestones in toddlers and preschoolers. Such a presentation can also be consistent with a developmental language disorder, in which delays are specific to the language domain and not global in nature, as in ID. Multidisciplinary assessment is indicated for proper differentiation, and formal audiological assessment is essential to rule out a contributing hearing loss. Young school-age children, who begin to struggle with academic demands in kindergarten and early elementary school, may be demonstrating a slower rate of learning associated with borderline intellectual functioning. Once again, multidisciplinary assessment is indicated to differentiate such children from those who are functioning in the average range of intelligence, but whose learning many be compromised by specific deficits consistent with a learning disability.

INTELLECTUAL LIMITATIONS

The primary characteristic of ID is cognitive limitation, indicated by an IQ below 70 to 75 (2 standard deviations below the mean of an intelligence test). In thinking about children, it is useful to consider their mental ages. Those with mild ID function at about two thirds of their chronological ages. Those with moderate, severe, and profound ID function at approximately one half, one third, and below one fourth of their chronological ages, respectively. Within the developmental disabilities field, individuals with IQs below 50 are often said to have "significant" or "severe" impairment. (The term "severe" can thus be used in a technical sense to indicate a particular classification level, or less technically, to refer to significant impairment.) IQs between approximately 70 and 79 (and sometimes between 70 and 84, depending on whether test norms or standard-deviation norms are used for classification), indicate borderline intelligence. Although they are not formally diagnosed with ID, children with borderline intelligence experience many of the same challenges as those with mild ID, and are at high risk of developing academic and behavior problems (6).

Children with ID reach plateaus beyond which further intellectual development is not anticipated. Sattler (4) indicated the approximate mental ages to be expected at adulthood: 8.3 to 10.9 years for mild, 5.7 to 8.2 years for moderate, 3.2 to 5.6 years for severe, and less than 3.2 years for profound ID. (See references 4, 20, and 21 for specific skills expected at different ages and levels of ID.)

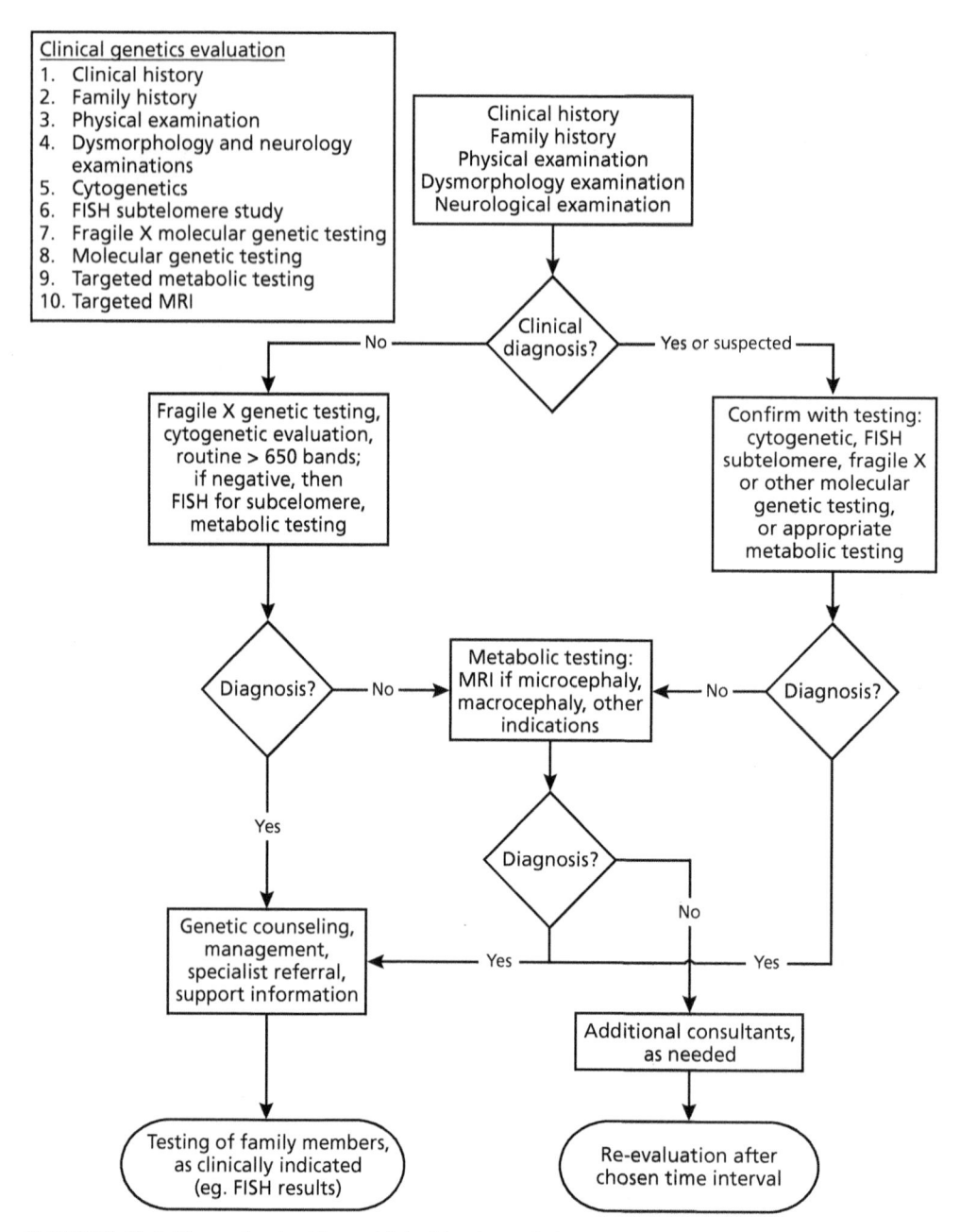

■ **FIGURE 12.1.** Diagnostic algorithm published by the AAP Committee. (Reprinted with permission from Moeschler JB, Shevell M, the Committee on Genetics. Clinical genetic evaluation of the child with mental retardation or developmental delays. *Pediatrics* 2006;117:2304–2316.

LEARNING AND INTERACTION STYLES

In addition to having subaverage intelligence and mental ages below their chronological ages, children with ID exhibit learning and interaction styles that differ from those of peers with typical development. During the preschool years, children with ID are apt to show less curiosity, less interest in discovering the function of objects, and more-restricted play than other children. They often experience difficulties establishing and developing friendships with other children, engage in higher levels of solitary play, and exhibit more negativity and discontent in peer interaction (22). Children of all ages with ID learn more slowly and forget more readily than other children. They may revert to earlier patterns and fail to use the new skills they have acquired. Children with ID do not generalize well and do not benefit from incidental learning opportunities. Teaching must be explicit and include frequent review. Children with ID may have trouble interpreting and prioritizing social information. Although eager for social approval, their judgment is apt to be poor, resulting in vulnerability to exploitation or maltreatment.

OTHER CHARACTERISTICS

Although some children with ID have dysmorphic features, many have an unstigmatized physical appearance. Most have adequate motor skills. It should be noted that, in assessment, failure of motor tasks may represent failure to comprehend cognitive aspects of the tasks. Many children with ID (particularly those with concurrent autism-spectrum symptoms) have isolated areas of stronger ability, often termed "savant" or "splinter" skills. (See reference 23 for a discussion of savant capacities.) Young children may be unusually good at labeling colors, shapes, letters, and numbers; some may read words. Older children may have well-developed calendar, mental-calculation, drawing, or musical talents. Although such achievements are impressive, they remain isolated and do not carry over into other aspects of cognitive ability.

Epilepsy in ID

The incidence of epilepsy in children with mental retardation is significantly higher than that in the general population (20% to 40% in children with ID and CP) (24–26); 8% to 18% in mild MR, and 30% to 36% in severe MR (27). The type of epileptic syndrome and the frequency and severity of seizures are related to the underlying cause of ID. The principles for management of epilepsy in individuals with ID are accurate diagnosis and classification of seizure type, consideration of associated medical conditions (e.g., tuberous sclerosis, cerebral palsy), use of appropriate medication and careful monitoring for side effects, and provision of information and support for the patient and family (27).

Seizures may exacerbate the functional deficits seen in individuals with ID. In the Isle of Wight study, up to 56% of children with MR and epilepsy exhibited comorbid psychiatric disorders as opposed to 30% in children with mental retardation alone (28). Matson et al. (29) stated that those individuals with ID and a diagnosis of seizure disorder were found to have significantly lower social and adaptive skills when compared with developmentally disabled controls with no seizures.

A number of epileptic syndromes are seen in association with ID. Lennox–Gastaut syndrome involves multiple types of intractable seizures and is associated with cognitive impairment (30). West syndrome involves the triad of infantile spasms, hypsarrhythmia on interictal EEG, and mental retardation, associated with a variety of etiologies and most commonly first seen in the first year of life (31).

Diagnosis of seizure disorder may be complicated in individuals with intellectual disability because of the presence of aberrant behavior, stereotypies, or involuntary movements that can be mistaken for seizures. Conversely, such movements/behaviors can be mistakenly assumed to be seizure related. In such cases, simultaneous EEG monitoring is indicated. Individuals with disabilities have more difficulty in achieving seizure control, greater likelihood of clusters of seizures, prolonged seizures, and status epilepticus. Despite lessening the frequency or intensity of seizures, antiepileptic medications have the potential to cause cognitive slowing or behavior disturbances or both, which significantly affect the quality of life. The new generation of antiepileptic drugs, such as lamotrigine, topiramate, zonisamide, levetiracetam, and oxcarbazepine, promise better seizure control with fewer idiosyncratic reactions and side effects. Nonetheless, careful monitoring and attention to potential interactions with medications prescribed for other purposes is indicated. For detailed discussions of the use of these medications, the reader is referred to reviews by Shields (24), Huber and Seidel (25), Pellock and Morton (26), and Santosh and Baird (27).

In instances in which medications do not achieve optimal control or in which side effects limit the effectiveness of pharmacotherapy, other treatment options such as ketogenic diet, vagus nerve stimulation (VNS), and epilepsy surgery can be considered. A ketogenic diet has been proven effective for medically refractory seizures (32,33). It has also been reported to improve sleep quality in children with therapy-resistant epilepsy (34). Vagus nerve stimulation has been reported effective in drug-resistant partial epilepsy (35) and in generalized and mixed forms (36). VNS avoids cognitive slowing, sedation, or behavioral effects. It is approved for patients older than 12 years and can be used as an adjunct to antiepileptic drug therapy. Effectiveness may be delayed for up to 1 to 2 years after implantation; effects on voice quality or swallowing are possible, and periodic readjustment of settings is required. A recent report suggests synergistic effects with the use of the ketogenic diet and VNS in children with medically refractory epilepsy (37).

A number of surgical procedures are considered for children with ID whose seizures are refractory to other treatments. Focal cortical resection can be successful in cases in which a defined epileptogenic zone can be safely removed without affecting the patient's functional status. It is most successful when performed early, after two or three failed attempts at control with medication (24). Advances in imaging techniques, EEG, and cortical mapping have contributed to the success of these procedures. Other surgical procedures to be considered include temporal lobectomy, hemispherectomy, callostomy, and subpial transection.

Dual Diagnosis

PREVALENCE

"Dual diagnosis" refers to the co-occurrence of intellectual disabilities and psychiatric disorders or behavior problems. Prevalence estimates of comorbid psychopathology vary widely, because of different ways of defining and measuring psychopathology, types of behavior problems included or excluded, characteristics of samples studied, and whether study participants reside in institutions or in the community (38–40). The prevalence of clinically significant behavior problems or psychiatric disorders in people with ID (including children) has been reported as 30% to 70% (41); 23% to 38% (42); 37% (43,44); 50% (45); 40% to 60% of children (39); 40% (46); 25% (47); more than 40% (48); 38% of preschool children (49); 39% of children and adolescents (3), 30% to 50% (50); and 37% of children (51). Higher rates are reported for children with ID than those for other children (3). Although the presence of comorbid psychopathology is well documented for children with ID, mental health services are not necessarily provided for them. In a study by Dekker and Koot (43), only 27% of children with a dual diagnosis received mental health services.

Autism

The overlap between ID and autism is well documented. In a large epidemiologic study of British children younger than 15 years, Wing (52) identified problems in socialization and communication, and repetitive or stereotyped behaviors consistent with autism in 82% of children with IQs below 20, 47% with IQs between 20 and 34, 40% with IQs between 35 and 49, and 2% with IQs between 50 and 69. Deb and Prasad (53) reported that 53% of Scottish children with IQs below 50 met criteria for autism. Nordin and Gillberg (54) found that 30% of Swedish children with IQs below 50 had autism-spectrum disorders (54). Conversely, ID was documented for 70% to 90% of children with autistic behavior (55), and 70% of adults previously diagnosed with autism during childhood (56). Volkmar et al. (57) reported IQs below 50 for 50% to 75% of children with autism.

Attention-deficit hyperactivity disorder

Attentional problems and hyperactivity are seen in children with ID. Because the children have lower mental ages, it is sometimes difficult to know whether ADHD symptoms are a problem in their own right or instead reflect functioning at an earlier developmental level. Walker and Johnson (58) cautioned that children with mild ID may exhibit attentional problems, but because their attention is consistent with their mental ages, they should not be given medication. Hastings et al. (59) compared rates of ADHD symptoms for children with ID and their siblings. Hyperactivity was identified in 60% of the children with ID and in fewer than 3% of their siblings. Children who were younger, had lower mental ages, or with concurrent autism had more symptoms of ADHD.

Symptoms and levels of intellectual impairment

Types of psychopathology vary with severity of intellectual impairment (60). Children with mild ID tend to have conventional psychiatric diagnoses (anxiety, mood, disruptive and antisocial behavior); those with more-severe impairment exhibit more stereotypies, aggression, autistic behaviors, self-injury, overactivity, and withdrawn behavior (38,45,48,61). The American Academy of Child and Adolescent Psychiatry Work Group (41) suggested that, although subjective feelings related to anxiety can be reported by people with mild ID, those with more-severe intellectual impairments may show their anxiety through avoidance or agitation, and their depression through aggressive behavior. Anorexia and bulimia are rare in people with moderate to severe ID (41). Eating disorders are apt to take the form of pica, rumination, regurgitation, rechewing food, and refusal to eat certain kinds of foods (6,41).

Children with significant ID who are ambulatory may exhibit more-severe behavior problems than nonambulatory children. In a study of children aged 4 to 11 years with IQ equivalents of 50 or below, Chadwick et al. (62) found that the most-severe behavior problems occurred for ambulatory, rather than for nonambulatory, children. Problems for ambulatory children included overactivity, running away, destructive behavior, scattering or throwing objects, temper tantrums, and attention seeking. Both ambulatory and nonambulatory children engaged in self-injury, screaming, making disturbing noises, sleep problems, lethargy, social withdrawal, and stereotypies.

Behavior Problems of Preschool Children

Children younger than 6 years with developmental delays experience more behavior problems than do those without delays. As with older children, types of problems vary with severity of delay. In a study of 3-year-olds with and without delays, Baker et al. (63) found that children with developmental quotients between 30 and 75 were 3 to 4 times more likely to have clinically significant behavior problems (particularly social withdrawal and attentional problems) than were age peers without delays. Based on a review of preschool children's records from a psychiatric inpatient facility, Crnic et al. (64) found that young children with borderline intelligence or mild ID had attention-deficit hyperactivity disorders and oppositional defiant disorders. Those with more-significant degrees of ID exhibited stereotypies, overactivity, self-injury, and sleep problems.

Many preschool children with ID have social-skills deficits. Studying children aged 3 to 5 years, with and without developmental delays, Merrell and Holland (65) found that children with delays were more likely to have social-skills deficits than were those without delays (prevalence of 27% and 6%, respectively). The children with delays had trouble initiating interaction with peers and working or playing independently. McIntyre et al. (66) found that young children with delays were 3 times more likely to have trouble with self-regulation and social skills than were children without delays. Children who could delay touching a toy at 36 and 60 months had fewer subsequent teacher-reported behavior problems than did children who did not delay gratification.

Psychopathology Associated with Genetic Syndromes

Many children with genetic syndromes associated with ID show specific kinds of psychopathology. For example, Handen and Gilchrist (67) described behavior problems seen in children with fragile X syndrome and mild to moderate ID: attentional deficits and hyperactivity, hand biting and flapping, perseverative speech, preoccupation with inanimate objects, shyness, and poor social interaction. Dykens and Hodapp (47) reported on behaviors seen in children with Prader–Willi syndrome: high rates of food seeking and food stealing; hyperphagia and impaired satiety; tantrums and outbursts; impulsivity; argumentativeness; and sadness. Obsessive–compulsive symptoms may include repetitive skin-picking; hoarding, ordering, redoing, or arranging; and need for symmetry or exactness. According to Dykens and Hodapp (47), children with Williams syndrome have more anxiety, fears and phobias, and attention-deficit hyperactivity disorders than do other children with ID. The children have high levels of "linguistic affect," involving prosody, narrative enrichment, and hyperverbal conversation. They are friendly and sociable, but may have indiscriminate sociability or social disinhibition. Although specific kinds of behavior problems have been associated with other genetic syndromes, children with Down syndrome are reported to have lower rates of psychopathology than do other children with ID (47,49,58).

Diagnostic Challenges

Diagnosing psychopathology in children with ID, particularly those with IQs below 50, can be a challenging process. "Diagnostic overshadowing" means that psychiatric disorders and behavior problems are erroneously attributed to ID, rather than being identified as problems in their own right (38,47,68). Because of their concrete thinking and limited communication skills, children with ID may have trouble conceptualizing and reporting their feelings, or linking feelings to major life events or precipitating factors (39). Psychiatric interviews requiring that children describe their feelings may not be useful (69). King et al. (70) emphasized the importance of context to the interpretation of behavior. For example, aggression in a nonverbal individual may represent mania if it occurs with insomnia, hyperactivity, hypersexuality, and irritability. If the aggressive behavior occurs in response to environmental stressors, it may instead represent anxiety.

Vulnerability to Maltreatment

Children with developmental disabilities, including ID, are disproportionately vulnerable to exploitation and maltreatment (61). A report of the National Center for Child Abuse and Neglect (71) indicated that children with disabilities were maltreated at 1.7 times the rate of children without disabilities. Rates of emotional neglect, physical abuse, sexual abuse, and physical neglect were 2.8, 2.1, 1.8, and 1.6 times higher, respectively, for children with disabilities. Verdugo et al. (72) studied 445 institutionalized children and adolescents with ID and found that 11.5% had experienced maltreatment. Within this group, physical neglect, emotional neglect, physical abuse, and sexual abuse were reported for 92%, 84%, 31%, and 2%, respectively.

Children with mild disabilities may experience higher rates of maltreatment than do those with more-severe disabilities (71,73). Because mild disabilities are less obvious, families and others may erroneously attribute challenging behavior to a child's character, rather than associating it with the disability (74). Horner-Johnson and Drum (75) noted that unique forms of maltreatment occur for individuals with ID, citing as an example the withholding of adaptive mobility and communication devices to control or isolate a person with ID.

Risk factors for maltreatment of children with ID are complex (see reference 74 for further discussion.) They include child factors (poor judgment, inability to protect themselves, desire for approval); family factors (stresses related to extra expenses and time needed for a child's clinical services, parental ID or psychopathology, frustration due to the child's behavior problems or failure to progress); and environmental factors (poverty, lack of services, social isolation).

Assessment

A diagnosis of ID is based on intellectual limitations and deficits in adaptive behavior. Intellectual limitations are generally defined as functioning more than 2 standard deviations below the mean of an intelligence test (IQ below 70 on tests having a standard deviation of 15). Intelligence tests are individually administered by a psychologist. Group tests of cognitive ability are sometimes used in research but cannot be used to diagnose ID. Adaptive behavior is usually assessed through the report of family members, caregivers, and teachers.

INTELLIGENCE TESTING

Intelligence tests assess key aspects of cognitive ability (verbal and nonverbal reasoning, memory, information processing, and problem-solving). Instructions are presented exactly the same way to all examinees. Rewording of instructions or provision of supplementary cues is not permitted and would be a violation of standardized testing procedures.

The Wechsler Intelligence Test for Children, Fourth Edition, for ages 6.0 to 16.11 years (76) and Stanford-Binet Intelligence Scale for Children, Fifth Edition (SB-5), for ages 2.0 to 85 years have strong psychometric properties and are frequently used to assess children and adolescents with ID (77). Both tests provide separate scores for language and nonverbal abilities, as well as a global IQ. Other intelligence tests include the Differential Ability Scales, Second Edition (DAS-II), for ages 2.6 to 17.11 years (78); the Kaufman Assessment Battery for Children, Second Edition (KABC-2), for ages 3.0 to 18.11 years (79); the Merrill-Palmer Revised Scales of Development, for ages 1 month to 6.6 years (80); and the Wechsler Preschool and Primary Scale of Intelligence, Third Edition (WPPSI-III), for ages 2.6 to 7.3 years (81). For examinees who do not have language, nonverbal tests include the Comprehensive Test of Nonverbal Intelligence (C-TONI), for ages 6.0 to 90 years (82); the Leiter International Performance Scale, Revised, for ages 2.0 to 20.11 years (83); and the Test of Nonverbal Intelligence, Third Edition (TONI-3), for ages 6.0 to 89 years (84).

Although these well-known tests are generally adequate for assessing the intelligence of children with mild impairments, they may lack sufficient "floor" (developmentally easier items) for children with more-severe impairments. Another challenge is that norms tables for many intelligence tests do not provide scores low enough to identify severe to profound ID. In such cases, the psychologist may have to document ID by using age equivalents available in infant tests, such as the Bayley Scales of Infant and Toddler Development (Bayley-III), for ages 1 to 42 months (85), or rely more heavily on a measure of adaptive behavior.

Testing procedures are sometimes modified for children with ID who have motor or sensory impairments. Cerebral palsy has been reported for 20% of children with ID (86) and for 43% of children with developmental disabilities and concurrent visual impairments (87). Estimates of hearing loss have ranged from 17% to 78% (61,88).

Many children with ID and cerebral palsy who have language can respond to verbal portions of conventional intelligence tests. If they do not have language, test formats may be modified so that children can indicate their response choices through eye gaze or use of adaptive devices.

For children with ID and visual impairments, verbal portions of tests can be administered if they do not require the presentation of pictures or other visual stimuli. Other modifications include presentation of test materials within specified fields of vision; use of materials offering high visual contrasts; and provision of magnification devices (89,90). No current, nationally standardized tests are available for children who are blind.

For deaf children, nonverbal tests and nonverbal portions of conventional tests are appropriate if instructions can be pantomimed. Sattler and Hardy-Braz (91) noted that children who are deaf should be tested by a psychologist who can communicate in a child's preferred modality or with the assistance of a sign interpreter.

ASSESSMENT OF ADAPTIVE BEHAVIOR

Adaptive behavior refers to skills of daily living and is thought to comprise conceptual, social, and practical areas (1). Adaptive behavior correlates strongly with intelligence, particularly at early developmental levels. For example, coefficients of 0.75, based on Vineland standard scores, and 0.89, based on age equivalents, were obtained in a study of preschool children by Vig and Jedrysek (92). For examinees who are not testable on intelligence tests, standard scores obtained on measures of adaptive behavior can be used to estimate levels of cognitive functioning.

The Vineland Adaptive Behavior Scales, Second Edition (Vineland-II), for ages 0 to 90 years (93) is frequently used to assess adaptive behavior. Through a semistructured interview, a parent, teacher, or caregiver provides information about a child's communication, daily living skills, socialization, and (for children younger than 6 years) motor skills. A maladaptive behavior scale is also available. Another instrument in current use is the Adaptive Behavior Assessment System, Second Edition (ABAS-II), for ages 0 to 89 years (94). Ten areas of adaptive behavior are assessed, with a motor scale available for young children.

Prognosis

ID is a lifelong condition. Infant development tests are not good predictors of future functioning because they measure gross motor and sensorimotor skills that have little association with cognitive ability. Once tests begin to measure cognition during the preschool years, IQs tend to remain stable over time. A number of longitudinal studies have documented IQ stability (95–98). The implication is that intervention can optimize children's functioning and provide information and support for their families, but is not expected to "cure" the ID.

Longitudinal studies have investigated adult functioning of individuals whose ID was identified during childhood. In a 40-year British follow-up study, investigators found that among people with mild ID (IQs 50 to 69), 67% had jobs, 73% were married, and 62% had children; more than 50% reported ongoing problems with reading, writing, and math (99). Keogh et al. (100) conducted a 20-year follow-up study of preschool children with delays. In early adulthood, the majority lived with their families or in group homes; most were unemployed or underemployed and had few friends.

Intervention

Intervention for children with ID includes supports and services for both the children and their families. An important first step is identification of the ID. Diagnostic labels can help others formulate realistic expectations for progress and behavior; protect children from maltreatment; and lead families to targeted information, resources, and support and advocacy groups.

Education

Federal legislation (PL94-142, reauthorized as IDEA or the Individuals with Disabilities Education Act) specifies that all children with disabilities are entitled to a free public education in the least restrictive environment and special services to meet their unique needs. A good deal of controversy has occurred about whether children with ID do better in special classes or in settings providing contact with peers who do not have ID. Because of their cognitive limitations and plateaus in development, children with ID cannot be expected to meet instructional goals developed for children without ID. In mainstream settings, instructional goals are modified, and special personnel are often assigned to assist the children.

For children with significant degrees of ID, specific skills are sometimes taught through a process of task analysis and systematic reward. Simple tasks are broken into component parts, and each new component is taught, reinforced, reviewed, and added to a previous component. For example, Sattler (4; p. 344) listed 22 component skills required for washing hands (wet hands under water, remove hands from water, direct hands toward soap dish, touch soap, etc.).

FUNCTIONAL BEHAVIORAL ASSESSMENT AND POSITIVE BEHAVIORAL SUPPORT

In addition to meeting the educational needs of children with ID, schools must address their behavior problems. The federal IDEA Amendments of 1997 (PL 105-17) specified that if a special education student has a behavior problem serious enough to impede learning, create a danger for self or others, require suspension for more than 10 days, or warrant inclusion in the student's Individual Education Plan (IEP), the IEP team must assess the behavior problem and develop an intervention plan based on that assessment (see reference 101 for a summary of legislative requirements). This kind of assessment is known as Functional Behavioral Assessment (FBA). Its purpose is to identify the function or cause of a behavior for a particular child and includes identification of triggers or antecedents as well as consequences that maintain the behavior. The intervention plan is often termed Positive Behavioral Support (PBS). Tasse (102) emphasized the need to collect observational data on an ongoing basis to monitor and revise understanding of functional relationships and efficacy of intervention strategies.

Psychopharmacology

Psychopharmacologic management should be considered as adjunctive therapy for behavioral disturbances in individuals with ID, along with educational and behavioral approaches. The expert consensus guidelines address the integration of these approaches in treatment of adults with ID, but the principles are applicable to children and adolescents as well (103).

As with any patient, thorough medical/family history and medical assessments, with particular attention to common associated conditions, such as seizure disorders, concomitant treatments for other medical conditions, and potential drug interactions must precede consideration of medication treatment. Genetic disorders (e.g., Prader–Willi, Lesch–Nyhan, Smith–Magenis, and fragile X syndromes) with particular behavioral concomitants and patterns of response to pharmacotherapy must be considered.

Establishment of the primary target symptom is essential in choosing first-line drug therapy. Hyperactive, aggressive, antisocial, stereotyped, and self-injurious behaviors are among those most commonly targeted in children with ID. Baseline assessments of behavior, abnormal movements, stereotypies, and mannerisms must be documented to distinguish pretreatment characteristics from medication side effects.

In their review of psychopharmacology in children and adolescents with mental retardation, Handen and Gilchrist (50) pointed out that most studies in ID tend to be open trials, case reports, or controlled studies with small samples. Their thorough literature review suggests that individuals with ID show similar responses to psychoactive medications as do the typically developing population, but that rates of response tend to be poorer and occurrence of side effects more frequent. The reader is referred to their excellent review, highlights of which are summarized later.

Attention-deficit hyperactivity disorder is cited as the most widely diagnosed psychiatric disorder in the ID population. Stimulants are recommended as a first-line treatment for hyperactive/impulsive symptoms. Side effects are similar to those reported in typically developing children, with a greater likelihood of developing tics and antisocial behavior. Pearson et al. (104) found significant improvement in behavior based on parent and teacher rating scales at methylphenidate doses of 0.6 mg/kg b.i.d., and did not find that these improvements were accompanied by increases in social anxiety, staring, or anxiety. Improvements in cognitive task performance were also demonstrated (105). Alternative treatments for hyperactive–impulsive symptoms, such as [ALPHA]-agonists clonidine and guanfacine, have been successfully used in treatment of hyperactivity and impulsivity, most recently reported by Posey et al. (106) in children with PDD. Tics and aggressive behaviors have also shown response to [ALPHA]-agonists. At the time of this writing, published data on the use of atomoxetine in ID are not available.

SSRIs have become the treatment of choice for depression and anxiety disorders in this population. SSRIs are recommended for the treatment of OCD, which may be related to stereotypic behavior and self-injury in the ID population. In a 1999 review, Aman et al. (107) documented decreases in SIB, irritability, and depressive symptoms in a majority of case reports and prospective open trials using fluoxetine in children with ID or pervasive developmental disorders or both (107). Side effects are similar to those reported in typically developing children and adolescents.

Antipsychotics are widely used in children and adolescents with ID. A relatively favorable side-effect profile as compared with typical antipsychotic medications has led to greater use of the atypical antipsychotics, risperidone being the most widely studied. In multiple trials, risperidone has been found to be beneficial in the treatment of disruptive behavior disorders (108,109), irritability, and self-injurious and repetitive behaviors. Monitoring for side effects such as weight gain, (predisposing to metabolic syndrome and type 2 diabetes), somnolence, headache, and extrapyramidal symptoms is recommended. Children and adolescents with ID were found to be at higher risk for the development of extrapyramidal reactions (110), including pseudo-parkinsonism, acute dystonic reactions, and akathisia, which can be mistaken for agitation and mistakenly treated with increased doses of medication. Individuals with ID are at risk for the development of neuroleptic malignant syndrome, with a higher mortality rate than in the general population (50).

Typical and atypical antipsychotics are also prescribed as mood stabilizers along with lithium and some antiepileptic drugs (valproic acid, divalproex sodium, carbamazepine, oxcarbazepine). This class of medications targets aggression, self-injurious behaviors, conduct problems, and symptoms associated with rapid-cycling bipolar disorder and mixed bipolar disorder, which are reported to occur with greater frequency in individuals with ID than in the general population (111,112). Lithium is reported to cause more side effects in children and adolescents with ID than in those who are typically developing (113,114). It has been described as the treatment of choice in the psychotic disorder associated with Prader–Willi syndrome (114). Valproic acid and divalproex sodium are reported effective in rapid-cycling bipolar disorder, aggression, and self-injurious behavior in children and adolescents, although these are still "off-label" uses (114). Fulminant hepatic failure and idiosyncratic hemorrhagic pancreatitis (most common in children with ID younger than 2 years) have been reported, as have blood disorders and polycystic ovary syndrome, rendering appropriate medical monitoring essential. Studies supporting the use of carbamazepine or oxcarbazepine in children and adolescents with ID are limited.

Psychotherapy

Psychotherapy can help children express emotions, enhance self-esteem, increase independence, and improve interactions with other people (70). Based on a consensus panel's review of 92 studies of treatment efficacy, conducted over a 30-year period, Prout and Nowak-Drabik (115) concluded that psychotherapy is moderately effective for people with ID. To participate in traditional forms of psychotherapy, children must have functional language, a capacity for insight, and sufficient cognitive ability to recognize causality and to relate feelings to causes. To respond to a cognitive–behavioral approach, they must be able to recognize relations between thoughts, affect, and behavior; monitor and test the validity of automatic thoughts; and substitute more-appropriate cognitions for distorted thoughts (116). Many children with ID do not have these capacities. Insight-oriented approaches may not be appropriate for them, and behavior modification or social-skills training may be more-effective choices.

Despite these concerns, several experts have described models of psychotherapeutic intervention for children with ID. In each, more-direct teaching, observation of behaviors, involvement of caregivers, restructuring of the environment, or a combination of these is present than might be used for children with typical development. Dosen (117) described developmental–dynamic relationship therapy, based on attachment theory. Within a framework of socioemotional development during the first 3 years of life, the child is helped to attain homeostasis, form an attachment with the therapist, and achieve a unique sense of self. By using an object-relations framework, Gaedt (118) described a psychodynamically oriented approach for children with ID and attachment problems. The therapist works with caregivers to create an emotional atmosphere within which the child can re-enter a disrupted developmental process. Juni (116) described a cognitive–behavioral therapeutic approach, incorporating indirect communication. The child "overhears" the therapist speaking "to no one in particular," gradually assimilates the therapist's dialogue, and indirectly improves the ability to manage emotions.

Working with Families

Although it is often assumed that raising a child with ID causes significant stress for families, this is not necessarily the case. A number of empirical investigations have shown that when family stress occurs, it is more apt to be due to a child's behavior problems than to the presence of ID (49,64,119,120,121). In a study by Plant and Sanders (122), parental stress correlated more strongly with difficult child behavior and difficulty of caregiving tasks than with the level of disability.

Siblings may be affected in special ways by their experience of living with a brother or sister who has ID. Rossiter and Sharpe (123) conducted a meta-analysis of 25 sibling studies and found a small, but statistically significant, negative effect for having a sibling with ID. Studies documenting negative effects indicated more depression, anxiety, and externalizing or internalizing behaviors in children who had a sibling with ID than in control children. Hannah and Midlarsky (124) studied helping behaviors in siblings of children with moderate to severe ID, comparing them with siblings of children with typical development. Compared with controls, siblings of children with ID provided more emotional support and assistance with activities of daily living. In working with families, it is important to recognize both psychological vulnerabilities and potential benefits of living with a sibling who has ID.

Families vary greatly in their desire for supports and services. Priorities change over time and at different stages of their child's development. Although professionals can inform families of the services available to them, they should be guided by the families' own choices.

Many families now use the Internet to obtain information about their child's disability, search for a second opinion, identify services, and join on-line support and advocacy groups (125). Zaidman-Zait and Jamieson (125) cautioned that some Web-based information is outdated, inaccurate, and not subject to peer review. Professionals can guide families to appropriate websites and other resources (Table 12.1).

Families should know that, at the age of 18, children with ID automatically become their own legal guardians unless the family makes other plans for them. Johnson and Walker (126) emphasized that families should develop long-term financial plans, including establishment of a Special Needs Will and Trust.

TABLE 12.1. RESOURCES
American Association on Intellectual and Developmental Disabilities (AAIDD) (formerly American Association on Mental Retardation) 444 North Capitol Street, NW, Suite 846, Washington DC 10001-1512 800-424-3688 www.aamr.org
The Arc of the United States 1010 Wayne Avenue, Suite 650, Silver Spring, MD 10910 800-433-5255 www.thearc.org
The Centers for Disease Control and Prevention (CDC) National Center on Birth Defects and Developmental Disabilities Mail-Stop E-88, 1600 Clifton Rd., Atlanta, GA 30333 www.cdc.gov
National Dissemination Center for Children with Disabilities (NICHCY) P.O. Box 1492, Washington, DC 20013 800-695-0285 www.nichcy.org

Conclusion

The accurate diagnosis of intellectual disability, as well as the identification of its causes and concurrent conditions, are essential components of intervention for children with ID. Subsequent provision of targeted clinical and educational services for children, information and support for their families, and systematic monitoring of progress, will optimize developmental outcomes.

Questions

1. Key elements of the definition of intellectual disability include all of the following except:
   A. Onset before age 18
   B. Discrepancy between intelligence and achievement
   C. Limitations in intellectual functioning
   D. Limitations in adaptive behavior

2. Characteristics of children with intellectual disability typically do not include:
   A. Deficits in gross motor skills
   B. Failure to benefit from incidental learning opportunities
   C. Tendency to forget skills previously mastered
   D. Poor social judgment

3. Characteristics of psychiatric or behavior problems in children with severe to profound intellectual disability include all of the following except:
   A. Hyperactivity
   B. Self-injurious behavior
   C. Social withdrawal
   D. Anorexia

4. The approximate mental age to be expected at adulthood for a child with moderate intellectual disability is:
   A. 8 to 11 years
   B. Less than 3 years
   C. 5½ to 8 years
   D. 3 to 5½ years

5. The medical assessment of individuals with intellectual disability should include all of the following except:

   A. Metabolic screen
   B. High-resolution chromosome analysis
   C. FISH for subtelomeric deletions
   D. Molecular analysis for fragile X

6. With appropriate intervention, children with formally diagnosed intellectual disabilities are expected to do all of the following except:

   A. Improve their social skills
   B. Increase their IQs
   C. Acquire new skills of daily living
   D. Ameliorate behavioral challenges

Answers

1. **B**
2. **A**
3. **D**
4. **C**
5. **A**
6. **B**

REFERENCES

1. Luckasson R, Borthwick-Duffy S, Buntinx WHE, et al. *Mental retardation: definition, classification, and systems of supports.* 10th ed. Washington, DC: American Association on Mental Retardation, 2002.
2. American Psychiatric Association. *Diagnostic and statistical manual of mental disorders.* 4th ed. text revision (DSM-IV-TR). Washington, DC: American Psychiatric Association, 2000.
3. Emerson E. Prevalence of psychiatric disorders in children and adolescents with and without intellectual disabilities. *J Intellect Disabil Res.* 2003;47: 51–58.
4. Sattler JM. *Assessment of children: behavioral and clinical applications.* 4th ed. San Diego: Jerome M. Sattler, 2002:189–211, 336–337.
5. Durkin MS, Stein ZA. Classification of mental retardation. In: Jacobson JW, Mulick JA, eds. *Manual of diagnosis and professional practice in mental retardation.* Washington, DC: American Psychological Association, 1996:67–73.
6. Gillberg C, Soderstrom H. Learning disability. *Lancet.* 2003;362:811–821.
7. Baroff GS. On the 2002 AAMR definition of mental retardation. In: Switzky HN, Greenspan S, eds. *What is mental retardation?* Washington, DC: American Association on Mental Retardation, 2006:29–38.
8. Srour MD, Mazer B, Shevell M: Analysis of clinical features predicting yield in the assessment of global developmental delay. *Pediatrics.* 2006;118: 139–145.
9. Van Karnebeek CDM, Jansweijer MCE, Leenders AG, et al. Diagnostic investigations in individuals with mental retardation: a systematic literature review of their usefulness. *Eur J Hum Genet.* 2005; 13:6–25.
10. Battaglia A, Carey JC. Diagnostic evaluation of developmental delay/mental retardation: an overview. *Am J Med Genet.* 2003:117C:3–14.
11. Curry CJ, Stevenson RE, Aughton D, et al. Evaluation of mental retardation: recommendations of a consensus conference. *Am J Med Genet.* 1997;72: 468–477.
12. Moeschler JB, Shevell M, the Committee on genetics. Clinical genetic evaluation of the child with mental retardation or developmental delays. *Pediatrics.* 2006;117:2304–2316.
13. Guttmacher AE, Collins FS. Genomic medicine: a primer. *N Engl J Med.* 2002;347:1512–1520.
14. Veltman JA. Genomic microarrays in clinical diagnosis. *Curr Opin Pediatr.* 2006;18:598–603.
15. Rauch A, Hoyer J, Guth S, et al. Diagnostic yield of various genetic approaches in patients with unexplained developmental delay or mental retardation. *Am J Med Genet.* 2006;140A:2063–2074.
16. Shevell M, Ashwal S, Donley D, et al. Practice parameter: evaluation of the child with global developmental delay. *Neurology.* 2003;60:367–380.
17. Knight, SJ, Flint J. Perfect endings: a review of subtelomeric probes and their use in clinical diagnosis. *J Med Genet.* 2001:109:440–451.
18. Biesecker LG. The end of the beginning of chromosome ends. *Am J Med Genet.* 2002;107:263–266.
19. DeVries BBA, White SM, Knight SJL, et al. Clinical studies on submicroscopic subtelomeric rearrangements: a checklist. *J Med Genet.* 2001;38: 145–150.
20. Berk H. Early intervention and special education. In: Smith R, ed. *Children with mental retardation: a parents' guide.* Rockville, MD: Woodbine House, 1993:173–207.
21. Editorial Board. Definition of mental retardation. In: Jacobson JW, Mulick JA, eds. *Manual of diagnosis and professional practice in mental retardation.* Washington, DC: American Psychological Association, 1996:13–53.
22. Zion E, Jenvey VB. Temperament and social behavior at home and school among typically developing children and children with intellectual disability. *J Intellect Disabil Res.* 2006;50:445–456.

23. Heaton P, Wallace GH. Annotation: the savant syndrome. *J Child Clin Psychol Psychiatry.* 2004; 45:899–911.
24. Shields WD. Management of epilepsy in mentally retarded children using the newer antiepileptic drugs, vagus nerve stimulation, and surgery. *J Child Neurol.* 2004;19:S58–S64.
25. Huber B, Siedel M. Update on treatment of epilepsy in people with intellectual disabilities. *Curr Opin Psychiatry.* 2006:19:492–496.
26. Pellock JM, Morton LD. Treatment of epilepsy in the multiply handicapped. *Mental Retard Dev Disabil Res Rev.* 2000;6:309–323.
27. Santosh P, Baird G. Psychpharmacotherapy in children and adults with intellectual disability. *Lancet.* 1999;354:233–242.
28. Richardson SA, Koller H. *Twenty two years.* Cambridge, Mass: Cambridge University Press, 1996: 1–328.
29. Matson JL, Bamburg JW, Mayville EA, et al. Seizure disorders in people with intellectual disability: an analysis of differences in social functioning, adaptive functioning and maladaptive behaviors. *J Intellect Disabil Res.* 1999;43:531–539.
30. Crumrine PK. Lennox-Gastaut syndrome. *J Child Neurol.* 2002;17(suppl 1):S70–S75.
31. Riikonen R. The latest on infantile spasms. *Curr Opin Neurol.* 2005;18:91–95.
32. Bough KJ, Rho JM. Anticonvulsant mechanisms of the ketogenic diet. *Epilepsia.* 2007;48:43–58.
33. Freeman JM, Kossoff EH, Hartman AL. The ketogenic diet: one decade later. *Pediatrics.* 2007;119: 535–543.
34. Hallbook T, Lundgren J, Rosen I. Ketogenic diet improves sleep quality in children with therapy-resistant epilepsy. *Epilepsia.* 2007;48:59–65.
35. Rychlicki F, Zamponi, N, Trignani R, et al. Vagus nerve stimulation: clinical experience in drug-resistant pediatric epileptic patients. *Seizure.* 2006; 15:483–490.
36. Saneto RP, Sotero de Menezes MA, Ojemann JG, et al. Vagus nerve stimulation for intractable seizures in children. *Pediatr Neurol.* 2006;35: 323–326.
37. Kossoff EH, Pyzik PL, Rubenstein JE, et al. Combined ketogenic diet and vagus nerve stimulation: rational polytherapy? *Epilepsia.* 2007;48:77–81.
38. Borthwick-Duffy SA. Epidemiology and prevalence of psychopathology in people with mental retardation. *J Consult Clin Psychol.* 1994;62:17–27.
39. Dosen A, Day K. Epidemiology, etiology, and presentation of mental illness and behavior disorders in persons with mental retardation. In: Dosen A, Day K, eds. *Mental illness and behavior disorders in children and adults with mental retardation.* Washington, DC: American Psychiatric Press, 2001:3–24.
40. Einfeld SL, Tonge BJ. Population prevalence of psychopathology in children and adolescents with disability, I: rationale and methods. *J Intellect Disabil Res.* 1996;40:91–98.
41. American Academy of Child and Adolescent Psychiatry Work Group on Quality Issues. Summary of practice parameters for the assessment and treatment of children, adolescents, and adults with mental retardation and comorbid mental disorders. *J Am Acad Child Adolesc Psychiatry.* 1999;38:1606–1610.
42. Blacher J, McIntyre LL. Syndrome specificity and behavioural disorders in young adults with intellectual disability: cultural differences in family impact. *J Intellect Disabil Res.* 2006;50: 184–198.
43. Dekker MC, Koot HM. DSM-IV disorders in children with borderline to moderate intellectual disability, I: prevalence and impact. *J Am Acad Child Adolesc Psychiatry.* 2003;42:915–922.
44. Dekker MC, Koot HM. DSM-IV disorders in children with borderline to moderate intellectual disability, II: child and family predictors. *J Am Acad Child Adolesc Psychiatry.* 2003;42:923–931.
45. Dekker MC, Koot HM, van der Ende J, et al. Emotional and behavioral problems in children with intellectual disability. *J Child Psychol Psychiatry.* 2002;41:407–417.
46. Dykens EM. Toward a positive psychology of mental retardation. *Am J Orthopsychiatry.* 2006; 76:185–193.
47. Dykens EM, Hodapp RM. Research in mental retardation: toward an etiologic approach. *J Child Psychol Psychiatry.* 2001;42:49–71.
48. Einfeld SL, Tonge BJ. Population prevalence of psychopathology in children and adolescents with intellectual disability, II: epidemiological findings. *J Intellect Disabil Res.* 1996;40: 99–109.
49. Eisenhower AS, Baker BL, Blacher J. Preschool children with intellectual disabilities: syndrome specificity, behaviour problems, and maternal well-being. *J Intellect Disabil Res.* 2005;49:657–671.
50. Handen B, Gilchrist R. Practitioner review: psychopharmacology in children and adolescents with mental retardation. *J Child Psychol Psychiatry.* 2006;47:871–882.
51. Stromme P, Diseth TH. Prevalence of psychiatric diagnoses in children with mental retardation: data from a population-based study. *Dev Med Child Neurol.* 2000;42:266–270.
52. Wing L. Language, social, and cognitive impairments in autism and severe mental retardation. *J Autism Dev Disord.* 1981;11:31–44.
53. Deb S, Prasad KBG. The prevalence of autistic disorder among children with a learning disability. *Br J Psychiatry.* 1994;165:395–399.
54. Nordin V, Gillberg C. Autism spectrum disorders in children with physical or mental disability or both, I: clinical and epidemiological aspects. *Dev Med Child Neurol.* 1996;38:297–313.
55. Myers BA. Misleading cues in the diagnosis of mental retardation and infantile autism in the preschool child. *Ment Retard.* 1989;27: 85–90.

56. Ballaban-Gill K, Rapin I, Tuchman RF, et al. Longitudinal examination of the behavioral, language, and social changes in a population of adolescents and adults with autistic disorder. *Pediatr Neurol.* 1996;15:217–223.
57. Volkmar FR, Burack JA, Cohen DJ. Deviance and developmental approaches in the study of autism. In: Hodapp RM, Burack JA, Zigler E, eds. *Issues in the developmental approach to mental retardation.* New York: Cambridge University Press, 1990:246–271.
58. Walker WO, Johnson CP. Mental retardation: overview and diagnosis. *Pediatr Rev.* 2006;27:204–212.
59. Hastings RR, Beck A, Daley D, et al. Symptoms of ADHD and their correlations in children with intellectual disabilities. *Res Dev Disabil.* 2005;26:456–468.
60. Brown EC, Aman MG, Lecavalier L. Empirical classification of behavioral and psychiatric problems in children and adolescents with mental retardation. *Am J Ment Retard.* 2004;109:445–455.
61. Dykens EM. Annotation: psychopathology in children with intellectual disability. *J Child Psychol Psychiatry.* 2000;41:407–417.
62. Chadwick O, Piroth N, Walker J, et al. Factors affecting the risk of behaviour problems in children with severe intellectual disability. *J Intellect Disabil Res.* 2000;44:108–123.
63. Baker BL, Blacher J, Crnic KA, et al. Behavior problems and parenting stress in families of three-year-old children with and without developmental delays. *Am J Ment Retard.* 2002;107:433–444.
64. Crnic K, Hoffman C, Gaze C, et al. Understanding the emergence of behavior problems in young children with developmental delays. *Infants Young Child.* 2004;17:223–235.
65. Merrell KW, Holland ML. Social-emotional behavior of preschool-age children with and without developmental delays. *Res Dev Disabil.* 1997;18:393–405.
66. McIntyre LL, Blacher J, Baker BL. The transition to school: adaptation in young children with and without intellectual disability. *J Intell Disabil Res.* 2006;50:349–361.
67. Handen BL, Gilchrist RH. Mental retardation. In: Mash EJ, Barkley RA, eds. *Treatment of childhood disorders.* 3rd ed. New York: Guilford, 2006:411–454.
68. Moss S, Bouras N, Holt G. Mental health services for people with intellectual disability: a conceptual framework. *J Intellect Disabil Res.* 2000;44:97–107.
69. Sullivan K, Hooper S, Hatton D. Behavioural equivalents of anxiety in children with fragile X syndrome: parent and teacher report. *J Intell Disabil Res.* 2007;51:54–65.
70. King BH, State MW, Shah B, et al. Mental retardation: a review of the past ten years: part I. *J Am Acad Child Adolesc Psychiatry.* 1997;36:1656–1663.
71. Jaudes PK, Shapiro LD. Child abuse and developmental disabilities. In: Silver JA, Amster BJ, Haecker T, eds. *Young children and foster care.* Baltimore: Paul Brookes, 1999:213–234.
72. Verdugo MA, Bermejo BG, Fuertes J. The maltreatment of intellectually handicapped children and adolescents. *Child Abuse Neglect.* 1995;19:205–215.
73. Benedict MI, White RB, Wulff LM, et al. Reported maltreatment in children with multiple disabilities. *Child Abuse Neglect.* 1990;14:207–217.
74. Vig S, Kaminer R. Maltreatment and developmental disabilities in children. *J Dev Phys Disabil.* 2002;14:371–386.
75. Horner-Johnson W, Drum CE. Prevalence of maltreatment of people with intellectual disabilities: a review of recently published research. *Ment Retard Dev Disabil Res Rev.* 2006;12:57–69.
76. Wechsler D. *Wechsler intelligence scale for children.* 4th ed. San Antonio: Psychological Corporation, 2003.
77. Roid GH. *Stanford-Binet intelligence scales.* 5th ed. Itasca, IL: Riverside, 2003.
78. Elliott CD. *Differential ability scales.* 2nd ed. San Antonio: Psychological Corporation, 2006.
79. Kaufman JC, Kaufman-Singer J, Kaufman NL. *Kaufman assessment battery for children.* 2nd ed. New York: Guilford, 2004.
80. Roid GH, Sampers JL. *Merrill-Palmer revised scales of development.* Wood Dale, IL: Stoelting, 2004.
81. Wechsler D. *Wechsler preschool and primary scale of intelligence.* 3rd ed. San Antonio: Psychological Corporation, 2002.
82. Hammill DD, Pearson NA, Wiederholt JL. *Comprehensive test of nonverbal intelligence.* San Antonio: Psychological Corporation, 1997.
83. Roid GH, Miller L. *Leiter international performance scale–revised.* Wood Dale, IL: Stoelting; 1997.
84. Brown L, Sherbenou RJ, Johnsen SK. *Test of nonverbal intelligence.* 3rd ed. San Antonio: Psychological Corporation, 1997.
85. Bayley N. *Bayley scales of infant and toddler development.* 3rd ed. San Antonio: Psychological Corporation, 2005.
86. Batshaw ML, Shapiro BK. Mental retardation. In: Batshaw ML, ed. *Children with disabilities.* 4th ed. Baltimore: Paul Brookes, 1997:335–359.
87. Mervis CA, Boyle CA, Yeargin-Allsopp M. Prevalence and selected characteristics of childhood vision impairment. *Dev Med Child Neurol.* 2002;44:538–541.
88. Evenhuis HM, Theunissen M, Denkers I, et al. Prevalence of visual and hearing impairment in a Dutch institutionalized population with intellectual disability. *J Intellect Disabil Res.* 2001;45:457–464.
89. Fewell RR. Assessment of visual functioning. In: Bracken BA, ed. *The psychoeducational assessment of preschool children.* 3rd ed. Needham Heights, MA: Allyn & Bacon, 2000:234–248.
90. Sattler JM, Evans CA. Visual impairments. In: Sattler JM, ed. *Assessment of children: behavioral*

and clinical applications. 4th ed. San Diego: Jerome M. Sattler, 2002:367–376.
91. Sattler JM, Hardy-Braz ST. Hearing impairments. In: Sattler JM, ed. *Assessment of children: behavioral and clinical applications.* 4th ed. San Diego: Jerome M. Sattler, 2002:377–389.
92. Vig S, Jedrysek E. Adaptive behavior of young urban children with developmental disabilities. *Ment Retard.* 1995;33:909–998.
93. Sparrow SS, Cichetti DV, Balla DA. *Vineland adaptive behavior scales.* 2nd ed. Circle Pines, MN: American Guidance Service, 2005.
94. Harrison PL, Oakland T. *Adaptive behavior assessment system.* 2nd ed. San Antonio: Psychological Corporation, 2003.
95. Bernheimer LP, Keogh BK. Stability of cognitive performance in children with developmental delays. *Am J Ment Retard.* 1988;92:539–542.
96. Carr J. Six weeks to twenty-one years old: a longitudinal study of children with Down's syndrome and their families. *J Child Psychol Psychiatry.* 1988;21:407–431.
97. Field M, Fox N, Radcliffe J. Predicting IQ changes in preschoolers with developmental disabilities. *Pediatrics.* 1990;11:184–189.
98. Keogh BK, Coots JJ, Bernheimer LP. School placement of children with nonspecific developmental delays. *J Early Intervent.* 1995;20:65–78.
99. Hall I, Strydom A, Richards M. Social outcomes in adulthood of children with intellectual impairment: evidence from a birth cohort. *J Intellect Disabil Res.* 2005;49:171–182.
100. Keogh BK, Bernheimer LP, Guthrie D. Children with developmental delays twenty years later: Where are they? How are they? *Am J Ment Retard.* 2004;3:219–230.
101. Drasgow E, Yell ML. Functional behavioral assessments: legal requirements and challenges. *School Psychol Rev.* 2001;30:239–251.
102. Tasse MJ. Functional behavioral assessment in people with intellectual disabilities. *Curr Opin Psychiatry.* 2006;19:475–480.
103. Aman MG, Crismon ML, Frances A. et al. *Treatment of psychiatric and behavioral problems in individuals with mental retardation, an update of the expert consensus guidelines.* Englewood, Colorado: Postgraduate Institute for Medicine, 2004.
104. Pearson DA, Santos CW, Roach JD, et al. Treatment effects of methylphenidate on behavioral adjustment in children with mental retardation and ADHD. *J Am Acad Child Adolesc Psychiatry.* 2003;42:209–216.
105. Pearson DA, Santos CW, Casat CD, et al. Treatment effects of methylphenidate on cognitive functioning in children with mental retardation and ADHD. *J Am Acad Child Adolesc Psychiatry.* 2004;43:677–685.
106. Posey DI, Litwiller M, Koburn A, Mc Dougle CJ. Paroxetine in autism. *J Am Acad Child Adolesc Psychiatry.* 1999;38:111–112.
107. Aman MG, Arnold LE, Armstrong SC. Review of serotonergic agents and perseverative behavior in patients with developmental disabilities. *Ment Retard Dev Disabil.* 1999;5:279–289.
108. Findling RL, Aman MG, Edrdekens M, et al. Risperidone disruptive behavior study group. *Am J Psychiatry.* 2004;161:677–684.
109. Croonenberghs J, Fegert JM, Findling RL, et al. Risperidone disruptive behavior study group. *J Am Acad Child Adolesc Psychiatry.* 2005;44:969–970.
110. Van Bellinghen M, De Troch C. Risperidone in the treatment of behavioral disturbances in children and adolescents with borderline intellectual functioning: a double-blind, placebo-controlled pilot trial. *J Child Adolesc Psychopharmacol.* 2001; 11:5–13.
111. Aman MG, Collier-Crespin A, Lindsay RL. Pharmacotherapy of disorders in mental retardation. *Eur Child Adolesc Psychiatry.* 2000;(suppl 1):198–207.
112. Vanstraelen M, Tyrer SP. Rapid cycling bipolar affective disorder in people with intellectual disability: a systematic review. *J Intellect Disabil Res.* 1999;43:349–359.
113. Green WH. *Child and adolescent clinical psychopharmacology.* Philadelphia: Williams & Wilkins, 2000.
114. Antochi R, Stavrakaki C, Emery PC. Psychopharmacological treatments in persons with dual diagnosis of psychiatric disorders and developmental disabilities. *Postgrad Med J.* 2003;9:130–146.
115. Prout HT, Nowak-Drabik KM. Psychotherapy with persons who have mental retardation: an evaluation of effectiveness. *Am J Ment Retard.* 2003;108:82–93.
116. Juni S. Indirect communication as an insight-oriented technique with the resistant and intellectually limited. *J Psychother Integr.* 2001;11:453–480.
117. Dosen A. Developmental-dynamic relationship therapy: an approach to more severely mentally retarded children. In: Dosen A, Day K, eds. *Treating mental illness and behavior disorders in children and adults with mental retardation.* Washington, DC: American Psychiatric Press, 2001:415–427.
118. Gaedt C. Psychodynamically oriented psychotherapy in mentally retarded children. In: Dosen A, Day K, eds. *Treating mental illness and behavior disorders in children and adults with mental retardation.* Washington, DC: American Psychiatric Press, 2001:401–414.
119. Baker BL, Blacher J, Olsson MB. Preschool children with and without developmental delays: behavior problems, parents' optimism, and well being. *J Intellect Disabil Res.* 2005;49:575–590.
120. Hassall R, Rose J, McDonald J. Parenting stress in mothers of children with an intellectual disability:

the effects of parental cognitions in relation to child characteristics and family support. *J Intellect Disabil Res.* 2005;49:405–418.
121. Baker BL, McIntyre LL, Blacher J, et al. Preschool children with and without developmental delays: behaviour problems and parenting stress over time. *J Intellect Disabil Res.* 2003;47:217–230.
122. Plant KM, Sanders MR. Predictors of care-giver stress in families of preschool children with developmental disabilities. *J Intellect Disabil Res.* 2007;51:109–124.
123. Rossiter L, Sharpe D. The siblings of individuals with mental retardation: a quantitative integration of the literature. *J Child Family Studies.* 2001;10:65–84.
124. Hannah ME, Midlarsky E. Helping by siblings of children with mental retardation. *Am J Ment Retard.* 2005;110:87–99.
125. Zaidman-Zait A, Jamieson JR. Providing web-based support for families of infants and young children with established disabilities. *Infants Young Child.* 2007;20:11–25.
126. Johnson CP, Walker WO. Mental retardation: management and prognosis. *Pediatri Rev.* 2006;27:249–256.

CHAPTER 13

Neurobehavioral Aspects of Traumatic Brain Injury in Children

ALEKSANDRA DJUKIC

Introduction

The tragedy of traumatic brain injuries (TBIs) begins with its sudden onset and selection of victims, generally children and young adults who have an expectation of long life and unlimited possibilities. The tragedy then encompasses families, whose coping abilities are stretched to the limit, patients who only dimly understand why their lives must be changed in such dramatic ways, and a professional community, which is responsible for their recovery and reintegration (1).

The burden of TBI in children is heavy. Each year, approximately 475,000 children younger than 14 years sustain TBI (2). For 5,000 of them, the outcome is fatal. TBI takes the lives of 6 times more U.S. children than those who die of HIV/AIDS (3). Of TBI survivors, 30,000 remain permanently disabled (4).

During the first days to week after the injury, the main focus of medical and surgical intervention is stabilization of the patient. As acute medical care has improved, the number of survivors has increased. These patients place increased and specific demands on the medical and educational communities to address their disabilities, which are often "silent."

Favorable initial physical recovery, which is usually quick, often leads to erroneous optimism based on assumptions that cognitive and behavioral recovery has been equally favorable. This misconception leads to the premature release of injured children to their prior, now inappropriate, school environments and other problems.

In reality, the acute TBI can become not only a chronic disease but also, because of the nature of development, a progressive one. Children grow out of certain disabilities caused by TBI but may grow into new ones. Functions that escaped damage by the impact can later pay the price of compensation for the recovery of those functions primarily damaged. To optimize long-term outcome, coordinated and lasting action by the medical, social, and educational communities is required.

Pathophysiology of TBI

Injury to the head can result in two categories of brain injuries: primary and secondary.

Primary injury occurs immediately after the impact and is related to instantaneous events caused directly by the blow. This injury results from tissue disruption that is often permanent and constitutes one of the most important limiting factors for a full recovery.

Secondary injuries are caused by a cascade of events triggered by the impact, such as vessel disruptions and hemorrhages, edema, seizures, increase in intracranial pressure, consequent decrease in the brain perfusion pressure, and brain shifts/herniations.

Mechanisms/Physics of the Primary Injury

The central event in any brain injury is movement of the brain within the skull (5). An understanding of the physics of TBI is a prerequisite for an understanding of the pathophysiology of brain injury, the basis of residual impairment, and possible treatment targets.

Two types of accelerating movement—linear and rotational—of the head and brain caused by the impact are pertinent. Each of them causes distinctive patterns of tissue damage (Fig. 13.1).

If the vector of the force passes through the center of gravity (CG) of the head, the head will assume linear acceleration along the direction of the force. All particles (cells) will travel with the same velocity and in the same direction: Hence they will sustain no intermolecular stress. As the accelerating head hits the ground, the skull suddenly decelerates, but the brain continues to move forward until it is stopped by one of the poles of the calvarium. This impact injures the brain at that pole and creates a negative pressure at the opposite one, which injures that pole of the brain (Fig. 13.2). Gyri, which are flat and have a large surface area, such as those in the frontal lobes, will be prone to extensive lesions. Injuries caused by the linear acceleration are mostly superficial (6).

Physics of the linear acceleration

- **Vector of the force passes through the center of gravity and causes linear acceleration**

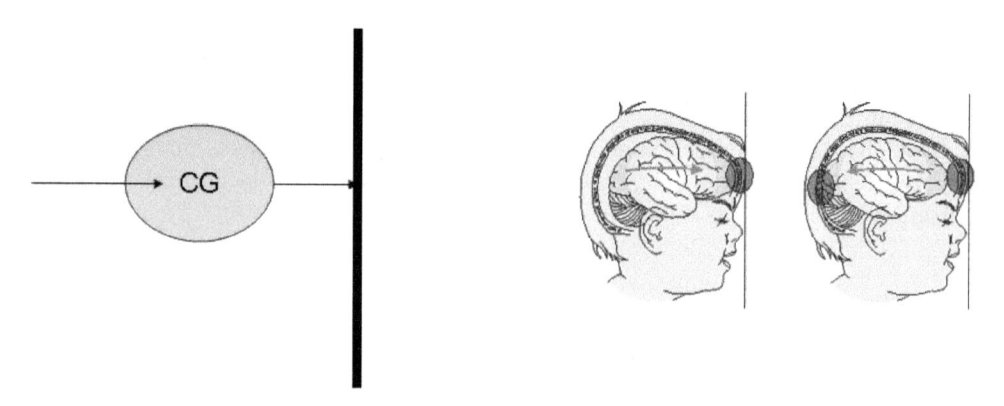

■ **FIGURE 13.1.** Linear acceleration causing crowding of the brain at the pole (coup) and creating negative pressure and cavitations at the antipole (contrecoup).

Physics of the rotational acceleration

- Rotation of the head around the center of gravity-stretching and shearing of nerve fibers

Diffuse axonal injury

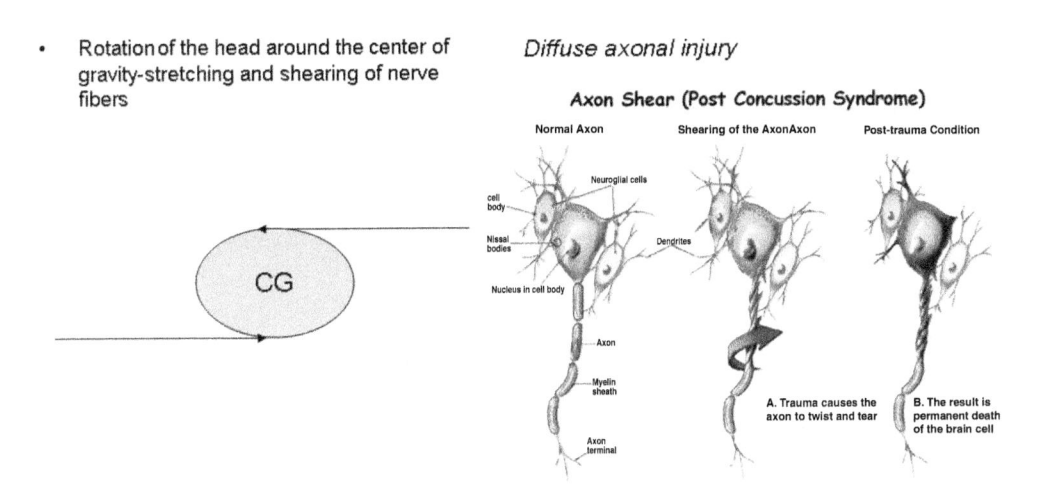

Axon Shear (Post Concussion Syndrome)

Normal Axon — Shearing of the Axon — Post-trauma Condition

A. Trauma causes the axon to twist and tear
B. The result is permanent death of the brain cell

FIGURE 13.2. Rotational acceleration leading to the widespread shearing injury.

When the vector of the force does not pass through the CG of the head, the head will assume rotational acceleration. Whereas the effect of linear acceleration depends on pressure changes and the impact of the brain against bony structures, rotational mechanisms produce *shearing strain*. Shearing-strain forces distort the shape of the brain, cause intermolecular stress, and lead to tearing of neural elements (7). Injuries caused by rotational forces are deep. The abundance of white matter lesions throughout the brain, indicative of widespread axonal injury (disconnection syndromes), is a pathologic hallmark of severely injured patients (Fig. 13.3). Axonal injury has a predilection for the gray–white matter junction, cerebellar peduncles, corpus callosum, fornices, and fiber tracts around the brain stem (8,9).

Asynchrony between the rotational movements of the brain and skull causes rubbing of the friable cortex against the rough surfaces of the skull base. Temporal and frontal parts of the brain and cingulate gyri, which are adjacent to the most prominent dural surfaces, are particularly vulnerable to injury. This disruption correlates with impairments of memory, frontal lobe functions, and emotional control.

In reality, most TBIs are produced by the combination of the two accelerating movements.

Imaging

Various neuroimaging techniques offer pertinent information concerning the diagnosis, clinical outcome, and recovery mechanisms after pediatric TBI. The main advantage of the computerized tomography (CT) is its availability and ability to detect lesions rapidly that require immediate surgical intervention, such as epidural hematomas and fractures. Magnetic resonance imaging (MRI) has a higher sensitivity in detecting intraparenchymal injuries, especially those associated with diffuse axonal injury. Diffusion tensor imaging (DTI) provides a quantitative assessment of the integrity of white matter tissue.

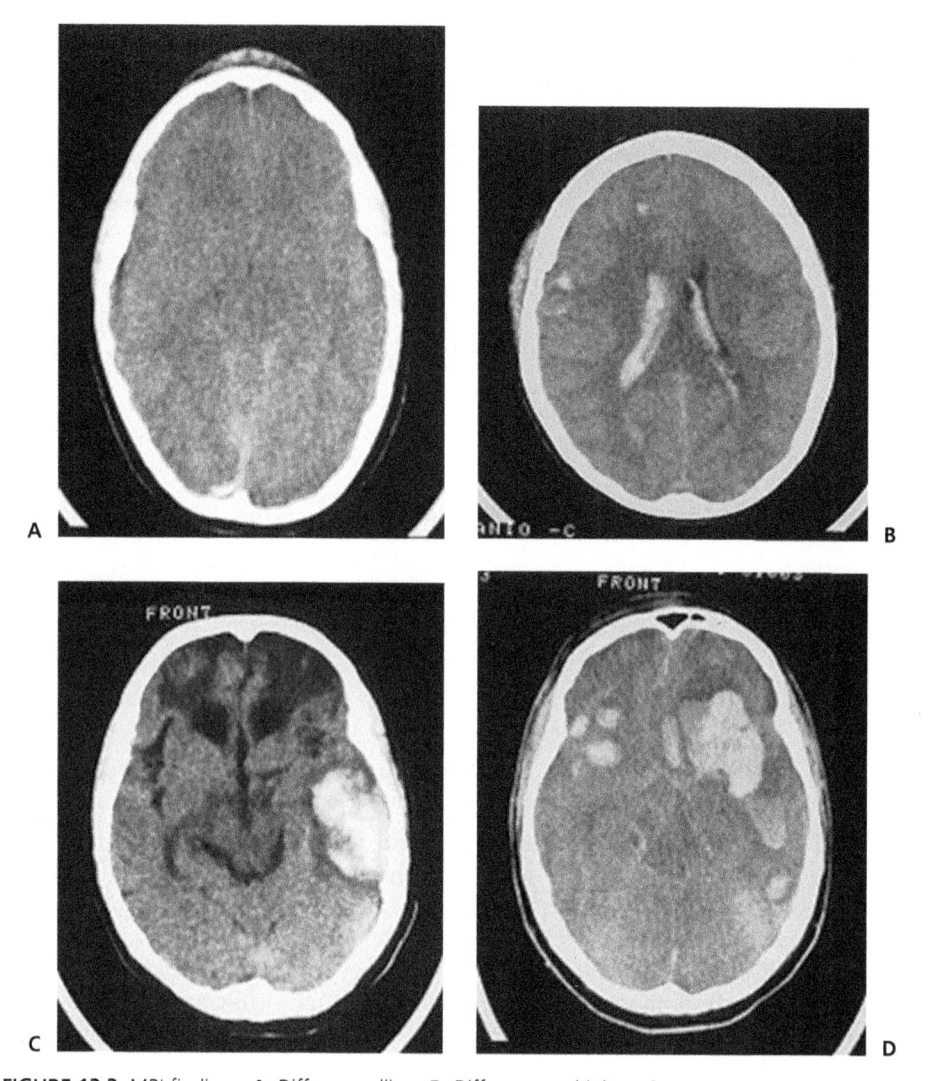

FIGURE 13.3. MRI findings. **A:** Diffuse swelling. **B:** Diffuse axonal injury. **C, D:** Frontotemporal contusions.

Newer imaging techniques, such as functional MRI, which records blood oxygen level–dependent signal in conjunction with conventional imaging, may in the future enable the clinician to understand plasticity and recovery processes. It also may facilitate the design of early-intervention and rehabilitation programs for children with TBI (10–12).

Clinical Course of TBI

Immediately after the injury, children may lose consciousness and remain comatose. If not comatose, injured children may show confusion, disorientation, and amnesia (Fig. 13.4). After the resolution of coma, pediatric patients recovering from severe TBI enter a state of anterograde amnesia (13). Behaviors characteristic of this period are restlessness, impulsive behaviors alternating with lethargy, irritability, and agitation. Restoration of memory

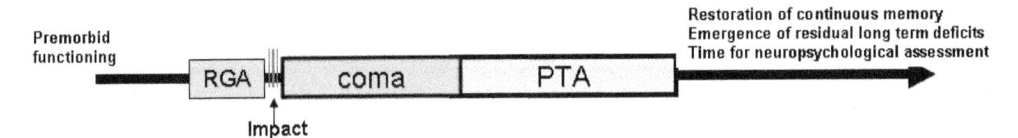

FIGURE 13.4. Restoration of cognitive functions after severe TBI. RGA, retrograde amnesia; PTA, post-traumatic, anterograde amnesia.

for ongoing events is not a continuous process. Patients regain "islands of memory," in which periods of confusion and amnesia alternate with those of good orientation. With time, lucid periods become longer and finally continuous. For confused TBI patients, the length of time elapsed until information is remembered on a day-to-day basis (i.e., the duration of post-traumatic amnesia) is a vital indicator of outcome (14).

Examples of different course scenarios in brain-injured patients who do not fully recover are the following:

1. There is gradual improvement of neurological functions, which is most prominent during the first months after injury but continues at a slower pace, especially with regard to cognitive recovery, which can occur over years.
2. Consequences become apparent after a delay. Damage to some areas of the brain, particularly the frontal lobes, in early childhood may not give rise to major problems until early or late adolescence, when normal maturation fails to occur (15,16).
3. Developmental functions that were not primarily injured eventually pay the price for the recovery of the injured functions. For example, young children who have injury to their language areas recover better than both older children and adults. In these young patients, "vicarious" areas of the contralateral hemisphere assume the functions of the damaged areas. However, these newly created and unnatural tasks eventually lead to overcrowding of the neural networks within the uninjured hemisphere. In addition to developing visuospatial skills, the nondominant hemisphere then becomes burdened with the task of organizing language. For example, visuospatial functions suffer as language functions recover (17,18).

Classification of TBI

The depth and duration of coma and length of time that children remain amnestic reflect the severity of brain damage. TBI is most often classified as mild, moderate, or severe, based on the Glasgow Coma Score (GCS) at presentation (Table 13.1) (19,20). A GCS of 13 to 15 defines mild TBI; 9 to 12, moderate TBI; and 8 or less, severe TBI. Although the GCS is a useful tool for the initial management, it has not been found to be an accurate predictor of cognitive outcome in children (21,22). For this purpose and for the prediction of residual deficits, especially those of interest to child psychiatrists, the duration of post-traumatic amnesia (PTA) is a more valuable index. As a rough guide, children with a GCS of 12 or below, those who have lost consciousness for more than 20 to 30 minutes, or those who have PTA of longer than 7 days are more likely to have psychological sequelae. These are children with moderate or severe injuries. This degree of brain injury warrants hospital admission and close medical surveillance after discharge. This group of patients might be of specific interest to child psychiatrists because it typically consists of

TABLE 13.1. GLASGOW COMA SCORE

Eye opening

Spontaneous	4
To loud voice	3
To pain	2
None	1

Verbal response

Oriented	5
Confused, disoriented	4
Inappropriate words	3
Incomprehensible sounds	2
None	1

Best motor response

Obeys	6
Localizes	5
Withdraws (flexion)	4
Abnormal flexion posturing	3
Extension posturing	2
None	1

children with pre-existing behavioral problems that worsen after the injury. These children are prone to recurrent injuries (23). Sports and bicycle accidents account for the majority of cases among 5- to 14-year-old children. Every attempt to reduce the likelihood of recurrent injury should be made because repeated TBIs may have an additive effect and lead to cognitive decline (24).

Immaturity of the Brain: Opportunities and Vulnerabilities

It was previously thought that infants would suffer minimal damage from TBI because of greater brain plasticity. Classic studies by Kennard (25,26) showed that the immaturity of the brain has a protective role regarding outcome. Optimistic clinical expectations that followed are summarized in the statement "It is better to have your injury early, if you can manage it" (27).

This concept has been challenged. Young children may be especially vulnerable to the diffuse nature of TBI and tend to have more global and profound consequences than do older children (28,29). Depending on the child's age, the same injury can lead to very different functional outcomes. A review of evidence for and against the argument that younger people show better recovery after brain injury can be found in Wilson (30).

In the report from the Traumatic Coma Data Bank, children younger than 4 years exhibited the poorest outcomes (28). The two main reasons for these observations are related to the nature of the injury and the specific tasks children encounter.

Because of the diffuse nature of rotational forces, all severe head injuries should be considered diffuse from the pathophysiological standpoint. The diffuse nature of injury associated with rotational forces decreases the ability of distant areas and surrounding areas to compensate (31).

With regard to the nature of the task, although adults may function well by relying on previously acquired knowledge, children cannot, because functions emerging at the time of TBI may suffer more than established ones (32). Thus depending of the developmental stage at the time of the injury, the same insult might have different outcomes (Table 13.2).

TABLE 13.2. PROGNOSTIC FACTORS RELEVANT FOR RECOVERY

Severity of insult
Number of insults
Age at time of insult
Premorbid cognitive functioning
Integrity of the rest of the brain
Motivation
Emotional factors
Family and psychosocial influences and coping abilities
Extent and quality of rehabilitation

According to Wilson (33), it is not only the kind of head injury that matters but also "the kind of head."

Neurobehavioral Outcome

Behavioral and cognitive problems as well as difficulties in adaptive functioning are common after TBI (34,35). Outcomes range from almost complete recovery to profound deficits that affect both the child and the family. Injury causes not only a direct loss of brain function but also indirect dysfunction. Sequelae develop as a result of emotional response to injury, exacerbation of pre-existing problems, and the fact that injured children have difficulty meeting the expectations of their peers.

Post-traumatic epilepsy is a serious clinical problem that can worsen functional outcome. The incidence of post-traumatic seizures ranges from 2% to 35%, with higher frequencies seen with more severe injury. The incidence of seizures after mild head injuries is not significantly greater than that in the general population. The seizure focus in 56% of patients is temporal, and in 36% of patients, frontal. Unfortunately, no efficacious preventive therapy for post-traumatic epilepsy has been established. Prophylactic use of antiepileptic drugs does not prevent post-traumatic epilepsy and may produce negative cognitive effects (36).

The incidence of *psychiatric disorders* is twice as high in children with TBI as in those with physical handicaps without cerebral involvement.

Behavioral manifestations differ during recovery from TBI. Altered consciousness, confusion, and inability to continuously remember ongoing events are behavioral hallmarks of the acute post-injury period.

Elements of post-traumatic stress disorder, with sleep disturbance, intrusive thoughts, nightmares, and avoidant and defiant behaviors characterize the subacute stage of the recovery. Intrusive thoughts related to the accident occur in the majority of children with moderate and severe injuries (37,38). However, such symptoms of post-traumatic stress disorders usually resolve within weeks.

The severity of head injury shows a positive correlation with the likelihood of chronic emotional and behavioral disorder. A 4-year follow-up study of children after TBI documented higher rate of behavior problems (36% in the severe and 22% in the moderate TBI group) compared with children with orthopedic injuries (10%) (39). The preinjury socioeconomic status, psychiatric status, family functioning, and the presence of the residual cognitive impairment in a child are also related to psychiatric morbidity (40).

Children who sustained mild TBI stand out as a group, primarily in regard to their premorbid behavior. In these children, the rate of premorbid behavioral disturbances is higher than in either those who sustain severe TBI or in those in a control group (41). Similarly, premorbid behavior in severely injured children did not differ from that of controls (42–44).

Before the injury, children with mild TBI are typically more impulsive, active, and prone to take risks leading to TBI. Exacerbation of a pre-existing psychiatric disturbance, rather than development of a new one, characterizes the behavioral outcome of the child with mild TBI (45,46).

The behavioral profile seen in injured children, which seems nonspecific, includes depression, anxiety, obsessive thoughts, and increased internalizing symptoms (37). Development of social disinhibition and inflexibility may create additional problems in peer relationships. Often in the new situation, injured children feel lonely (47). Behavioral and cognitive impairments form a two-way causal relation.

In terms of post-traumatic psychotic disorders, the prevalence of schizophrenia increased by two- to threefold over a 10- to 20-year period in large groups of subjects with family histories of psychiatric diagnoses (48–50).

Understanding the long-term impact of TBI on cognitive and behavioral functioning requires an assessment of the child's level of functioning, cognitive profile, and the family dynamics, before as well as after the injury.

Cognitively, the main problems are related to loss of skills, failure to make age-appropriate progress, and slower rate of learning.

Mean intelligence quotient scores after TBI are significantly related to both the severity of the injury and the age of the child. Children in younger age groups (2 to 8 years) show more severe deficits in intelligence testing scores, even when the length of coma was relatively short, than did those in older age groups (9 to 18 years). Brain-injured infants show lower scores compared with both school-aged children and adolescents (51–53).

In children who had been comatose for at least 24 hours, IQ scores below 85 were common at least 6 months after injury (54). However, progressive improvement in performance on IQ tests was noted up to 5 years after injury in children with mild to moderate TBI (55).

In regard to memory, the medial temporal lobe structures (hippocampus and hippocampal gyrus), which are responsible for learning new information and stabilizing recently acquired memories, are particularly vulnerable. Thus damage to these structures leads to inability to consolidate temporary engrams into long-term memory storage. Even if correctly perceived, incoming information cannot be stored beyond immediate use unless the hippocampus is intact (56,57). In contrast, long-term memories and engrams, which have been already stored before the injury, can be retrieved without problems.

For this reason, soon after an injury, children appear to have had little damage as they begin to regain skills, draw on their fund of knowledge, and remember details from their prior everyday life, such as their address, telephone number, and friends' names. However, once injured children are expected to acquire new information and make academic progress, problems with memory slowly emerge. Over time, the gap between injured children and their peers increases (58,59).

In comparison with adults with the same residual memory deficit, children are relatively more handicapped because integration of new knowledge into their existing knowledge base is their main daily task. Adults, who have lost the larger quantity of well-stored engrams before injury, are functionally protected and can therefore function better with the same cognitive deficit.

Executive functions include the ability to approach, initiate, plan, and carry out tasks, maintain motivation, monitor performance, inhibit irrelevant actions, use strategies, and retain cognitive flexibility. They are especially sensitive to TBI (60).

Executive functions undergo later maturation (61). Therefore damage to relevant areas of the brain in early childhood may not give rise to major problems until early or late adolescence, when the frontal lobes become fully functional (62,63).

Executive functioning deficits are most likely to be seen in increased levels of emotional lability, impulsivity, rigidity, and perseveration. Impairment in psychosocial adjustment has been extensively documented in children after TBI (64). Adolescents especially have social and executive skill impairments, which are late-developing skills. They report more-labile emotions, less-effective regulation of emotions, and more depressive symptoms—all of which have an impact on adaptive functioning (65–67). In comparison with adults who sustained injury with similar localization, prefrontal lesions in children are more likely to cause maladaptive and antisocial behaviors (68,69). Adults who sustained orbitofrontal and ventromedial frontal lesions before age 2 years have been found to exhibit an increased incidence of disruptive behaviors, failure to follow rules, deficient empathy, and lack of moral reasoning (69).

The relation of attention-deficit hyperactive disorder (ADHD) and TBI is especially interesting. Whereas developmental ADHD affects approximately 6% of children, in groups of children who sustain TBI, its incidence in the preinjury period is 10% to 20%. In addition, as a part of executive dysfunctioning, approximately 20% of children who sustain TBI exhibit the onset of ADHD after their injury. This posttraumatic, novel disorder is called "secondary ADHD" (70,71).

Ubiquitous traumatic axonal injury and focal lesions within the frontal lobes pose a significant risk for disruption in the development of frontally guided "managerial functions."

LANGUAGE

Although classical aphasia syndromes are infrequent in children, language pathology is common after pediatric head trauma. Up to 3 years of age, even if injury is sustained earlier, lexical production and comprehension is delayed. Despite normal scores on the Verbal scale of the Wechsler tests and normal conversational speech, subtle nonaphasic language deficits—word finding, object naming, and difficulties understanding abstractions—may persist. Difficulties vary with age: syntax and grammar are more vulnerable in preschoolers; higher-level language functions are more vulnerable in teenagers (72). Written language is more affected in children than in adolescents with head injury of comparable severity. Perhaps this discrepancy results from older children having learned to read. Such a well-learned skill is less vulnerable than the ability to acquire skills *de novo* (73–75).

The long-term follow-up of children with TBI showed that when the injury is located mainly in the left hemisphere, children exhibit subsequent deficits in tests of both verbal and nonverbal skills relative to neurologically normal children and adult patients with similar injuries.

Because of the diffuse nature of TBI, recovery in this group of children is less complete than recovery in childhood stroke and other focal lesions.

Other cognitive skills, such as visuoconstructive spatial orientation, are usually less severely and less frequently affected (34).

Impairments in *academic achievement* that develop after TBI are a consequence of a variety of mutually interactive cognitive psychological and social factors. In a study of children injured between 5 and 15 years of age, the slopes of growth curves of academic achievement showed significant changes over time (76). Even the most severely injured children who emerge from coma exhibit some recovery. However, the duration of this positive trend is limited and followed by deceleration. In children with mild to moderate injury, the shape of the curve of their improvement is more linear, and the duration of their recovery longer (77). By 2 years after injury, cognitive scores appear to be more impaired if a left hemisphere injury was sustained before the child was 5 years of age (78).

Overall, long-term follow-up studies demonstrate that even 10 years after a severe or moderate TBI, up to 50% of children had not made normal progress in school. Kleinpeter

(79) and Klonoff (80) reported that about a fourth of children younger than 9 years at injury, including those with relatively mild to moderate injuries, had failed a grade or required special educational provisions.

Postacute Treatment

The aim of postacute rehabilitation programs is to facilitate the most efficient coping with life demands. To promote restoration of patient's abilities to the highest level of physical, psychological, and social adaptation, the postacute rehabilitation protocols must meet the following requirements:

1. They must be comprehensive and include collaboration among different health professionals. Successful postacute child rehabilitation programs coordinate pharmacotherapy, social skills training, behavioral management, and cognitive/academic strategies (81–83).
2. They must establish close partnership with families. Work with both the child and family should aim to compensate for residual deficits, understand and treat cognitive and behavioral impairments, identify and acknowledge the role of these impairments in functional disabilities, and enable achievement of optimal social integration (81). The child must learn to cope with a new situation. Families learn to avoid placing excessive demands on their child. It is imperative to clarify expectations for the child.
3. They must take into account interactions among the nature of the TBI, the individual's developmental course, and the type of the response in the community (84).

Comprehensive neuropsychological and psychosocial assessment represents a necessary prerequisite to any meaningful rehabilitation planning. Children with TBI may exhibit problems as a result of primary brain injury (e.g., impulsivity, inattention, hyperactivity) or secondary to hospitalization, family separation, and adjustment to residual disabilities (e.g., anxiety, depression, social isolation). Primary impairment in cognitive functioning may lead to a broader, secondary psychological dysfunction if not addressed appropriately, and emotional status can clearly have an impact on academic functioning. Understanding the contribution of each of these problems in each patient is a prerequisite to any treatment planning (85).

Nonpharmacological treatment methods include environmental modification and behavioral interventions (group therapy, individual counseling, and behavior management). The methods draw heavily on established principles of psychotherapy, behavioral modification, and cognitive rehabilitation. The choice of treatment strategy is based on the patient's developmental level, stage of recovery, and severity and type of symptoms.

In the absence of placebo-controlled, randomized clinical trials of pharmacologic treatment of the behavioral sequelae of TBI in children, pharmacological treatment still heavily relies on findings from trials on adult TBI or learning disability and from individual case reports (86).

The use of typical neuroleptics has been standard in the treatment of agitation and delirium after TBI. Medications that may be helpful for intermittent explosive disorder include stimulants, carbamazepine, risperidone, lithium, amantadine, and bromocriptine. Melatonin has been useful for chronic sleep-onset disturbance that does not respond to behavioral management. In some patients with post-traumatic daytime sleepiness, stimulants have been useful. Preliminary studies suggest that stimulants may be effective in treating post-traumatic ADHD. However, a review of the literature indicates that a smaller proportion of the children with preinjury ADHD were treated with stimulants after the injury compared with a national survey of school-age children with developmental ADHD. In comparison with the 39% of patients with preinjury ADHD who received stimulant medications after TBI, less than 7% of children with secondary ADHD were treated during the 2 years after TBI. Cyproterone acetate, medroprogesterone acetate (antiandrogens), and goserlin, a luteinizing hormone–releasing factor analogue, have been used for problems related to sexual disinhibition.

In general, medications with significant sedative, antidopaminergic, and anticholinergic properties should be avoided or used sparingly. Children with TBI may be particularly susceptible to adverse effects of psychopharmacologic medications. Sedating medications can interfere with their overall cognitive recovery and may provoke paradoxical hyperactivity.

Any medication program should be accompanied by intensive counseling to help children overcome their emotional issues and move ahead in their rehabilitation program.

Despite significant advances in the understanding of pediatric TBI sequelae, the postacute rehabilitation continues to lag. The importance of the "latent and silent" deficits remains underestimated in the medical community. Di Scala et al. (87) followed up 24,021 children and adolescents hospitalized for TBI and reported that 27% of their sample had evidence of functional impairment on discharge. However, 75% of these children were discharged home with no active rehabilitation program, and only 1.8% were referred for educational assistance.

Recovery and brain reorganization after pediatric brain injury involve complex interactions between endogenous factors (injury location and age at injury) and exogenous ones (environmental influences that include a variety of therapeutic strategies). Early injury may have a cumulative effect on ongoing development. Additional deficits may emerge through childhood as more functions are expected to mature (88). Fortunately, the immature brain has a robust ability to benefit from environmental stimulation throughout development. Therefore postinjury rehabilitation should be intensive, comprehensive, and open-ended.

Summary

The burden of deficits caused by pediatric TBI is great. Its survival rates have increased significantly because of increasingly effective emergency care and specialized treatment facilities (89).

Problems with cognitive, behavioral, and emotional functioning can be debilitating. They are "invisible disabilities" that affect interpersonal relationships, education, and employment (90).

The traditional view that children are relatively resistant to brain injury has clearly been overstated. Evidence exists that younger children may have even more severe and long-lasting cognitive sequelae from diffuse injury in comparison with older children and adults. Rapidly developing skills seem to be more adversely affected than already consolidated skills. Consequences may be subtle and delayed.

Residual cognitive, behavioral, and emotional problems are predominately influenced by both "injury variables" and "child variables." The important injury variables are its cause and severity. The important child variables are the premorbid functioning, age, and developmental level of the child both at injury and at assessment.

Comprehensive rehabilitation programs should integrate the compensatory approaches of neuropsychological, occupational, speech, physical therapy, psychiatry, social work, and neurology to address the array of difficulties experienced by the children with TBI (91).

Questions

1. Which brain structures are especially vulnerable to the effects of TBI?
   A. The corpus callosum and deep white matter
   B. Temporal lobes
   C. Frontal lobes
   D. All of the above

2. Which of the following statements is incorrect?
   A. In groups of children who sustain TBI, the incidence of ADHD in the preinjury period is 10% to 20%.
   B. In groups of children who sustain TBI, the incidence of ADHD in the preinjury period is the same as that in the general population.
   C. The incidence of ADHD is higher in children with mild TBI than in the more severely injured groups.
   D. The post-traumatic novel disorder called "secondary ADHD" develops in 20% of children who sustain TBI.

3. What is the role of antiepileptic medications in the treatment of the brain-injured child?
   A. All patients should be aggressively treated to prevent the occurrence of seizures.
   B. Treatment should be initiated in patients as soon as seizures occur and maintained until the patient has 2 seizure-free years.
   C. Prophylactic use of antiepileptic drugs does not prevent post-traumatic epilepsy.

4. When should a teenager who has sustained a concussion without LOC but with confusion lasting about 30 minutes be permitted to return to sports?
   A. When the child has remained symptom free for 2 weeks, regardless of the imaging findings.
   B. Not during the same season if imaging shows any abnormality.
   C. At 4 to 6 weeks after the injury, if the child reports no subjective symptoms and the neurological examination is normal.
   D. When the parent reports that the child has fully returned to his baseline and has no post-concussion symptoms.

5. Posttraumatic psychiatric morbidity is significantly related to:
   A. The preinjury socioeconomic status
   B. Family functioning
   C. Presence of the residual cognitive impairment
   D. Severity of injury
   E. All of the above

Answers

1. A
2. B
3. C
4. B
5. E

REFERENCES

1. Ylvisaker M, ed. *Head injury rehabilitation: children and adolescents.* Boston: College Hill Press, 1985:xv.
2. Langlois J, Rutland-Brown W, Thomas K. *Traumatic brain injury in the United States: emergency department visits, hospitalizations, and deaths.* Atlanta: Centers for Disease Control and Prevention, National Center for Injury Prevention and Control, 2004.
3. Bishop NB. Traumatic brain injury: a primer for primary care physicians. *Curr Probl Pediatr Adolesc Health Care.* 2006;36:318–331.
4. Keenan HT, Bratton SL. Epidemiology and outcomes of pediatric traumatic brain injury. *Dev Neurosci.* 2006;28:256–263.
5. Denny-Brown DE, Russell WR. Experimental cerebral concussion. *Brain.* 1941;64:93–164.

6. Pang D. Pathophysiological correlates of neurobehavioral syndromes following closed head injury. In: Ylvisaker M, ed. *Head injury rehabilitation: children and adolescents.* Boston: College Hill Press, 1985:3–70.
7. Strich SJ. Shearing of nerve fibers as a cause of brain damage due to head injury. *Lancet.* 1961;2:443–448.
8. Strich SJ. The pathology of brain damage due to blunt injury. In: Walker AE, Caveness WF, Critchley M, eds. *The late effects of head injury.* Springfield, IL: Charles C Thomas, 1969: 501–524.
9. Jellinger K, Setelberger F. Protracted posttraumatic encephalopathy-pathology, pathogenesis and clinical implications. *J Neurol Sci.* 1970;10: 51–94.
10. Ashwal S, Holshouser BA, Shu SK, et al. Predictive value of proton magnetic resonance spectroscopy in pediatric closed head injury. *Pediatr Neurol.* 2000;23:114–125.
11. Holshouser BA, Ashwal S, Shu S, et al. Proton MR spectroscopy in children with acute brain injury: comparison of short and long echo time acquisitions. *J Magn Reson Imaging.* 2000;11: 9–19.
12. Stiles J. Neural plasticity and cognitive development. *Dev Neuropsychol.* 2000;18:237–272.
13. Crovitz HF. Techniques to investigate posttraumatic and retrograde amnesia after head injury. In: Levin HS, Grafman J, Eisenberg HM, eds. *Neurobehavioral recovery from brain injury.* New York: Oxford University Press, 1987:330–340.
14. Corkin HS, Hurt RW, Twitchell TE, et al. Consequences of nonpenetrating and penetrating head injury: retrograde amnesia, posttraumatic amnesia and lasting effects on cognition. In: Levin HS, Grafman J, Eisenberg HM, eds. *Neurobehavioral recovery from brain injury.* New York: Oxford University Press, 1987:318–329.
15. Levin HS, Hanten G. Executive functions after traumatic brain injury in children. *Pediatr Neurol.* 2005;33:79–93.
16. Gualtieri T, Cox DR. The delayed neurobehavioral sequelae of traumatic brain injury. *Brain Inj.* 1991;5:219–232.
17. Goldman PS. Functional recovery after lesions of the nervous system, 3: developmental processes in neural plasticity: recovery of function after CNS lesions in infant monkeys. *Neurosci Res Progr Bull.* 1974;12:217–222.
18. De Bellis MD, Keshavan MS, Clark DB, et al. Developmental traumatology, part II: brain development. *Biol Psychiatry.* 1999;45:1271–1284.
19. Teasdale G, Jennett B. Assessment of coma and impaired consciousness: a practical scale. *Lancet.* 1974; 2:81–84.
20. Reilly PL, Simpson DA, Sprod R, et al. Assessing the conscious level in infants and young children: a pediatric version of the Glasgow Coma Scale. *Childs Nerv Syst.* 1988;4:30–33.

21. Lieh-Lai MW, Theodorou AA, Sarnaik AP, et al. Limitations of the Glasgow Coma Scale in predicting outcome in children with traumatic brain injury. *J Pediatr.* 1992;120:195–199.
22. Michaud LJ, Rivara FP, Grady MS, et al. Predictors of survival and severity of disability after severe brain injury in children. *Neurosurgery.* 1992;31:254–264.
23. Max JE, Lansing AE, Koele SL, et al. Attention deficit hyperactivity disorder in children and adolescents following traumatic brain injury. *Dev Neuropsychol.* 2004;25:159–177.
24. Ropper AH, Gorson KC. Concussion. *N Engl J Med.* 2007;356:166–172.
25. Finger S. Margaret Kennard and her "principle" in historical perspective. In: Finger S, et al. *Brain injury: theoretical and controversial issues.* New York: Plenum Press, 1988:117–132.
26. Kennard MA. Reorganization of motor function in the cerebral cortex of monkeys deprived of motor and premotor areas in infancy. *J Neurophysiol.* 1938;1:477–496.
27. Teuber HL. Recovery of function after brain injury in man. In: *Outcome of severe damage to the central nervous system: Ciba foundation symposium. 34.* Amsterdam: Elsevier, 1975:159–186.
28. Levin HS, Aldrich EF, Saydjari C, et al. Severe head injury in children: experience of the Traumatic Coma Data Bank. *Neurosurgery.* 1992;31: 435–443.
29. Kochanek PM. Pediatric traumatic brain injury: quo vadis? *Dev Neurosci.* 2006;28:244–255.
30. Wilson BA, Vizor A, Bryant T. Predicting severity of cognitive impairment after severe head injury. *Brain Inj.* 1991;5:189–197.
31. Kolb B, Wishaw IQ. Brain plasticity and behavior. *Annu Rev Psychol.* 1998;49:43–64.
32. Kolb B, Gibb R. Early brain injury, plasticity and behavior. In: Nelson CA, Luciana M, eds. *Handbook of developmental cognitive neuroscience.* London: Bradford, 2001:175–190.
33. Wilson BA. Recovery of cognitive functions following nonprogressive brain Injury *Curr Opin Neurobiol.* 1998;8:281–287.
34. Middleton JA. Practitioner review: psychological sequelae of head injury in children and adolescents. *J Child Psychol Psychiatry.* 2001;42: 165–180.
35. Arsanow RF, Satz P, Light R. Behavioral problems and adaptive functioning in children with mild and severe closed head injury. *J Pediatr Psychol.* 1991;16:543–557.
36. Statler KD. Pediatric posttraumatic seizures: epidemiology, putative mechanisms of epileptogeneis. *Dev Neurosci.* 2006;28:354–363.
37. Di Gallo A, Barton J, Parry-Jones WL. Road traffic accidents: early psychological consequences in children and adolescents. *Br J Psychiatry.* 1997; 170:358–362.
38. Max JE, Castillo CS, Robin DA, et al. Posttraumatic stress symptomatology after childhood

38. ...traumatic brain injury. *J Nerv Ment Dis.* 1998;186: 589–596.
39. Max JE, Koele S L, Smith WL, et al. Psychiatric disorders in children and adolescents after severe traumatic brain injury: a controlled study. *J Am Acad Child Adolesc Psychiatry.* 1998;37:832–840.
40. Rivara JB, Jaffe KM, Polissar NL, et al. Family functioning and children's academic performance and behavior problems in the year following traumatic brain injury. *Arch Phys Med Rehabil.* 1994;75:369–379.
41. Rutter M, Chadwick O, Shaffer S, et al. A prospective study of children with head injuries, 1: design and methods. *Psychol Med.* 1980;10: 633–645.
42. Yeates KO, Taylor HG, Drotar D, et al. Preinjury family environment as a determinant of recovery from traumatic brain injuries in school-age children. *J Int Neuropsychol Soc.* 1997;3:617–630.
43. Fletcher JM, Ewing-Cobbs L, Francis DJ, et al. Variability in outcomes after traumatic brain injury in children: a developmental perspective. In: Broman SH, Michel ME, eds. *Traumatic brain injury in children.* Oxford: Oxford University Press,1995:3–21.
44. Levin HS, Ewing-Cobbs L, Eisenberg HM. Neurobehavioral outcome of pediatric closed head injury. In: Broman SH, Michel ME, eds. *Traumatic brain injury in children.* Oxford: Oxford University Press, 1995:70–94.
45. Dunbar G, Lewis Hill R. Control processing and road-crossing skills. *Psychologist.* 1999:12: 398–399.
46. West R, Train H, Junger M, et al. Accidents and problem behavior. *Psychologist.* 1999;12:395–397.
47. Warschausky S, Cohen EH, Parker JG, et al. Social problem-solving skills of children with traumatic brain injury. *Pediatr Rehabil.* 1997;1:77–81.
48. Malaspina D, Goetz R, Friedman JH, et al. Traumatic brain injury and schizophrenia in members of schizophrenia and bipolar disorder pedigrees. *Am J Psychiatry.* 2001;158:440–446.
49. Violon A. Post-traumatic psychoses. *Acta Neurochir Suppl.* (Wien) 1988;44:67–69.
50. Davison K, Bagley CR. Schizophrenia-like psychoses associated with organic disorders of the central nervous system. In: Herrington RN, ed. *Current problems in neuropsychiatry.* Ashford, Kent, England: 1969:113–184.
51. Brown G, Chadwick OFD, Shaffer D, et al. A prospective study of children with head injuries in adulthood, III: psychiatric sequelae. *Psychol Med.* 1981;11:63–78.
52. Chadwick O. Psychological sequelae in head injury in children. *Dev Med Child Neurol.* 1985;27: 72–75.
53. Taylor HG, Yeates KO, Wade SL, et al. A prospective study of short-and long-term outcomes after traumatic brain injury in children behavior and achievement. *Neuropsychology.* 2002;16:15–27.
54. Levin H S, Ewing-Cobbs L, Eisenberg HM. Neurobehavioral outcome of pediatric closed head injury. In: Broman SH, Michel ME, eds. *Traumatic brain injury in children.* Oxford: Oxford University Press, 1995:70–94.
55. Brink JD, Garrett AL, Hale WR, et al. Recovery of motor and intellectual function in children sustaining severe head injuries. *Dev Med Child Neurol.* 1970;12:565–571.
56. Levin HS, Eisenberg HM. Neuropsychological impairment after closed head injury in children and adolescents. *J Pediatr Psychol.* 1979;4: 389–402.
57. Ewing-Cobbs L, Fletcher JM, Levin HS. Neuropsychological sequelae following pediatric head injury: memory functions. In: Ylvisaker M, ed. *Head injury rehabilitation: children and adolescents.* Boston: College Hill Press, 1985:77.
58. Tasker RC. Changes in white matter late after severe traumatic brain injury in childhood. *Dev Neurosci.* 2006;28:302–308.
59. Craig GN, Campbell S, Kuehn M, et al. Medical and cognitive outcome in children with traumatic brain injury *Can J Neurol Sci.* 2004;31: 213–219.
60. Fletcher JM, Ewing-Cobbs L, Miner ME, et al. Behavioral changes after closed head injury in children. *J Consult Clin Psychol.* 1990;58:93–98.
61. Luciana M, Nelson CA. The functional emergence of prefrontally guided working memory systems in four- to eight-year-old children. *Neuropsychologia.* 1998;36:273–293.
62. Goldman PS. Functional recovery after lesions of the nervous system: developmental processes in neural plasticity: recovery of function after CNS lesions in infant monkeys. *Neurosci Res Progr Bull.* 1974;12:217–222.
63. Diamond A. Normal development of prefrontal cortex from birth to young adulthood: cognitive functions, anatomy, and biochemistry. In: Stuss DT, Knight RT, eds. *Principles of frontal lobe function.* London: Oxford University Press, 2002: 466–503.
64. Ewing-Cobbs L, Prasad MR, Landry SH, et al. Executive functions following traumatic brain injury in young children: a preliminary analysis. *Dev Neuropsychol.* 2004;26:487–512.
65. Silk JS, Steinberg L, Morris AM. Adolescents' emotion regulation in daily life: links to depressive symptoms and problem behavior. *Child Dev.* 2003;74:1869–1880.
66. Eisenberg N, Fabes RA, Murphy B, et al. The role of emotionality and regulation in children's social functioning: a longitudinal study. *Child Dev.* 1995;66:1360–1384.
67. Eisenberg N, Guthrie IK, Fabes RA, et al. Prediction of elementary school children's externalizing problem behaviors from attentional and behavioral regulation and negative emotionality. *Child Dev.* 2000;71:1367–1382.

6. Pang D. Pathophysiological correlates of neurobehavioral syndromes following closed head injury. In: Ylvisaker M, ed. *Head injury rehabilitation: children and adolescents*. Boston: College Hill Press, 1985:3–70.
7. Strich SJ. Shearing of nerve fibers as a cause of brain damage due to head injury. *Lancet.* 1961;2:443–448.
8. Strich SJ. The pathology of brain damage due to blunt injury. In: Walker AE, Caveness WF, Critchley M, eds. *The late effects of head injury.* Springfield, IL: Charles C Thomas, 1969: 501–524.
9. Jellinger K, Setelberger F. Protracted posttraumatic encephalopathy-pathology, pathogenesis and clinical implications. *J Neurol Sci.* 1970;10: 51–94.
10. Ashwal S, Holshouser BA, Shu SK, et al. Predictive value of proton magnetic resonance spectroscopy in pediatric closed head injury. *Pediatr Neurol.* 2000;23:114–125.
11. Holshouser BA, Ashwal S, Shu S, et al. Proton MR spectroscopy in children with acute brain injury: comparison of short and long echo time acquisitions. *J Magn Reson Imaging.* 2000;11: 9–19.
12. Stiles J. Neural plasticity and cognitive development. *Dev Neuropsychol.* 2000;18:237–272.
13. Crovitz HF. Techniques to investigate posttraumatic and retrograde amnesia after head injury. In: Levin HS, Grafman J, Eisenberg HM, eds. *Neurobehavioral recovery from brain injury.* New York: Oxford University Press, 1987:330–340.
14. Corkin HS, Hurt RW, Twitchell TE, et al. Consequences of nonpenetrating and penetrating head injury: retrograde amnesia, posttraumatic amnesia and lasting effects on cognition. In: Levin HS, Grafman J, Eisenberg HM, eds. *Neurobehavioral recovery from brain injury.* New York: Oxford University Press, 1987:318–329.
15. Levin HS, Hanten G. Executive functions after traumatic brain injury in children. *Pediatr Neurol.* 2005;33:79–93.
16. Gualtieri T, Cox DR. The delayed neurobehavioral sequelae of traumatic brain injury. *Brain Inj.* 1991;5:219–232.
17. Goldman PS. Functional recovery after lesions of the nervous system, 3: developmental processes in neural plasticity: recovery of function after CNS lesions in infant monkeys. *Neurosci Res Progr Bull.* 1974;12:217–222.
18. De Bellis MD, Keshavan MS, Clark DB, et al. Developmental traumatology, part II: brain development. *Biol Psychiatry.* 1999;45:1271–1284.
19. Teasdale G, Jennett B. Assessment of coma and impaired consciousness: a practical scale. *Lancet.* 1974; 2:81–84.
20. Reilly PL, Simpson DA, Sprod R, et al. Assessing the conscious level in infants and young children: a pediatric version of the Glasgow Coma Scale. *Childs Nerv Syst.* 1988;4:30–33.
21. Lieh-Lai MW, Theodorou AA, Sarnaik AP, et al. Limitations of the Glasgow Coma Scale in predicting outcome in children with traumatic brain injury. *J Pediatr.* 1992;120:195–199.
22. Michaud LJ, Rivara FP, Grady MS, et al. Predictors of survival and severity of disability after severe brain injury in children. *Neurosurgery.* 1992;31:254–264.
23. Max JE, Lansing AE, Koele SL, et al. Attention deficit hyperactivity disorder in children and adolescents following traumatic brain injury. *Dev Neuropsychol.* 2004;25:159–177.
24. Ropper AH, Gorson KC. Concussion. *N Engl J Med.* 2007;356:166–172.
25. Finger S. Margaret Kennard and her "principle" in historical perspective. In: Finger S, et al. *Brain injury: theoretical and controversial issues.* New York: Plenum Press, 1988:117–132.
26. Kennard MA. Reorganization of motor function in the cerebral cortex of monkeys deprived of motor and premotor areas in infancy. *J Neurophysiol.* 1938;1:477–496.
27. Teuber HL. Recovery of function after brain injury in man. In: *Outcome of severe damage to the central nervous system: Ciba foundation symposium. 34.* Amsterdam: Elsevier, 1975:159–186.
28. Levin HS, Aldrich EF, Saydjari C, et al. Severe head injury in children: experience of the Traumatic Coma Data Bank. *Neurosurgery.* 1992;31: 435–443.
29. Kochanek PM. Pediatric traumatic brain injury: quo vadis? *Dev Neurosci.* 2006;28:244–255.
30. Wilson BA, Vizor A, Bryant T. Predicting severity of cognitive impairment after severe head injury. *Brain Inj.* 1991;5:189–197.
31. Kolb B, Wishaw IQ. Brain plasticity and behavior. *Annu Rev Psychol.* 1998;49:43–64.
32. Kolb B, Gibb R. Early brain injury, plasticity and behavior. In: Nelson CA, Luciana M, eds. *Handbook of developmental cognitive neuroscience.* London: Bradford, 2001:175–190.
33. Wilson BA. Recovery of cognitive functions following nonprogressive brain Injury *Curr Opin Neurobiol.* 1998;8:281–287.
34. Middleton JA. Practitioner review: psychological sequelae of head injury in children and adolescents. *J Child Psychol Psychiatry.* 2001;42: 165–180.
35. Arsanow RF, Satz P, Light R. Behavioral problems and adaptive functioning in children with mild and severe closed head injury. *J Pediatr Psychol.* 1991;16:543–557.
36. Statler KD. Pediatric posttraumatic seizures: epidemiology, putative mechanisms of epileptogeneis. *Dev Neurosci.* 2006;28:354–363.
37. Di Gallo A, Barton J, Parry-Jones WL. Road traffic accidents: early psychological consequences in children and adolescents. *Br J Psychiatry.* 1997; 170:358–362.
38. Max JE, Castillo CS, Robin DA, et al. Posttraumatic stress symptomatology after childhood

traumatic brain injury. *J Nerv Ment Dis.* 1998;186: 589–596.
39. Max JE, Koele S L, Smith WL, et al. Psychiatric disorders in children and adolescents after severe traumatic brain injury: a controlled study. *J Am Acad Child Adolesc Psychiatry.* 1998;37:832–840.
40. Rivara JB, Jaffe KM, Polissar NL, et al. Family functioning and children's academic performance and behavior problems in the year following traumatic brain injury. *Arch Phys Med Rehabil.* 1994;75:369–379.
41. Rutter M, Chadwick O, Shaffer S, et al. A prospective study of children with head injuries, 1: design and methods. *Psychol Med.* 1980;10: 633–645.
42. Yeates KO, Taylor HG, Drotar D, et al. Preinjury family environment as a determinant of recovery from traumatic brain injuries in school-age children. *J Int Neuropsychol Soc.* 1997;3:617–630.
43. Fletcher JM, Ewing-Cobbs L, Francis DJ, et al. Variability in outcomes after traumatic brain injury in children: a developmental perspective. In: Broman SH, Michel ME, eds. *Traumatic brain injury in children.* Oxford: Oxford University Press,1995:3–21.
44. Levin HS, Ewing-Cobbs L, Eisenberg HM. Neurobehavioral outcome of pediatric closed head injury. In: Broman SH, Michel ME, eds. *Traumatic brain injury in children.* Oxford: Oxford University Press, 1995:70–94.
45. Dunbar G, Lewis Hill R. Control processing and road-crossing skills. *Psychologist.* 1999:12: 398–399.
46. West R, Train H, Junger M, et al. Accidents and problem behavior. *Psychologist.* 1999;12:395–397.
47. Warschausky S, Cohen EH, Parker JG, et al. Social problem-solving skills of children with traumatic brain injury. *Pediatr Rehabil.* 1997;1:77–81.
48. Malaspina D, Goetz R, Friedman JH, et al. Traumatic brain injury and schizophrenia in members of schizophrenia and bipolar disorder pedigrees. *Am J Psychiatry.* 2001;158:440–446.
49. Violon A. Post-traumatic psychoses. *Acta Neurochir Suppl.* (Wien) 1988;44:67–69.
50. Davison K, Bagley CR. Schizophrenia-like psychoses associated with organic disorders of the central nervous system. In: Herrington RN, ed. *Current problems in neuropsychiatry.* Ashford, Kent, England: 1969:113–184.
51. Brown G, Chadwick OFD, Shaffer D, et al. A prospective study of children with head injuries in adulthood, III: psychiatric sequelae. *Psychol Med.* 1981;11:63–78.
52. Chadwick O. Psychological sequelae in head injury in children. *Dev Med Child Neurol.* 1985;27: 72–75.
53. Taylor HG, Yeates KO, Wade SL, et al. A prospective study of short-and long-term outcomes after traumatic brain injury in children behavior and achievement. *Neuropsychology.* 2002;16:15–27.
54. Levin H S, Ewing-Cobbs L, Eisenberg HM. Neurobehavioral outcome of pediatric closed head injury. In: Broman SH, Michel ME, eds. *Traumatic brain injury in children.* Oxford: Oxford University Press, 1995:70–94.
55. Brink JD, Garrett AL, Hale WR, et al. Recovery of motor and intellectual function in children sustaining severe head injuries. *Dev Med Child Neurol.* 1970;12:565–571.
56. Levin HS, Eisenberg HM. Neuropsychological impairment after closed head injury in children and adolescents. *J Pediatr Psychol.* 1979;4: 389–402.
57. Ewing-Cobbs L, Fletcher JM, Levin HS. Neuropsychological sequelae following pediatric head injury: memory functions. In: Ylvisaker M, ed. *Head injury rehabilitation: children and adolescents.* Boston: College Hill Press, 1985:77.
58. Tasker RC. Changes in white matter late after severe traumatic brain injury in childhood. *Dev Neurosci.* 2006;28:302–308.
59. Craig GN, Campbell S, Kuehn M, et al. Medical and cognitive outcome in children with traumatic brain injury *Can J Neurol Sci.* 2004;31: 213–219.
60. Fletcher JM, Ewing-Cobbs L, Miner ME, et al. Behavioral changes after closed head injury in children. *J Consult Clin Psychol.* 1990;58:93–98.
61. Luciana M, Nelson CA. The functional emergence of prefrontally guided working memory systems in four- to eight-year-old children. *Neuropsychologia.* 1998;36:273–293.
62. Goldman PS. Functional recovery after lesions of the nervous system: developmental processes in neural plasticity: recovery of function after CNS lesions in infant monkeys. *Neurosci Res Progr Bull.* 1974;12:217–222.
63. Diamond A. Normal development of prefrontal cortex from birth to young adulthood: cognitive functions, anatomy, and biochemistry. In: Stuss DT, Knight RT, eds. *Principles of frontal lobe function.* London: Oxford University Press, 2002: 466–503.
64. Ewing-Cobbs L, Prasad MR, Landry SH, et al. Executive functions following traumatic brain injury in young children: a preliminary analysis. *Dev Neuropsychol.* 2004;26:487–512.
65. Silk JS, Steinberg L, Morris AM. Adolescents' emotion regulation in daily life: links to depressive symptoms and problem behavior. *Child Dev.* 2003;74:1869–1880.
66. Eisenberg N, Fabes RA, Murphy B, et al. The role of emotionality and regulation in children's social functioning: a longitudinal study. *Child Dev.* 1995;66:1360–1384.
67. Eisenberg N, Guthrie IK, Fabes RA, et al. Prediction of elementary school children's externalizing problem behaviors from attentional and behavioral regulation and negative emotionality. *Child Dev.* 2000;71:1367–1382.

68. Price BH, Daffner KR, Stowe RM, et al. The compartmental learning disabilities of early frontal lobe damage. *Brain.* 1990;113:1383–1393.
69. Anderson SW, Bechara A, Damasio H, et al. Impairment of social and moral behavior related to early damage in human prefrontal cortex. *Nat Neurosci.* 1999;2:1032–1037.
70. Gerring JP, Brady KD, Chen A, et al. Premorbid prevalence of ADHD and development of secondary ADHD after closed head injury. *J Am Acad Child Adolesc Psychiatry.* 1998;37:647–654.
71. Schachar R, Levin HS, JE HS, et al. Attention deficit hyperactivity disorder symptoms and response inhibition after closed head injury in children: do preinjury behavior and injury severity predict outcome? *Dev Neuropsychol.* 2004;25:179–198.
72. Lees J. Recovery of speech and language deficits after head injury in children. In: Johnson DA, Uttley D, Wyke MA, eds. *Children's head injury: who cares?* Brighton, England: Falmer Press, 1989: 80–95.
73. Ewing-Cobbs L, Barnes M. Linguistic outcomes following traumatic brain injury in children. *Semin Pediatr Neurol.* 2002;9:209–217.
74. Ewing-Cobbs L, Levin HS, Eisenberg F, et al. Language functions following closed-head injury in children and adolescents. *J Clin Exp Neuropsychol.* 1897;9:575–592.
75. Chapman SB, Culhane KA, Levin HS, et al. Narrative discourse after closed head injury in children and adolescents. *Brain Lang.* 1992;43:42–65.
76. Ewing-Cobbs L, Barnes M, Fletcher JM, et al. Modeling of longitudinal academic achievement scores after pediatric traumatic brain injury. *Dev Neuropsychol.* 2004;25:107–133.
77. Taylor HG, Yeates KO, Wade SL, et al. A prospective study of short- and long-term outcomes after traumatic brain injury in children: behavior and achievement. *Neuropsychology.* 2002;16:15–27.
78. Ewing-Cobbs L, Fletcher JM, Levin H. Neuropsychological sequelae following pediatric head injury: academic sequelae. In: Ylvisaker M, ed. *Head injury rehabilitation: children and adolescents.* Boston: College Hill Press, 1985:75–76.
79. Kleinpeter U. Social integration after brain trauma in childhood. *Acta Paedopsychiatric.* 1975;32:68–75.
80. Klonoff H, Low MD, Clark C. Head injuries in children: a prospective five year follow-up. *J Neurol Neurosurg Psychiatry.* 1977;40:1211–1219.
81. Limond J, Leeke R. Practitioner review: cognitive rehabilitation for children with acquired brain injury. *J Child Psychol Psychiatry.* 2005;46:339–352.
82. Teeter PA. Neurocognitive interventions for childhood and adolescent disorders: a transactional model. In: Reynolds CR, Fletcher-Janzen E, eds. *Handbook of clinical child neuropsychology.* London: Plenum Press, 1997.
83. Ylvisaker M. *Traumatic brain injury rehabilitation: children and adolescents.* Boston: Butterworth-Heinemann, 1998.
84. Luiselli JK, Gardner R, Arons M, et al. Comprehensive community-based education and neurorehabilitation for children and adolescents with traumatic brain injury. *Behav Intervent.* 1998;13:181–200.
85. Anderson V, Catroppa C. Advances in postacute rehabilitation after childhood-acquired brain injury: a focus on cognitive, behavioral, and social domains. *J Phys Med Rehabil.* 2006;85:767–778.
86. Bjorklund DF, Miller PH, Coyle TR, et al. Instructing children to use memory strategies: evidence of utilization deficiencies in practitioner review: cognitive rehabilitation for children with acquired brain injury-memory training studies. *Dev Rev.* 1997;7:411–441.
87. Perrott SB, Taylor HG, Montes JL. Neuropsychological sequelae, familial stress, and environmental adaptation following pediatric head injury. *Dev Neuropsychol.* 1991;7:69–86.
88. Bates G. Medication in the treatment of the behavioral sequelae of traumatic brain injury. *Dev Med Child Neurol.* 2006;48:697–701.
89. Di Scala C, Osberg RC. Children hospitalized for traumatic brain injury: transition to post-acute care. *J Head Trauma Rehabil.* 1997;12:1–10.
90. Giza CC, Prins ML. Is being plastic fantastic? Mechanism of altered plasticity after developmental traumatic brain injury. *Dev Neurosci.* 2006;28:364–379.
91. Chamberlain MA. Head injury: the challenge: principles and practice of service organization. In: Chamberlain MA, Neumann V, Tennant A, eds. *Traumatic brain injury rehabilitation.* London: Chapman & Hall Medical, 1995.

Neuropsychiatric Aspects of Pediatric HIV Infection

MARYLAND PAO AND LUCY ANN CIVITELLO

Introduction

Since the first descriptions of pediatric AIDS in the 1980s, neurodevelopmental abnormalities have been a well-known complication of human immunodeficiency virus (HIV) infection in children, causing significant morbidity and mortality (1–3). Over the last several years, significant progress has been made in the early diagnosis of HIV-infected infants and children. Treatment is being initiated earlier, with multiple drug regimens according to Centers for Disease Control (CDC) guidelines. For example, all infants younger than 12 months with documented HIV infection are being started on multidrug regimens (4). Additionally, progress has been made in the treatment of HIV infection, including the use of highly active antiretroviral therapy (HAART). As a result, infants, children, and adolescents with HIV infection are living longer, and the prevalence and natural history of neurological illnesses in these patients have changed and, in many cases, improved.

The central nervous system (CNS) manifestations of HIV infection can be subdivided into two main groups: (a) those directly attributable to HIV brain infection, and (b) those indirectly related to the effects of HIV disease on the brain, such as CNS opportunistic infections (OIs), malignancies, and cerebrovascular disease.

Peripheral nervous system (PNS) abnormalities occur relatively frequently in adult HIV-infected patients and are usually related to antiretroviral therapy, HIV disease, or OIs (5–8). Although much less common in infants and children, neuropathies and myopathies do occur, with similar etiologies (9,10).

Primary HIV-Related CNS Disease

HIV-related CNS disease is a prominent feature in pediatric patients. Early in the epidemic, it was recognized that the frequent neurological abnormalities seen in these children were due to the direct effects of HIV infection on the brain and not due to OIs or malignancies (1–3). HIV was isolated from the brain and cerebrospinal fluid (CSF) in 1985 (11). Soon after, HIV antigens were detected in the brain; viral particles were visualized in brain macrophages by electron microscopy; HIV nucleic acids were detected in brain tissue by *in situ* hybridization; and intrathecal anti-HIV antibodies were observed (12–15).

Epidemiology

The prevalence of HIV-related CNS disease in children was estimated at 50% to 90% in early studies (16–18). By the mid-1990s, the prevalence was estimated to be between 20% and 50% (19–22). Since the advent of HAART, a decrease in the prevalence of CNS disease has been documented in adults in the Multicenter AIDS Cohort Study (23). In another study, the incidence of moderate or severe dementia in adults was noted to decrease from 7% in 1989 to 1% in 2000. Changes in the type of dementia in adults have also occurred; most patients with dementia now have a more-static form (24). The prevalence of encephalopathy has also decreased in children, from 40.7% in children born before 1996 to 18.2% in children born after 1996, as documented in a retrospective study of 146 vertically infected children followed up at one institution. In this study, the prevalence of progressive encephalopathy decreased from 29.6% in children born before 1996 compared with 12.1% in those born after 1996 (25). In New York, Chiriboga et al. (26) also documented a decrease in the rate of progressive encephalopathy from 31% in 1992 to 1.6% in 2000.

In general, children younger than 3 years have higher rates of CNS disease than do older children and adolescents (19–21), and patients with more advanced degrees of immune suppression have higher rates of encephalopathy (27), a trend that remains true in the post-HAART era. Of 62 children first seen with HIV infection before the age of 3 years in London, 22% had abnormal neurological signs, and 40% had significant developmental delays. Children with more-severe immune dysfunction had more neurological abnormalities and developmental delays (28).

It also is important to note that HIV-related CNS disease may be the presenting manifestation of HIV infection in as many as 18% of pediatric patients (29). This is an unusual occurrence in adults.

Early onset of HIV infection (i.e., infection occurring *in utero*) increases a child's risk for poor neurodevelopmental outcome within the first 30 months of life (30). Early onset of neurological symptoms and signs in HIV-infected infants (before the age of 1 year) seems to have a different significance and pathophysiology than those occurring later on in children and adults (31). When pediatric patients from the French Perinatal Cohort were compared with the French SEROCO Cohort of adults, the cumulative incidence of encephalopathy was higher in children than in adults only during the first year after infection (9.9% vs. 0.3%) and during the second year (4.2% vs. 0), but was similar afterward (less than 1% per year in each group). The cumulative incidence at 7 years reached 16% in children and 5% in adults. The early encephalopathy was not prevented by zidovudine (ZDV) use during pregnancy. In addition, the infants who went on to develop early CNS symptoms had significantly smaller head sizes and weights at birth than did their counterparts without neurological symptoms. These findings suggest a prenatal onset of HIV brain infection in this subgroup of infants with early onset of neurological disease. It also suggests that the course and pathophysiology of CNS disease in older children and adolescents is more similar to the dementia and motor cognitive dysfunction seen in adults, which may have important therapeutic and preventive implications.

Clinical Manifestations

The well-described classic triad of HIV-related encephalopathy identified in the mid-1980s and early 1990s included developmental delays (particularly motor and expressive language), acquired microcephaly, and pyramidal tract motor deficits (1–3). In the past, pediatric patients were classified with either the presence or absence of encephalopathy.

However, it is evident that a broad spectrum of clinical manifestations and severity of CNS disease exists in infants and children. This has become increasingly obvious with the decreased prevalence of severe encephalopathy in the HAART era. These observations have led to the development of a new classification system for pediatric HIV-related CNS disease that is currently used at the National Cancer Institute (NCI) of the National Institutes of Health (NIH). This system is used to track the CNS status of children on different treatment protocols and natural history studies. Patients are classified as having encephalopathy, as having CNS compromise, or as not apparently being affected.

Patients with encephalopathy have more severe and pervasive CNS dysfunction that affects their day-to-day functioning than do patients without encephalopathy (Table 14.1). Encephalopathy can be either progressive (subtypes include plateau and the more severe subacute) or static.

The subacute progressive type is often seen in infants and young children who are naive to antiretroviral therapy (1–3,16,17,32,33). The hallmarks of this disorder are loss of previously acquired milestones, particularly motor and expressive language, with progressive nonfocal motor dysfunction (spastic quadriplegia or hypotonia in young infants and spastic diplegia or hypotonia in older infants and children) (33). The course is usually slower, developing over weeks to months, and more insidious than the course observed with OIs, tumor, or stroke. Children with HIV encephalopathy may have prominent oromotor dysfunction, facial diparesis, and abnormal eye movements (particularly nystagmus and impaired upgaze) (17). Impaired brain growth leads to acquired microcephaly. Progressive

TABLE 14.1 CLINICAL MANIFESTATIONS OF HIV-RELATED ENCEPHALOPATHY

Progressive encephalopathies

Subacute progressive
Loss of milestones
Progressive motor dysfunction
Oromotor dysfunction
Acquired microcephaly
Cognitive deterioration
Apathy
Progressive long-tract signs
Movement disorders (uncommon)
Cerebellar signs (uncommon)
Seizures (uncommon)
More-rapid course (weeks to months)

Plateau
No loss of skills
No or slower acquisition of skills
Decline in rate of cognitive development
Motor dysfunction (nonprogressive)
Acquired microcephaly
More indolent course

Static encephalopathy
Fixed deficits
No loss of skills
Skills acquired at a stable but slow rate
Deficient, but stable IQ
Motor dysfunction (nonprogressive)
Static course
Many potential etiologies

cognitive deterioration occurs along with social regression and apathy. Extrapyramidal movement disorders (particularly bradykinesia, which can be responsive to L-dopa), cerebellar signs and symptoms, and seizures occur less commonly (34). Seizures may occur in about 16% of children with HIV-related CNS disease (17). About half of seizures seen are provoked by febrile illnesses. Recurrent unprovoked seizures (epilepsy) are rarely due to HIV CNS disease; more often they are due to other factors (e.g., complications of prematurity, CNS OIs). Rarely, infants and toddlers also exhibit generalized subcortical myoclonus that clinically resembles myoclonic seizures (infantile spasms). However, EEGs are typically normal, and myoclonus resolves with treatment of HIV CNS disease alone. In the school-aged child, the first complaints may be a decline in academic achievement, change in behavior, and psychomotor slowing. Eventually, progressive cognitive impairment and new pyramidal tract signs (hyperreflexia and gait disturbances) occur.

The course of the plateau type of progressive encephalopathy is more indolent, with either the absence of acquisition of new developmental skills or a slower rate of acquisition of skills than previously. The rate of cognitive development declines, as does the rate of brain growth. Motor involvement is common, particularly spastic diplegia.

Children with static encephalopathy tend to have fixed neurodevelopmental deficits with no loss of skills. Development continues at a stable but slow rate. IQs are stable but low. Motor dysfunction is common, but not progressive. Whereas the etiology of progressive encephalopathy is thought to be related to the direct effects of HIV brain infection, the etiology of static encephalopathy can be varied and can include *in utero* exposure to drugs, alcohol, infections, or a combination of these; prematurity; and perinatal difficulties. Other factors to consider include genetic influences and nutritional, endocrinologic, and metabolic factors. Environmental and psychosocial factors may also affect development. Finally, HIV brain infection may play a role as well.

Children with HIV-related CNS compromise have less-severe CNS dysfunction and usually function normally (i.e., attend school, interact normally). They typically have normal overall cognitive functioning, but they may have had a significant decline in one or more neuropsychological tests (but are still functioning above the delayed range), or they may have significant impairments in selective neurodevelopmental functions. Alternatively, they may have a mildly abnormal neurological examination (pathologically brisk deep tendon reflexes with extensor plantar responses) that does not affect their day-to-day functioning. Patients who were functioning in the average cognitive range at baseline and who have shown improvement after institution of or change in antiretroviral therapy are also classified in this category.

The specific domains of neuropsychological impairment seen in children with HIV disease include expressive (greater than receptive) language, attention, adaptive functioning (socialization, behavior, quality of life), and memory (35–39). In children treated with HAART, specific deficits in executive function and processing speed have been described (40).

Children are classified as apparently not affected when their cognitive functioning is at least within normal limits and when no evidence is apparent of a decline in functioning or of neurological deficits that affect their day-to-day functioning. In addition, no therapy-related improvements in cognitive or motor functioning should occur.

Adolescents who are not vertically infected with HIV, but are infected through drug use or sexual practices, may display neurocognitive changes more similar to those of adults (41). In adults, the features of HIV dementia consist of the new onset of progressive disabling cognitive impairment (memory loss, psychomotor slowing), usually with motor dysfunction (gait disturbance, tremor, hyper-reflexia, fine motor impairments, and apraxia) and behavioral change (apathy). Neuropsychological testing usually shows impairment in frontal lobe functioning, psychomotor speed, and nonverbal memory, which has been termed a subcortical dementia. Typically in adults, HIV dementia develops when the patient has profound immune suppression. Risk factors include low CD4 counts, anemia, increased age, female gender, and injection-drug use. Before HAART, the course of adult HIV dementia was progressive over 3 to 9 months, resulting in severe neurological deficits and death, which appeared similar to the progressive encephalopathy in children. Since HAART, several subtypes of dementia have developed, including (a) a subacute progressive dementia seen in untreated patients similar to that of the pre-HAART era, (b) a chronic active dementia, seen in patients receiving HAART with poor adherence or viral resistance, and (c) a chronic inactive dementia, seen in patients receiving HAART who have had some neurological recovery and are stable (24,42). Minor cognitive/motor disorder (MCMD) is a more subtle form of HIV-related CNS disease seen in adults, which seems to be similar to CNS compromise seen in children.

Non–HIV-Related CNS Impairments

Some CNS impairments are thought possibly to be due to exposure to prenatal cocaine or multiple substances (43), as well as the quality of the child's environment (44,45). Additional contextual factors such as poverty, nutrition, caregiver stability, caregiver psychiatric illness, and ongoing drug use on child development, regardless of prenatal drug exposure and HIV disease status (46), may play a role in the etiology of CNS impairment as well.

Neuroradiologic Findings

Neuroradiologic studies provide essential information for the evaluation and management of HIV-related CNS disease. The most common abnormalities seen on CT scans in symptomatic, treatment-naive, HIV-infected children are ventricular enlargement, cortical atrophy, white-matter attenuation, and basal ganglia calcifications (47). Calcifications are seen primarily in vertically infected children or premature babies who were given transfusions in the neonatal period. They are not typically seen in adults (48). Therefore calcifications may indicate a selective vulnerability of the basal ganglia of the developing brain to HIV infection.

In general, greater degrees of CT brain scan abnormalities are seen with more-advanced stages of HIV disease (49). In addition, the severity of CT brain abnormalities has been correlated with lower levels of general cognitive abilities and language functioning in children with symptomatic HIV infection (27,35,50).

A correlation also exists between cortical atrophy, but not calcifications and CSF RNA viral concentrations (51). This finding supports the hypothesis that active HIV replication in the CNS is at least partially responsible for the development of cortical atrophy. Intracerebral calcifications appear to have a different pathophysiologic mechanism and may not be related to active HIV replication but rather may indicate the timing and location of initial viral entry into the immature brain.

A decreased prevalence of CT-scan abnormalities has been found in children treated with combination nucleoside analogue antiretroviral therapy, even before the availability of protease inhibitors (52).

Ventricular enlargement, cortical atrophy, white-matter attenuation, and basal ganglia calcifications are seen also on magnetic resonance imaging (MRI) scans, although calcifications are not as well seen as on CT scans. White-matter abnormalities are more readily seen on MRIs. Mild white-matter MRI changes in children are not necessarily correlated with cognitive dysfunction, although extensive white-matter changes may be associated with cognitive impairments (53,54).

Proton magnetic-resonance spectroscopy (MRS) studies in adults have revealed decreased levels of N-acetyl aspartate (NAA) (indicating neuronal loss) and increased levels of choline (Cho; indicating cell membrane turnover), and myoinositol (MI) (a glial marker), particularly in the white matter (55,56). These changes have been correlated with clinical CNS disease. MRS studies in encephalopathic HIV-infected children have shown a decrease in NAA and an increase in MI, indicating neuronal loss. Decreased NAA/Cr ratios with lactate peaks (indicative of anaerobic metabolism) were reversed by ZDV in at least two children with HIV-related CNS disease (57,58). Abnormal spectra have been seen in children with normal structural imaging. The abnormalities on MRS (low NAA-to-Cho ratio) correlated with poor neuropsychological performance in these children (59). In general, MRS findings in adults and children are consistent with neuronal cell loss and inflammation, some of which can be reversed by antiretroviral treatment.

CSF Studies

Routine CSF studies may show nonspecific abnormalities, such as a mild pleocytosis or elevated protein level, but are usually normal. In adults, an aseptic meningitis is often seen at the time of seroconversion, but this has seldom been documented in the pediatric population.

Children and adults with abnormal brain function have increased levels of HIV RNA in the CSF as compared with those patients with normal brain function (60–63). As noted previously, RNA viral load in the CSF is correlated with cortical atrophy on CT scans in children (51). Therefore CSF viral load may be predictive of CNS status. In support of this notion is a study showing that elevated baseline CSF HIV RNA levels in adults significantly predicted progression to neuropsychological impairment at follow-up 1 year later (64). In addition, markers of immune activation in the CSF (and serum) such as tumor-necrosis factor, [BETA]$_2$-microglobulin, neopterin, quinolinic acid, and certain chemokines (such as MCP-1) have been correlated with CNS disease in both adults and children. These observations may be important in neuropathogenesis (65–69).

Diagnosis of HIV-Related CNS Disease

The diagnosis of HIV-related CNS disease remains a clinical diagnosis, based on history, physical and neurological examinations, and age-appropriate neuropsychological testing, which can be compared with prior testing, if available. Other causes of CNS disease should be ruled out, including CNS OIs, malignancies, cerebrovascular disease, and non–HIV-related conditions (static encephalopathies due to effects of prematurity; maternal drug use; other congenital infections; genetic, nutritional, and endocrinologic factors, etc.). Neuroimaging should also be part of the workup to rule out OIs, malignancies, and cerebrovascular disease, as well as to identify the characteristic features of HIV-related CNS disease. CSF studies should be done primarily to rule out OIs.

Neuropathology

The prominent neuropathologic findings in both children and adults with HIV-related CNS disease include cortical atrophy, microglial nodules, multinucleated giant cells, myelin pallor, and astrocytosis.

HIV "encephalitis" consists of perivascular inflammatory cell infiltrates (microglial nodules) composed of microglia, macrophages, and multinucleated giant cells (70,71). These infiltrates occur in the subcortical white matter, the deep gray nuclei (putamen, globus pallidus), and pons. The characteristic finding in pediatric CNS disease, not seen in adults, is a calcific basal ganglia vasculopathy, which consists of vascular and perivascular mineralization, sometimes extending into the white matter.

HIV leukoencephalopathy consists of myelin loss and reactive astrocytosis. In adults, neuronal loss is seen in the hippocampi as well as in the orbitofrontal and temporal cortex, along with loss of dendritic arborizations. These features are difficult to appreciate in pediatric patients because few standards exist for neuronal cell counts (72).

Neuropathogenesis

HIV enters the brain early during the course of infection in adults, either as free viral particles or within infected monocytes, which then set up residence in the brain as macrophages (73,74). Evidence suggests that the blood–brain barrier (BBB) is disrupted in HIV CNS disease. Matrix metalloproteinases (MMPs) (which degrade collagen type IV, a component of the BBB) and their inhibitors, both of which are produced and secreted by microglia and macrophages, may be involved in the development of CNS disease (75,76). MMP-9 has been shown to be present in the CSF of HIV-infected children with abnormal neurological findings (77).

Only two brain cell types, the microglia/macrophage and the astrocyte, have clearly been shown to be infected by HIV (78–83). In microglia, a productive and cytopathic infection results, but in astrocytes, a latent or restricted infection results. Despite the prominent neuronal cell loss and evidence of neuronal apoptosis, neurons were previously not thought to be directly infected by HIV. However, in a recent study, HIV-infected neurons were detected in the cortical gray matter in two children with progressive CNS disease (84). In another study, HIV-1 DNA was identified in neural progenitor cells of four pre–HAART era pediatric AIDS patients, suggesting that neurons may be infected even *in utero* (85). The immune systems of infants and children are not as well developed as those in adults; viral loads tend to be higher in younger patients. These observations suggest that immature neurons and other brain cells in children may be more susceptible to HIV-1 infection than are those in adults, resulting in some of the differences seen between pediatric and adult neuroAIDS.

These observations lead to several important considerations. First, because glial cells outnumber neurons by 10:1 in the CNS, potentially a large number of infected cells exist in the CNS. The brain may act as an important viral reservoir and theoretically may even reseed the periphery. Second, this suggests that products released from HIV-infected glial cells may be responsible for causing neurotoxicity (78,79,83). These products may be derived from the virus or from the host and can set up a chain of events leading to a significant amount of potentially irreversible neuronal dysfunction at sites distant from infected cells.

Infected, activated glial cells release viral proteins (gp120, tat), as well as a number of host-derived soluble factors, which are toxic to neurons (86,87). These factors include the proinflammatory cytokines [tumor-necrosis factor (TNF–α), interleukin-1 (IL-1), IL-6, interferon (IFN)-γ and -α, arachidonic acid and its metabolites, quinolinic acid (an agonist of excitatory amino acid receptors), and nitric oxide (65–68,88–91). Chemokines are also released, resulting in an influx of monocytes from peripheral blood into the brain, resulting in an increase in inflammation as well as an increase in the number of target cells for the virus in the brain (92). The chemokine, monocyte chemoattractant protein-1 (MCP-1) is present in high levels in the CSF and brains of adult patients with HIV dementia (69). In addition, in children, MCP-1 is present in the CSF and declines in parallel with CSF HIV RNA with antiretroviral treatment (77). Macrophage inflammatory protein-1α (MIP-1-α) and MIP-1-β may be important in CNS disease as well (63). The possibility also exists that some chemokines have an anti-inflammatory effect (for example, IL-10) and may be neuroprotective (93).

In addition, chemokine receptors have been identified as important co-receptors for HIV entry into target cells. Astrocytes express the CXCR4 chemokine receptor, and evidence indicates that this expression may be related to neuronal damage (94). Microglia express the CCR5 chemokine receptor (95). Individuals with defective CCR5 alleles seem to exhibit resistance to HIV-1 infection. Children with the CCR5-wt/Delta 32 genotype had significantly delayed disease progression, including less neurocognitive impairment (96). In adults, the E4 isoform for apolipoprotein E has been associated with dementia severity in some studies (24). This suggests that host factors influencing the host's immune response may be important in the development of CNS HIV disease and that a genetic predisposition may exist to the development of neurological impairment. Alternatively, other genetic factors also may protect the host from developing CNS disease.

This entire process of HIV CNS infection is amplified by cell-to-cell interactions between HIV-infected macrophages and astrocytes, which initiate a self-perpetuating cascade of neurotoxic events in the brain. These events ultimately lead to an increase in the extracellular concentration of the excitatory amino acid glutamate, which, through activation of the N-methyl-D-aspartate (NMDA) receptor and non-NMDA excitatory amino acid receptors leads to increases in intracellular calcium concentrations and eventually disruption of mitochondrial function, generation of nitric oxide and other free radicals, and eventual activation of apoptotic and other cellular pathways (78,79,83,97–99).

Therapeutic approaches to HIV-related CNS disease will be most successful if they are based on knowledge of these mechanisms and target both active HIV replication in the brain and the associated indirect neurotoxic events.

Secondary CNS Disorders

These disorders are not directly attributable to HIV brain infection but are related to the effects of immune suppression and other unknown factors.

OPPORTUNISTIC INFECTIONS OF THE CNS

Children with HIV infection have fewer problems with CNS OIs compared with adults, probably because OIs represent reactivation of previous, relatively asymptomatic infections. Nevertheless, CNS OIs can present significant problems in children, and their incidence may increase because children with HIV disease are living longer.

Generally, OIs are seen in patients with severe immunosuppression (CD4$^+$ lymphocyte counts less than 200 cells per microliter) and in older children and adolescents. They may also occur in infants and younger children as a result of congenital infection.

The most common CNS OI in children is cytomegalovirus (CMV) infection, which may appear as a subacute or chronic encephalitis/ventriculitis, an acute ascending radiculomyelitis, or as an acute or subacute neuritis (100–103). Other viruses [herpes simplex virus (HSV), varicella-zoster virus (VZV)] may also cause an acute or subacute encephalitis (104). Progressive multifocal leukoencephalopathy (PML), caused by the JC virus (a papovavirus), has rarely been reported in the pediatric AIDS population (105).

Fungal infections (*Candida* and *Aspergillus*) are the second most common CNS OI in children. (100). Cryptococcal meningitis, although seen in 5% to 10% of adult AIDS patients, was reported in less than 1% of pediatric AIDS patients followed up at the NCI over a period of 8 years (106).

Toxoplasma encephalitis, a protozoan CNS infection, is the most common cause of intracranial mass lesions in adults with AIDS, occurring in 10% to 50% of patients (107). However, it has been reported in only about 1% of HIV-infected children (108).

Bacterial CNS infections are also relatively uncommon in children with HIV infection (16,109). Unusual bacterial pathogens must be considered in these immunocompromised hosts such as *Mycobacterium tuberculosis,* atypical mycobacteria, syphilis, *Bartonella, Listeria monocytogenes,* and *Nocardia asteroides* (106,110).

NEOPLASMS

Primary CNS lymphoma is the most common cause of CNS mass lesions in pediatric AIDS patients and is the second most common cause of focal neurological deficits after stroke (111,112). This contrasts with the adult AIDS population, in which toxoplasmosis is the most common cause of CNS mass lesions. These are usually high-grade, multifocal B-cell tumors, which appear with subacute onset of change in mental status or behavior, headache, seizures, and new focal neurological signs. The tumors have a predilection for the deep gray matter (basal ganglia and thalamus). On neuroimaging studies, they enhance with contrast and have edema and mass effect. Treatment options include steroids, radiation therapy, and systemic chemotherapy.

CEREBROVASCULAR DISEASE

Strokes are the most common cause of focal neurological deficits in children with HIV infection (111,113). Strokes may be secondary to hemorrhage (related to coagulopathies) or ischemia. Ischemic strokes may be embolic or may be related to an infectious vasculitis (for example, VZV) (114). In AIDS patients, a hypercoagulable state may be related to acquired protein C or S deficiencies or both. In addition, a characteristic vasculopathy is seen in HIV-infected children, resulting in aneurysmal dilatation of vessels of the circle of Willis with or without associated ischemic infarction or hemorrhage (115–117). The etiology of this vasculopathy is unclear, but it may be related to direct viral invasion of the vessel walls (117).

Treatment of HIV-Related CNS Disease

The three main types of therapy for HIV CNS disease are as follows: (a) antiretroviral, (b) neuroprotective, and (c) symptomatic, including psychiatric disorders.

ANTIRETROVIRAL THERAPY

Ample evidence indicates that HIV encephalopathy is at least in part related to active viral replication in the brain (60–62). Evidence also suggests that the CNS is a separate compartment from the rest of the body in HIV disease (63,118–122). Plasma viral loads do not necessarily reflect the degree of viral replication in the brain. The brain may also serve as a viral reservoir and may theoretically reseed the plasma (120), potentially with species of pathophysiologic significance (for example, with drug-resistance mutations). At times of high plasma viral load, virus trafficking into the CNS may occur through a disrupted BBB. If HIV CNS disease is a concern, patients should be treated with drugs able to cross the BBB and reach effective concentrations in the CSF and brain. Some evidence suggests that HIV CNS disease may be worse when the peripheral viral load is high, perhaps because of continued seeding of the CNS from the periphery. Aggressive efforts to decrease the peripheral viral load may therefore also have beneficial effects on CNS HIV disease.

The earliest regimens consisted of single-agent therapy with nucleoside analogue reverse transcriptase inhibitors (NRTIs). Of these agents, zidovudine (AZT, ZDV, Retrovir) and stavudine (d4T, Zerit) have relatively good CSF penetration (122,123). Both continuous-infusion ZDV and oral intermittent ZDV have been shown to be clinically beneficial in pediatric patients with HIV-related encephalopathy, but in general, the effects were not long-lasting (124,125). Early epidemiologic studies in Europe demonstrated a decreased prevalence of dementia in adult AIDS patients after ZDV was introduced into that population (126). Limited studies document the clinical efficacy of d4T in CNS disease in pediatric patients (127).

Other NRTIs, didanosine (ddI, Videx) and zalcitabine (ddC, Hivid), have less CSF penetration (122,123). One study of pediatric patients suggested clinical benefits of ddI in HIV-related encephalopathy (128). When either ZDV or ddI was given alone in a recent study of adult HIV-infected patients, motor abnormalities improved (129). Lamivudine (3TC, Epivir) has some CSF penetration as well.

Combination therapy with NRTIs was introduced in the 1990s. One study, conducted between 1991 and 1995, demonstrated that combination therapy with ZDV and ddI was more effective than either ZDV or ddI alone against HIV encephalopathy in treatment-naive children. In this study, long-term benefits for ZDV did not appear, compared with ddI monotherapy (130). In adults, combinations containing either d4T or ZDV have been found to be equally efficacious in improving motor function (131).

A more recently developed NRTI, abacavir (ABC, Ziagen) crosses the BBB and offers the potential for good CNS coverage in children and adults (122). However, most studies of the efficacy of abacavir in HIV-related CNS disease have occurred with combinations of other antiretroviral agents. One such study, done in 14 children with HIV-associated encephalopathy, used high-dose abacavir in combination with two or three other antiretroviral drugs. Good virologic and immunologic responses ensued, and children younger than 6 years also demonstrated neuropsychological improvement (132).

Of the non-nucleoside reverse transcriptase inhibitors (NNRTIs), nevirapine (NVP, Viramune) has the best potential for treatment of CNS disease. NVP has been studied more extensively than the other NNRTIs in children. It was found to be effective in combination with ZDV and ddI in children with advanced HIV disease (133). Efavirenz (EFU, Sustiva, Stocrin) and delavirdine (DLV, Rescriptor) have less CSF penetration than nerivrapine.

Protease inhibitors (PIs) were studied clinically in the mid-1990s. As a rule, PIs have poor CSF penetration, with indinavir (Crixivan) having the best penetration in this group of drugs (122). Indinavir was shown to be present in the CSF in therapeutic concentrations with a reduction in CSF viral load in 25 adult patients in a Swedish study published in 1999 (134). In addition, a reduction in CSF viral load was seen in the indinavir-treated patients compared with control patients. Ritonavir (Norvir) and indinavir were the first two PIs used in pediatric clinical trials (135,136). Full-scale IQs significantly improved from baseline to 6 to 7 months and to 18 to 24 months with either drug (used in combination with two NRTIs), but then appeared to plateau at 36 months, possibly because of the development of drug resistance (52). Other commonly used PIs include nelfinavir (Viracept), saquinavir (Invirase, Fortovase), and amprenavir (AMP, Agenerase). Kaletra is the combination of Lopinavir and low-dose Ritonavir.

Because the CSF penetration of PIs is so poor, *in vitro* models are being used to study the transport of PIs across the BBB. These studies show that PIs are mainly transported across the BBB in an active process by a plasma membrane–localized drug transporter, Pgp (P-glycoprotein). Substances that inhibit Pgp could increase the concentrations of PIs in the brain by decreasing their efflux out of the brain and therefore may be helpful in treating HIV-related brain injury (137).

HAART, introduced in 1996, is defined as the combination of at least three drugs, usually including a PI. HAART has been found to be beneficial in the treatment of HIV CNS disease in many studies in adults. In a French study, HAART improved subcortical cognitive functions in adults with HIV-related CNS dysfunction (138). These patients demonstrated continued improvement in performance on psychomotor tests, with a plateau in improvement on memory tasks, suggesting that sustained HAART therapy may be necessary to produce optimal neurocognitive benefits. In a large retrospective study in Germany ($n = 563$), the prevalence of AIDS dementia and neuropathy as well as toxoplasma encephalitis has significantly decreased since the introduction of HAART. CD4 counts were significantly higher as well (139).

In three separate studies, both clinical and proton-MRS abnormalities improved in adult HIV-infected patients with mild cognitive impairment who were treated with HAART (140–142). In the most recent study, both viral loads and CD4 counts improved at 3 months, but cerebral metabolite concentrations and clinical test measures did not show any improvement until 9 months after the institution of HAART (142).

Few studies of the effect of HAART on cognitive function in HIV-infected children have been reported, other than the previously mentioned NCI study (52). Two case reports exist of improvement of HIV-related encephalopathy in children treated with HAART (143,144). Combination antiretroviral therapy was associated with a decline in CSF HIV RNA and an improvement in neurological status in 25 children (7 months to 10 years of age) who were studied in Panama (145). However, by week 48 of treatment, 67% of the children had new mutation patterns in the CSF, and discordant evolution of virus in the CSF and plasma appeared to occur.

Somewhat disturbing is a recent report documenting neuropsychological outcome in 489 HIV-infected children who were enrolled in two large multicenter protocols. These studies included children who were not naive to treatment and who were clinically and immunologically stable. They were treated with varying antiretroviral combinations including PIs. Neuropsychological test scores were lower than normal at baseline for this cohort of children, with a mean cognitive score of 83.5. After 48 weeks of PI-containing regimens, even though plasma viral loads improved, no significant improvement was found in neuropsychological test scores, except for a vocabulary score (146).

Also disturbing is a report from NCI documenting discordant decline in cognitive function in four children treated with HAART, despite clinical, immunologic, and virologic stability in the periphery (147). This again brings up the possibility of discordant evolution of the virus in plasma and CSF, with the possible emergence of drug-resistant strains in the CSF.

Currently, HAART, including one NRTI or NNRTI with good CSF penetration, is indicated in the treatment of children with HIV-related CNS disease. ZDV, d4T, abacavir, and nevirapine have the best CSF penetration among the NRTIs and NNRTIs. The choice of individual drugs would depend on the patient's history of prior antiretroviral use and on drug-resistance patterns. No clear-cut evidence suggests that regimens containing multiple CSF-penetrating drugs are superior to those with single CSF-penetrating drugs (132). The latter option would be preferred if possible to decrease the development of resistance mutations to multiple drugs.

NEUROPROPHYLAXIS

Once CNS disease is present, antiretroviral regimens may improve neurocognitive dysfunction. However, because an improved survival rate occurs for patients with HIV disease who are treated with HAART, it is possible that CNS disease is being delayed and not prevented. It is possible that CNS disease is present but is not so severe, making the diagnosis more elusive. Therefore the prophylactic value of antiretroviral therapy on the CNS is becoming more important. ZDV appears to have some beneficial prophylactic effects for HIV CNS disease (126,148). The MAC study, conducted in the United States, documented the decreasing incidence of CNS disease in adults since the advent of HAART (23).

In addition, a neuroprotective effect of early antiretroviral treatment seems to occur in children with vertical HIV infection. Children treated with antiretroviral therapy before the onset of neurological symptoms showed delayed presentation of HIV-related progressive encephalopathy (0.6 years in the nontreated group vs. 2.5 years in the treated group), and the survival of children in the treated group was significantly longer (149).

The prophylactic value of HAART for HIV CNS disease appears to occur in a subgroup of adult patients with subclinical psychomotor slowing and with clinical motor signs. However, this prophylactic effect appears to be time limited, which again may be related to the development of drug resistance over time. HAART may not have prophylactic effects for patients with more-sustained subclinical psychomotor slowing (150).

In an autopsy series of 436 adult HIV+ patients who died between 1985 and 1999, the incidence of severe encephalopathy decreased over time, but the relative incidence of mild to moderate encephalopathy increased in the HAART era (1996–1999) (151). This perhaps indicates that HAART can successfully prevent or treat severe forms of dementia and encephalopathy but may not prevent milder cases.

NEUROPROTECTION

Neuroprotective strategies (adjunctive therapies) are directed toward the effects of viral proteins and other cellular "toxins" such as cytokines on neuronal function. These strategies are largely investigational at this time and are not recommended for general use in pediatric patients.

Steroids have the potential to downregulate cytokine production, but no large studies have examined these drugs in the HIV-infected patient (152,153). Neither pentoxifylline nor thalidomide, TNF-α antagonists, have had beneficial effects in adults with CNS disease (152,154). Nimodipine, a calcium channel blocker, may be of some benefit in adults who are also receiving ZDV (155). Memantine is an analogue of the antiviral drug amantadine and acts as an uncompetitive antagonist of the NMDA receptor. Memantine is now being studied as a potential neuroprotective agent in HIV-infected adults with cognitive impairment (156). L-Deprenyl (selegeline), an antioxidant and putative antiapoptotic agent, has been shown to reverse *in vitro* mitochondrial dysfunction in human fetal neurons exposed to CSF from HIV-infected patients with dementia (157). Clinical trials are in progress. Other antioxidants [thioctic acid (α-lipoic acid), didox, imidate, etc.] are being studied both *in vitro* and in clinical trials (158). Minocycline, an antibiotic, has anti-inflammatory properties and has been shown to improve CNS disease in the SIV (simian immunodeficiency virus) model (24,93).

Additional potential agents for drug development and clinical trials are other antioxidants, other cytokine antagonists, antichemokine agents, other NMDA-receptor antagonists, nitric oxide synthase inhibitors, inhibitors of arachidonic acid metabolites, and inhibitors of apoptosis (78).

SYMPTOMATIC TREATMENT

Symptomatic treatment includes pharmacologic treatment of pain, movement disorders, seizures, spasticity, attention-deficit hyperactivity disorder (ADHD), and other psychiatric/behavioral disorders in children with HIV-related CNS disease. Because the full gamut of developmental and childhood psychiatric disorders is seen in children and adolescents with HIV/AIDS, only the most commonly seen clinical disorders will be highlighted. Adult psychiatric syndromes of adjustment disorder, major depression, anxiety, and delirium are seen in children as well. As in adults (159), treatment of psychiatric syndromes in children and adolescents may improve outcomes.

In youth with HIV infection, changes in mental status or the emergence of new cognitive or psychiatric disorders requires collaboration with the medical team to rule out any reversible and treatable causes. Therefore psychiatrists treating HIV+ youth should be familiar with assessments of basic immune function and viral load and have a low threshold for ordering additional medical evaluations such as head imaging and CSF examination and even antiretroviral drug resistance testing. Then, to make the best diagnosis and to institute treatment, a thorough psychiatric assessment based on multiple brief examinations of the child or adolescent and information gathered from additional sources, including family, staff, and teachers, is needed. A child's biologic predisposition to depression and anxiety is suggested by: (a) a family history of a mood or anxiety disorder, or other psychiatric disorder; and (b) previous psychiatric symptoms or psychiatric treatment. Precipitating and perpetuating factors for psychiatric disorders should also be identified. Although many children cope well and adapt, symptoms of depression such as fatigue, cognitive impairment, decreased social interaction and exploration, and anorexia may be in part derived from a cytokine/immunologic response to HIV and its treatments. It may be possible only to determine that antiretroviral medication is causing psychiatric side effects by evaluating the time course of psychiatric symptoms in relation to starting HIV medications regimens and by trials of stopping treatment. See Table 14.2 (160) for common psychiatric side effects of antiretroviral medications.

In general, one can use the same psychotropic medications in the HIV-infected child as in the general population. However, bone marrow suppression, liver disease and pancreatitis may cause treatment-limiting toxicities and affect metabolism of antiretrovirals, particularly PIs. Psychotropic medications do not replace comprehensive, multidisciplinary care and multimodal treatment but may improve the quality of life for pediatric HIV/AIDS patients by decreasing discomfort and increasing functioning. Important determining factors for pharmacologic intervention are severity and duration of psychiatric symptoms and overall level of functional impairment.

Children with severe neurodevelopmental deficits may require physical, occupational, and speech therapy. Children with static encephalopathies resulting in spastic diplegia have been shown to benefit from botulinum toxin injections (161). A case report details the successful use of intrathecal baclofen in a girl with HIV-related encephalopathy and a spastic paraparesis (162). Educational remediation is indicated for children with ADHD or learning disabilities or both. Optimal nutrition is extremely important in the care of these children. Other causes of neurodevelopmental disorders, such as endocrinologic and metabolic disturbances, such as hypothyroidism and vitamin and cofactor deficiencies, should be carefully sought out and treated.

Psychiatric Disorders in HIV

The prevalence of psychiatric disorders in pediatric HIV/AIDS has been difficult to determine and has been limited by small and diverse demographic samples, lack of consistent testing measurements, frequent subthreshold *Diagnostic and Statistical Manual of Mental Disorders* (DSM)-IV diagnoses, lack of appropriate control groups, and differences between pre- and post-HAART samples (163). A recent review of reported DSM psychiatric diagnoses in pediatric HIV/AIDS found average prevalence rates of attention-deficit

TABLE 14.2 NEUROPSYCHIATRIC SIDE EFFECTS OF THERAPEUTIC DRUGS FOR HIV

Agent	Effects
Anti-infective	
Abacavir	Depressed mood, headache, anxiety
Acyclovir	Depressed mood, agitation, auditory and visual hallucinations, depersonalization, tearfulness, confusion, hyperesthesia, hyperacusis, insomnia, thought insertion, headache
Amphotericin-B	Delirium
Amprenavir	Depression, headache
Atazanavir	Headache
Cephalosporins	Confusion, disorientation, paranoia
Cycloserine	Anxiety, confusion, depression, disorientation, hallucinations, paranoia, loss of appetite, fatigue
Dapsone	Agitation, hallucinations, insomnia
Didanosine	Mania
Efavirenz	Depression, hallucinations, nightmares, insomnia, poor concentration, aggressive behavior, suicidal ideation, mania
Enfurvirtide	Anxiety, insomnia, depression
Ethambutol	Headache, dizziness, confusion, visual disturbances
Ethionamide	Depression, drowsiness, hallucinations, neuritis
5-Flucytosine	Delirium, headache, persisting neurocognitive impairment
Foscarnet	Seizures, headache
Indinavir	Insomnia
Isoniazid	Depression, agitation, hallucinations, paranoia
Ketoconazole	Dizziness, headache, photosensitivity
Lamivudine	Possible depressed mood
Lopinavir/ritonavir	Headache, insomnia
Metronidazole	Depression, agitation, delirium, seizures
Nelfinavir	Anxiety, possible depressed mood, insomnia
Nevirapine	Headache, insomnia, delirium, delusions, hallucinations
Pentamidine	Delirium, hallucinations
Quinolones	Psychosis, delirium, seizures, anxiety, insomnia, depression
Rifampin	Headache, fatigue, loss of appetite
Ritonavir	Agitation, anxiety, confusion, hallucinations, possible depressed mood
Saquinavir	Anxiety, irritability, hallucinations
Stavudine	Headache, anxiety, mania
Sulfonamides	Headache, neuritis, insomnia, loss of appetite, photosensitivity
Tenofovir	Headache, depression, dizziness
Thiabendazole	Hallucinations
Trimethoprim-sulfamethoxazole	Delirium, mutism, depression, loss of appetite, insomnia, apathy, headache, neuritis
Zalcitabine	Agitation, anxiety, mania, hallucinations
Zidovudine	Depressed mood, agitation, headache, myalgia, insomnia, mania
Antineoplastic	
Methotrexate	Delirium
Procarbazine	Mania
Vinblastine	Depression, loss of appetite, headache, neuritis
Vincristine	Ataxia, headache, hallucinations, neuritis
Interferon-α	Depression, weakness, anergic–apathetic states
Other	
Amantadine	Visual hallucinations
Barbiturates	Excitement, hyperactivity, hallucinations, depression
Benzodiazepines	Delirium, drowsiness, amnesia, excitement
Corticosteroids	Confusion, depression, hallucinations, mania, paranoia
Meperidine	Delirium
Metoclopramide	Depression, mania, akathisia
Morphine	Delirium, agitation
Phenytoin	Confusion, delirium, euphoria
Tricyclic antidepressants	Drowsiness, mania, delirium, insomnia

Modified with permission from Grant I, Atkinson JH. Neuropsychiatric aspects of HIV infection and AIDS. In: Sadock BJ, Sadock VA eds. *Kaplan and Sadock's comprehensive textbook of psychiatry*, 7th ed. Philadelphia: Lippincott Williams & Wilkins, 2000:320.

hyperactivity disorder at 28.6%, anxiety disorders at 24.3%, and depression at 25% (164). The review included a study of HIV-infected youth aged 6 to 15 that suggests that depression (47%) and attentional disorders (29%) are most common and that depression may be associated with encephalopathy and worsening immune function (165). A higher rate of psychotropic medication use and of psychiatric hospitalizations in HIV-infected children compared with HIV-uninfected controls has been reported (166). In addition, a high rate of use of psychotropic medication (45%) in an HIV clinic cohort (N = 64; mean age, 15.3 years) is reported, with psychostimulants and antidepressants being most commonly prescribed, and 30% of the sample taking two or more psychotropic medications (167).

ATTENTION-DEFICIT HYPERACTIVITY DISORDER

Attention-deficit hyperactivity disorder (ADHD) is a childhood-onset (before age 7 years) disorder frequently diagnosed in children with HIV/AIDS, characterized by sustained impulsivity, poor attention, and hyperactivity (168). Short attention span, disorganization, forgetfulness, and difficulty staying seated (in younger children) are often described. In older children and adolescents, attention-deficit disorder (ADD) may be diagnosed as the symptoms of hyperactivity wane. On neuropsychological tests, poor processing speed is frequently noted. The differential diagnoses include anxiety, cognitive disorders, language disorders, medication toxicity, psychosocial stressors, and progressive HIV disease.

Psychostimulants are often used to treat ADHD/ADD in children with HIV, although dosing is not well established, and efficacy is variable. Often, higher doses of stimulants are required to achieve scholastic benefit but must be balanced against appetite loss, growth retardation, and insomnia, which are often significant issues for children with HIV. Clonidine, bupropion, and atomoxetine use has been described as well (167,169).

BEHAVIORAL DISORDERS

In young children with HIV, oppositional defiant disorder (ODD) is often diagnosed. ODD is characterized by a recurrent pattern of losing one's temper, frequent arguing with adults or authority, refusing to follow rules, blaming others for one's mistakes, and being angry or vindictive for at least 6 months and of sufficient severity to cause impairment (168). These behaviors are often seen in children from disrupted or unstable environments and must be distinguished from underlying cognitive or language difficulties as well as mood and anxiety disorders.

Conduct disorder is a repetitive and persistent pattern of aggressive behaviors, serious violation of rules, and destruction of property (168) and is occasionally seen in adolescents with HIV; it may be more common in those who acquire HIV as adolescents. The new onset of conduct-disordered behaviors in an adolescent should lead immediately to screening for mood, learning, and substance-abuse disorders.

Treatment for these behavioral disorders is directed at behavioral and parenting interventions. Medications, such as low doses of atypical antipsychotics or mood stabilizers, are considered if behavioral dyscontrol is severe (167).

MOOD DISORDERS

Major depression

Major depression is marked by depressed mood or irritability in children daily for at least 2 weeks (168). Vegetative symptoms such as decreased appetite, difficulty sleeping, and poor energy are difficult to assess in youth with HIV because they are frequent complaints and may be secondary to HIV and its treatment. Increased somatic complaints such as headaches and fatigue, as well as withdrawal from peers and family, are often seen in depressed children. Anhedonia, or the lack of enjoyment of activities, may also be seen. A diagnosis of major depression is seen with increasing frequency in adolescents with HIV. Whether this is due, in part, to developmental aspects of mood neurobiology, to increased cognitive abilities in understanding one's situation, or to chronic HIV infection is not clear. Differential diagnoses include worsening medical status, age-appropriate nonadherence, bereavement, adjustment disorder, and dysthymia. One case report of abacavir-induced depression in pediatric HIV that resolved with discontinuation of the medication has been described (170).

For treatment of depression in HIV+ youth, clinicians should follow current treatment guidelines for the management of depression in children. Antidepressants including tricyclic antidepressants (TCAs), as well as selective serotonin reuptake inhibitors (SSRIs) and bupropion, have been used empirically, and off-label in many cases, in youth with HIV (167). No evidence indicates that one SSRI is more effective than another in youth. Citalopram or mirtazapine may be used because of fewer side effects and less-problematic drug–drug interactions. Mirtazapine may be used to promote weight gain and treat insomnia. Methylphenidate, which may also potentiate opiate treatment, may be useful for pain and depression in HIV (171).

Bipolar disorder

Pediatric bipolar disorder may be difficult to distinguish from ADHD and is frequently comorbid with ADHD and substance-abuse disorder. No evidence indicates that higher rates of pediatric bipolar disorder are associated with pediatric HIV infection, as in adults. Treatment options include divalproex sodium (Depakote), when neutropenia is not a concern, other mood stabilizers such as lamotrigine, and, rarely, lithium (172). Similarly, drug–drug interactions, neutropenia, and hepatotoxicity are clinical management concerns.

Anxiety disorders

Separation anxiety

Separation anxiety is common in pediatric HIV, because it may be precipitated by a life stress such as moving, death of a pet, or parental illness. Cognitive behavioral therapy may be helpful; in severe cases of school refusal, treatment with SSRIs and TCAs has been reported.

Post-traumatic stress disorder

Post-traumatic stress disorder from traumatic events, including those arising from the hospital environment and invasive medical treatments, may be seen in children with HIV/AIDS. Symptoms include hypervigilence, flashbacks of the trauma, intrusive thoughts, nightmares, difficulty sleeping, and irritability or mood lability. Benzodiazepines, such as lorazepam, used in low doses in conjunction with nonpharmacologic distraction techniques and psychotherapy, may be appropriate for procedures that provoke significant anxiety in children. Clonazepam is longer acting and may be helpful with more-pervasive and prolonged anxiety symptoms. Benzodiazepines can cause sedation, confusion, and behavioral disinhibition and should be carefully monitored, especially in those patients with CNS dysfunction.

Benzodiazepine withdrawal precipitated by abrupt discontinuation occurs most frequently on transfer out of intensive-care settings.

Antihistamines have been used to sedate anxious children but are not recommended for treatment of persistent anxiety; their anticholinergic properties can precipitate or worsen delirium.

Delirium

Delirium is marked by impaired attention and fluctuating consciousness. In children, disorientation, sleep disturbance, irritability, confusion, apathy, agitation, exacerbation at night, and impaired responsiveness are often observed. Hallucinations or other perceptual disturbances, paranoia, and memory impairment, although frequently seen in adult delirium, are less common in younger children (173). Underlying medical causes such as medication intoxication should be evaluated. Certain antiretroviral agents such as efavirenz have been associated with a number of significant CNS effects, including dizziness, sleep disturbances, and mood alterations, which often resolve after the first few weeks of therapy but also may persist (174).

Treatment should focus on reorienting children in developmentally appropriate ways and by enhancing environmental cues (lights on during the day, off at night; or by positioning near a window for natural light). Benzodiazepines and anticholinergic agents may aggravate delirium and should be avoided. Very low doses of an atypical antipsychotic medication may be considered. However, Scharko et al. (164) described a case in which risperidone was not effective, and haloperidol was required to treat a delirium in the context of HIV dementia.

Dementia

The previous case report (164) suggests that HIV-associated dementia (HAD), well described in adults, may also be seen in HIV+ adolescents who become treatment resistant or discontinue treatment. This clinical presentation is becoming more common, and low-dose typical and atypical antipsychotic medications may be useful.

Substance abuse

Clinicians should be aware that in adolescents with HIV/AIDS, substance-abuse disorders may develop despite their medical condition. What may begin as developmentally appropriate experimentation can become a disorder as youth find that substances help them escape the reality of having a chronic life-threatening illness or may treat underlying pain, anxiety or mood disorders or both. In addition, a genetic or environmental predisposition to substance abuse may exist. Treatment must be initiated immediately and closely monitored.

Pain disorders

Children living with HIV commonly experience pain (175–177), including abdominal pain of unclear etiology, myositis, tension headaches, and neuropathic pain that is difficult to manage. Discomfort related to invasive procedures, toxicities and adverse drug reactions, invasive secondary infections, pancreatitis, and erosive esophagitis may be treated pharmacologically. Pain has been found to be associated with more-severe immunosuppression and increased likelihood of death (177).

No published studies examine the relation between chronic pain and psychological distress in HIV-infected children. Nevertheless, children fear pain, and pain is made worse by emotional distress. The treatment goal must be to minimize pain and oversedation when possible. Pediatric pain-management principles with age-appropriate assessment of all developmental ages should be applied and include a repertoire of nonpharmacologic (such as distraction, relaxation, psychotherapies, and hypnosis) and pharmacologic treatments (178,179).

Confidentiality

Knowledge of a psychiatrist's obligations with regard to confidentiality of HIV-positive patients' diagnosis and an understanding of a provider's responsibilities with regard to duty to warn and duty to protect the rights of others from harm are essential. Laws differ from state to state; therefore practitioners have an obligation to know the law in the state in which they practice and to be aware that the law may differ greatly, even within a small geographic area. Additional information concerning treatment of adolescents with psychiatric conditions with regard to consent, confidentiality, and competence may also vary from state to state (180).

Developmental and Psychosocial Issues

How a school-age child copes with his or her illness depends on many factors including age and developmental stage (including cognitive abilities, parental adaptation, social skills, and his or her psychological makeup) (181). It also is important to assess the disclosure status and stage of illness because all these factors determine the meaning the illness carries for the child and the kind of psychological and intellectual resources available to cope with the disease and to meet each challenge.

Because of the stigma associated with this disease, parents' anxiety associated with informing school personnel about their child's diagnosis is tremendous (182). Most parents keep an HIV/AIDS diagnosis from the school for as long as possible. If the family decides it is in the child's best interest to share the diagnosis with the school, the health care team can assist families with the school process.

In adolescence, developmental tasks such as struggles for independence, experimenting with adult behaviors, impulsivity, risk-taking and a sense of invulnerability, coupled with awakening sexuality, put adolescents at particular risk for acquiring HIV (183). The risk of acquiring HIV/AIDS during adolescence comes from high-risk sexual behavior and intravenous drug use. Youth with mental health problems may be at greater risk of exposure to HIV (184,185). Gay and lesbian youth may be at increased risk for mental health concerns (186) and for sexual risk-taking behaviors that place them at particular risk for acquiring HIV (187). Throughout adolescence, for those with vertically acquired HIV, pubertal development and sexuality, fear of contagion and transmissibility, and a need for adherence to complex and often toxic regimens become primary concerns (188). As these adolescents and young adults mature, pregnancy will occur (189), so health care providers must review safer sexual behaviors and make barrier protection available.

Disclosure

The question of when and how to disclose the diagnosis of HIV to one's child or others or both can cause significant psychological distress for children, adolescents, and parents/caregivers. The gamut of emotional reactions seen after disclosure range from no reaction to acute panic or anxiety to acceptance. Delayed reactions are common. Parents may report the onset of new psychosomatic complaints, nightmares, emotional lability, and regressive behavior (181). The American Academy of Pediatrics (190) published guidelines that endorsed disclosure of HIV to older children and adolescents as beneficial and ethically appropriate. Factors associated with a parent's decision to disclose the HIV diagnosis to his or her child, predictors of disclosure, and the psychological impact of disclosure have been described (191–199). Disclosure of an HIV diagnosis to children is an individualized and dynamic process that should take place in a supportive atmosphere of cooperation between health professionals and parents and should be conceived of as a process rather than as a single event (200,201). It is also critical to obtain a clear understanding of the family's cultural background and the factors that might influence responses to an HIV diagnosis or disclosure of the diagnosis to the child (202,203); clear and effective language-interpretation services are essential (204). Cognitive impairment must be assessed as well and may change over the course of time.

Medication Adherence

Adherence in children and adolescents living with HIV is a growing significant clinical issue (205–208). Side effects of HIV treatment such as diarrhea, nausea, skin rashes, unusual deposits of body fat, and lipodystrophy are additional barriers to adolescent adherence (209). Other factors that contribute to poor adherence include impulsivity, short attention spans, and a desire to fit in with peers. Adolescents with advanced HIV disease, who are out of school and have higher alcohol use and depression, are less likely to be adherent (205,208). A social crisis such as a breakup with a girlfriend or boyfriend, a family fight, a problem in school or on the job, or a death can lead to brief periods of nonadherence with taking medications and other health-related behaviors. Assessment for grief, depression, anxiety, and other mental health problems should be considered if nonadherence suddenly occurs. Because developmentally appropriate resistance of authority and experimentation with nonadherence may lead to an increased risk of HIV viral resistance, it may be wise to defer treatment with a protease inhibitor until the treatment team believes the teen will be able to adhere to the regimen. Adolescents are most adherent when they are well informed about their treatment and believe that taking medications is their own decision (181). The goals for these young adults with HIV/AIDS are to increase self-care behaviors such as medical adherence and health-related interactions, to reduce secondary transmission, and to enhance their quality of life (210).

End of Life

In HIV, often no clearly defined moment exists when treatment has failed; rather, the end of life usually occurs as a result of overwhelming opportunistic infections in the face of severe prolonged immunosuppression. The optimum timing and pace of conversations about Advanced Care Planning between adolescents and their families is not known but the Institute of Medicine has recommended that such conversations be initiated at the time of diagnosis and updated periodically during ongoing treatment (211). Before initiating any discussions about end-of-life care with adolescents, it is important to evaluate for depression, bereavement, anxiety, pain, and even unrecognized delirium. Psychiatric illnesses such as depression and anxiety disorders can be identified even in the midst of terminal illnesses, and treatment may alleviate many symptoms and improve quality of life. Meetings with the family to discuss options and to explore palliative care are often most helpful if staff members who have been most intimately involved with the child can be present. Open communication, pain control, involvement with friends and family, distractions, and the maintenance of familiar routines all convey a sense of security that is important in reassuring the dying child (212).

Other Nervous System Abnormalities

MYELOPATHIES

Vacuolar myelopathy, seen in up to 30% of adult AIDS patients at autopsy in the past, is rarely seen in children (213). Spinal corticospinal tract degeneration is one of the characteristic features seen in pediatric AIDS patients at autopsy, but this is not usually a clinical diagnosis (214). Myelopathies can also be due to OIs (HSV, CMV, VZV) or tumors.

PERIPHERAL NEUROPATHIES

Peripheral neuropathies are less common in children than in adults with HIV infection. Several patterns of neuropathy, similar to adult patients, were seen in a retrospective review of 50 children who were referred for nerve-conduction velocities (10) because of clinical concerns. The most common pattern was a distal sensory or axonal neuropathy, possibly related to antiretroviral use or HIV disease itself or both. Carpal tunnel syndrome was less common. A subacute demyelinating neuropathy due to HIV infection was seen in one child, and a lumbosacral polyradiculopathy related to VZV infection was seen in one adolescent. Paresthesias and pain were the most common presenting complaints, followed by weakness or loss of motor milestones.

Symptoms and signs of peripheral neuropathy were seen in one third of 39 children in a recent study conducted in Brazil. The most common clinical findings were diminished vibration sense and diminished ankle jerks. Nerve-conduction studies revealed axonal changes. In general, the features in these children were less severe than those described in adults (215).

Antiretrovirals that have been implicated in peripheral neuropathy include but are not limited to the NRTIs ddI, ddC, and d4T. Peripheral neuropathies due to these agents can be severe and may require discontinuation of the drug.

MYOPATHIES

Numerous muscle disorders have been described in adults with HIV infection, including HIV myopathy, ZDV- and d4T-induced mitochondrial myopathy, and secondary myopathies (due to OIs or lymphoma) (216,217). Typically these patients appear with progressive proximal muscle weakness, sometimes with pain and elevated creatine phosphokinase (CPK). These muscle disorders can occur in children, but are less common.

Summary

Evidence indicates that the incidence of HIV-related CNS disease has declined since the advent of HAART. However, it is possible that more slowly evolving, less-severe CNS disease may become more prevalent in the future as life expectancy increases and as drug resistance occurs. HAART does improve neurocognitive dysfunction in at least a subset of patients with CNS disease. However, nervous system involvement, when it does occur, can have a profound impact on quality of life as well as on survival.

HIV-related CNS disease such as encephalopathy is a common presentation in children as compared with adults, in whom dementia is a late manifestation of HIV disease. Neuropathies and myopathies are less common in children. Early onset of neurological symptoms and signs in HIV-infected infants (before the age of 1 year), such as impaired brain growth and acquired microcephaly, predicts worse neurodevelopmental outcome and seems to have a different significance and pathophysiology than those occurring later in children and adults. The course and pathophysiology of CNS disease in older children and adolescents is more similar to the dementia and motor cognitive dysfunction seen in adults. Children with HIV infection have fewer problems with CNS OIs and are more likely to have CNS neoplasms as the most common cause of mass lesions compared with adults. Also, HIV-infected children have a characteristic vasculopathy, resulting in aneurysmal dilatation of vessels of the circle of Willis with or without associated ischemic infarction or hemorrhage that is not seen in adults. These variations may have important therapeutic and preventive implications.

Behavioral and psychiatric manifestations, especially ADHD and depression, are common in children and adolescents with HIV. In addition, the vicissitudes of coping and living with a stigmatizing disease presents many opportunities for mental health clinicians to support HIV+ children and their families.

The accurate diagnosis and management of neurological and psychiatric disease in pediatric patients remains a challenge. Ongoing and future studies of neuroprophylaxis and neuroprotection are essential in this disease, as well as the development of newer antiretroviral agents with improved CSF penetration.

Questions

1. HIV CNS disease as the first manifestation of HIV disease occurs in children:
   A. more than half of the time.
   B. commonly, about 90% of the time.
   C. HIV never is initially seen as CNS disease in children.
   D. approximately 20% of the time.
   E. HIV rarely appears as CNS disease in children (<1%).

2. The classic triad of HIV encephalopathy is
   A. peripheral neuropathies, cognitive delays, motor delays.
   B. language delay, behavioral abnormalities, peripheral neuropathies.
   C. motor deficits, acquired microcephaly, language delay.
   D. microcephaly, myopathy, myelopathy.

3. Abnormalities seen on computed tomography in treatment-naïve, symptomatic HIV-infected children do NOT include
   A. cortical atrophy.
   B. brain stem infarcts.
   C. white matter attenuation.
   D. basal ganglia calcifications.
   E. ventricular enlargement.

4. The most common CNS opportunistic infection (OI) in children is
   A. herpes simplex virus.
   B. cytomegalovirus.
   C. Cryptococcal meningitis.
   D. varicella zoster virus.
   E. JC virus (papovavirus).

5. All of the following have good CNS penetration except
   A. efavirenz.
   B. zidovudine.
   C. stavudine (d4T).
   D. abacavir.
   E. nevirapine.

6. Psychiatric assessment of new-onset change in behavior in an HIV+ child includes
   A. lumbar puncture.
   B. interview of the child and family.
   C. head CT.
   D. blood tests for CD4 and viral load.
   E. all of the above.

Answers

1. D
2. C
3. B
4. B
5. A
6. E

REFERENCES

1. Belman AL, Ultmann MH, Horoupian D, et al. Neurological complications in infants and children with AIDS. *Ann Neurol.* 1985;8:560–566.
2. Epstein LG, Sharer LR, Joshi VV, et al. Progressive encephalopathy in children with AIDS. *Ann Neurol.* 1985;17:488–496.
3. Epstein LG, Sharer LR, Oleske JM, et al. Neurologic manifestations of HIV infection in children. *Pediatrics.* 1986;78:678–687.
4. Centers for Disease Control and Prevention. Guidelines for the use of antiretroviral agents in pediatric HIV infection. *MMWR Morb Mortal Wkly Rep.* 1998;47:1.
5. Cornblath Dr, McArthur JC. Predominantly sensory neuropathy in patients with AIDS and AIDS-related complex. *Neurology.* 1988;38:794–796.
6. So YT, Holtzman DM, Abrams DI, Olney RK. Peripheral neuropathy associated with acquired immunodeficiency. *Arch Neurol.* 1988;45:945–948.
7. Miller RG. Neuromuscular complications of HIV. *West J Med.* 1994;160:447–454.
8. Simpson SM, Olney RK. Peripheral neuropathies associated with HIV infection. *Neurol Clin.* 1992;10:685–711.
9. Raphael SA, Price ML, Lischner HW, et al. Inflammatory demyelinating polyneuropathy in a child with symptomatic HIV infection. *J Pediatr.* 1991;118:242–245.
10. Floeter MK, Civitello LA, Everett CR, et al. Peripheral neuropathy in children with HIV infection. *Neurology.* 1997;49:207–212.
11. Levy JA, Shimabukuro J, Hollander H, et al. Isolation of AIDS-associated retroviruses from CSF and brain of patients with neurological symptoms. *Lancet.* 1985;11;586–588.
12. Epstein LG, Goudsmit J, Paul DA, et al. Expression of HIV in CSF of children with progressive encephalopathy. *Ann Neurol.* 1987;21:397–401.
13. Koenig S, Gendelman HE, Orenstein JM, et al. Detection of AIDS viruses in macrophages in brain tissue from AIDS patients with encephalopathy. *Science.* 1986;233:1089–1093.
14. Shaw GM, Harper MR, Hahn BH, et al. HTLV-III infection in brains of children and adults with AIDS encephalopathy. *Science.* 1985;227:177–181.
15. Resnick L, DiMarzo-Veronese F, Schupbach J, et al. Intrablood-brain–barrier synthesis of HTLV-III–specific IgG in patients with neurologic symptoms associated with AIDS or AIDS-related complex. *N Engl J Med.* 1985;313:1498–1504.
16. Belman AL, Diamond G, Dickson D, et al. Pediatric AIDS: neurologic syndromes. *Am J Dis Child.* 1988;142:29–35.
17. Civitello LA, Brouwers P, Pizzo PA. Neurologic and neuropsychologic manifestations in 120 children with symptomatic HIV infection. *Ann Neurol.* 1993;34:481.
18. Epstein LG, Sharer LR. Neurology of HIV infection in children. In: Rosenblum ML, Levy RM, Bredesen DE, eds. *AIDS and the nervous system.* New York: Raven Press, 1998:79–101.
19. England JA, Baker CJ, Raskino C, et al. Clinical and laboratory characteristics of a large cohort of symptomatic HIV-infected infants and children. *Pediatr Infect Dis J.* 1996:15:1025–1036.
20. Blanche S, Newell M, Mayaux M, et al. Morbidity and mortality in European children vertically infected by HIV-l. *Acquir Immune Defic Syndr Hum Retrovirol.* 1997;14:442–450.
21. Lobato MN, Caldwell MB, Ng P, Oxtoby MJ. Encephalopathy in children with perinatally acquired HIV infection. *J Pediatr.* 1995;126:710–715.
22. The European Collaborative Study. Neurologic signs in young children with HIV infection. *Pediatr Infect Dis J.* 1990;9:402–406.
23. Sacktor N, Lyles RH, Skolasky R, et al. HIV-associated neurologic disease incidence changes: Multicenter AIDS Cohort Study, 1990-1998. *Neurology.* 2001;56:257–260.
24. McArthur JC, Brew BJ, Nath A. Neurological complications of HIV infection. *Lancet Neurol.* 2005;4:543–555.
25. Shanbhag M, Rutstein R, Zaoutis T, et al. Neurocognitive functioning in pediatric HIV infection. *Arch Pediatr Adolesc Med.* 2005;159:651–656.
26. Chiriboga CA, Fleishman S, Champion S, et al. Incidence and prevalence of HIV encephalopathy in children with HIV infection receiving HAART. *J Pediatr.* 2005;146:402–407.
27. Brouwers P, Tudor-Williams G, DiCarli C, et al. Relation between stage of disease and neurobehavioral measures in children with symptomatic HIV disease. *AIDS.* 1995;9:713–720.
28. Foster CJ, Biggs Rl, Melvin D, et al. Neurodevelopmental outcomes in children with HIV infection under 3 years of age. *Dev Med Child Neurol.* 2006;48:677–682.
29. Vincent J, Bash M, Shanks D, et al. Neurologic symptoms as the initial presentation of HIV infection in pediatric patients. Fifth International Conference on AIDS, Montreal, June 1989 (abst TBP 176).
30. Smith R, Malee K, Charurat M, et al. Timing of perinatal HIV-1 infection and rate of neurodevelopment. *Pediatr Infect Dis J.* 2000;19:862–871.
31. Tardieu M, Le Chenadec J, Persoz A, et al. HIV-l–related encephalopathy in infants compared with children and adults. *Neurology.* 2000;54:1089–1095.
32. Mintz M. Clinical features and treatment interventions for HIV-associated neurologic disease in children. *Semin Neurol.* 1999;19:165–176.
33. Belman AL, Taylor F, Nachman S, Milazzo M. HIV-1–associated CNS disease syndromes in infants and children. *Neurology.* 1994;44:168–169.
34. Mintz M, Tardieu M, Hoyt L, et al. Levodopa therapy improves motor function in HIV-infected children. *Neurology.* 1996;47:1583–1585.

35. Wolters P, Brouwers P, Moss H, Pizzo P. Differential receptive and expressive language functioning of children with symptomatic HIV disease and relation to CT-scan brain abnormalities. *Pediatrics.* 1995;95:112–119.
36. Whitt JK, Hooper SR, Tennison MB, et al. Neuropsychologic functioning of HIV-infected children with hemophilia. *J Pediatr.* 1993;122:52–59.
37. Moss H, Brouwers P, Wolters PL, et al. The development of a Q-sort behavioral rating procedure for pediatric HIV patients. *J Pediatr Psychol.* 1994;19:27–46.
38. Nicholas, Dazord A, Manificat S. Evaluation of life quality for children infected by HIV: validation of a method and preliminary results. *Pediatr AIDS HIV Infect.* 1996;7:254–260.
39. Klaas P, Wolters P, Civitello L, et al. Verbal learning and memory in children with HIV-1. International Neuropsychological Society Meeting, Stockholm Sweden, February 2002:14–17.
40. Martin SC, Wolters PL, Toledo-Tamula MA, et al. Cognitive functioning in school-aged children with vertically-acquired HIV infection being treated with HAART. *Dev Neuropsychol.* 2006;30:633–657.
41. Willen EJ. Neurocognitive outcomes in pediatric HIV. *MRDD Res Rev.* 2006;12:223–228.
42. McArthur J. HIV dementia: an evolving disease. *J Neuroimmunol.* 2004;157:3–10.
43. Lester BM, ElSohly M, Wright LL, et al. The maternal lifestyle study: drug use by meconium toxicology and maternal self-report. *Pediatrics.* 2001;107:309–317.
44. Brown JV, Bakeman R, Coles CD, et al. Prenatal cocaine exposure: a comparison of 2-year-old children in parental and nonparental care. *Child Dev.* 2004;75:1282–1296.
45. Frank DA, Augustyn M, Knight WG, et al. Growth, development, and behavior in early childhood following prenatal cocaine exposure: a systematic review. *JAMA.* 2001;285:1613–1625.
46. Coles CD, Black MM. Impact of prenatal substance exposure on children's health, development, school performance, and risk behavior. *J Pediatr Psychol.* 2006;31:1–4.
47. DeCarli C, Civitello LA, Brouwers P, Pizzo PA. The prevalence of computed axial tomographic abnormalities in 100 consecutive children symptomatic with the human immunodeficiency virus. *Ann Neurol.* 1993;34:198–205.
48. Civitello L, Brouwers P, DeCarli C, Pizzo P. Calcification of the basal ganglia in children with HIV infection. *Ann Neurol.* 1994;36:506.
49. Brouwers P, Tudor-Williams G, DeCarli C, et al. Interrelations among patterns of change in neurocognitive, CT brain imaging, and CD4 measures associated with antiretroviral therapy in children with symptomatic HIV infection. *Adv Neuroimmunol.* 1994;4:223–231.
50. Brouwers P, DeCarli C, Civitello L, et al. Correlation between computed tomographic brain scan abnormalities and neuropsychological function in children with symptomatic HIV disease. *Arch Neurol.* 1995;52:39–44.
51. Brouwers P, Civitello L, DeCarli C, et al. Cerebrospinal fluid viral load is related to cortical atrophy and not to intracerebral calcifications in children with symptomatic HIV disease. *J Neurovirol.* 2000;6:390–397.
52. Civitello LA, Wolters P, Serchuck L, et al. Long-term effect of protease inhibitors on neuropsychological function and neuroimaging in pediatric HIV disease. *Ann Neurol.* 2000;48:513.
53. Tardieu M, Blanche W, Brunelle F. Cerebral magnetic resonance imaging studies in HIV-1 infected children born to seropositive mothers. [Abstract] in: Neuroscience of HIV-1 Infect. Satellite Conference on AIDS, Padova, Italy, 1991:60.
54. Brouwers P, van der Vlugt H, Moss H, et al. White matter changes on CT brain scans are associated with neurobehavioral dysfunction in children with symptomatic HIV disease. *Child Neuropsychol.* 1995;1:93–105.
55. Menon DK, Ainsworth JG, Cox IJ, et al. Proton MR spectroscopy of the brain in AIDS dementia complex. *J Comput Assist Tomogr.* 1992;16:538–542.
56. Lauenberger J, Haussinger D, Bayer S, et al. HIV-related metabolic abnormalities in the brain: depiction with proton MR spectroscopy with short echo times. *Radiology.* 1996;199:805–810.
57. Lu D, Pavlakis S, Frank Y, et al. Proton MR spectroscopy of the basal ganglia in healthy children and children with AIDS. *Radiology.* 1996;199:423–428.
58. Pavlakis SG, Lu D, Frank Y, et al. Brain lactate and N-acetylaspartate in pediatric AIDS encephalopathy. *AJNR Am J Neuroradiol.* 1998;19:383–385.
59. Gabis L, Belman A, Huang W, et al. Clinical and imaging study of HIV-1 infected youth receiving HAART:pilot study using MRS. *J Child Neurol.* 2006;21:486–490.
60. Sei S, Stewart SK, Farley M, et al. Evaluation of HIV-1 RNA levels in cerebrospinal fluid and viral resistance to zidovudine in children with HIV-encephalopathy. *J Infect Dis.* 1996;174:1200–1206.
61. McArthur JC, McClernon DR, Cronin MF, et al. Relationship between HIV-associated dementia and viral load in CSF and brain. *Ann Neurol.* 1997;42:689–698.
62. McClernon DR, Lanier R, Gartner S, et al. HIV in the brain: RNA levels and patterns of zidovudine resistance. *Neurology.* 2001;57:1396–1401.
63. DeLuca A, Ciancio BC, Larussa D, et al. Correlates of independent HIV-1 replication in the CNS and of its controls by antiretrovirals. *Neurology.* 2002;59:342–347.
64. Ellis RJ, Moore DJ, Childers ME, et al. Progression to neuropsychologic impairment in HIV infection predicted by elevated CSF levels of HIV RNA. *Arch Neurol.* 2002;59:923–928.
65. Mintz M, Rapaport TR, Oleske JM, et al. Elevated levels of tumor necrosis factor are associated

with progressive encephalopathy in children with AIDS. *Am J Dis Child.* 1989;143:771–774.
66. Zakum D, Orav J, Korengay J, et al. Correlation of ribonucleic acid polymerase chain reaction acid-dissociated p24 antigen, and neopterin with progression of disease: a retrospective, longitudinal study of vertically-acquired HIV-I infection in children. *J Pediatr.* 1997;130:898–905.
67. McArthur JC, Nance-Sproson TE, Griffin DE, et al. The diagnostic utility of elevation in CSF beta-2-microglogulin in HIV-1 dementia. *Neurology.* 1992;42:1707–1712.
68. Brouwers P, Heyes MP, Moss HA, et al. Quinolinic acid in the CSF of children with symptomatic HIV type 1 disease: relationship to clinical status and therapeutic response. *J Infect Dis.* 1993;168:1380–1386.
69. Cinque P, Vago L, Mengozzi M, et al. Elevated CSF levels of monocyte chemotactic protein-1 correlate with HIV-1 encephalitis and local viral replication. *AIDS.* 1998;12:1327–1332.
70. Sharer LR, Mintz M. Neuropathology of AIDS in children. In: Scaravilli F, ed. *The neuropathology of HIV infection.* Berlin: Springer-Verlag, 1993:201–214.
71. Sharer LR. Neuropathologic aspects of HIV-1 infection in children. In: Gendelman HE, Lipton SA, Epstein L, et al., eds. *The neurology of AIDS.* New York: Chapman & Hall, 1998;408–418.
72. Everall IP, Luthert PJ, Lantos PL. Neuronal loss in the frontal cortex in HIV infection. *Lancet.* 1991;337:1119–1121.
73. Davis L, Hjelle BL, Miller VE, et al. Early viral brain invasion in iatrogenic HIV infection. *Neurology.* 1992;42:1736–1739.
74. Nottett HS, Shawan S. HIV-1 entry into brain: mechanisms for the infiltration of HIV-1 infected macrophages across the blood-brain barrier. In: Gendelman HE, Lipton SA, Epstein L, et al., eds. *The neurology of AIDS.* New York: Chapman & Hall, 1998;49–60.
75. Conant K, Irani D, Sjulson L, et al. A potential role for matrix metalloproteinases in the development of HIV dementia: 6th Conference on Retroviruses and Opportunistic Infections. Chicago, 1999 (abst 282).
76. Ghorpade A, Che M, Labenz C, et al. Mononuclear phagocytes secrete metalloproteinases that affect the neuropathogenesis of AIDS dementia: 6th Conference on Retroviruses and Opportunistic Infections, Chicago, 1999 (abst 283).
77. Mccoig C, Castrejon MM, Saavedra-Lozano J, et al. CSF and plasma concentrations of proinflammatory mediators in HIV-infected children. *Pediatr Infect Dis J.* 2004;23:114–118.
78. Nath A. Pathobiology of HIV dementia. *Semin Neurol.* 1999;19:113–127.
79. Zheng J, Gendelman HE. The HIV-1 associated dementia complex: a metabolic encephalopathy fueled by viral replication in mononuclear phagocytes. *Curr Opin Neurol.* 1997;10:319–325.
80. Tornatore C, Chandra R, Berger JR, Major EO. HIV-1 infection of subcortical astrocytes in the pediatric central nervous system. *Neurology.* 1994;44:481–487.
81. Strizki JM, Albright AV, Sheng H, et al. Infection of primary human microglia and monocyte-derived macrophages with acute HIV-1 isolates: evidence of differential tropism. *J Virol.* 1996;70:7564–7662.
82. Basagra O, Lavi E, Bobroski L, et al. Cellular reservoirs of HIV-1 in the CNS of infected individuals: identification by combination of in situ PCR and immunohistochemistry. *AIDS.* 1996;10:573f–585f.
83. Brew BJ, Wesselngh SL, Gonzabeg M, et al. How HIV leads to neurological disease. *Med J Aust.* 1996;164:233–234.
84. Canto-Nogues C, Sanchez-Ramon S, Alvarez S, et al. HIV-1 infections of neurons might account for progressive HIV-1 associated encephalopathy in children. *J Mol Neurosci.* 2005;27:79–89.
85. Schwartz L, Laurence D, Cavert W, et al. Infection of nestin-positive neural progenitor cells in archival pediatric brain tissue: 12th Conference on Retroviruses and Opportunistic Infections, Boston, Massachusetts, February 2005.
86. Nath A, Haughey NJ, Jones M, et al. Synergistic neurotoxicity by HIV proteins Tat and gp120: protection by memantine. *Ann Neurol.* 2000;47:186–194.
87. Magnuson DS, Knudson BE, Geiger JD, et al. HIV type 1 Tat activates non-N-methyl-D-aspartate excitatory amino acid receptors and causes neurotoxicity. *Ann Neurol.* 1995;37:373–383.
88. Selmaj KW, Rane CS. Tumor necrosis factor mediates myelin and oligodendrocyte damage in vitro. *Ann Neurol.* 1988;23:339.
89. Talley AK, Dewhurst S, Perry SW, et al. Tumor necrosis factor alpha-induced apoptosis in human neuronal cells: protection by the antioxidant N-acetylcysteine and the genes bcl-2 and cmA. *Mol Cell Biol.* 1995;15:2359–2366.
90. Genis P, Jett M, Bernton EW, et al. Cytokines and arachidonic metabolites produced during HIV-infected macrophage-astroglia interactions: implications for the neuropathogenesis of HIV disease. *J Exp Med.* 1992;176:1703–1718.
91. Bukrinsky MI, Nottet HS, Schmidtmayerova H, et al. Regulation of nitric oxide synthase activity in HIV-1 infected monocytes: implications for HIV-associated neurologic disease. *J Exp Med.* 1995;181:735–745.
92. Sanders VJ, Pittman CA, White MG, et al. Chemokines and receptors in HIV encephalitis. *AIDS.* 1998;12:1021–1026.
93. Mitchell CD. HIV-1 encephalopathy among perinatally infected children: neuropathogenesis and response to HAART. *MRDD Res Rev.* 2006;12:216–222.
94. Zheng J, Thylan MR, Ghorpade A, et al. Linkages between intracellular CXCR4 signaling, neuronal apoptosis, and the neuropathogenic mechanisms for HIV-1-associated dementia: 6th Conference on Retroviruses and Opportunistic Infections, Chicago, 1999 (abst 288).

95. Samson M, Libert F, Doranz BJ, et al. Resistance to HIV-1 infection in Caucasian individuals bearing mutant alleles of the CCR5 chemokine receptor gene. *Nature.* 1996;382:722–725.
96. Singh KK, Barroga CF, Hughes MD, et al. Genetic influence of CCR5, CCR@, and SDF-1 variants on HIV-1-related disease progression and neurological impairment in children with symptomatic HIV-1 infection. *J Infect Dis.* 2003;188:1461–1472.
97. Petito CK, Roberts B. Evidence of apoptotic cell death in HIV encephalitis. *Am J Pathol.* 1995;146:1121–1130.
98. Lipton SA. Similarity of neuronal cell injury and death in AIDS dementia and focal cerebral ischemia: potential treatment with NMDA open-channel blockers and nitric-oxide-related species. *Brain Pathol.* 1996;6:507–517.
99. Ferrarese C, Aliprandi A, Tremolizzo L, et al. Increased glutamate in CSF and plasma of patients with HIV dementia. *Neurology.* 2001;57:671–675.
100. Kozlowski PB, Sher JH, Dickson DW, et al. CNS in pediatric HIV infection: a multicenter study. In: Kozlowski PB, Snider DA, Vietze PM, et al., eds. *Brain in pediatric AIDS.* Basel: Karger, 1990:132–146.
101. Kalayjian RC, Cohen ML, Bonomo RA, et al. CMV ventriculoencephalitis in AIDS. *Medicine.* 1993;72:67–77.
102. Holland NR, Power C, Matthews VP, et al. CMV encephalitis in AIDS. *Neurology.* 1994;44:507–514.
103. Fuller GN, Guilof RJ, Scaravilli F, et al. Combined HIV-CMV encephalitis presenting with brainstem signs. *J Neurol Neurosurg Psychiatry.* 1989;52:975–979.
104. Annunziato PW, Gershon AA. Herpesvirus infections in children infected with HIV. In: Wilfert CM, Pizzo PA, eds. *Pediatric AIDS: the challenge of HIV infection in infants, children and adolescents.* Baltimore: Williams & Wilkins, 1998:205–225.
105. Berger JRF, Scott G, Albrecht J, et al. PML in HIV-1 infected children. *AIDS.* 1992;6:837–842.
106. Walsh TJ, Muller FM, Groll A, et al. Fungal infections in children with HIV. In: Wilfert CM, Pizzo PA, eds. *Pediatric AIDS: the challenge of HIV infection in infants, children and adolescents.* Baltimore: Williams & Wilkins, 1998:183–204.
107. American Academy of Neurology. Evaluation and management of intracranial mass lesions in AIDS. *Neurology.* 1998;50:21–26.
108. Simonds RJ, Gonzalo O. *Pneumocystis carinii* pneumonia and toxoplasmosis. In: Wilfert CM, Pizzo PA, eds. *Pediatric AIDS: the challenge of HIV infection in infants, children and adolescents.* Baltimore: Williams & Wilkins, 1998:251–265.
109. NICHD IVIG Study Group. IVIG for the prevention of bacterial infections in children with symptomatic HIV infection. *N Engl J Med.* 1991;325:73–80.
110. Cohen BA, Berger JR. Neurologic opportunistic infections in AIDS. Gendelman HE, et al., eds. New York: Chapman and Hall; 1998:303–332.
111. Dickson DW, Llen AJF, Werdenheim KM, et al. CNS pathology in children with AIDS and focal neurologic signs: stroke and lymphoma. In: Kozlowski PB, Snider DA, Vietze PM, et al., eds. *Brain in pediatric AIDS.* Basel: Karger, 1990:147–157.
112. Epstein LG, DiCarlo FJ, Joshi VV, et al. Primary lymphomas of the CNS in children with AIDS. *Pediatrics.* 1988;82:355–363.
113. Park YD, Belman AL, Kim TS, et al. Stroke in pediatric AIDS. *Ann Neurol.* 1990;28:303–311.
114. Frank Y, Lim W, Kahn E, et al. Multiple ischemic infarcts in a child with AIDS, varicella-zoster infection and cerebral vasculitis. *Pediatr Neurol.* 1989;5:64–67.
115. Husson RN, Saini R, Lewis LL. Cerebral artery aneurysms in children infected with HIV. *J Pediatr.* 1992;121:927–930.
116. Mazzoni P, Chiriboga CA, Millar WS, Rogers A. Intracerebral aneurysms in HIV infection: case report and literature review. *Pediatr Neurol.* 2000;23:252–255.
117. Kure K, Park YD, Kim TS, et al. Immunohistochemical localization of an HIV epitope in cerebral aneurysmal arteriopathy in pediatric AIDS. *Pediatr Pathol.* 1989;9:655–667.
118. Pialeux G, Fournier S, Moulignier A, et al. CNS as a sanctuary for HIV-1 infection despite treatment with zidovudine, lamivudine and indinavir. *AIDS.* 1997;11:1302–1303.
119. Gisslen M, Norkrans G, Svennerholm B. HIV-1 RNA detectable with ultrasensitive PCR in plasma but not in CSF during combination treatment with zidovudine, and indinavir. *AIDS.* 1998;12:114–115.
120. Pomerantz RJ. Residual HIV-1 infection during antiretroviral therapy: the challenge of viral persistence. *AIDS.* 2001;15:1201–1211.
121. Stingele K, Haas J, Zimmermann T, et al. Independent HIV replication in paired CSF and blood viral isolates during antiretroviral therapy. *Neurology.* 2001;56:355–361.
122. McArthur JC, Sacktor N, Selnes O. HIV-associated dementia. *Semin Neurol.* 1999;19:129–150.
123. Enting RH, Hoetelmans MW, Lange JMA, et al. Antiretriviral drugs and the CNS. *AIDS.* 1998;12:1941–1955.
124. Pizzo P, Eddy J, Falloon J, et al. Effect of continuous IV infusion of zidovudine in children with symptomatic HIV infection. *N Engl J Med.* 1988;319:889–896.
125. McKinney RE, Maha MA, Connor EM, et al. A multicenter trial of oral zidovudine in children with HIV infection. *N Engl J Med.* 1991;324:1018–1025.
126. Portegies P, de Gans J, Lange JM, et al. Declining incidence of AIDS dementia complex after introduction of zidovudine treatment. *Br Med J.* 1989;299:819–821.

127. Kline MW, Dunkle LM, Church JA, et al. A phase I/II evaluation of stavudine (d4T) in children with HIV infection. *Pediatrics.* 1995;96:247–252.
128. Butler KM, Husson RN, Balis FM, et al. Dideoxyinosine in children with symptomatic HIV infection. *N Engl J Med.* 1991;324:1018–1025.
129. Arendt G, Giesen HV, Hefter H, and Theisen A. Therapeutic effects of nucleoside analogues on psychomotor slowing in HIV infection. *AIDS.* 2001;15:493–500.
130. Englund JA, Baker CJ, Raskino C, et al. A trial comparing zidovudine, didanosine, and combination therapy for initial treatment of symptomatic HIV-infected children. *N Engl J Med.* 1997;336:1704–1712.
131. Sacktor N, Tarwater PM, Skolasky MA, et al. CSF antiretroviral drug penetrance and the treatment of HIV-associated psychomotor slowing. *Neurology.* 2001;57:542–544.
132. Saavadra-Lozano J, Ramos JT, Sanz F, et al. Salvage therapy with abacavir and other reverse transcriptase inhibitors for HIV-1-associated encephalopathy. *Pediatr Infect Dis J.* 2006;25:1142–1152.
133. Luzuriaga K, Bryson Y, Krogstad P, et al. Combination treatment with zidovudine, didanosine, and nevirapine in infants with HIV-1 infection. *N Engl J Med.* 1997;336:1343–1349.
134. Martin C, Sonnerborg A, Svensson JO, Stahle L. Indinavir-based treatment of HIV-1 infected patients: efficacy in the central nervous system. *AIDS.* 1999;13:1227–1232.
135. Mueller BU, Nelson RP Jr, Sleasman J, et al. A phase I/II study of the protease inhibitor ritonavir in children with HIV infection. *Pediatrics.* 1998;101:335–343.
136. Mueller BU, Sleasman J, Nelson RP Jr, et al. A phase I/II study of the protease inhibitor indinavir in children with HIV infection. *Pediatrics.* 1998;102:101–109.
137. van der Sandt ICJ, Vos CMP, Nabulsi L, et al. Assessment of active transport of HIV protease inhibitors in various cell lines and the in vitro blood-brain barrier. *AIDS.* 2001;15:483–491.
138. Suarez S, Baril L, Stankoff B, et al. Outcome of patients with HIV-1-related cognitive impairment on HAART. *AIDS.* 2001;15:195–200.
139. Maschke M, Kastrup O, Esser S, et al. Incidence and prevalence of neurological disorders associated with HIV since the introduction of HAART. *J Neurol Neurosurg Psychiatry.* 2000;69:376–380.
140. Chang L, Ernst T, Leonido-Yee M, et al. HAART reverses brain metabolite abnormalities in mild HIV dementia. *Neurology.* 1999;53:782–789.
141. Stankoff B, Tourbah A, Suarez S, et al. Clinical and spectroscopic improvement in HIV-associated cognitive impairment. *Neurology.* 2001;56:112–115.
142. Chang L, Witt M, Miller E, et al. Cerebral metabolite changes during the first nine months of HAART. *Neurology.* 2001;56(suppl 3):A474.
143. Tepper VJ, Farley H, Rothman MI, et al. Neurodevelopmental/neuroradiologic recovery of a child infected with HIV after treatment with combination antiretroviral therapy using the HIV-specific protease inhibitor, ritonavir. *Pediatrics.* 1998;101:e7.
144. Rosenfeldt R, Henrik N, Valerius H, Paerregaard A. Regression of HIV-associated progressive encephalopathy of childhood during HAART. *Scand J Infect Dis.* 2000;32:571–574.
145. McCoig C, Castrejon MM, Castano E, et al. Effect of combination antiretroviral therapy on CSF HIV RNA, HIV resistance, and clinical manifestations of encephalopathy. *J Pediatr.* 2002;141:36–44.
146. Jeremy R, Kim S, Nozyce M, et al. Neuropsychological functioning and viral load in stable antiretroviral therapy-experienced HIV-infected children. *Pediatrics.* 2005;115;380–387.
147. Tamula MA, Wolters PL, Walsek C, et al. Cognitive decline with immunologic and virologic stability in four children with HIV disease. *Pediatrics.* 2003;112:679–684.
148. Simpson DM. HIV-associated dementia: review of pathogenesis, prophylaxis and treatment studies of zidovudine therapy. *Clin Infect Dis.* 1999;29:19–34.
149. Sanchez-Ramon S, Resino S, Bellon Cano JM, et al. Neuroprotective effects of early antiretrovirals in vertical HIV infection. *Pediatr Neurol.* 2003;29:218–221.
150. Geisen HJ, Hefter H, Jablonski H, Arendt G. HAART is neuroprophylactic in HIV-1 infection. *J Acquir Immune Defic Syndr.* 2000;23:380–385.
151. Neuenberg JK, Brodt HR, Herndier BG, et al. HIV-related neuropathy, 1985-1999: rising prevalence of HIV encephalopathy in the era of HAART. *J Acquir Immune Def Syndr.* 2002;31:171–177.
152. Chao CC, Hu S, Close K, et al. Cytokine release from microglia: differential inhibition by pentoxifylline and dexamethasone. *J Infect Dis.* 1992;166:847–853.
153. Steihm ER, Bryson YS, Frenhal LM, et al. Prednisone improves HIV encephalopathy in children. *Pediatr Infect Dis J.* 1992;11:49.
154. Peterson PK, Hu S, Sheng WS, et al. Thalidomide inhibits TNF-alpha production by lipopolysaccharide and lipoarabine mannah-stimulated human microglial cells. *J Infect Dis.* 1995;172:1137–1140.
155. Galgani S, Balestra P, Narciso P, et al. Nimodipine plus zidovudine versus zidovudine alone in the treatment of HIV-1-associated cognitive deficits. *AIDS.* 1997;11:1520–1521.
156. Navia BA, Yiannoutsos CT, Chang L, et al. ACTG 301: a phase II randomized double-blind, placebo-controlled trial of memantine for AIDS dementia complex. *Neurology.* 2001;56(suppl):A474–A475.
157. Turchan JT, Gairola C, Schifitto G, et al. CSF from HIV demented patients causes mitochondrial dysfunction reversible by novel antioxidants. *Neurology.* 2001;56(suppl 3):475.

158. Dana Consortium. On the therapy of HIV dementia and related cognitive disorders: a randomized, double-blind, placebo-controlled trial of deprenyl and thioctic acid in HIV-associated cognitive impairment. *Neurology.* 1998;50:645–651.
159. Angelino AF, Treisman GJ. Management of psychiatric disorders in patients infected with human immunodeficiency virus. *Clin Infect Dis.* 2001;33:847–856.
160. Grant I, Atkinson JH. Neuropsychiatric aspects of HIV infection and AIDS. In: Sadock BJ, Sadock VA, eds. *Kaplan and Sadock's comprehensive textbook of psychiatry,* 7th ed. Philadelphia: Lippincott Williams & Wilkins, 2000:320.
161. Antoni N, Perez-Duenas B, Fortuny C, et al. Botulinum toxin in the treatment of spasticity in HIV-infected children affected with progressive encephalopathy. *AIDS.* 1004;18:352–353.
162. Kolaski K. Use of intrathecal baclofen in a child with spastic paraparesis related to HIV infection: a case report. *Arch Phys Med Rehabil.* 2006;87:1001–1003.
163. Lourie KJ, Pao M, Brown LK, Hunter H. Psychiatric issues in pediatric HIV/AIDS. In: Citron K, Brouillette MJ, Beckett A, eds. *HIV and psychiatry: a training and resource manual.* 2nd ed. Cambridge, UK: Cambridge University Press, 2005:81–195.
164. Scharko AM. DSM psychiatric disorders in the context of pediatric HIV/AIDS. *AIDS Care.* 2006;18:441–445.
165. Misdrahi D, Vila G, Funk-Brentano I, et al. DSM-IV mental disorders and neurological complications in children and adolescents with human immunodeficiency virus type 1 infection (HIV-1). *Eur Psychiatry.* 2004;19:182–184.
166. Gaughan DM, Hughes MD, Oleske JM, et al. Psychiatric hospitalizations among children and youths with human immunodeficiency virus infection. *Pediatrics.* 2004;113:e544–e551.
167. Wiener L, Battles H, Ryder C, Pao M. Psychotropic medication use in HIV-infected youth receiving treatment in a single institution. *J Child Adolesc Psychopharmacol.* 2006;16:741–753.
168. American Psychiatric Association. *Diagnostic and statistical manual of mental disorders.* 4th ed. Washington, DC: American Psychiatric Association, 1994.
169. Cesena M, Lee DO, Cebollero AM, et al. Behavioral symptoms of pediatric HIV-1 encephalopathy successfully treated with clonidine. *J Am Acad Child Adolesc Psychiatry.* 1995;34:302–306.
170. Palacin PS, Aramburo A, Moraga FA, et al. Neuropsychiatric reaction induced by abacavir in a pediatric human immunodeficiency virus-infected patient. *Pediatri Infect Dis J.* 2006;25:382.
171. Walling VR, Pfefferbaum B. The use of methylphenidate in a depressed adolescent with AIDS. *J Dev Behav Pediatr.* 1990;11:195–197.
172. Kowatch RA, Delbello MP. Pediatric bipolar disorder: emerging diagnostic and treatment approaches. *Child Adolesc Psychiatry Clin North Am.* 2006;15:73–108.
173. Turkel SB, Tavaré CJ. Delirium in children and adolescents. *J Neuropsychiatry Clin Neurosci.* 2003;15:431–435.
174. Treisman GL, Kaplin AI. Neurologic and psychiatric complications of antiretroviral agents. *AIDS.* 2002;16:1201–1215.
175. Hirschfeld S, Moss H, Dragisic K, et al. Pain in pediatric human immunodeficiency virus infection: incidence and characteristics in a single-institution pilot study. *Pediatrics.* 1996;98:449–452.
176. Lolekha R, Chanthavanich P, Limkittikul K, et al. Pain: a common symptom in human immunodeficiency virus–infected Thai children. *Acta Paediatr.* 2004;93:891–898.
177. Gaughan DM, Hughes MD, Seage GR 3rd, et al. The prevalence of pain in pediatric human immunodeficiency virus/acquired immunodeficiency syndrome as reported by participants in the Pediatric Late Outcomes Study (PACTG 219). *Pediatrics.* 2002;109:1144–1152.
178. Duff AJA. Incorporating psychological approaches into routine paediatric venipuncture. *Arch Dis Child.* 2003;88:931–937.
179. Greco C, Berde C. Pain management for the hospitalized pediatric patient. *Pediatr Clin North Am.* 2005;52:995–1027.
180. Campbell AT. Consent, competence, and confidentiality related to psychiatric conditions in adolescent medical practice. *Adolesc Med.* 2006;17:25–47.
181. Wiener L, Havens J, Ng W. Psychosocial problems in pediatric HIV infection. In: Shearer WT, ed. *Medical management of AIDS in children.* Philadelphia: WB Saunders, 2003;373–394.
182. Cohen J, Reddington C, Jacobs D, et al. School-related issues among HIV-infected children. *Pediatrics.* 1997;100:e8.
183. Samples CL, Goodman E, Woods E. Epidemiology and medical management of adolescents. In: Pizzo PA, Wilfert C, eds. *Pediatric AIDS,* 3rd ed. Baltimore: Lippincott Williams & Wilkins, 1998:615.
184. Brown LK, Danovsky MB, Lourie KJ, et al. Adolescents with psychiatric disorders and the risk of HIV. *J Am Acad Child Adolesc Psychiatry.* 1997;36:1609–1617.
185. Donenberg GR, Emerson E, Bryant FB, et al. Understanding AIDS-risk behavior among adolescents in psychiatric care: links to psychopathology and peer relationships. *J Am Acad Child Adolesc Psychiatry.* 2001;40:642–653.
186. Fergusson DM, Horwood J, Beautrais AL. Is sexual orientation related to mental health problems and suicidality in young people? *Arch Gen Psychiatry.* 1999;56:876–880.
187. Garofalo R, Wolf RC, Kessel S, et al. The association between health risk behaviors and sexual orientation among a school-based sample of adolescents. *Pediatrics.* 1998;101:895–902.

188. Grubman S, Gross E, Lerner-Weiss N, et al. Older children and adolescents living with perinatally acquired human immunodeficiency virus infection. *Pediatrics.* 1995;95:657–663.
189. Centers for Disease Control and Prevention. Pregnancy in perinatally HIV-infected adolescents and young adults: Puerto Rico, 2002. *MMWR.* 2003;52:149–151.
190. American Academy of Pediatrics Committee on Pediatrics AIDS. Disclosure of illness status to children and adolescents with HIV infection. *Pediatrics.* 1999;103:164–166.
191. Nehring WM, Lashley FR, Malm K. Disclosing the diagnosis of pediatric HIV infection: mother's views. *J Soc Pediatr Nurs.* 2000;5:5–14.
192. Gerson AC, Joyner M, Fosarelli P, et al. Disclosure of HIV diagnosis to children: when, where, why, and how. *J Pediatr Health Care.* 2001;15:161–167.
193. Mellins CA, Brackis-Cott E, Dolezal C, et al. Patterns of status disclosure to perinatally HIV-infected children and subsequent mental health outcomes. *Clin Child Psychol Psychiatry.* 2002;7:10–114.
194. Lester P, Chesney M, Cooke M, et al. When the time comes to talk about HIV: factors associated with diagnostic disclosure and emotional distress in HIV-infected children. *Acquir Immune. Defic Syndr.* 2002;31:309–317.
195. Sherman BF, Bonanno GA, Wiener L, Battles HB. When children tell their friends they have AIDS: possible consequences for psychological well-being and disease progression. *Psychosom Med.* 2000;62:238–247.
196. Instone SL. Perceptions of children with HIV infection when not told for so long: implications for diagnosis disclosure. *J Pediatr Health Care.* 2000;14:235–243.
197. Wiener L, Battles H, Heilman N. Factors associated with parents' decision to disclose their HIV diagnosis to children. *Child Welfare.* 1998;LXXVII:115–135.
198. Bachanas P, Kullgren K, Schwartz K, et al. Predictors of psychological adjustment in school-age children infected with HIV. *J Pediatr Psychol.* 2001;26:343–352.
199. Howland LC, Gortmaker SL, Mofenson LM, et al. Effects of negative life events on immune suppression in children and youth infected with human immunodeficiency virus type 1. *Pediatrics.* 2000;106:540–546.
200. Lipson M. What do you say to a child with AIDS? *Hastings Cent Rep.* 1993;23:6–12.
201. Lipson M. Disclosure of diagnosis to children with human immunodeficiency virus or acquired immunodeficiency syndrome. *J Dev Behav Pediatr.* 1994;15:S61–S65.
202. Mason HRC, Marks G, Simoni JM, et al. Culturally sanctioned secrets: Latino men's nondisclosure of HIV infection to family, friends, and lovers. *Health Psychol.* 1995;14:6–12.
203. Mettler MA, Borden K, Lopez E, et al. Racial and ethnic patterns of disclosure to children with HIV. Presented at the American Psychological Association's annual conference, Chicago, IL, 1997.
204. Munet-Vilaro F. Delivery of culturally competent care to children with cancer and their families: the Latino experience. *J Pediatr Oncol Nurs.* 2004;21:155–159.
205. Wiener L, Riekert K, Ryder C, Wood L. Assessing medication adherence in adolescents with HIV when electronic monitoring is not feasible. *AIDS Patient Care STDS.* 2004;18:31–43.
206. Van Dyke RB, Lee S, Johnson GM, et al. Reported adherence as a determinant of response to highly active antiretroviral therapy in children who have human immunodeficiency virus infection. *Pediatrics.* 2002;109:e61.
207. Hammami N, Nostlinger C, Hoeree T, et al. Integrating adherence to highly active antiretroviral therapy into children's daily lives: a qualitative study. *Pediatrics.* 2004;114:591–597.
208. Murphy DA, Belzer M,. Durako SJ, et al. Longitudinal antiretroviral adherence among adolescents infected with human immunodeficiency virus. *Arch Pediatr Adolesc Med.* 2005;159:764–770.
209. Santos CP, Felipe YX, Braga PE, et al. Self-perception of body changes in persons living with HIV/AIDS: prevalence and associated factors. *AIDS.* 2005;19:S14–S21.
210. Rotheram-Borus MJ, Miller S. Secondary prevention for youths living with HIV. *AIDS Care.* 1998;10:17–34.
211. Field MJ, Behrman RE, eds. *When children die: improving palliative and end-of-life care for children and their families.* Washington, DC: The National Academies Press, 2003.
212. Wiener L, Hersh SP, Kazak A. Psychiatric and psychosocial support for child and family. In: Pizzo PA, Poplack DG, eds. *Principles and practice of pediatric oncology.* 5th ed. Philadelphia: Lippincott, 2005;1414–1445.
213. Petito CK, Navia BA, Cho ES, et al. Vacuolar myelopathy pathologically resembling subacute combined degeneration in patients with AIDS. *N Engl J Med.* 1985;312:874–879.
214. Dickson DW, Belman AL, Tin TS, et al. Spinal cord pathology in pediatric AIDS. *Neurology.* 1989;39:227–235.
215. Prufer de QC, Araujo A, Nascimento OJM, et al. Distal sensory polyneuropathy in a cohort of HIV-infected children over five years of age. *Pediatrics.* 2000;106:1–4.
216. Dalakas M, Illa I, Pezeshkpour GH, et al. Mitochondrial myopathy caused by long-term zidovudine therapy. *N Engl J Med.* 1990;322:1098–1105.
217. Walter EB, Drucker RP, McKinney RE, et al. Myopathy in HIV-infected children receiving long-term zidovudine therapy. *J Pediatr.* 1991;119:152–155.

CHAPTER 15

Pediatric Multiple Sclerosis

LAUREN B. KRUPP

Multiple sclerosis (MS) is an immune-mediated inflammatory demyelinating disorder of the central nervous system (CNS). MS can develop in children and adolescents, although usually it affects young and middle-aged adults. An estimated 2% to 3% of patients with MS are younger than 18 years (1,2). They represent an underserved, understudied MS subgroup. Although much of our understanding of the pathogenesis, clinical and radiologic features, and treatment of MS is based on studies of adult patients, the clinical and research experience with children has grown. The study of pediatric MS has the potential to provide insights into the nature of MS for all affected individuals.

MS is now a treatable disease, whereas, prior to 1993, no therapies to alter the disease course were available. The ability to treat MS has accelerated the need to establish an accurate diagnosis quickly, particularly in children, because treatment is most effective when started early in the disease course (3). Fortunately, magnetic resonance imaging (MRI) has facilitated the diagnosis.

Definition

To facilitate clinical research and establish uniform criteria for the diagnosis, an operational and consensus-based definition for pediatric MS was developed. Although it still must be tested in prospective longitudinal studies (4), the definition is a first step in recognizing the key elements of the pediatric MS diagnosis. The criteria for the diagnosis require:

1. Multiple episodes of CNS demyelination disseminated in time and space with no lower age limit.
2. MRI findings can be applied to meet dissemination-in-space criterion if they show three of the following four features (a) nine or more white matter lesions or one gadolinium-enhancing lesion, (b) three or more periventricular lesions, (c) one juxtacortical lesion, and (d) an infratentorial or spinal cord lesion.
3. The combination of an abnormal cerebral spinal fluid (CSF) and two lesions on the MRI, of which one must be in the brain, can also be used to meet dissemination-in-space criterion; the CSF must show either oligoclonal bands (OCBs) or an elevated immunoglobulin G (IgG) index.
4. MRI can be used to satisfy criteria for dissemination in time after the initial clinical event, even in the absence of a new clinical demyelinating event. A new gadolinium-enhancing lesion or new T_2 lesion 3 months after the clinical event can be a surrogate for another clinical event.

The diagnosis of MS relies on the clinical features of the disease. CSF can help exclude other conditions, such as lymphoma or Lyme disease, and can provide additional confirmation by the presence of either OCBs (immunoglobulins whose antigenic target still remains unclear) or an elevated IgG index (the relative amount of IgG in the CSF compared with the serum). In some instances of MS, the CSF may be negative for OCBs and the IgG index. Typically, the cell count in the CSF is less than 50 cells per milliliter. Evoked-potential testing also is useful for identifying silent lesions but is less sensitive than MRI.

Demographic Features

The exact prevalence of pediatric MS is unknown. The studies that suggest a prevalence of 3% to 5% among children younger than 16 years are all retrospective (5). Nonetheless, if approximately 4% of the MS population is younger than 18 years, it can be estimated that worldwide, 100,000 or more children have MS. The frequency of MS steadily increases with age, such that in a fraction of a percentage, MS develops during early childhood, whereas among teens, the frequency is closer to 3%.

The disease usually begins with a mean age at onset between 8 and 14 years, depending on whether the cohort has a cut-off below 16 or 18 years (1,2,6). The distribution of boys and girls varies according to age. For children age 10 years or older, girls outnumber boys by approximately 2.5:1 (1,2,7,8). For children younger than 10 years, the ratio of girls and boys is approximately 0.5:1 (9,10). The increase in girls during puberty is recapitulated in adult MS. Whereas more women than men with MS are among the 20- to 40-year-old age group, in older age groups (consistent with the menopausal age range), men begin to equal women in frequency. These demographic features suggest that sex hormones play a role in MS pathogenesis. Additional evidence pointing to the role of sex hormones comes from a pilot clinical trial of MS in men that showed protective effects of testosterone (11).

Clinical Findings

SYMPTOMS AND SIGNS

Presenting symptoms of MS often depend on the location of the white-matter lesions. Initial symptoms typically include optic neuritis (unilateral or bilateral), motor weakness, balance problems, sensory disturbance, loss of coordination, bladder dysfunction, or problems related to brainstem involvement (facial numbness, diplopia). In different clinical series, motor, visual, or sensory disturbances are the most common presentation (5). A polysymptomatic onset has been described in 8% to 67% of the patients (1,2,5,7).

At presentation, children compared with adults tend to have more brainstem and cerebellar symptoms, encephalopathy, or optic neuritis (12,13). Among those younger than 6 years, seizures, marked alteration in consciousness, a polysymptomatic onset, and atypical MRIs are more frequent (9,12).

MRI FINDINGS

The MRI is extremely valuable in the diagnosis of MS. In contrast to other demyelinating disorders of childhood, MS lesions predominantly involve the white matter (Fig. 15.1). Cortical or central gray matter involvement is uncommon (6). The lesions tend to be discrete, often associated with gadolinium enhancement, and are usually periventricular (7). Although it is less true of the youngest pediatric MS group, many older children have MRI

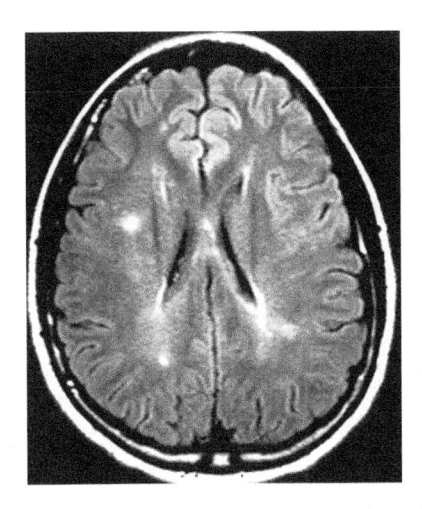

■ **FIGURE 15.1** This MRI from a 15-year-old girl with MS shows, in this axial flare image, typical discrete hyperintense white-matter lesions in the patient's right corona radiata, posterior periventricular areas, and body of the corpus callosum.

findings that are similar to those of adults. In adults, criteria for a "positive MRI" include three of the four requirements: (a) one gadolinium-enhancing lesion or nine lesions involving the white matter, (b) three or more periventricular lesions, (c) an infratentorial, and (d) a juxtacortical lesion. A lesion involving the spinal cord can be used as either one of the nine lesions or instead be of an infratentorial location. If a child or teenager with possible MS meets the MRI criteria established for adults with MS, then the MRI findings are highly supportive of the MS diagnosis. Moreover, these children tend to have a worse prognosis than do those whose MRIs are less specific.

Some children with MS who lack typical MRI findings can have large tumefactive lesions associated with edema, rarely a mass effect, or deep grey-matter involvement (14). In these cases, the diagnosis can be more challenging.

DISEASE COURSE

The course in more than 93% to 98% of pediatric MS cases (5) is characterized by relapses and remissions. Relapses are defined as the development of new neurological symptoms and signs lasting at least 24 hours that subsequently improve or stabilize. A progressive course without relapses is rare and usually suggests an alternative diagnosis. Over time (sometimes decades), most children with MS accumulate neurological impairments. However, this progression occurs more gradually in children than in adults with the disease (12,13). Less commonly, pediatric MS can have an aggressive course, and severe deficits during childhood can develop (15).

The classification of MS subtypes refers to the different patterns of the disease course. Although this classification was developed for adult MS cases, it also applies to pediatric ones. The relapsing–remitting MS (RRMS) subtype is the most common type. Residual deficits may or may not develop from the relapse. Over time, most adults and children with MS will have a transition from a relapsing–remitting course to progression, defined as secondary progressive MS. During the progressive phase of the disease, patients simply insidiously and gradually accumulate increasing deficits. A much less common MS subtype—estimated in most series of children to occur in fewer than 3%—is primary progressive MS. In this subtype, no relapses occur at the onset, but instead, patients follow a steadily progressive course from the beginning. In primary progressive MS, symptoms and signs accumulate over time, and relapses never occur. Another even more rare MS subtype is progressive relapsing MS. In these patients, the initial course is one of gradual progression; however, these individuals subsequently have occasional relapses, and such individuals are classified as having progressive relapsing MS.

Patients with relapsing–remitting disease will make a transition to a secondary progressive course at different rates. Among adults, the transition typically occurs 7 to 10 years after diagnosis. In contrast, children progress more gradually, and a secondary progressive form of the disease develops approximately 20 years after the diagnosis. During the same time period, in more than half of children with MS, permanent deficits will develop (8,12,13). Hence, the majority of children and adolescents will grapple with the more disabling aspects of their disease during young adulthood. However, compared with an adult onset, those with a pediatric onset will have permanent deficits, including inability to ambulate independently, at a significantly younger age (2,8,12,13).

Prognostic Factors

It is extremely difficult to predict the disease course in any one individual child or adult with MS. Some individuals show minimal signs of the disease throughout their course and experience few relapses. Others relapse frequently and rapidly progress to requiring a wheel chair.

Some features help to determine whether, at the time of a child's first demyelinating event, a likelihood of a subsequent event exists. Risk for the development of subsequent relapses—making a diagnosis of MS much more likely—was addressed in a prospective study of 168 children who had their first demyelinating event. An increased risk for a subsequent event was found if the initial event was optic neuritis or if the child was older than 10 years (16). A decreased risk for a second event was noted in children first seen with spinal cord symptoms or alteration in mental status (16).

The factors predicting the disease course can be more difficult to define than those features associated with a second clinical episode. Those with an initial progressive course without any associated relapses (primary progressive MS) consistently do worse than those with a relapsing–remitting course (12,13,17). Studies of adults with MS have identified prognostic features related to relapses and development of impairments. The degree of recovery from the initial event, time to the second event, and the number of clinical events in the first 5 years have been identified as prognostic indicators of subsequent disability (18). Among children, besides a progressive course at onset, female gender, short interval between the first and second attacks, clinical symptoms of sphincter dysfunction, number of relapses within the first 2 years, absence of encephalopathy, and typical MS MRI findings predict more-pronounced disease (12,13,17,19). Although factors can be linked to more or less severe disease, for any one patient it is extremely difficult to predict the subsequent course.

Psychosocial Features

BEHAVIORAL ISSUES

Many aspects of pediatric MS pose challenges to families beyond those associated with chronic illness. The condition is rare, its course is uncertain, its manifestations are unpredictable and varied, and therapies are incomplete. Behavioral problems include denial, difficulty with family and peers, and noncompliance with therapy (20). A further concern is that perceived stress can increase the probability of another MS relapse (21).

Young people with MS or other chronic diseases may be at a particularly high risk for additional psychological problems (22) because of the effects of the disease on the brain, as well as the psychological reaction to the chronic illness. In adults with MS, depression is associated with an increased lesion burden in the inferior–medial frontal–temporal areas (23). Similar findings might be expected to apply to children with MS.

AFFECTIVE DISORDERS

In our experience of 13 children with MS, unselected for psychiatric illness and who underwent psychiatric interviews, six (46%) had affective disorders including major depression, anxiety disorder, and panic attacks. Much more information on psychiatric complications of MS comes from studies of adults. All show that affective disorders are frequent (24) and are more common compared with other neurological diseases with similar levels of disability.

More than 25% of adults with MS from community samples have depression (25). The lifetime prevalence of major depression in clinical samples is even higher—approximately 40% to 50% (26,27). Although more studies have addressed the depression associated with MS, anxiety disorders are another frequent and disabling problem. In various samples, 34% have anxiety, and 25% need treatment for it (24).

PSYCHOSOCIAL CONCERNS

Because of the low prevalence of pediatric MS, most youngsters will not have met anyone else in their community with the diagnosis. Until recently, most of the available support programs were geared to adults, so that children and families often felt isolated and frustrated. Fortunately, the National Multiple Sclerosis Society (NMSS) is currently developing programs that reach out to affected children. Other problems with psychosocial implications (severe fatigue, cognitive dysfunction, and visible neurological deficits) are inherent to the disease. These symptoms can all interfere with both social and school-related functions. However, many of these problems can be treated.

The clinician who treats individuals with pediatric MS must balance the effects of chronic illness, the high frequency of denial, and the disruption of family relations with the realities of clinical management. The only effective available disease-modifying therapies as of 2008 require either injections or infusions. Fortunately, many children and teenagers are remarkably resilient and handle their treatments well.

COGNITIVE AND ACADEMIC FUNCTIONING

More than one third of children with MS have cognitive deficits attributable to the disease. The most vulnerable areas are memory, perceptual and visual motor skills, executive functioning, cognitive processing speed, and global IQ (20,28–31). A similar range of deficits is also observed in adults. The rate of progression of cognitive loss is not known. One small sample of patients followed up longitudinally suggested that worsening could be identified within 1 to 2 years (28).

Declines in academic functioning can be mitigated by educating school personnel, providing special accommodations, such as reduced work load due to fatigue, and teaching compensatory strategies to assist with memory loss (20,28–32). Despite the disruption in daily activities that can be associated with cognitive dysfunction, most children will be able to graduate from high school. Some, but not all, will be able to go on to higher education.

Pathology and Pathogenesis

ENVIRONMENT

Both genetic and environmental factors contribute to MS. The prevalence of MS increases the greater the distance from the equator (33). Another factor pointing to an environmental role is timing of birth. The ratio of children born in May versus November is significantly higher among those with MS than in the normal population (34). Another potential environmental influence associated with MS risk is the amount of sunlight exposure during childhood. Less exposure to sunlight during childhood has been associated with an increased MS risk (35). The association between sunlight exposure and MS may be mediated by vitamin D levels, which have been shown to be low in white MS patients compared with healthy controls (36). Studies of migration suggest that during childhood, the place of residence is more closely associated with MS risk than is the place of birth (37,38).

GENETICS

Although clearly a role exists for environmental effects on MS pathogenesis, genetics also plays a role (5). A monozygotic twin sibling of an MS patient has a 20% to 30% risk for the disease in contrast to the reduced risk of a dizygotic twin of an individual with MS. The gene most closely associated with MS risk is *HLA-DR1B*. This genetic marker shows an increased frequency in adults as well as in children with the disease (5,39).

Recently, an association of the genes coding for the receptors of the cytokines interleukin (IL)-7 and IL-2 have been identified in adult MS (40,41). These cytokines play a role in T- and B-cell development. Both T and B cells contribute to the pathogenesis of MS. However, the exact role of the cytokines is still under investigation.

Pathology

The immune-mediated pathogenesis is supported by the pathological findings of inflammatory infiltrates consisting of monocytes, CD4 and CD8 cells, immune complex deposition, and other cells of the immune system. The animal model of MS and the benefits of immune-modulating and immunosuppressive treatments also support the role of the immune system in the disease (42).

Pathologically, the bulk of the disease process is within the cerebral white matter, where demyelination develops as a result of the inflammatory infiltrate. Within the MS plaque, a loss is noted of oligodendrocytes, the myelin-producing cell within the CNS. The type of immunopathology can vary between patients, as can the degree of axonal degeneration. Over time, areas of acute inflammation develop gliosis and, in contrast to active plaques, lose signs of ongoing myelin breakdown (43).

The event triggering the development of the immune attack against CNS myelin is unknown. The hypothesis is that, in a genetically predisposed individual exposed to certain viral antigens or other environmental triggers, the immune system is activated. As a result of molecular mimicry, the immune activation becomes directed against CNS myelin. These steps lead to an immune cascade, resulting in migration of inflammatory cells across the blood–brain barrier where damage to the CNS occurs (42).

Because a well-defined and narrow interval exists between potential environmental exposures and the development of MS in children, pediatric MS represents a novel opportunity to examine environmental influences. For example, an international investigation of more than 100 children with MS identified a greater than expected frequency of remote

Epstein–Barr virus (EBV) infection in MS cases compared with controls (44). Additional research examining other disease-related exposures during childhood has the potential to benefit individuals of all ages affected by MS.

Differential Diagnosis

The differential diagnosis of MS is large and includes other inflammatory disorders of the white matter, infections, neoplasms, vasculitis, hereditary disorders of the white matter, metabolic disorders, mitochondrial disorders, and vitamin deficiencies (45). Examples of several entities within each category are listed later.

ACUTE DISSEMINATED ENCEPHALOMYELITIS (ADEM)

The most challenging differential diagnostic problem in the management of acute demyelinating disorders of the CNS is distinguishing ADEM, a self-limited inflammatory immune-mediated disorder, from MS, a chronic condition. Although the two disorders can overlap in presentation, certain features are more typical of ADEM than of MS (Table 15.1) (46).

The typical clinical features of ADEM not usually found in MS are fever and encephalopathy (manifested by stupor, severe lethargy, seizures, confusion, and rarely coma). Focal and multifocal signs of cerebral white-matter dysfunction that mimic MS include optic neuritis (bilateral or unilateral), pyramidal signs (hemiparesis, paraparesis, or monoparesis), sensory loss, or brainstem and cerebellar signs. The MRI in ADEM typically shows large poorly defined lesions that involve the white matter but can also affect deep grey structures such as the basal ganglia. OCBs are present in 25% or fewer of ADEM cases (7,32,46,47). In contrast, the frequency of OCBs in MS is higher, ranging from 55% to 95%, in MS patients across different studies (12,48). Although several differences exist between ADEM and MS, the clearest is the disease course over the next few years. Three or more recurrent episodes after the initial 3 months of illness generally indicate MS. In ADEM, unlike MS, the vast majority of patients recover partially or fully from the initial event and do not develop subsequent demyelinating events or a chronic disorder.

INFECTIONS

Among the infections that bear some clinical similarity to MS are meningitis, encephalitis, and brain abscess (45). In particular, Lyme disease and HIV can, in many of their features, mimic MS. However, MRI abnormalities will often distinguish MS from most infections.

NEOPLASMS

Occasionally MS patients can have a single tumefactive lesion that resembles a lymphoma or other neoplasm. Most often in neoplasms, grey-matter involvement will lead to a diagnosis

TABLE 15.1 CLINICAL DIFFERENCES BETWEEN ADEM AND MS

Features	ADEM	MS
Typical age group	<10 yr	≥10 yr
Encephalopathy	Required in definition	Rare
Seizures	Occasional	Rare
Grey-matter involvement on MRI	Often	Rare
CSF pleocytosis >50 mm/mL	Often	Rare
OCB	Occasional	Often

other than MS. CSF might show abnormal cytology suggesting malignancy. At times, the only way to be sure of the diagnosis is biopsy.

VASCULITIS

Systemic lupus erythematosus, Behçet disease, sarcoidosis, CNS vasculitis, Sjögren syndrome, and other systemic immune-mediated disorders can have manifestations that can be mistaken for those of MS.

NEUROGENETIC LEUKOENCEPHALOPATHIES

Metabolic and genetic leukoencephalopathies that involve the cerebral white matter can have MRI appearances that resemble those in MS. However, their progressive course, the presence of developmental delay, and the onset during infancy or childhood distinguish them from MS. This group of disorders includes but is not limited to adrenoleukodystrophy (ALD); metachromatic leukodystrophy (MLD), Pelizaeus-Merzbacher and Refsum diseases; and adult- and juvenile-onset Alexander disease.

Cerebral autosomal dominant arteriography with subcortical infarcts and leukoencephalopathy (CADASIL) is a disorder of the white matter, the MRIs of which can be at times difficult to distinguish from MS. Migraine and strokelike episodes are typical features of CADASIL, which often is first seen with a family history. In contrast to MS, in CADASIL, the CSF usually lacks OCBs, and genetic testing can establish the diagnosis.

MITOCHONDRIAL DISORDERS

Mitochondrial disorders can also cause signs and symptoms in cerebral white matter that can be difficult to distinguish from MS. However, they typically are first seen with systemic manifestations, muscle disease, and the involvement of grey matter on the MRI. A particular challenge is Leber hereditary optic neuritis, which causes visual loss and optic neuritis, but its progressive course and genetic testing can establish the diagnosis.

VITAMIN DEFICIENCIES

A number of vitamin deficiencies can have symptoms that overlap with those of MS. For example, deficiency in vitamin B_{12} can cause optic neuropathy, fatigue, cognitive impairments, myelopathy, and peripheral neuropathy. The MRI may show some similarities to MS. Abnormalities in folate metabolism can produce myelopathic symptoms as well as ataxia. For these disorders, the presence of neuropathy, anemia, and abnormal red blood cell morphology can lead to the correct diagnosis. Vitamin E deficiency can cause ataxia, myelopathy, and neuropathy and can develop with malabsorption syndromes or as an autosomal recessive disorder (45).

Although the differential diagnosis of MS is large, attention to the primary clinical, radiologic, and laboratory features of MS will facilitate the diagnosis. The nature of the disease course, the evolution of the MRI, and the lack of other laboratory or systemic abnormalities will usually help establish the presence or absence of MS.

Treatment

The first principle of MS therapy for patients of all age groups is education and reassurance. Because of the low frequency of the pediatric MS diagnosis, affected individuals and their families are often even more overwhelmed than is an adult with MS. The majority of support systems, informational materials, and MS-related web sites remain geared to adults with the disease. However, in recent years, the NMSS is adding information related to children. Additional web sites related to current pediatric MS centers also include educationally related content.

TREATMENT OF RELAPSES

Management of acute relapses includes neurological evaluation and initiation of steroid therapy for relapses that affect daily functioning, with the goal of decreasing the duration of the relapse and enhancing the rate of recovery (49,50). Because no clinical trials for relapse management have been completed in pediatric MS, treatment follows the approach used for adults. High doses of parenteral methylprednisolone (typically 1 g) appear more effective than smaller oral doses (51). Treatment regimens vary from 3 to 5 days. In our experience, children respond to doses ranging from 20 to 30 mg per kilogram. In adults, high doses of oral methylprednisolone have been substituted for parenteral therapy (52). Complications can develop with steroid therapy and include gastrointestinal upset, irritability, insomnia, and, at their most extreme, psychosis. It is not easy to predict which patients will be at greatest risk for behavior-related side effects.

On occasion, in children with MS treated with high doses of steroids followed by an oral taper, steroid dependence develops (inability to wean off therapy because of recurrence of symptoms). Sometimes these children fail to respond to steroid therapy. In the event of steroid dependence, the weaning period can be managed with pulse intravenous immunoglobulin therapy. Although this strategy is commonly used and seemingly effective, no clinical trials have tested its efficacy. Intravenous immunoglobulin has been found to be effective for patients who do not respond to steroid therapy (53). Alternatively, patients failing to improve with steroids may respond to plasmapheresis (54).

DISEASE-MODIFYING THERAPIES

Disease-modifying therapies (DMTs) constitute the principal approach to altering the course of MS. These treatments have been shown to be useful only in relapsing–remitting MS or in adults with a single relapse who are at high risk for a subsequent event. The medications are most effective in decreasing the frequency and severity of relapses. To a lesser degree, DMTs lessen the accumulation of neurological impairments or disability. The most commonly used agents (in order of their timing of FDA approval) are interferons β1b subcutaneous (s.q.; Betaseron) at a dose of 250 µg every other day; interferon β1a intramuscular (Avonex) at a dose of 30 µg once a week; glatiramer acetate (Copaxone) s.q. at a dose of 20 mg daily; and interferon β1a s.q. (Rebif) at a dose of 44 µg 3 times per week) (Table 15.2). The interferons and glatiramer acetate affect the immune system by slightly different mechanisms. However, each of these therapies has its own advantages and disadvantages, largely based on adverse-event profile, convenience, and relative effect on MRI. Psychiatric complications have been anecdotally associated with the interferon therapies. However, in the pivotal clinical trials including the most recent, the frequency of mood disorder was not significantly different from that with placebo (3).

Natalizumab (Tysabri), mitoxantrone (Novantrone), and cyclophosphamide (Cytoxan), which are administered intravenously, are usually prescribed when first-line agents fail. Although both mitoxantrone and cyclophosphamide can be used as induction therapies, only preliminary studies at the time of this writing support this approach.

TABLE 15.2 CURRENT DISEASE-MODIFYING THERAPIES USED IN MS

	Dose and frequency
First-line treatments	
Interferon β1a intramuscular (Avonex)	30 mg once per wk
Interferon β1a subcutaneous (Rebif)	44 μg 3 times per wk
Interferon β1b (Betaseron)	250 μg every other day
Glatiramer acetate (Copaxone)	20 mg daily
Second-line treatments	
Natalizumab (Tysabri)	300 mg in normal saline, monthly infusions
Novantrone (Mitoxantrone)	12 mg/kg i.v. every 3 mo to a maximum of 144 mg/kg
Cyclophosphamide (Cytoxan)	600–800 mg/kg monthly for 3–6 mo followed by biannual pulses

SYMPTOMATIC THERAPY

A major principle of therapy is symptomatic management (49,55). Among the many MS symptoms, the high frequency of depressed affect and perceived stress merits emphasis (24). If mood-related problems are not treated, they tend to worsen. Overall, treatment studies of depression in MS support the use of antidepressant therapy and cognitive behavioral therapy. In choosing antidepressants, it is important to be aware of the many symptoms of MS that might be aggravated by antidepressant therapy, such as bladder dysfunction and excessive fatigue. Cognitive behavioral therapy emphasizing active coping skills, as well as antidepressant therapies, can also help the depression associated with MS (24).

Symptomatic therapy also includes management of MS-induced pain, including painful spasms. A variety of benefits have been associated with exercise and physical therapy. Medications that treat spasticity unresponsive to exercise or stretching include baclofen, a γ-aminobutyric acid (GABA) agonist, and tizanidine, a central α-adrenergic agonist. These agents can be effective as monotherapy or in combination.

Another very frequent problem is fatigue. Fatigue is intrinsic to MS as well as a consequence of its comorbid depression, sleep disturbance, and pain. Management includes steps to conserve energy, exercise, and medication. Medications considered effective and also found to be well tolerated in children include amantadine, which is an N-methyl-D-aspartate (NMDA) receptor antagonist, and modafinil (49).

In addition to a neurologist, ideally familiar with MS in children, professionals from physical therapy, neuropsychology, nursing, and psychiatry are often needed to address the issues associated with the disease—we hope in a multidisciplinary setting. A recreational program for teenagers with MS is also available through the Teen Adventure Program. This activity helps them meet peers in a pleasant, nonmedical setting. As progress in the management of MS grows, individuals can expect better and more convenient treatment options.

Summary

MS can develop in children and adolescents. Teenagers are affected more frequently than younger children. The disease is almost always relapsing–remitting at its onset and hence treatable. Psychosocial comorbidities are frequent and likely result from changes in the cerebral white matter as well as the consequences of chronic illness. MS responds best to multidisciplinary treatment, including modifying the disease course with immune-modulating therapies and treating ongoing symptoms, such as mood disorders.

Questions

1. What is the estimated frequency of pediatric MS?
   A. <1%
   B. 2% to 3%
   C. 5%
   D. ≥5%

2. What are the main clinical features of pediatric MS?
   A. progressively severe visual impairments, ataxia, paresis, and sensory disturbances
   B. relapsing and remitting visual impairments, ataxia, paresis, and sensory disturbances
   C. development of dementia
   D. epilepsy

3. Which is the best description of the MRI findings in MS?
   A. diffuse demyelination of cerebral and spinal cord white matter
   B. discrete grey-matter lesions in the cerebrum, optic nerves, and spinal cord
   C. nine or more lesions of the white matter, often in periventricular location
   D. none of the above

4. Which psychiatric comorbidities have been identified in children with MS?
   A. attention-deficit hyperactivity disorder
   B. learning disabilities
   C. autistic-spectrum disorder symptoms
   D. depression, anxiety disorder, adjustment disorder, and panic attacks

5. Which of the following is not a principle of MS therapy?
   A. immunomodulation
   B. specific treatment of psychiatric comorbidities
   C. exercise
   D. increasing immunologic surveillance

6. What evidence points to environmental and genetic contributors to the disease process?
   A. The frequency of MS decreases with distance from the equator.
   B. The incidence of MS increases in proportion to sunlight exposure during childhood.
   C. Migration studies show that place of birth is a more powerful predictor than childhood residence in determining MS risk.
   D. The association of MS with the gene for *HLA-DRB1* is strong.

Answers

1. B. In approximately 2% to 3% of the 400,000 individuals with MS in the United States, MS developed before they were 18 years old.

2. B. In children, the main clinical features, which relapse and remit, are optic neuritis–induced visual impairments, balance problems, motor deficits, and sensory impairments.

3. C. MRI findings in pediatric as well as adult MS include nine or more lesions of the white matter, gadolinium-enhancing lesions, lesions with a periventricular location, infratentorial and spinal cord lesions, and lesions that are juxtacortical.

4. D. Children with MS have comorbid depression, anxiety disorder, adjustment disorder, and panic attacks.

5. D. MS therapy consists primarily of treatments that alter the disease course and reduce symptoms. First-line therapies modify the disease course by decreasing relapse frequency and accumulation of MRI lesions. All require injections and work by modifying the immune system. Symptomatic management includes addressing depression, pain, sleep disturbance, and spasticity. In addition to pharmacologic interventions, exercise is a mainstay of therapy.

6. D. The frequency of MS increases with the distance from the equator. The lack of sunlight exposure during childhood and low vitamin-D serum levels have been linked to MS risk. Migration studies indicate that childhood residence is more important than place of birth in determining MS risk. Although the genetic contribution is supported by the higher concordance of monozygotic compared with dizygotic twins, the strongest genetic association is with the gene *HLA-DRB1*.

REFERENCES

1. Duquette P, Murray TJ, Pleines J, et al. Multiple sclerosis in childhood: clinical profile in 125 patients. *J Pediatr.* 1987;111:359–363.
2. Ghezzi A, Deplano V, Faroni J, et al. Multiple sclerosis in childhood: clinical features of 149 cases. *Mult Scler.* 1997;3:43–46.
3. Kappos L, Polman CH, Freedman MS, et al. Treatment with interferon beta-1b delays conversion to clinically definite and McDonald MS in patients with clinically isolated syndromes. *Neurology.* 2006;67:1242–1249.
4. Krupp LB, Banwell B, Tenembaum S, et al. Consensus definitions proposed for pediatric multiple sclerosis and related disorders. *Neurology.* 2007;68:S7–S12.
5. Ness JM, Chabas D, Sadovnick A, et al. Clinical features of children and adolescents with multiple sclerosis. *Neurology.* 2007;68:S37–S45.
6. Banwell B, Shroff M, Ness JM, et al. MRI features of pediatric multiple sclerosis. *Neurology.* 2007;68:S46–S53.
7. Mikaeloff Y, Adamsbaum C, Husson B, et al. MRI prognostic factors for relapse after acute CNS inflammatory demyelination in childhood. *Brain.* 2004;127:1942–1947.
8. Boiko A, Vorobeychik G, Paty D, et al. Early onset multiple sclerosis: a longitudinal study. *Neurology.* 2002;59:1006–1010.
9. Ruggieri M, Polizzi A, Pavone L, et al. Multiple sclerosis in children under 6 years of age. *Neurology.* 1999;53:478–484.
10. Haliloglu G, Anlar B, Aysun S, et al. Gender prevalence in childhood multiple sclerosis and myasthenia gravis. *J Child Neurol.* 2002;17:390–392.
11. Sicotte NL, Giesser BS, Tandon V, et al. Testosterone treatment in multiple sclerosis: a pilot study. *Arch Neurol.* 2007;64:683–688.
12. Renoux C, Vukusic S, Mikaeloff Y, et al. Natural history of multiple sclerosis with childhood onset. *N Engl J Med.* 2007;356:2603–2613.
13. Simone IL, Carrara D, Tortorella C, et al. Course and prognosis in early-onset MS: comparison with adult-onset forms. *Neurology.* 2002;59:1922–1928.
14. Hahn CD, Shroff MM, Blaser SI, et al. MRI criteria for multiple sclerosis: evaluation in a pediatric cohort. *Neurology.* 2004;62:806–808.
15. Ruggieri M, Iannetti P, Polizzi A, et al. Multiple sclerosis in children under 10 years of age. *Neurol Sci.* 2004;25:S326–S35.
16. Mikaeloff Y, Suissa S, Vallee L, et al. First episode of acute CNS inflammatory demyelination in childhood: prognostic factors for multiple sclerosis and disability. *J Pediatr.* 2004;144:246–252.
17. Ghezzi A, Pozzilli C, Liguori M, et al. Prospective study of multiple sclerosis with early onset. *Mult Scler.* 2002;8:115–118.
18. Confavreux C, Vukusic S, Adeleine P. Early clinical predictors and progression of irreversible disability in multiple sclerosis: an amnesic process. *Brain.* 2003;126:770–782.
19. Mikaeloff Y, Caridade G, Assi S, et al. Prognostic factors for early severity in a childhood multiple sclerosis cohort. *Pediatrics.* 2006;118:1133–1139.
20. MacAllister WS, Boyd JR, Holland NJ, et al. The psychosocial consequences of pediatric multiple sclerosis. *Neurology.* 2007;68:S66–S69.
21. Mohr DC, Goodkin DE, Bacchetti P, et al. Psychological stress and the subsequent appearance of new brain MRI lesions in MS. *Neurology.* 2000;55:55–61.
22. Hoare P, Mann H. Self-esteem and behavioural adjustment in children with epilepsy and children with diabetes. *J Psychosom Res.* 1994;38:859–869.
23. Feinstein A, Roy P, Lobaugh N, et al. Structural brain abnormalities in multiple sclerosis patients with major depression. *Neurology.* 2004;62:586–590.
24. Siegert RJ, Abernethy DA. Depression in multiple sclerosis: a review. *J Neurol Neurosurg Psychiatry.* 2005;76:469–475.
25. Patten SB, Beck CA, Williams JV, et al. Major depression in multiple sclerosis: a population-based perspective. *Neurology.* 2003;61:1524–1527.
26. Joffe RT. Depression and multiple sclerosis: a potential way to understand the biology of major depressive illness. *J Psychiatry Neurosci.* 2005;30:9–10.
27. Sadovnick AD, Remick RA, Allen J, et al. Depression and multiple sclerosis. *Neurology.* 1996;46:628–632.
28. MacAllister WS, Belman AL, Milazzo M, et al. Cognitive functioning in children and adolescents with multiple sclerosis. *Neurology.* 2005;64:1422–1425.
29. Kalb RC, DiLorenzo TA, LaRocca NG, et al. The impact of early-onset multiple sclerosis on cognitive and psychosocial indices. *Int J MS Care.* 1999;1:2–17.

30. Bye AM, Kendall B, Wilson J. Multiple sclerosis in childhood: a new look. *Dev Med Child Neurol.* 1985;27:215–222.
31. Banwell BL, Anderson PE. The cognitive burden of multiple sclerosis in children. *Neurology.* 2005;64:891–894.
32. Dale RC, de Sousa C, Chong WK, et al. Acute disseminated encephalomyelitis, multiphasic disseminated encephalomyelitis and multiple sclerosis in children. *Brain.* 2000;123:2407–2422.
33. Kurtzke JF, Hyllested K. Multiple sclerosis in the Faroe Islands, I: clinical and epidemiological features. *Ann Neurol.* 1979;5:6–21.
34. Sadovnick AD, Duquette P, Herrera B, et al. A timing-of-birth effect on multiple sclerosis clinical phenotype. *Neurology.* 2007;69:60–62.
35. van der Mei IA, Ponsonby AL, Dwyer T, et al. Past exposure to sun, skin phenotype, and risk of multiple sclerosis: case-control study. *Br Med J.* 2003;327:316.
36. Munger KL, Levin LI, Hollis BW, et al. Serum 25-hydroxyvitamin D levels and risk of multiple sclerosis. *JAMA.* 2006;296:2832–2838.
37. Pugliatti M, Riise T, Sotgiu MA. Evidence of early childhood in the susceptibility period in multiple sclerosis: space-time cluster analysis in a Sardinian population. *Am J Epidemiol.* 2006;164:326–333.
38. Ascherio A, Munger KL. Environmental risk factors for multiple sclerosis, Part II: noninfectious factors. *Ann Neurol.* 2007;61:504–513.
39. Sotgiu S, Pugliatti M, Sanna A, et al. Multiple sclerosis complexity in selected populations: the challenge of Sardinia, insular Italy. *Eur J Neurol.* 2002;9:329–341.
40. Hafler DA, Compston A, Sawcer S, et al. Risk alleles for multiple sclerosis identified by a genomewide study. *N Engl J Med.* (in press).
41. Gregory SG, Schmidt S, Seth P, et al. Interleukin 7 receptor alpha chain (IL7R) shows allelic and functional association with multiple sclerosis. *Nat Genet.* 2007 (in press).
42. Hafler DA, Slavik JM, Anderson DE, et al. Multiple sclerosis. *Immunol Rev.* 2005;204:208–231.
43. Pittock SJ, Lucchinetti CF. The pathology of MS: new insights and potential clinical applications. *Neurologist.* 2007;13:45–56.
44. Banwell B, Krupp L, Kennedy J, et al. Clinical features and viral serologies in children with multiple sclerosis: results of a multinational study. *Lancet Neurol.* 2007 (in press).
45. Hahn JS, Pohl D, Rensel M, et al. Differential diagnosis and evaluation in pediatric multiple sclerosis. *Neurology.* 2007;68:S13–S21.
46. Tenembaum S, Chitnis T, Ness J, et al. Acute disseminated encephalomyelitis. *Neurology.* 2007;68:S23–S36.
47. Leake JA, Albani S, Kao AS, et al. Acute disseminated encephalomyelitis in childhood: epidemiologic, clinical and laboratory features. *Pediatr Infect Dis J.* 2004;23:756–764.
48. Pohl D, Rostasy K, Reiber H, et al. CSF characteristics in early-onset multiple sclerosis. *Neurology.* 2004;63:1966–1967.
49. Pohl D, Waubant E, Banwell B, et al. Treatment of pediatric multiple sclerosis and variants. *Neurology.* 2007;86:S54–S65.
50. Brusaferri F, Candelise L. Steroids for multiple sclerosis and optic neuritis: a meta-analysis of randomized controlled clinical trials. *J Neurol.* 2000;247:435–442.
51. Oliveri RL, Valentino P, Russo C, et al. Randomized trial comparing two different high doses of methylprednisolone in MS: a clinical and MRI study. *Neurology.* 1998;50:1833–1836.
52. Miller D, Weinstock-Guttman B, Béthoux F, et al. A meta-analysis of methylprednisolone in recovery from multiple sclerosis exacerbations. *Mult Scler.* 2000;6:267–273.
53. Sahlas DJ, Miller SP, Guerin M, et al. Treatment of acute disseminated encephalomyelitis with intravenous immunoglobulin. *Neurology.* 2000;54:1370–1372.
54. Weinshenker BG, O'Brien PC, Petterson TM, et al. A randomized trial of plasma exchange in acute central nervous system inflammatory demyelinating disease. *Ann Neurol.* 1999;46:878–886.
55. Krupp LB, Rizvi SA. Symptomatic therapy for underrecognized manifestations of multiple sclerosis. *Neurology.* 2002;58:S32–S39.

CHAPTER 16

The Development and Neuropsychology of Visual Impairment

RICK O. GILMORE, JOEL M. WEINSTEIN,
AND REBECCA VON DER HEIDE

Introduction

At least half of the human brain responds to visual stimulation, and so the study of vision has dominated the field of behavioral neuroscience since the 1950s. Moreover, whereas many scientists studying vision do not focus on how visual perception changes over development, most clinicians do share these concerns, in large part because the most common diseases of vision tend to occur early (e.g., strabismus) or late (e.g., glaucoma) in life. In this chapter, we summarize what is known about the normal development of the visual system and its disorders, with an emphasis on infancy and childhood. The reader interested in more-thorough summaries of the issues we discuss should consult volumes by Daw (1), Simons (2), Atkinson (3), or Rakic (4).

The chapter is divided into three sections, including this introduction. Section 1 describes the visual system and its normal developmental patterns; Section 2 describes the most common diseases and disorders of visual development; Section 3 provides a brief conclusion.

Normal Development

In comparison to the auditory or somatosensory systems, the visual system is relatively immature at birth. Newborns do not see details well, are insensitive to low levels of contrast, and are sensitive to color and motion over much narrower ranges than are adults. Vision develops rapidly over the first 6 months after birth, followed by a somewhat slower rate of change into the preschool years. It was once thought that visual capacities were largely mature by the time children entered school at 5 or 6 years of age, but recent tests with very sensitive measures have shown that changes in basic visual processing continue into adolescence. In this section, we briefly review some of the essential facts concerning normal development of the visual system.

ANATOMY AND PHYSIOLOGY OF THE DEVELOPING VISUAL SYSTEM

The eye

The formation of a focused, undistorted visual image on the retinal surface is the first step in the process of visual perception. The eye consists of a family of structures that contribute

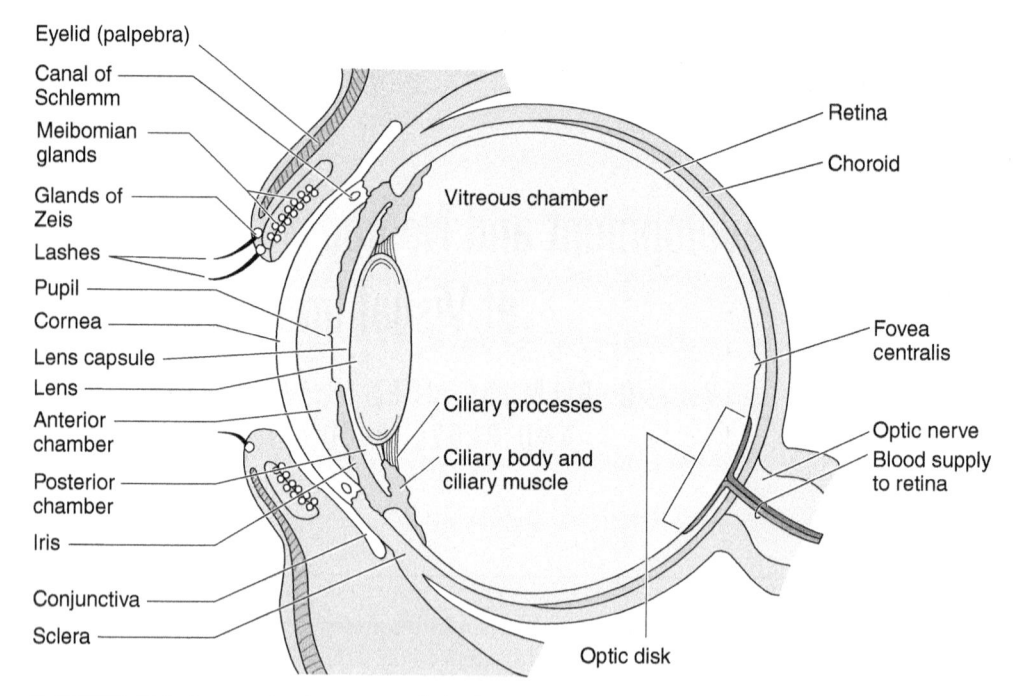

FIGURE 16.1 Cross-sectional anatomy of the human eye. (Reprinted with permission from Willis MC. *Medical terminology: the language of health care, 2nd ed.* Baltimore: Lippincott Williams & Wilkins, 2006.)

to the formation of this image: the cornea, lens, and iris/pupillary system (Fig. 16.1). The retina itself is functionally segregated and composed of two broad classes of photoreceptors: rods and cones. Rods subserve achromatic vision at low light levels and are concentrated in the peripheral portions of the retina. Cones subserve color or chromatic perception and are the only photoreceptors in the central portion of the fovea, the 1- to 2-degree region of the visual field where daytime visual acuity is best. Both classes of photoreceptors synapse on retinal bipolar cells, which signal information from photoreceptors to ganglion cells. Approximately 1 million ganglion cells in each eye receive input from this retinal network and send action potentials along the optic nerve and tract to the brain.

The eye and retina undergo prolonged patterns of pre- and postnatal development. Retinal cells appear to be generated during an extended period in embryonic development that begins in the first half of gestation and continues up to the time of birth, even though cell formation has long ended in the downstream structures, such as visual cortex. Roughly 60% of the initially produced retinal ganglion cells are lost by the time of birth because of programmed cell death.

Many features of the retinal architecture appear to develop early are largely independent of functional activity (but see 9). For example, the distribution of rods and cones in the fetal retina appears roughly adult-like before the onset of functional synaptic contacts with horizontal or bipolar cells. Conversely, the newborn retina does not have the dense packing of photoreceptors in the central foveal region characteristic of adults, and the outer, light sensitive segments of photoreceptors do not reach their mature length for several months after birth. Large-scale photoreceptor migration toward the fovea and increases in outer segment length occur during the first year of life (5), but other subtle morphological changes occur up to the age of 4 years.

Furthermore, the eye itself undergoes changes in size and shape. Although proportionately large at birth relative to head size, considerable growth occurs in the size of the globe. The distance from the cornea to the retina increases by about 25% by 1 year of age and increases another 25% by adolescence (6).

The visual brain

Despite the complexity of its circuitry, the retina is only the first stage in visual processing in the human. We now turn to a discussion of the subcortical and cortical structures that support visual functions (Fig. 16.2).

Subcortical structures

The critical subcortical components of the visual system consist of the optic nerve and tract, and its associated structures, the superior colliculus (SC) and associated structures, the hypothalamus, and the lateral geniculate nucleus (LGN) of the thalamus. Projections from the retina to the SC mature early and may form the main basis of neonatal visual perception and visually guided action, according to one model of visual development (3,7,8). Conversely, projections from the retina to the hypothalamus may not make functional connections until 3 to 4 months after birth. This could account, at least in part, for the difficulties parents of young infants have in helping their children keep a consistent schedule of nighttime sleep because the hypothalamus helps maintain the body's circadian rhythm by means of projections to the pineal gland, among other structures.

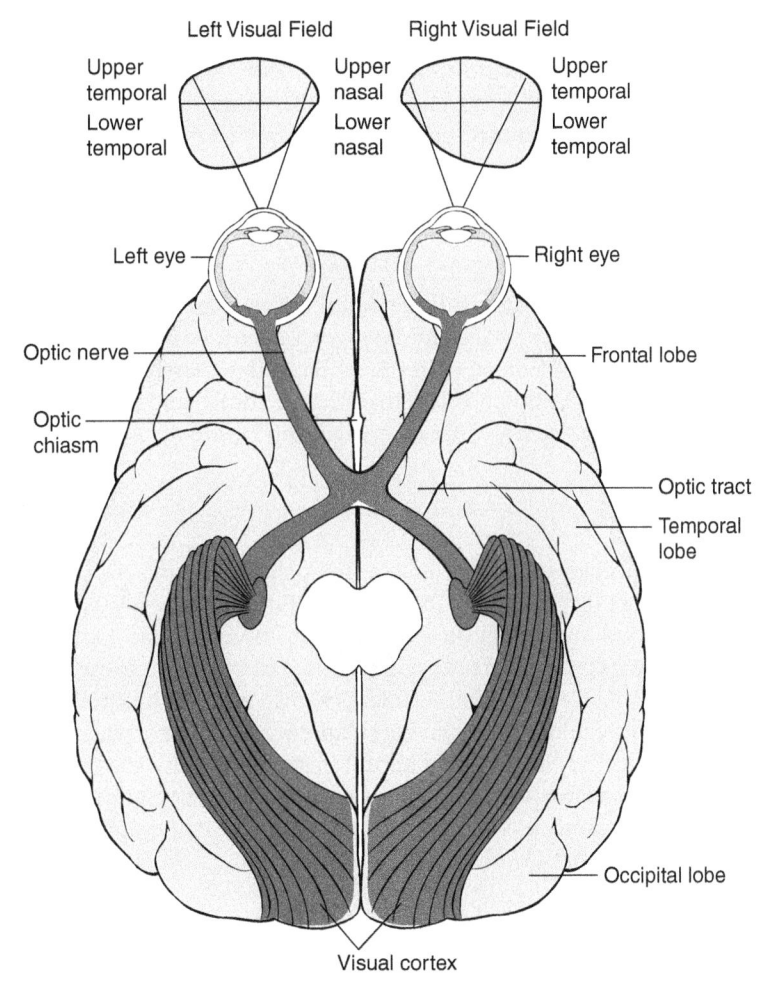

■ **FIGURE 16.2** Projection patterns from the retinae, through the optic chiasm, to the lateral geniculate nucleus (LGN), via the optic radiations to visual cortex in the occipital lobe. (Reprinted with permission from Weber J, Kelley J. *Health assessment in nursing*, 2nd ed. Philadelphia: Lippincott Williams & Wilkins, 2003.)

Cortical structures

Visual information activates as much as half of the primate cerebral cortex, but the most crucial structures are located in the occipital lobe, the site of primary visual cortex (V1) and associated regions V2 to V4, with additional higher-order systems located in the parietal, temporal, and frontal lobes (11,12). The best available evidence suggests that visual cortex undergoes substantial postnatal development in the human (10,13–16).

The development of visual behavior

Much of what is known about the development of the human visual system early in life comes from systematic studies of visual behavior. In this section, we briefly discuss changes in the size of the visual field, increases in visual acuity, and changes in visual behaviors thought to be specifically related to the dorsal and ventral visual-processing streams.

Field size

Neonates have binocular visual fields that are only 15% to 25% of the 160- to 170-degree values typical of the average human adult (17), and field size does not reach adult values until 12 to 24 months. Monocular field size has a somewhat more rapid developmental time course, approaching adult levels by approximately four months (18). Moreover, field size for static targets develops more rapidly in the temporal visual field than in the nasal field. Field sizes to moving targets grow more slowly; adult levels are not reached until approximately the end of the first year of life (19). Differences between the nasal and temporal hemifields have been attributed both to peripheral factors, such as differential timing in retinal maturation, and to central factors, such as the anatomy of crossed versus uncrossed projections.

Visual acuity

The ability to resolve detailed features of the visual image is critical for the recognition of form. In the adult, visual acuity is close to the theoretic limit imposed by the optics of the eye, sampling density of photoreceptors in the retina, and processing in the cortex. Visual acuity in infants and young children is less than that in adults, and is even below the theoretic limit, but both grating and vernier acuity develop rapidly in the first 6 to 8 months of life (20–22).

Binocular vision

Humans depend on mechanisms that compare the disparity or offset of images between the two eyes to estimate distance from the observer. For binocular visual mechanisms to work properly, both eyes must align on a single point in visual space, and circuits in V1 and higher-order systems must be able to compute retinal disparity. These systems are immature in the neonate but develop rapidly. Infants show visual evoked potentials (VEPs or brain electrical patterns evoked by visual stimulation) activated by binocular correlation between 8 and 20 weeks (23) and a rather abrupt onset of disparity sensitivity between 12 and 20 weeks (24). Thereafter, the minimal retinal disparity that can be detected appears to increase rapidly. Some authors have speculated that the formation of ocular dominance columns allows stereoacuity (25).

Motion perception

Motion perception is critical both for perceiving objects moving relative to the environment and for determining where and how fast the observer is moving (26,27). Primitive capacities to detect and respond to visual motion have been observed in newborns. By 7 to 8 weeks, direction-selective VEPs are observed (28), and behavioral measures show gradual development in direction selectivity up to 18 to 20 weeks (27). Development in motion sensitivity outside the infancy period is poorly understood, but recent evidence suggests that it has a prolonged developmental time course, continuing well into the early school-age years.

Color, shape, and form

In general, young infants do not discriminate colors well, and evidence indicates that sensitivity to shorter (i.e., blue) wavelengths may be especially impaired. Sensitivity to red–green differences appears to emerge in the second month after birth, and discrimination of blue–yellow differences sometime later (29).

However, most vision scientists agree that the detection of an object's overall shape is an important first step in the complex, and poorly understood, process of form perception. Selectivity for the orientation of static or moving-line segments, a characteristic of neurons in V1, undoubtedly plays an important role. Newborns can discriminate large changes in orientation (30), and sensitivity to smaller changes in orientation appears to develop gradually over the first several months after birth (3). Thus although considerable postnatal development occurs, the neonatal visual system is well disposed to extracting crude information about shape and form.

Abnormal Development

We now turn to a discussion about disorders and diseases of the eye and visual system. When dealing with visual disorders in children, it is important to recognize the plasticity of the developing visual system. Children who do not receive appropriate visual stimulation early in life will not develop the neural circuitry required for normal vision and will have some form of visual developmental delay. These defects may or may not be remediable, depending on the child's chronological age, the intensity of the visual rehabilitation program, and unknown factors that govern the "critical period" for the development of neurovisual circuitry. A large body of clinical and experimental evidence suggests that different critical periods exist for the development of various components of visual perception (1). As discussed earlier in this chapter, motion detection, two-dimensional binocular vision, and three-dimensional depth perception (stereopsis) all begin and end their maturation at different ages. Although the clinical and experimental literature refer to "critical periods" for the development of these cognitive faculties, in practice, neither the duration of the critical period nor the extent of plasticity has been precisely defined for any of these functions. Undoubtedly both the duration and extent of the critical periods are dependent on both genetic factors and prior environmental conditioning.

Because of the neural plasticity inherent in the infant visual system, the distinction between "congenital" and "acquired" visual defects may be less important in the first 2 years of life than the nature of the visual impediment. For example, severe unilateral congenital cataracts (an opacity in one or both ocular lenses), which are not removed in the first 2 months of life, are likely to result in severe and irreversible visual loss, despite heroic effects at rehabilitation at a later age. Infantile esotropia (eye misalignment), conversely, is compatible with excellent vision and some degree of stereopsis after surgical alignment in the first year or even 18 months of life. Nevertheless, it is safe to state that, for most pediatric visual disorders, the earlier the treatment, the better the outcome.

DISORDERS OF THE EYE

Congenital and developmental cataracts

Cataracts may occur as an isolated disorder or as part of a multisystem genetic or metabolic disease. The association between cataract and various systemic diseases has been reviewed elsewhere (32). This discussion is limited to the diagnosis and visual rehabilitation of children with cataracts, irrespective of the etiology of the cataracts.

Isolated cataracts in childhood are usually genetically determined and are most commonly inherited in an autosomal-dominant pattern. As with other autosomal-dominant conditions, penetrance may be incomplete (i.e., not all carriers may show the phenotype and, when present, its severity may vary). Cataracts occurring in documented autosomal-dominant pedigrees are almost always bilateral. However, sporadic unilateral cataracts occur quite commonly.

Early diagnosis of congenital and juvenile cataracts is imperative to avoid severe amblyopia (impaired or dim vision without obvious defect or change in the eye, see later). Surgery after the age of 3 months rarely results in vision better than 20/200. Early diagnosis and treatment, conversely, is compatible with an excellent visual outcome if no other ocular anomalies are present, such as microphthalmos, corneal opacity, or retinal or optic nerve dysplasia. The visual outcome in children with cataracts has improved greatly over the past 15 to 20 years because of advances in surgical technique and technology, better contact lenses, and, in selected cases, the use of intraocular lenses (33). Nevertheless, parents of children with congenital or developmental cataracts must understand that surgery is only the first step in a long process that will require a major expenditure of time and energy on the part of parents and patients. Amblyopia is common, and intensive patching is the rule rather than the exception. Eye examinations under anesthesia may be needed several times annually to check refraction, rule out retinal abnormalities, and monitor for glaucoma, which occurs in about 30% of children after cataract surgery.

Although in most children with congenital cataracts, useful vision develops, acuity is rarely at the norm for the age, and a few patients, especially those who have delayed surgery, never develop good vision. The psychosocial impact of poor vision in infancy is protean. Many aspects of development—gross and fine motor, cognitive, psychosocial, and interpersonal skills—depend on vision. An approach to children with severe visual disability is discussed in greater detail later. In addition to the psychosocial impact of visual impairment, quality of life in children with congenital cataracts is affected by the necessity for recurrent surgeries, amblyopia therapy, and frequent medical visits. Quality-of-life scores, according to one report, may be comparable to those reported in children with severe systemic diseases, such as cancer (34).

Congenital/juvenile glaucoma

Glaucoma, an excessive intraocular pressure causing retinal degeneration, may occur in childhood as an isolated anomaly (primary congenital or juvenile glaucoma), in association with systemic abnormalities, such as Sturge–Weber and Lowe syndromes or the mucopolysaccharidoses, or may be associated with other ocular abnormalities, such as aniridia (congenital underdevelopment of the iris). Ho and Walton (35) reviewed the systemic associations. Most cases of isolated primary congenital and juvenile glaucoma are inherited, and several gene loci have been isolated. However, genotype–phenotype correlation has not been close (i.e., the same gene defect may result in widely disparate severity and manifestation within the same family) (35).

The typical patient with primary congenital glaucoma (PCG) is first seen sometime during the first year of life with symptoms related to corneal edema, including tearing, photophobia, and discomfort, often manifested as eye rubbing. The cornea is usually cloudy and enlarged, giving rise to the term "buphthalmus" (ox eye). The most severe form of primary congenital glaucoma is seen at birth with diffuse corneal opacification and enlargement. If corneal enlargement is not appreciated and the corneal clouding is mild, the child may be incorrectly diagnosed with nasolacrimal duct obstruction, and definitive surgery may be delayed.

Surgery is the primary treatment of choice for congenital glaucoma, though supplemental medication may be useful (35,36). After surgery, children with PCG require repeated eye examinations under anesthesia to check intraocular pressure and monitor for optic disc damage. Myopia is frequent due to elongation of the globe. Asymmetric myopia may lead to amblyopia and the need for patching therapy. With early diagnosis and intervention, visual prognosis is very good. However, at least 20% of children will require more than one surgical procedure (36).

The visual outcome in children with congenital glaucoma is variable. Multiple surgeries are not infrequent, and prolonged intensive therapy for amblyopia may be necessary. In children with a poor visual outcome, cognitive, psychosocial, and motor development may all be delayed because of visual impairment. Children with severe visual impairment require an extensive support network, including psychological support for both child and parents. These considerations are discussed at greater length later in the chapter. In addition, children with recurrent surgeries, hospitalizations, and visits to doctors may have the same quality-of-life issues that have been well documented in children with rheumatologic disease and cancer (33). Psychiatric support is essential in helping these children to overcome the handicaps of low vision and of multiple medical and surgical procedures.

Strabismus and amblyopia

Strabismus, a misalignment of the eyes, and amblyopia, an acquired loss of monocular function, are major public health problems, occurring in 2% to 5% of children even in developed countries (37). These disorders begin in infancy or early childhood and have a profound effect on subsequent visual development, including both monocular and binocular vision. In addition, the psychosocial stigma of "crossed eyes" and of wearing an occlusive eye patch may damage self-esteem and other aspects of emotional development. Early recognition of strabismus and amblyopia are important for minimizing their visual and psychosocial consequences. The alternative to early diagnosis and treatment is frequently a scenario involving prolonged patching, multiple surgeries, amblyopia, impaired binocular vision (depth perception), and a life-long suboptimal cosmetic outcome. Childhood strabismus may cause exotropia (one eye turning outward toward the ear), esotropia (one eye turning inward toward the nose), or, more rarely, hypertropia (one eye turning upward).

A number of studies demonstrated the negative psychosocial impact of strabismus in both adults and children (38–44). A negative attitude toward strabismus seems to emerge in nonstrabismic children at approximately 5 to 6 years of age (40). Therefore both children and adults with strabismus may have poor self-esteem, a higher incidence of dysfunctional interpersonal relationships, and poorer prospects for employment (42). It appears that negative attitudes toward strabismus are directed more frequently toward girls and women than toward boys and men. In addition, mothers of children with strabismus express more dissatisfaction with their maternal role and may become depressed and dysfunctional (43). The psychiatrist can actively assist parents and children in overcoming these obstacles.

Mounting evidence indicates that surgery for strabismus can result in significant improvement in both psychological and visual function (44). Parents may be unaware of this benefit and may have been told by friends, family, or the primary physician that surgery would have none. Although it is not the psychiatrist's role to recommend strabismus surgery, he or she can help the parent and child explore all issues that may affect the child's self-esteem.

Infantile esotropia

Formerly called "congenital esotropia," infantile esotropia is first seen with one eye that deviates inwardly from the other. It has its onset during the first 6 months of life. In one half to two thirds of these children, the esotropia is alternating. For example, the child alternates from minute to minute between fixation with the right eye (left esotropia) and fixation with the left eye (right esotropia). Although many normal infants have a small-angle intermittent deviation in the first 3 months of life, a constant or large-angle deviation beyond the fourth month of life will almost always persist indefinitely in the absence of treatment (45).

The majority of children with infantile esotropia are otherwise developmentally normal. Groups at higher risk for infantile esotropia include children with Down syndrome (trisomy 21), intraventricular hemorrhage, hydrocephalus, cerebral palsy, or prematurity of less than 32 weeks of gestation.

As discussed earlier, the cortical circuits for binocular vision develop rapidly between the ages of 3 and 6 months. Children with infantile esotropia will not develop any form of binocular vision without intervention to realign the visual axes (46). These children function in an essentially monocular mode. Information from the fixating eye (the eye that is targeted on the object of interest) is processed normally, whereas information from the deviated eye, which presents conflicting visual information, is largely suppressed and ignored by the visual cortex. Precise depth perception, which requires binocular information, is not possible if either eye is misaligned. In addition, if the child does not alternate—if he has a strong preference for fixation with one eye and never, or rarely, uses the other eye—the visual cortex will not develop the circuits required to decode the incoming message from the chronically deviated eye. The result will be poor vision in that eye (i.e., amblyopia).

Several retrospective longitudinal studies have demonstrated that the long-term outcome in children with infantile esotropia strongly correlates with duration of misalignment (47,48). The eyes of children who undergo surgical realignment after less than 3 months of constant esotropia have a lower incidence of amblyopia, better binocular vision, and better long-term stability of alignment; fewer require repeated surgery for recurrent strabismus. A consensus exists among pediatric ophthalmologists that children with infantile esotropia should have surgery before the age of 9 months (49).

Accommodative esotropia

Accommodative esotropia usually is first seen between the ages of 18 months and 5 years and is associated with moderate to severe farsightedness (hyperopia) (50). This type of esotropia is caused by excessive use of the "near reflex," which consists of the triad of accommodation, convergence, and miosis. In children who are excessively farsighted (hyperopic), parallel light rays from infinity do not converge on the retina, and additional focusing activity (accommodation) is needed (Fig. 16.3). In turn, accommodation is ac-

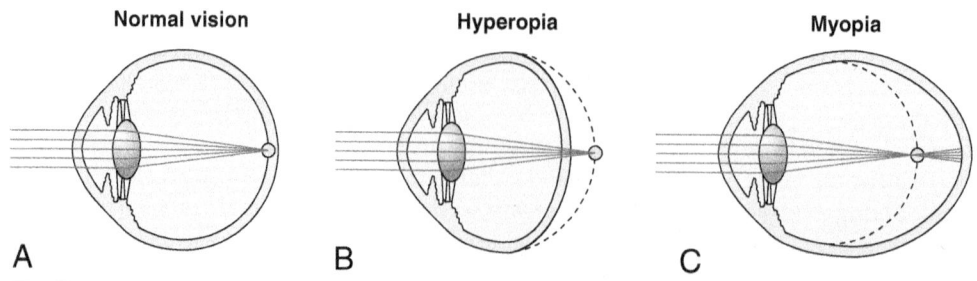

■ **FIGURE 16.3** Optics of hyperopia. In a normal eye, parallel light rays emanating from infinity are focused to a point on the retina. In a hyperopic eye, refracting power is insufficient, and light rays are directed to a virtual focus behind the retina. (Reprinted with permission from Willis MC. *Medical terminology: the language of health care, 2nd ed.* Baltimore: Lippincott Williams & Wilkins, 2006.)

complished by invoking the near reflex, which results in inappropriate convergence. The child then has clear vision, because of accommodation, but misaligned visual axes because of inappropriate convergence. In children, this misalignment leads to suppression of information from the deviated eye and lack of binocular vision.

If the child does not alternate fixation—if the same eye always turns inward and the deviation is chronic—amblyopia will result (see later). In this situation, circuits for monocular vision will fail to develop or, if present, will be actively disassembled.

The treatment for accommodative esotropia is glasses, which provide focusing power and substitute for the near reflex with its inappropriate convergence (Fig. 16.4). Contact lenses may be used in lieu of glasses in older children and teenagers. Like infantile

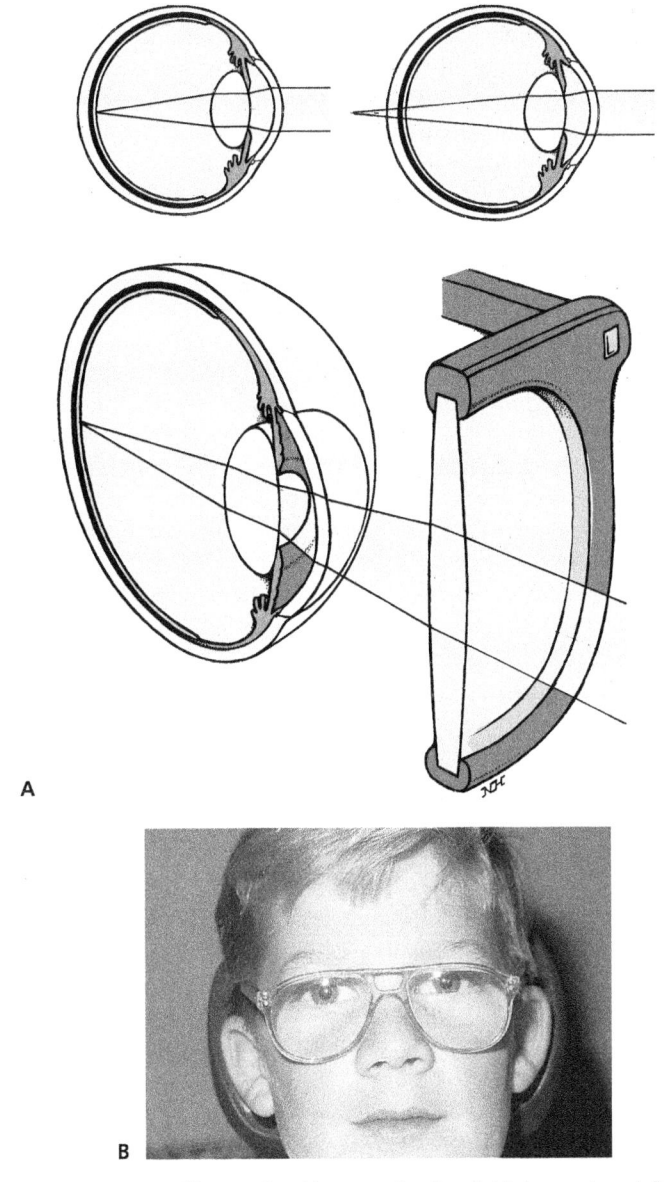

■ **FIGURE 16.4 A:** Correction of hyperopia with spectacles. Parallel light rays from infinity are "pre-bent" by the spectacle lens, enabling the hyperopic eye to bring them to a focus on the retina. (Illustration by Neil O. Hardy, Westpoint, CT.) **B:** Child with accommodative esotropia without glasses demonstrating left esotropia. (Reprinted with permission from Tasman W, Jaeger E. *The Wills Eye Hospital Atlas of Clinical Ophthalmology*, 2nd ed. Philadelphia: Lippincott Williams & Wilkins, 2001.

esotropia, accommodative esotropia requires early intervention. Duration of misalignment is negatively correlated with quality of both monocular and binocular vision (stereopsis), as well as with risk for future deterioration of alignment, which may require surgery (50).

Exotropia

Exotropia, or the outward deviation of the eye, is slightly less common than esotropia in childhood. Its onset is usually between 18 months and 4 to 5 years. Exotropia, unlike esotropia, usually remains intermittent, and patients with this disorder usually have normal, or near-normal, binocular vision when their eyes are not crossed. Also, because the deviation is usually intermittent, amblyopia is absent or mild.

Many children with exotropia do not require intervention because their deviation occurs intermittently and only rarely (51). Patching may be useful to break the suppression that occurs when one eye is deviated (i.e., patching of the deviated eye may promote "diplopia awareness" and a conscious effort to realign the eyes). Surgery is recommended for children whose deviation occurs frequently, disrupts activities requiring normal binocular vision, and is unresponsive to conservative measures (52).

Amblyopia

Amblyopia (Greek *amblus*, dim and *op-*, eye) may have several causes, and more than one cause may exist in the same child. In all cases, cortical suppression of the affected eye represents an adaptation to conflicting visual information from the two eyes. The visual cortex resolves this conflict by suppression of information from one eye during binocular viewing. Chronic binocular suppression eventually leads to loss of monocular cortical circuits and decreased visual acuity (i.e., amblyopia). Strabismic amblyopia occurs when one eye is misaligned. Refractive or anisometropic amblyopia occurs in children with asymmetric refractive errors between the two eyes. In these children, one eye is chronically defocused. Deprivation amblyopia occurs with partial or complete occlusion of one eye (e.g., by a cataract or severe ptosis).

Patching of the sound eye is the mainstay of amblyopia therapy. The mechanism of action of sound-eye occlusion has been studied extensively in both human and animal experiments (53). It appears that, during the "critical period" of visual cortical development, the two eyes compete for synapses on visual cortical cells. In children with a poorly formed image in one eye (due to defocus, occlusion, or misalignment), cortical connections from the sound eye will predominate. Occlusion of the sound eye eliminates this competition and permits establishment of connections related to the amblyopic eye. In many cases, part-time patching, for as little as 2 hours daily, may be as effective as full-time patching in the treatment of amblyopia. In children with anisometropia without strabismus, glasses alone may be sufficient to treat amblyopia.

A series of recent randomized clinical trials showed that, in many circumstances, the use of atropine eyedrops to blur the sound eye is as effective as patching (54). However, treatment for amblyopia must be highly individualized. The decision about whether to use patching or atropine drops depends on expected compliance with either therapy. A major advantage of atropine is that, once the drop is instilled, it works for several days to a week or more. This eliminates the common scenario of negotiation between child and parent to discontinue patching early. Atropine also avoids the social stigma of patching, a major cause of noncompliance in school-aged children. In children with severe amblyopia, however, vision in the sound eye after atropinization may not be sufficient to permit schoolwork and other essential activities.

Amblyopia therapy is often prolonged. Therapy for dense amblyopia often requires atropine or patching for up to a year. If amblyopia is severe or has been present for a long time, the final vision rarely reaches 20/20, but can often be improved substantially with prolonged therapy. Recurrent amblyopia after discontinuation of therapy occurs in about 30% of children and is treated with reinstitution of patching or atropine treatment (54).

A number of studies have documented the psychosocial aspects of amblyopia and its therapy in young children (55–58). Quality-of-life surveys have demonstrated that a significant number of children believe that amblyopia interferes with schoolwork and generally affects their social interactions (55,56). Patients with amblyopia have a higher degree of somatization, obsessive–compulsive behavior, depression, anxiety, and interpersonal sensitivity than control subjects or children with strabismus who have not undergone patching for amblyopia (57,58). Psychiatrists must focus on these issues to minimize the impact of amblyopia and amblyopia therapy on self-image as well as academic performance and interpersonal relationships.

Compliance with amblyopia therapy is often a source of parent–child conflict. However, compliance is essential if amblyopia therapy is to be successful. For many reasons, children may fail to comply with patching, including the visual difficulty of dealing with enforced monocular vision and using an eye that sees poorly, as well as the physical discomfort of wearing a patch. The most serious obstacle in many children is the social stigma of wearing a patch, along with negative perceptions and negative behavior from peers. Parents may also be subject to pressure from family members and friends, who may encourage them to discontinue patching until the child is older and presumably emotionally stronger. Unfortunately, this often results in permanent discontinuation of patching, and attempts to regain vision at a later age are likely to be unsuccessful because the critical period for amblyopia therapy has passed. However, treatment must go forward to reverse amblyopia and restore visual acuity. The psychiatrist can play an important role in helping both children and parents overcome the psychosocial barriers to successful therapy.

Retinopathy of prematurity and ophthalmic complications of prematurity

Retinopathy of prematurity (ROP) is a disorder of the immature retina that affects low-birth-weight, primarily premature, infants. The disorder affects 65% of premature infants of birth weight less than 1,250 g. In most cases, the disorder is self-limited, although about 6% of these infants require treatment (47,59). However, in some children, progression may lead to retinal detachment, glaucoma, and a blind, sometimes painful eye (60). Early intervention with laser or cryotherapy can prevent or minimize these complications. A series of prospective, masked, randomized clinical trials has defined a "threshold" of ROP severity that, if untreated, frequently leads to irreversible visual loss (61). Treatment at threshold significantly decreases the incidence of vision-threatening complications.

Several studies have demonstrated the increased risk of other vision-threatening complications in preterm and, to a lesser extent, low-birth-weight children. These threats include strabismus, amblyopia, high myopia, and cerebral visual impairment (CVI) (62). Because of the high incidence of these complications, premature children should be screened throughout the first 5 years of life (63). Unfortunately, follow-up of premature infants has been notoriously problematic once they leave the nursery. Clinical experience suggests that spotty follow-up appears to be largely a function of the same socioeconomic factors that frequently lead to prematurity and low birth weight: poverty, teenage pregnancy, difficulty with access to medical care, and lack of a supportive family environment.

Despite active intervention and therapy, some children with ROP have a poor visual outcome. In the absence of other neurological or cognitive deficits, management of the psychosocial impact of visual impairment is similar in this group to the management of other children with impaired vision (see later section). Unfortunately many children with

ROP have other cognitive and neurological deficits that complicate their management. A complete discussion of the management of multiply handicapped children is beyond the scope of this chapter, but basic guidelines are also discussed later.

DISORDERS OF THE VISUAL BRAIN

Cerebral visual impairment (CVI)

A variety of visual defects involving both primary and higher visual function may occur in infants with damage to the cerebral visual pathways. Central visual acuity is often subnormal because of white-matter and cortical damage (64). Visual field defects are common and tend to involve the inferior visual field (65). Optic-disc structure is often affected because of loss of optic nerve fibers after trans-synaptic degeneration of the optic radiations. Severe degeneration of the optic radiations may result in excavated optic cups, simulating glaucoma—a pseudo-glaucomatous appearance (65).

Disorders of higher visual function, also are common (66), including impaired simultaneous perception, impaired perception of movement, difficulty recognizing faces, and problems with spatial perception and route finding. Recognition of these specific deficits is essential to understanding the child's visual experience and to planning effective educational and cognitive rehabilitation.

Both CVI and ROP are associated with prematurity and low birth weight and may coexist. In the setting of prematurity, cerebral visual loss is usually associated with periventricular leukomalacia (PVL). PVL is caused by white-matter ischemia due to an immature, dysplastic cerebral vasculature, resulting in areas of white-matter infarction in both the anterior and posterior periventricular areas (67). Ischemia to the posterior periventricular area results in damage to the optic radiations, whereas more-anterior ischemia results in cerebral palsy and spastic diplegia. Hypoxic/ischemic damage to the periventricular area may also affect cortical development. "Subplate neurons," residing in the periventricular zone, play a crucial role in synaptogenesis and cortical development. It appears, therefore, that both white-matter tracts and the developing cortex are highly vulnerable to hypoxic/ischemic changes in the developing brain (67).

Delayed visual maturation

The term *delayed visual maturation* has been applied to infants with poor vision without nystagmus, eye-movement abnormalities, evidence on magnetic resonance imaging (MRI) of a cerebral lesion affecting the visual pathways, and a normal ophthalmologic examination. Behavioral assessment of visual acuity in these infants depends on the integrity of the fixation and following reflex. In infants with apparently poor vision, the clinician must first establish that the child is able to generate saccadic eye movements. If eye movements are not present with the vestibulo-ocular stimulation ("doll's eye" reflex), impaired visual behavior is probably due to inability to generate eye movements.

The vast majority of infants with "isolated" delayed visual maturation achieve normal visual acuity (68). In the absence of other clinical or radiologic signs of neurological damage, the prognosis for normal vision is excellent. However, in a large proportion of these infants, neurological dysfunction, including seizures, cerebral palsy, autism, psychiatric disorders, learning disabilities, and attention-deficit disorder, later develops (68). It seems obvious, therefore, that infants with delayed visual maturation require continued monitoring of neurological function despite apparent recovery of vision.

Conversely, the term *delayed visual maturation* is misleading, in that no evidence exists of true delay in the anatomic or physiologic development of any of the primary or secondary visual pathways in these infants. Physiologic measures, such as VEP, of both retinal and cortical function have been uniformly normal. Hoyt (68) suggested that the primary defect in these infants is a form of visual inattention.

Brain tumors involving the visual pathways

Craniopharyngioma and optic-pathway glioma are the two most common brain tumors affecting the visual pathways in children. However, children with such tumors rarely are first seen with visual symptoms. They most often appear with symptoms of increased intracranial pressure, such as lethargy, headache, and disturbances in behavior and mood. Unfortunately, these symptoms are nonspecific. Severe visual loss and advanced tumor growth are the rule rather than the exception.

Craniopharyngioma is most common in the 4- to 12-year-old age group (69). The suprasellar location of this tumor often results in endocrine dysfunction, most frequently delayed growth and delayed puberty. In advanced cases, these tumors are difficult to excise completely, and adjunctive radiation may be necessary.

Optic-pathway gliomas may affect the optic nerve, chiasm, or optic tract. These tumors are histologically benign grade I or II pilocytic astrocytomas. About 50% of these children have neurofibromatosis type I (NFI) (70). Management is somewhat controversial, but the majority of these tumors are nonaggressive. Visual loss, if present, tends to be mild and stable, although severe visual loss can occur. Multifocal tumors, including ones affecting both optic nerves, imply a diagnosis of NFI. If visual loss is progressive or if the tumor expands in size to compress vital structures, such as the hypothalamus, chemotherapy, usually vincristine and carboplatin, is the treatment of choice in children younger than 6 or 7 years. Although radiation may be considered in older children (70), it cannot be administered to younger children because of the potentially damaging effect of radiation to the frontal lobes, resulting in significant cognitive dysfunction.

In addition to visual impairment, children with brain tumors often have severe neurological and neuropsychiatric handicaps. Visual impairment, if severe, can exacerbate delays in motor and psychosocial development, resulting in a vicious circle of developmental delay and psychosocial dysfunction. Significant alterations of the sleep–wake cycle are also common (71). These deficits often adversely affect the quality of life. It is, therefore, not surprising that the majority of parents of children with brain tumors report significant difficulty caring for their child (72). Psychiatric input is essential in the complex medical, social, and psychiatric treatment of the associated nonvisual disorders. The management of these patients and their families must be individualized and requires a multidisciplinary team approach, including specialists in the areas of ophthalmology, psychiatry, social work, neurology/neurosurgery rehabilitation medicine, and others (72,73).

DISORDERS INVOLVING BOTH THE EYE AND THE CEREBRAL VISUAL PATHWAYS

Metabolic disorders

Many metabolic disorders affect the ocular structures, and a complete discussion of the ocular manifestations of these disorders is beyond the scope of this chapter. Metabolic disorders may affect the cornea (e.g., mucopolysaccharidoses), the lens (e.g., galactosemia), the retina (e.g., Bardet–Biedl syndrome), or optic nerve (e.g., papillorenal syndrome). In some cases, visual signs or symptoms may be the first indication of the disease (e.g., cataract in galactosemic infants). More frequently, visual symptoms or signs are discovered in the course of investigating a multisystem disorder. Treatment is directed at the underlying metabolic disturbance. In some cases, when the posterior segment of the eye is unaffected, cataract extraction or corneal transplantation may be beneficial.

Ocular albinism

Albinism may affect only the ocular structures ("isolated" ocular albinism) or may affect both the eye and the skin (oculocutaneous albinism). Patients with "isolated" ocular albinism often have lighter skin than their parents and siblings, and skin biopsy demonstrates abnormal melanocytes. However, clinical symptoms are limited to vision. Patients with oculocutaneous albinism usually have poor central vision, approximately 20/200, but essentially normal peripheral vision. Vision is limited not only by the absence of melanin in the eye but also by hypoplasia of the fovea, abnormal chiasmal connections, and abnormal optic disks (74). Patients with all forms of albinism tend to be photosensitive.

Children with isolated ocular albinism tend to have slightly better vision than those with the oculocutaneous form. Acuity may be anywhere from 20/25 to 20/200, with 20/50 to 20/100 being the norm. These children may have brown or green irides, and usually, but not always, nystagmus. They are often misdiagnosed because of the subtlety of their ocular abnormalities.

Optic nerve hypoplasia and the septo-optic dysplasia syndrome

Optic nerve hypoplasia, which may be unilateral or bilateral, may occur as an isolated finding or in conjunction with other central nervous system malformations. Patients with isolated optic nerve hypoplasia (i.e., without accompanying CNS malformations) may have vision anywhere from 20/20 to no light perception.

The septo-optic dysplasia syndrome consists of optic nerve hypoplasia (usually bilateral), agenesis of the septum pellucidum, and hypopituitarism (75). Children with this syndrome may be first seen in the neonatal period with hypoglycemia due to hypopituitarism. They may also appear later in childhood with failure to grow, hypothyroidism, delayed puberty, or, rarely, precocious puberty. Vision ranges from 20/25 to no light perception, but generally tends to be poor (i.e., worse than 20/200 in each eye). These children may also have cortical migration abnormalities—schizencephaly and cortical heterotopia (76)—with associated developmental delay.

NONORGANIC VISUAL DISORDERS

The terms *functional* or *hysterical* visual loss have been applied to a variety of clinical situations in which no organic basis for the patient's visual defect is found. In practice, nonorganic visual symptoms may arise for a variety of reasons. Successful treatment depends on uncovering the underlying psychological factors that motivate the child's symptoms. The approach to the problem involves three distinct steps:

1. The diagnosis of nonorganic visual loss must be made with absolute certainty. Physicians should demonstrate to the child's parents by physical examination and, if necessary, ancillary tests that the child's symptoms and physical findings are incompatible with a known disease process and have a nonorganic nature. If physicians or parents have a lingering fear that an organic problem has been overlooked, they will not work in earnest to eliminate the psychological factors that are causing the problem.
2. Underlying psychological stressors must be identified. These may include sibling rivalry, emotional and physical abuse (including sexual abuse or harassment), or other family conflict. Problems at school, including both academic failure and peer conflict, are also a frequent cause of nonorganic visual loss.
3. A rational and systematic plan for eliminating stressors must be devised. It is of paramount importance to enlist the help of the parents in this process. In most cases, the psychological stressors are temporary and the situation can be remediated. However,

children who have repeated episodes of nonorganic visual loss or other nonorganic physical symptoms will require more specialized care by a psychologist or psychiatrist (77–79). Sletteberg et al. (77), reporting on the results of hysterical visual impairment in adults, children, and adolescents, stated

> the most important finding in this study is the difference in prognosis related to age at the onset of symptoms.... The younger patients seem to have a much better prognosis for later social and visual function than those who are older at the onset of symptoms.

They concluded, "The need for psychiatric intervention is small among children and adolescents, who have a favorable prognosis without any specific treatment." This view is supported by Rada et al. (78), who did not find a hysterical personality in most children with visual conversion disorders. The lack of entrenched psychopathology in children is also supported by the study of Turgay (79), who reported a large series of children and adolescents who underwent psychiatric intervention for a variety of conversion disorders, including visual symptoms. Only three of 89 patients required more than 4 weeks of integrative child and family therapy for full recovery.

Clinical presentation

The typical child with a nonorganic visual defect is between the ages of 7 and 16, with girls outnumbering boys. The disability is often inconsistent with the child's behavior. For example, a child claiming visual loss to avoid school may remain surprisingly adept at video games. The child may have had repeated examinations by ophthalmologists or optometrists, and, despite normal findings, vision seems to decrease after each examination. Laboratory and radiologic tests, if they have been performed, are all normal. Onset of the visual defect may be sudden, in which case it is often related to an emotionally traumatic event, such as serious illness or death of a close family member. In general, both eyes are affected symmetrically. Complaints of bilateral but asymmetric visual loss merit a thorough search for organic disease. Prompt recognition of the nonorganic nature of visual loss along with the appropriate supportive management is a great relief to fearful parents. Prompt diagnosis also avoids prolonged anguish and uncomfortable, sometimes risky procedures.

Nonorganic visual symptoms may take several forms, each representing a very different psychopathology, and each requiring a different form of treatment. These clinical scenarios are listed later.

Conversion disorder

Conversion disorder, sometimes called hysteria, is characterized by the absence of conscious awareness, on the part of the patient, that his or her problem is psychological and not organic (80). No conscious intent exists to deceive the family or the doctor. Children who manifest hysterical visual loss sometimes have a history of other nonorganic symptoms, such as recurrent abdominal pain, etc. Hysterical visual loss is most common in 9- to 12-year-old children, with girls far outnumbering boys. Serious family conflict is a common contributing factor, and sexual abuse should always be kept in mind. True conversion disorders in children are usually easy to diagnose. However, they may be difficult to treat because of the severe underlying emotional disturbance.

Malingering

Malingers are children and adults who intentionally simulate a visual deficit to achieve a secondary gain. Malingering, for example, to avoid school failure, is more frequently seen in the preteen and teenage years, whereas feigned poor vision to obtain glasses is typically seen in 7- to 10-year-old girls. Most children with visual malingering do not have serious underlying psychological disorders, although repeated malingering may be a sign of more-serious stress, anxiety, depression, or adjustment reaction (80). Whether repeated malingering in children may be a precursor to more serious psychosocial adjustment disorders is unknown because long-term studies have not been done.

Depression

Nonorganic visual complaints in children, like other nonorganic somatic complaints, may be a symptom of underlying depression. Evaluation of these children should include an assessment of mood as well as an inquiry into disturbances of sleep and appetite.

Nonorganic visual loss associated with an underlying organic visual disorder

Patients with true organic visual loss often have superimposed nonorganic symptoms (80). An example might be a child with a simple refractive error who behaves as if nearly blind. Motivation for such behavior may vary from child to child. In some children, the behavior seems to be motivated by a concern that the underlying organic disorder will not be acknowledged. In general, the nonorganic symptoms disappear once the organic pathology is recognized and adequately treated.

Munchausen and Munchausen-by-Proxy syndromes

Although Munchausen syndrome is rare in children, some children are victims of the Munchausen-by-proxy syndrome perpetrated by a parent or a caregiver. Ocular (or nonocular) injuries are inflicted on the child in a pattern that may simulate an organic disorder. Caregivers who are involved in the Munchausen-by-proxy syndrome often have some medical knowledge and have become adept at deceiving physicians (81). It is important to remember, however, that self-abuse, including ocular abuse, may be part of some metabolic disorders, including Lesch–Nyhan syndrome, Riley–Day syndrome, and forms of autism (82).

VISUAL HALLUCINATIONS

Visual hallucinations are uncommon in children but may be encountered in a variety of clinical settings. Several characteristics help differentiate visual hallucinations related to occipital epilepsy, migraine, or toxic encephalopathy from those occurring in the setting of psychosis. Clinical criteria are not absolute, however, and electroencephalogram (EEG) and MRI may be needed to make a definitive determination. In general, visual hallucinations due to nonpsychiatric disorders are emotionally neutral, whereas those due to psychiatric disorders often have a strong affective component. In addition, visual hallucinations related to psychosis are often accompanied by an auditory component, unlike most visual hallucinations due to nonpsychiatric disorders. The characteristics of various types of childhood visual hallucinations are described later.

Migraine

Both young children and teenagers may experience visual hallucinations as part of a migraine diathesis (83). The visual aura in migraine usually lasts between 5 minutes and 1 hour. The aura is often preceded by irritability, lethargy, or other atypical behavior. Younger children may be unable to describe the visual aura other than to indicate that they cannot see well. In some case, they may describe "polka dots," "wavy lines," or other obscurations. When the obscuration is hemianopic (confined to one visual field), the child may describe it as monocular and occurring in the eye on the side of the hemianopia.

Older children and teenagers may generally describe a more characteristic progressive visual obscuration consistent with "classic" migraine (i.e., migraine with visual aura). This may consist of a typical scintillating, C-shaped, slowly moving scotoma with jagged edges ("fortification scotoma"), sometimes with faintly colored lines along the zigzag borders. As in adults, other "nonclassic" forms of obscuration are common, including obscurations described as "TV interference," or looking through turbulent water. The visual obscuration is characteristically followed by a period of lethargy, sometimes with somnolence. Headache, which may be mild, moderate, or severe, usually begins near the end of the visual obscuration. At onset, it is often hemicranial and may progress to become a holocephalic distribution. Light and sound sensitivity may be prominent. Nausea, sometimes progressing to vomiting, is also common. Often a family history of migraine is known. On occasion, migraine may occur in the absence of headache (acephalgic migraine) and may be difficult to differentiate from occipital epilepsy (also, see Chapter 7).

Occipital epilepsy

Visual hallucinations associated with occipital epilepsy may occur in a variety of settings (84). Benign and malignant tumors, as well as congenital structural malformations of the occipital lobe, including polymicrogyria and other cortical dysplasias, may give rise to epilepsy. Occipital epilepsy also has been described in mitochondrial myopathies, including mitochondrial encephalopathy and lactic acid syndrome (MELAS) and mitochondrial encephalopathy and ragged red fibers (MERRF). Unrelated to those congenital structural occipital malformations, a distinct form of epilepsy has been described in association with bilateral occipital calcifications. A large number of these patients have had overt or subclinical celiac disease. Finally, occipital epilepsy may occur in the absence of structural cerebral abnormalities.

Taylor et al. (84) divided the syndrome of "benign childhood occipital seizures" (BCOSs) into three types: early-onset childhood epilepsy with occipital spikes, late-onset childhood epilepsy with occipital spikes, and idiopathic photosensitive occipital epilepsy. The first two syndromes are characterized by abnormal interictal EEG, whereas the third is characterized by a normal interictal EEG with a paroxysmal photic response at a wide range of flash frequencies.

The differentiation of the visual syndromes of occipital epilepsy from the visual aura of migraine has been reviewed in detail by several authors (84–86). According to Panayiotopoulos et al. (85), the visual hallucinations associated with occipital seizures are characteristically "frequent, brief, predominantly multicolored, with circular or spherical patterns" (85). The difficulty of differentiation is underscored by the fact that some patients with BCOSs may have a normal interictal EEG (see also Chapter 5, "Epilepsy" and Chapter 19, "The Diagnostic Approach to Neuropsychiatric Presentations").

Charles Bonnet syndrome

The Charles Bonnet syndrome, which occurs in children as well as adults, consists of recurrent visual hallucinations occurring in patients with profound visual impairment (87). The visual loss either may be due to local ocular disease or may involve the cerebral visual pathways. The syndrome may be produced by profound visual loss involving only one hemifield. Nevertheless, affected individuals have normal cognitive function. This curious visual phenomenon resembles, in some respects, the "phantom limb" phenomenon that occurs in individuals who have lost a limb. In patients with the Charles Bonnet syndrome, sensory deprivation may enhance activity in intact areas of the visual system (e.g., temporal lobe), which gives rise to conscious visual hallucinations. Their hallucinations, characteristically formed and complex, generally consist of animate figures (e.g., people or animals), often appearing in a dynamic, cartoon-like fashion.

Hallucinogen perception disorder

The hallucinogenic properties of various "psychedelic" drugs, such as LSD, are well known. Of particular interest is the unique ability of LSD to produce recurrent episodes of the symptoms that occurred during the intoxication phase of the drug. This recurring syndrome often includes, or may be limited to, visual hallucinations. The symptoms have been classified in the literature as short-term flashbacks, consisting of brief, nondistressing, recurrent episodes, often accompanied by a pleasant affect, and "hallucinogen perception disorder" (HPD), which is characterized by long-term, distressing, recurrent, and sometimes pervasive hallucinations, often with an unpleasant affect. Palinopsia, or persistence of visual images for several seconds, may also be seen in this disorder. Lerner (88) reviewed the diagnosis and treatment of HPD. The next section describes the visual side effects of drugs commonly used in psychiatric practice.

DRUG-INDUCED VISUAL SIDE EFFECTS

A variety of ocular and neuro-ophthalmologic side effects have been described in association with drugs commonly used in psychiatric practice. Visual abnormalities have been described in conjunction with use of antidepressants, neuroleptics, benzodiazepines, carbamazepine, lithium, topiramate, and others (89–91). A brief discussion of the major drug-induced side effects follows.

Tricyclic antidepressants are often accompanied by significant anticholinergic side effects (92) that may include pupillary dilation with accompanying light sensitivity, and cycloplegia with accompanying impairment of accommodation. The accommodative insufficiency is most often symptomatic in presbyopic or prepresbyopic adults (i.e., those older than 40 to 45 years), but it may also affect children. The impaired accommodation may result in reading difficulties that are incorrectly attributed to other causes, such as lack of motivation and emotional disability. Parents of children using these antidepressants should be informed of their side effects. If problems with reading or near work arise, an ophthalmologist should be consulted.

Topiramate, a sulfamate-substituted monosaccharide, is an antiepileptic drug that also suppresses migraine and neuropathic pain. It has also been used for weight reduction, depression, and bipolar disorder. Acute myopia, a side effect of topiramate (93), is probably caused by a disturbance of the osmotic state of the lens with resulting alteration of lens thickness and refractive index. This side effect has been described in both children and adults and is completely reversible with discontinuation of the drug. In contrast, acute angle-closure glaucoma, another side effect, has thus far been described only in adults (94). It probably occurs primarily in adults who are predisposed to angle-closure glaucoma because of pre-existing narrow angles. Angle-closure glaucoma of any etiology constitutes a vision-threatening emergency and should prompt urgent referral to an ophthalmologist. Although angle closure due to topiramate has not been described in children, topiramate should probably not be used in children with known preexisting malformations of the anterior segment of the eye.

Ocular side effects are not common in patients taking serotonin reuptake inhibitors (SSRIs). However, macular lesions have been reported as a toxic effect of sertraline (95). Thus patients started on sertraline should be informed of this potential risk and should be examined regularly by an ophthalmologist.

Nefazodone may produce an unusual derangement of motion-perception impairment (akinetopsia) (96) and sometimes a sense of visual shimmering, or "ghost images." These phenomena are similar to visual hallucinations seen by some subjects during LSD abuse, described previously (70).

Vigabatrin is an effective antiepileptic drug available in the United States only on a "compassionate use" basis. Nevertheless, it has found fairly widespread use in children with intractable seizures, especially those with structural anomalies (e.g., tuberous sclerosis). In nearly 50% of adult patients taking vigabatrin, visual-field defects primarily involving peripheral vision develop, but some may have mild to moderate loss of central vision (visual acuity) as well as color-vision defects (72). In preverbal and nonverbal children, vigabatrin retinal toxicity is monitored by electroretinography, and these children must have electroretinograms at 4- to 6-month intervals. The defects are usually asymptomatic but appear to be irreversible.

Pseudotumor cerebri is a well-documented, although uncommon, side effect of lithium carbonate (97) (see Chapter 7, Headaches in Children and Adolescents). Patients in whom this side effect develops may experience headaches due to increase in intracranial pressure, diplopia due to sixth nerve palsy, and blurred vision, sometimes with transient episodes of uni- or bilateral visual loss due to papilledema. Prolonged papilledema may result in significant loss of vision. Fortunately, the syndrome resolves with discontinuation of lithium.

Phenothiazines may produce retinal pigmentary changes (73). In general, these are mild and have minimal effect on retinal function. More severe involvement, usually resulting from many years of use, may cause decreased central and/or peripheral vision. Patients who take phenothiazines for more than a year should undergo annual ophthalmologic examinations to monitor for phenothiazine retinal toxicity. Phenothiazines may also cause corneal deposits and cataract (98).

THE PSYCHOSOCIAL IMPACT OF VISUAL IMPAIRMENT ON PARENTS AND CHILDREN

The prevalence of isolated severe visual disability in otherwise healthy children has decreased in developing countries, whereas the prevalence of multiply handicapped children has increased significantly (35). Many of these children, especially those who are born prematurely, have both visual and neurological disabilities. As outlined later, visually handicapped children, with or without other neurological disabilities, require a highly individualized, multispecialty program of educational, cognitive, and motor rehabilitation if they are to achieve their full potential. Ideally, a rehabilitation program should begin as soon as the diagnosis of visual impairment is made.

In children with normal vision, development proceeds more or less spontaneously as the infant visually explores his or her environment. In children with impaired vision, this interaction does not proceed spontaneously and must be actively encouraged. Strong reinforcement of visual exploratory behavior, at the appropriate stage of developmental readiness, is critical to minimize delays in the child's visual maturation. Various stimulation programs, devised for visually impaired infants (37), require ongoing assessment of the infant's visual development and readiness for new forms of visual stimulation.

The education of visually impaired children is a highly specialized discipline (38). The plan for each student must take into account his or her ocular disorder, neurological impairment, cognitive disability, and other health issues. Relevant parameters of visual function that may affect presentation of educational material include visual acuity at distance, near acuity, color vision, and presence of hemianopia. In children with cerebral visual impairments (CVIs), visual information must be presented in a simple, uncomplicated form with as little distraction as possible to prevent visual and cognitive "overloading" (38). Children with purely ocular disorders, conversely, benefit from enrichment of the visual environment, with multiple shapes, sizes, and (if not color deficient) colors.

Early visual loss has a profound effect on motor development (39). Moderately or severely visually impaired infants tend to be relatively passive and may not be mobile unless encouraged. If they are not encouraged to explore manually, all aspects of their motor and cognitive development may be impaired. This assistance includes not only gross and fine motor development, but also language and communicative skills (40,41). In the absence of visual information, language development may be grossly delayed because language concepts are based primarily on visual and auditory experience. Knowledgeable, timely intervention can minimize the impact of visual deprivation on language and cognition.

Learning Braille is an important part of the rehabilitation of not only children with poor vision but also of those with normal vision who have illnesses that will eventually cause visual loss. In those cases, Braille should be taught at an early age, while vision is at least partially intact. Learning Braille is much easier for younger children because of the plasticity of their language skills (99).

Emotional development is also strongly affected by infantile and childhood visual impairment (42–45). Visually impaired infants may not respond and smile to human faces and may be misjudged as indifferent to social contact. This inability may adversely affect parental bonding. Early intervention can help overcome this obstacle by emphasizing verbal contact and touch. Older children may be unable to judge the emotional reactions of peers and adults. This can lead to a sense of isolation, an exaggerated need for predictability, and a rigid personality. Assistance during play by a knowledgeable and sympathetic adult can often overcome this sense of isolation.

It is essential that parents come to terms with the emotional issues related to parenting a visually disabled child. During the first few months after the diagnosis is made, parents are most vulnerable to fear, anxiety, and development of negative attitudes. They may feel isolated and helpless in dealing with the formidable responsibility of caring for their disabled infant. If they are to develop a positive, constructive approach, they must have the support of a team of experienced professionals who can guide them. Contact with similarly affected families through parent support groups can be extremely helpful in dealing with these obstacles.

Conclusion

In this chapter, we summarized the vast literature on the development and functioning of the eye and visual brain. We also described the most prevalent disorders affecting the eye, ocular movements, visual brain, and other, related neural systems. We summarized disorders that may cause visual hallucinations and vision-related side effects of common psychiatric medications, concentrating on pediatric and adolescent patients.

Although many unanswered questions remain, substantial progress has been made over the past three decades in characterizing the normal development of the eye and visual brain. Most important, we know that the visual system is especially sensitive to perturbations caused by disease or congenital defect during infancy and early childhood. The early onset of visual injury accentuates the importance of early diagnosis and treatment for achieving the best possible outcomes.

Toward this end, the practical-minded reader may come to the end of this chapter wondering which of the many disorders we describe are most likely to occur in typical clinical practice and which of them merit the greatest attention. Any definitive answer is clearly subjective, but we list below the top ten visual conditions clinicians are apt to encounter most often in practices involving children and adolescents:

1. Cerebral visual impairment associated with prematurity
2. Cerebral visual impairment associated with other central nervous system disease (e.g., stroke, tumor)
3. Severe visual impairment associated with local ocular disease (e.g., congenital glaucoma, retinopathy of prematurity)
4. Psychosocial adjustment problems of children dealing with severe visual impairment
5. Psychosocial adjustment problems of parents dealing with a child with severe visual impairment

6. Nonorganic visual loss (i.e., "malingering," "hysterical visual loss,")
7. Munchausen or Munchausen-by-proxy syndromes
8. Cosmetic deformities or other issues related to strabismus (crossed eyes)
9. Noncosmetic issues related to strabismus (e.g., impaired depth perception with decreased performance in sports or activities of daily life)
10. Issues related to patching for amblyopia (psychosocial issues related to stigma of wearing a patch, parental control issues related to compliance with patching, etc.)

Although this list is unlikely to change substantially in subsequent years, clinicians should anticipate that even more focused and effective therapies will emerge from ongoing research into the normal and abnormal patterns of visual development over the next decade.

Questions

1. The largest number of retinal photoreceptors are called _____. These cells are located in the _____ portions of the retina and contribute to vision in _____ conditions.
   A. cones; peripheral; daylight
   B. rods; peripheral; night-time
   C. cones; central; night-time
   D. rods; central; daylight

2. After a head injury, a child loses the ability to recognize faces or objects but shows normal visual acuity and visual-field size. She likely sustained damage to what part of the visual-processing system?
   A. the ventral ("what") stream, projecting toward temporal cortex
   B. the dorsal ("where/how") stream, projecting toward parietal cortex
   C. the primary visual cortex
   D. the fovea

3. Treatment for amblyopia may include which of the following?
   A. glasses
   B. patching of the sound eye
   C. atropine drops for the sound eye
   D. any of the above

4. The first step in dealing with a child with nonorganic visual loss should be
   A. determining whether the parents believe that the child's visual loss may be nonorganic.
   B. making sure that organic visual loss has been ruled out with certainty.
   C. identifying underlying psychological stressors.
   D. devising a rational plan for eliminating all possible stressors.

5. Nonorganic visual loss in children is characterized by
   A. peak incidence in the 3- to 5-year age group.
   B. frequent association with concurrent organic visual pathology.
   C. male preponderance.
   D. generally poor prognosis for recovery.

6. Munchausen-by-proxy syndrome is characterized by
   A. injuries that may closely mimic a nontraumatic disease process.
   B. injuries often inflicted by parents or caregivers.
   C. injuries inflicted by perpetrators with specialized medical knowledge.
   D. all of the above.

7. The following might be a clue to nonorganic diplopia:
   A. diplopia that resolves when one eye is covered
   B. diplopia that is present only when gazing to the left
   C. diplopia that is worse when fatigued
   D. diplopia that occurs only with viewing specific objects (e.g., animals)

8. The most common ocular side effect of tricyclic antidepressants is
   A. flashing lights.
   B. myopia.
   C. blurred near vision.
   D. diplopia.

9. In children, topiramate may cause
   A. myopia.
   B. angle-closure glaucoma.
   C. diplopia.
   D. pseudotumor cerebri.

10. Vigabatrin may cause
    A. peripheral vision loss.
    B. myopia.
    C. diplopia.
    D. glaucoma.

11. Pseudotumor cerebri has been associated with
    A. phenothiazines.
    B. topiramate.
    C. lithium.
    D. tricyclics.

12. Which of the following may be delayed in infants with severely impaired vision?
    A. fine motor development
    B. language development
    C. cognitive development
    D. any or all of the above

Answers

1. B
2. A
3. D
4. B
5. B
6. D
7. D
8. C
9. A
10. A
11. C
12. D

REFERENCES

1. Daw NW. *Visual development*. New York: Plenum Press, 1995.
2. Simons K, ed. *Early visual development, normal and abnormal*. Oxford: Oxford University Press, 1993.
3. Atkinson J. *The developing visual brain*. Oxford: Oxford University Press, 2000.
4. Rakic P. An overview: development of the primate visual system: from photoreceptors to cortical modules. In: Lent R, ed. *The visual system: from genesis to maturity*. Boston: Birkhauser, 1992:1–17.
5. Hendrickson AE. Morphological development of the primate retina. In: Simons K, ed. *Early visual development, normal and abnormal*. Oxford: Oxford University Press, 1993:287–295.
6. Hirano S, Yamamoto Y, Takayama H, et al. Ultrasonic observation of eyes in premature babies: Part 6. Growth curves of ocular axial length and its components. *Acta Soc Ophthalmol Jpn*. 1979;83:1679–1693.
7. Bronson GW. Structure, status and characteristics of the nervous system at birth. In: Stratton P, ed. *Psychobiology of the human newborn*. Chichester: Wiley & Sons, 1982:109–118.
8. Johnson MH. Cortical maturation and the development of visual attention in early infancy. *J Cogn Neurosci*. 1990;2:81–95.
9. Shatz CJ. Emergence of order in visual system development. *Proc Natl Acad Sci U.S.A.* 1996;93:602–608.
10. Huttenlocher PR, de Courten C, Garey LG, Van der Loos H. Synaptogenesis in human visual cortex: evidence for synapse elimination during normal development. *Neurosci Lett*. 1982;33:247–252.
11. Hubel DH, Wiesel TN. Receptive fields and functional architecture of monkey striate cortex. *J Physiol*. 1967:195:215–243.
12. Ungerleider LG, Mishkin M. Two cortical visual systems: separation of appearance and location of objects. In: Ingle DL, Goodale MA, Mansfield RJW, eds. *Analysis of visual behavior*. Cambridge, MA: MIT Press, 1982:549–586.
13. Dehay C, Kennedy H, Bullier J, Berland M. Absence of interhemispheric connections of area 17 during development in the monkey. *Nature*. 1988;331:348–350.
14. Conel JL. *The postnatal development of the human cerebral cortex*. Vols. I–VIII. Cambridge, Mass: Harvard University Press, 1939–1967.

15. Huttenlocher PR, Dabholkar AS. Regional differences in synaptogenesis in human cerebral cortex. *J Comp Neurol.* 1997;387:167–178.
16. Chugani HT, Phelps ME, Mazziotta JC. Positron emission tomography study of human brain functional development. *Ann Neurol.* 1987;22:487–497.
17. Sireteanu R. Development of the visual field: results from human and animal studies. In: Vital-Durand F, Atkinson J, Braddick OJ, eds. *Infant vision.* Oxford: Oxford University Press, 1996:17–31.
18. Lewis TL, Maurer D. The development of the temporal and nasal visual fields during infancy. *Vis Res.* 1992;32:903–911.
19. Mohn G, van Hof-van Duin J. Development of the binocular and monocular visual fields during the first year of life. *Clin Vis Sci.* 1986;1:51–64.
20. Teller DY, McDonald MA, Preston K, et al. Assessment of visual acuity in infants and children: the Acuity card procedure. *Dev Med Child Neurol.* 1986;28:779–789.
21. Westheimer G. Visual hyperacuity. *Progr Sens Physiol.* 1981:1:1–30.
22. Skoczenski AM, Norcia AM. Development of VEP vernier acuity and grating acuity in human infants. *Invest Ophthalmol Vis Sci.* 1999;40:2411–2417.
23. Braddick OJ, Wattam-Bell J, Atkinson J. The onset of binocular function in human infants. *Hum Neurol.* 1983;2:65–69.
24. Birch EE, Gwiazda J, Held R. Stereoacuity development for crossed and uncrossed disparities in human infants. *Vis Res.* 1982;22:507–513.
25. Held R. Binocular vision: behavioral and neuronal development. In: Mehler J, Fox R, eds. *Neonate cognition: beyond the blooming, buzzing confusion.* Hillsdale, NJ: Lawrence Erlbaum, 1985:152–158.
26. Banton T, Bertenthal BI. Multiple developmental pathways for motion processing. *Optom Vis Sci.* 1997;74:751–760.
27. Gilmore RO, Baker TJ, Grobman KH. Stability in infants' discrimination of optic flow. *Dev Psychol.* 2004;40:259–270.
28. Wattam-Bell JRB. Development of visual motion processing. In: Vital-Durand F, Atkinson J, eds. *Infant vision.* Oxford: Oxford University Press, 1996:79–94.
29. Teller DY. First glances: the vision of infants. *Invest Opthamol Vis Sci.* 1997;38:2183–2203.
30. Atkinson J, Hood B, Wattam-Bell J, et al. Development of orientation discrimination in infancy. *Perception.* 1988;17:587–595.
31. Johnson MH, Morton J. *Biology and cognitive development: the case of face recognition.* Oxford: Blackwell, 1991.
32. Amaya L, Taylor D, Russell-Eggitt I, et al. The morphology and natural history of childhood cataracts. *Surv Ophthalmol.* 2003;48:125–144.
33. Forbes BJ, Guo S. Update on the surgical management of pediatric cataracts. *J Pediatr Ophthalmol Strabismus.* 2006;43:143–151.
34. Chak M, Rahi JS. British Congenital Cataract Interest Group: the health-related quality of life of children with congenital cataract: findings of the British Congenital Cataract Study. *Br J Ophthalmol.* 2007;91:922–926. Epub 2007 Jan 23.
35. Ho CL, Walton DS. Primary congenital glaucoma: 2004 update. *J Pediatr Ophthalmol Strabismus.* 2004;41:271–288.
36. Ho CL, Walton DS. Management of childhood glaucoma. *Curr Opin Ophthalmol.* 2004;15:460–464.
37. Attebo K, Mitchell P, Cumming R, et al. Prevalence and causes of amblyopia in an adult population. *Ophthalmology.* 1998;105:154–159.
38. Akay AP, Cakaloz B, Berk AT, Pasa E. Psychosocial aspects of mothers of children with strabismus. *JAAPOS.* 2005;9:268–273.
39. Menon V, Saha J, Tandon R, et al. Study of the psychosocial aspects of strabismus. *J Pediatr Ophthalmol Strabismus.* 2002;39:203–208.
40. Baker JD. The value of adult strabismus correction to the patient. *JAAPOS.* 2002;6:136–140.
41. Paysse EA, Steele EA, McCreery KM, et al. Age of the emergence of negative attitudes toward strabismus. *JAAPOS.* 2001;5:361–366.
42. Coats DK, Paysse EA, Towler AJ, Dipboye RL. Impact of large angle horizontal strabismus on ability to obtain employment. *Ophthalmology.* 2000;107:402–405.
43. Olitsky SE, Sudesh S, Graziano A, et al. The negative psychosocial impact of strabismus in adults. *JAAPOS.* 1999;3:209–211.
44. Smith LK, Thompson JR, Woodruff G, Hiscox F. Factors affecting treatment compliance in amblyopia. *J Pediatr Ophthalmol Strabismus.* 1995;32:98.
45. Fu VL, Stager DR, Birch EE. Progression of intermittent, small-angle, and variable esotropia in infancy. *Invest Ophthalmol Vis Sci.* 2007;48:661–664.
46. Tychsen L. Can ophthalmologists repair the brain in infantile esotropia? Early surgery, stereopsis, monofixation syndrome, and the legacy of Marshall Parks. *JAAPOS.* 2005;9:510–521.
47. Birch EE, Fawcett S, Stager DR. Why does early surgical alignment improve stereoacuity outcomes in infantile esotropia? *JAAPOS.* 2000;4:10–14.
48. Birch EE, Stager DR Sr, Berry P, Leffler J. Stereopsis and long-term stability of alignment in esotropia. *JAAPOS.* 2004;8:146–150.
49. Hutcheson KA. Childhood esotropia. *Curr Opin Ophthalmol.* 2004;15:444–448.
50. Fawcett SL, Birch EE. Risk factors for abnormal binocular vision after successful alignment of accommodative esotropia. *JAAPOS.* 2003;7:256–262.
51. Romanchuk KG, Dotchin SA, Zurevinsky J. The natural history of surgically untreated intermittent exotropia-looking into the distant future. *JAAPOS.* 2006;10:225–231.
52. Asjes-Tydeman WL, Groenewoud H, van der Wilt GJ. Timing of surgery for primary exotropia in children. *Strabismus.* 2006;14:191–197.
53. Hoyt CS. Amblyopia: a neuro-ophthalmic view. *J Neuroophthalmol.* 2005;25:227–231.

54. Holmes JM, Repka MX, Kraker RT, Clarke MP. The treatment of amblyopia. *Strabismus*. 2006;14:37–42.
55. Koklanis K, Abel LA, Aroni R. Psychosocial impact of amblyopia and its treatment: a multidisciplinary study. *Clin Experiment Ophthalmol*. 2006;34:743–750.
56. Williams C, Harrad R. Amblyopia: contemporary clinical issues. *Strabismus*. 2006;14:43–50, review.
57. Jackson S, Harrad RA, Morris M, Rumsey N. The psychosocial benefits of corrective surgery for adults with strabismus. *Br J Ophthalmol*. 2006;90:883–888.
58. Woodruff G, Hiscox F, Thompson JR, Smith LK. Factors affecting the outcome of children treated for amblyopia. *Eye*. 1994;8:627–631.
59. Palmer EA, Flynn JT, Hardy RJ, et al. Incidence and early course of retinopathy of prematurity. The Cryotherapy for Retinopathy of Prematurity Cooperative Group. *Ophthalmology*. 1991;98(11):1628–1640.
60. Good WV, Hardy RJ, Dobson V, et al. Early treatment for retinopathy of Prematurity Cooperative Group: the incidence and course of retinopathy of prematurity: findings from the Early Treatment for Retinopathy of Prematurity study. *Pediatrics*. 2005;116:15–23.
61. Good WV. Early treatment for retinopathy of Prematurity Cooperative Group. Final results of the Early Treatment for Retinopathy of Prematurity (ETROP) randomized trial. *Trans Am Ophthalmol Soc*. 2004;102:233–248.
62. O'Keefe M, Kafil-Hussain N, Flitcroft I, Lanigan B. Ocular significance of intraventricular haemorrhage in premature infants. *Br J Ophthalmol*. 2001;85:357–359.
63. O'Connor AR, Stewart CE, Singh J, Fielder AR. Do infants of birth weight less than 1500 g require additional long term ophthalmic follow up? *Br J Ophthalmol*. 2006;90:451–455.
64. Brodsky MC. Semiology of periventricular leucomalacia and its optic disc morphology. *Br J Ophthalmol*. 2003;87:1309–1310.
65. Brodsky MC, Fray KJ, Glasier CM. Perinatal cortical and subcortical visual loss: mechanisms of injury and associated ophthalmologic signs. *Ophthalmology*. 2002;109:85–94.
66. Dutton GN, Saaed A, Fahad B, et al. Association of binocular lower visual field impairment, impaired simultaneous perception, disordered visually guided motion and inaccurate saccades in children with cerebral visual dysfunction: a retrospective observational study. *Eye*. 2004;18:27–34.
67. McQuillen PS, Ferriero DM. Perinatal subplate neuron injury: implications for cortical development and plasticity. *Brain Pathol*. 2005;15:250–260.
68. Hoyt CS. Constenbader lecture: delayed visual maturation: the apparently blind infant. *JAAPOS*. 2004;8:215–219.
69. May JA, Krieger MD, Bowen I, Geffner ME. Craniopharyngioma in childhood. *Adv Pediatr*. 2006;53:183–209.
70. Opocher E, Kremer LC, Da Dalt L, et al. Prognostic factors for progression of childhood optic pathway glioma: a systematic review. *Eur J Cancer*. 2006;42:1807–1816. Epub 2006 Jun 30.
71. Palm L, Nordin V, Elmqvist D, et al. Sleep and wakefulness after treatment for craniopharyngioma in childhood: influence on the quality and maturation of sleep. *Neuropediatrics*. 1992;23:39–45.
72. Freeman K, O'Dell C, Meola C. Childhood brain tumors: parental concerns and stressors by phase of illness. *J Pediatr Oncol Nurs*. 2004;21:87–97.
73. Pedreira CC, Stargatt R, Maroulis H, et al. Health related quality of life and psychological outcome in patients treated for craniopharyngioma in childhood. *J Pediatr Endocrinol Metab*. 2006;19:15–24.
74. Russell-Eggitt I. Albinism. *Ophthalmol Clin North Am*. 2001;14:533–546.
75. Brodsky MC, Glasier CM. Optic nerve hypoplasia: clinical significance of associated central nervous system abnormalities on magnetic resonance imaging. *Arch Ophthalmol*. 1993;111:66–74.
76. Miller SP, Shevell MI, Patenaude Y, et al. Septo-optic dysplasia plus: a spectrum of malformations of cortical development. *Neurology*. 2000;54:1701–1703.
77. Sletteberg O, Bertelsen T, H¿vding G. The prognosis of patients with hysterical visual impairment. *Acta Ophthalmol*. (Copenh) 1989;67:159–163.
78. Rada RT, Meyer GG, Krill AE. Visual conversion reaction in children, I: diagnosis. *Psychosomatics*. 1969;10:23–28.
79. Turgay A. Treatment outcome for children and adolescents with conversion disorder. *Can J Psychiatry*. 1990;35:585–589.
80. Lim SA, Siatkowski RM, Farris BK. Functional visual loss in adults and children patient characteristics, management, and outcomes. *Ophthalmology*. 2005;112:1821–1828.
81. Dhanda D, Raymond MR, Hutnik CM, Probst LE. Ocular Munchausen's syndrome: a costly disorder. *Can J Ophthalmol*. 1999;34:226–228.
82. Ashkenazi I, Shahar E, Brand N, et al. Self-inflicted ocular mutilation in the pediatric age group. *Acta Paediatr*. 1992;81:649–651.
83. Lewis DW. Pediatric migraine. *Pediatr Rev*. 2007;28:43–53.
84. Taylor I, Scheffer I, Berkovic S. Occipital epilepsies: identification of specific and newly recognized syndromes. *Brain*. 2003;126:753–769.
85. Panayiotopoulos CPJ. Elementary visual hallucinations in migraine and epilepsy. *J Neurol Neurosurg Psychiatry*. 1994;57:1371–1374.
86. Panayiotopoulos CP, Ahmed Sharoqi I, Agathonikou A. Occipital seizures imitating migraine aura. *J Royal Soc Med*. 1997;90:255–257.
87. Mewasingh L, Kornreich C, Christiaens F, et al.

Pediatric phantom vision (Charles Bonnet) syndrome. *Pediatr Neurol.* 2002;26:143–145.
88. Lerner AG, Gelkopf M, Skladman I, et al. Flashback and hallucinogen persisting perception disorder: clinical aspects and pharmacological treatment approach. *Isr J Psychiatry Relat Sci.* 2002;39:92–99.
89. Santaella RM, Fraunfelder FW. Ocular adverse effects associated with systemic medications: recognition and management. *Drugs.* 2007;67:75–93.
90. Mejico LJ, Bergloeff J, Miller NR. New therapies with potential neuro-ophthalmologic toxicity. *Curr Opin Ophthalmol.* 2000;11:389–394.
91. Oshika T. Ocular adverse effects of neuropsychiatric agents: incidence and management. *Drug Saf.* 1995;12:256–263.
92. Bartlett JD, Jaanus SD. Drugs affecting the pupil. In: Bartlett JD, Jaanus SD, eds. *Clinical ocular pharmacology*. Boston: Butterworth-Heinemann, 1995:972–973.
93. Sen HA, O'Halloran HS, Lee WB. Case reports and small case series: topiramate-induced acute myopia and retinal striae. *Arch Ophthalmol.* 2001;119:775–777.
94. Levy J, Yagev R, Petrova A, et al. Topiramate-induced bilateral angle-closure glaucoma. *Can J Ophthalmol.* 2006;41:221–225.
95. Sener EC, Kiratli H. Presumed sertraline maculopathy. *Acta Ophthalmol Scand.* 2001;79:428–430.
96. Horton JC, Trobe JD. Akinetopsia from nefazodone toxicity. *Am J Ophthalmol.* 1999;128:530–531.
97. Ames D, Wirshing WC, Cokely HT, et al. The natural course of pseudotumor cerebri in lithium-treated patients. *J Clin Psychopharmacol.* 1994;14:286–287.
98. Yasuhara T, Nishida K, Uchida K, et al. Corneal endothelial changes in schizophrenic patients with long-term administration of major tranquilizers. *Am J Ophthalmol.* 1996;121:84–88.
99. Cohen LG, Weeks RA, Sadato N, et al. Period susceptibility for cross-modal plasticity in the blind. *Ann Neurol.* 1999;45:451–460.

CHAPTER 17

Challenges of Congenital Hearing Loss

WENDY OSTERLING

Introduction

Congenital hearing loss or deafness, occurring in 1 to 3 per 1,000 infants, is the most common human birth defect in the United States (1). An average of 33 babies are born with a hearing loss each day, which totals approximately 12,000 children annually. These statistics do not include those who develop sensorineural hearing loss later in childhood.

Normal hearing is critical for language development. Hearing loss alone does not have direct behavioral or developmental consequences (2). Growing up with a lack of hearing in a heavily auditory environment does, however, have indirect consequences on the development of language, academic performance, and psychosocial interactions. Children with hearing loss face potential life-long communication barriers. Various physical abnormalities and mental retardation, often in distinct syndromes, may accompany hearing loss.

At various stages of development, affected children and their families cope, react, and adapt differently to this disability. Like children with other chronic illnesses or disabilities, children with hearing loss have an increased risk of developing comorbid psychiatric disorders.

The diagnosis of hearing loss or deafness is heterogeneous with respect to severity, age at onset, and cause. Amplification, communication mode, and language fluency also influence the child's development and identity (3).

Anatomy of Hearing

Under normal circumstances, hearing begins when sound waves enter the external ear, travel down the ear canal, and strike the tympanic membrane. Sound waves striking the membrane trigger bone conduction through the three ossicles—stapes, incus, and malleus—in the middle ear cavity. The sound waves vibrate the ossicles, which amplify and convert the sound energy into mechanical, conduction energy that, in turn, resonates in the fluid-filled cavities of the inner ear cochlea.

Hair cells in the cochlea then convert the mechanical, conduction energy into electrical, sensorineural energy. Each hair cell connects with its own auditory nerve receptor. The mammalian inner ear contains 15,000 to 20,000 hair cells that make up the organ of Corti. Once these hair cells are damaged, they cannot recover or regenerate.

The sensorineural activity travels through the auditory division of the eighth cranial nerve to the superior olive, inferior colliculus, and medial geniculate nucleus of the thalamus. Pathways then bring it in the form of cortical auditory evoked potentials (CAEPs) to the auditory cortices. The primary auditory cortex, Brodmann areas 40 and 41, is located in the temporal lobe near the lateral sulcus of the temporal gyrus (the Heschl gyri). This cortical region is also adjacent to Wernicke's area, which is the site of word comprehension, and near the Broca's area, the site of language production. Other auditory cortices lie in the frontal and parietal lobes.

Varieties of Hearing Loss

PERIPHERAL HEARING LOSS

Peripheral hearing loss can be divided into three varieties: conductive, sensorineural, and mixed. Conductive hearing loss (CHL), the most common variety, results from interrupted sound transmission in the external ear or impaired middle ear bone conduction. Fluid in the middle ear, often from otitis media causing an effusion, is the most common cause of CHL. An effusion in the middle ear can cause a temporary 25-decibel (dB) hearing loss, which is equivalent to wearing earplugs. Other causes of CHL include atresia, stenosis, otosclerosis, middle-ear cholesteatoma, and obvious mechanical factors, such as impacted cerumen, a foreign body in the ear canal, or tympanic membrane perforation.

Children with CHL can hear speech, but the resultant distorted sound quality leads to difficulties with early language discrimination. These children are at risk for speech, language, and learning problems. They require more intervention than just watchful waiting and follow-up auditory testing. For children with an effusion, the initial treatment is generally a 10- to 14-day trial of antibiotics to combat any underlying ear infection. If that strategy fails, a consultation with otolaryngology surgery is usually solicited for evaluation for tympanostomy or pressure equilibrating (PE) tubes. Persistent middle-ear effusion during a child's first 3 years can result in decreased scores, at 7 years of age, in tests of speech, language, and cognitive abilities (4).

Sensorineural hearing loss (SNHL), which accounts for most cases of congenital deafness, results in severe hearing loss affecting high-frequency sounds. Maldevelopment of the cochlea, from neuronal changes, synaptic abnormalities, or altered connectivity, causes most cases of SNHL. In additional to children with congenital SNHL, in two to three per 1,000 others, SNHL develops. Causes of acquired SNHL include genetic mutations, infection, ototoxic medications, noise, and anatomic anomalies.

CENTRAL HEARING LOSS

Children who have impaired ability to perceive or process sounds in the auditory cortex are said to have "central hearing loss." In practical terms, these children have normal hearing but difficulty in a variety of auditory tasks, particularly listening selectively in noisy environments, properly combining sound input from both ears, integrating auditory information, or processing speech.

Development of Hearing

Biobehavioral research has established a "critical period" of learning and development that ends at approximately 7 years of age. The central auditory pathways have maximal plasticity during the first 3.5 years of life (5). If stimulation is delivered within this critical period, CAEP latencies reach age-normal values within 3 to 6 months. In contrast, if stimulation is withheld for longer than 7 years, CAEP latencies and plasticity decrease, and the auditory nerves undergo atrophy. Therefore the best time for intensive therapy with auxiliary aids (hearing aids or cochlear implant) is before or during the first 3.5 years.

Lack of hearing can seriously impair cognitive organization, language development, and speech perception. Restricted development of neural connections in animal models suggests that the primary auditory cortex may be functionally decoupled from the higher-order auditory cortex in situations of less sensory input (6). However, higher-order cortex for other sensory modalities, such as vision and sensory perception, may compensate for lack of auditory stimulation. For example, deaf people tend to have heightened peripheral visual acuity. Studies have shown that they are more easily distracted by peripheral field stimuli and less by central field stimuli compared with hearing people (7). This follows the theory of "cross-modal plasticity" (changes in auditory cortex responses to visual stimuli), in which the multimodal associative cortex combines information and is more sensitive to these functioning sensory modalities (8). Studies with functional magnetic resonance imaging (fMRI) and cognitive behavioral tests show evidence of neuroplasticity in the auditory area, the superior temporal sulcus, recruiting more visual, tactile, and signed input in deaf individuals (9). This cognitive reorganization does not appear to affect intellectual function: the deaf have a distribution similar to that of hearing individuals (10,11).

Neurobiologists are currently looking for biomarkers for CAEP to determine the developmental integrity of the central auditory pathways as a way to evaluate the acoustic amplification and stimulation for normal development (5). Monitoring CAEP biomarkers should allow a study of the maturation of the central auditory pathways and help guide the decision regarding hearing aids or cochlear implant.

"Auditory–verbal advocates" support wearing hearing aids or undergoing cochlear implantation or both as soon as hearing loss is diagnosed to maximize auditory stimulation. Even marginal stimulation, these advocates state, helps preserve nerve functioning and prevents their atrophy even in *prelingual deafness* (hearing loss occurring before the development of language). Continued auditory stimulation is equally important to maintain the neural integrity in *postlingual deafness* (hearing loss occurring after the development of language).

Etiologies

Approximately 50% of cases of deafness are inherited, with 80% in an autosomal-recessive, 18% in an autosomal-dominant, and 2% in an X-linked recessive pattern. More than 100 genes are associated with hearing loss. Genetic causes of hearing loss are sometime identifiable by their accompanying distinctive physical features, such as low-set ears, light-colored hair, white forelock, hypertelorism, thin lips, and broad nasal bridge (12). When hearing loss is regularly associated with these features, it is termed a *syndromic* hearing loss. About 30% of the genetic causes occur as one of the 350 forms of syndromic hearing loss (Table 17.1).

Conversely, 50% to 70% of cases of genetic hearing loss occur as isolated deficits. Because these cases lack associated distinctive clinical features, they are termed *nonsyndromic* hearing loss. Physicians can often identify them by their pattern of inheritance, age at the onset of the hearing loss, progression, audiologic characteristics, and accompanying otologic findings, such as vestibular dysfunction.

The most common hereditary cause of hearing loss is a mutation in the gap-junction gene (*GJB*). More than one half of infants with nonsyndromic hearing loss will have identifiable mutations in one of two gap-junction genes, *GJB2* (connexin 26) (30% to 50%) and *GJB6* (connexin 30). The gap junctions are responsible for recycling potassium ions from the hair cells to the stria vascularis (one of the three fluid-filled compartments of the cochlea) and actively pumping them back into the cochlear endolymph. Sound perception

TABLE 17.1 FREQUENTLY OCCURRING SYNDROMES INVOLVING ASSOCIATED HEARING LOSS AND THE RELATIVE FREQUENCY

Alport syndrome: 1%
  (progressive renal failure, progressive late-onset high-frequency HL)
Alström syndrome: common in Acadians of Nova Scotia and Louisiana
  (childhood truncal obesity, progressive retinal dystrophy, progressive SNHL)
Bartter syndrome (type 4): most common in consanguineous Middle Easterners
  (polyhydramnios, metabolic acidosis)
Biotinidase deficiency: 1/60,000
  (seizures, hypotonia, ataxia, organic acidemia, SNHL)
Branchio-oto-renal (BOR) syndrome: 2%
  (HL, preauricular pits, malformed pinnae)
Fabry disease: 1/40,000
  (vascular skin lesions, abdominal pain, nephropathy, renal failure)
Jervell and Lange-Nielson syndrome: 0.25% to 0.5%
  (SNHL, prolongation of QT interval, syncope)
Nance deafness: >1%
  (congenital fixation of stapes footplate with mixed HL)
Pendred syndrome: 4% to 10%
  (SNHL, goiter, cochlear malformation)
Treacher–Collins syndrome: 1%
  (CHL, malformed ossicles, microtia, cleft palate, micrognathia)
Usher syndrome: 4% to 6%
  (SNHL, vestibular symptoms, retinitis pigmentosa)
Waardenburg syndrome: 1% to 4%
  (patches of eye, skin, hair hypopigmentation)

From Morton CC, Nance WE. Newborn hearing screening: a silent revolution. *N Engl J Med* 2006;354:20, 2151–2164, with permission.

depends on the maintenance of high endocochlear potential within the cochlea, which fails in malformed gap junctions (13). Many children and adults with this hearing loss have residual hearing that can be amplified with hearing aids, which indicates the presence of a few remaining normal hair cells among the impaired gap junctions.

With this genetic information, medical professionals have shifted from the simple detection of hearing loss to the identification of its cause (14). Genetic information offers patients and families guidelines regarding disease prevention, therapy, and interpretation of the results of early intervention. Understanding the etiology of the child's disease offers psychological benefits and helps prepare for the child's future.

About 50% of the infants born with SNHL have one of a group of known risk factors for neonatal hearing loss (Table 17.2), but the other 50% have none of them. Thus newborn hearing screening is as important for infants who have no risk factors as for those who do.

TABLE 17.2 RISK FACTORS FOR NEONATAL HEARING LOSS

Family history of sensorineural hearing loss
Congenital infection
Presence of craniofacial anomalies
Birth weight <1,500 g
Neonatal jaundice necessitating an exchange transfusion
Ototoxic medications (e.g., furosemide, aminoglycosides)
Bacterial meningitis
Apgar scores at 5 min of ≤3
Syndrome associated with hearing loss

From Joint Committee on Infant Hearing. Year 2000 Position Statement: principles & guidelines for early hearing detection & intervention programs. *Pediatrics* 2000;106:798–817, with permission.

TABLE 17.3 AMERICAN ACADEMY OF PEDIATRICS RECOMMENDS INFANTS AND CHILDREN SHOULD BE SCREENED IN THE FOLLOWING SITUATIONS

Parental concerns regarding hearing/language development
History of bacterial meningitis
Confirmed neonatal infections associated with hearing loss (e.g., CMV)
History of significant head trauma, especially with temporal bone fracture
Presence of syndrome associated with hearing loss
Exposure to ototoxic medications (e.g., gentamicin)
Presence of neurodegenerative disorder
Confirmed incidence of infectious diseases (e.g., mumps, measles)

From Cunningham M, Cox EO, the Committee on Practice and Ambulatory Medicine and the Section on Otolaryngology and Bronchoesophagology. Hearing assessment in infants and children: recommendations beyond neonatal screening. *Pediatrics* 2003;111:2, 436–440, with permission.

Other important environmental causes of hearing loss are prematurity, prenatal and postnatal infections, anoxia, head trauma, subarachnoid hemorrhage, and pharmacologic ototoxicity. Ototoxic drugs, aminoglycoside antibiotics and chemotherapeutic agents, particularly cisplatin and carboplatin, can cause permanent hearing loss. Ten percent of patients have mutations in mitochondrial genes that make them susceptible to aminoglycoside ototoxicity due to impaired metabolism (15).

Commonly used antidepressants and antipsychotics are not known to affect hearing, except for one report that valproate induced hearing loss and tinnitus (16). Teratogens, such as antineoplastic and antiepileptic drugs, may result in multiple fetal anomalies, including atresia of the ear canal, lobes, low-set ears, and malformation of the inner ear. The Food and Drug Administration (FDA) strongly advises pregnant women not to use category C and D medications.

In utero rubella infection was historically the most common infectious cause of congenital deafness, but, since the introduction of the rubella vaccine, the incidence of rubella deafness has decreased significantly. Currently, the majority of infectious causes of congenital deafness are *in utero* cytomegalovirus (CMV) and toxoplasmosis infections. *In utero* CMV infection causes about 10% of cases of congenital hearing loss and 35% of those with moderate-to-severe late-onset loss (17). However, because 84% of newborns with congenital CMV infection lack distinctive clinical findings, this virus infection is usually not recognized as the cause of congenital hearing loss in many children. Although the development of *Haemophilus* and pneumococcal vaccinations has also reduced the incidence of bacterial meningitis leading to hearing loss, bacterial meningitis still occurs and causes deafness in about 10% of cases.

In contrast to congenital hearing loss, progressive early-onset hearing loss, which is not present at birth, can result from infection, ototoxic drugs, autoimmune disease of the inner ear, enlargement of the vestibular aqueduct, injury, or other genetic mutations. The Joint Committee of Infant Hearing has identified 10 risk indicators that should prompt monitoring of hearing status, even if the results of newborn screening are normal (18) (Table 17.3).

Newborn Hearing Screening and Diagnosis

Prior to the 1990s, hearing loss was diagnosed in infants around 18 months of age. During the first few months of life, deaf babies with babbling and gestural behaviors can develop similarly to hearing babies. Their hearing loss can be subtle and difficult to diagnose in reciprocal parent–child interactions based on smiling, cooing, and visual tracking before 6 months of age. From 6 months onward, parents may suspect a hearing problem if the child fails to respond to his or her name, imitate sounds, or produce words by 12 months of age. A hearing loss should not affect fine or gross motor development, but primarily language development, which can contribute to other psychosocial consequences. The presence of other disorders such as seizures, intellectual disability, or cerebral palsy has been associated with increased prevalence of language delay, psychosocial challenges, and adjustment problems (19).

The Colorado Newborn Screening program showed that infants who were diagnosed and received intervention within the first 6 months of life were more likely to have better language, social, and emotional development than were those diagnosed later. This observation was consistent, regardless of the mode of communication—speaking or signing (20). Early identification and early intervention influence prognosis, development, language acquisition, and educational outcome (21). Interestingly, deaf children born to deaf parents acquire native fluency in American Sign Language (ASL) and achieve the same parallel language milestones in ASL as do children with no hearing loss (22).

Hearing loss can have detrimental effects on brain development. Once the diagnosis of deafness is confirmed, physicians should look for comorbidities, including language deficits, cognitive dysfunction, learning disabilities, speech disability, mental retardation, and psychiatric disturbances. If the child has a syndromic hearing loss, neurological components may be present, such as epilepsy, tics, attention-deficit disorder, mental retardation, ataxia, and balance problems. A deaf child can appear autistic or mentally retarded simply because he or she cannot interact with others. This can result in a misdiagnosis of the deaf child as having learning disability or attention deficit disorder. If an in utero infection or toxicity caused the hearing loss, depending on the timing of embryologic development, the insult may also result in blindness, mental retardation, and delayed gross motor skills. Similarly, perinatal trauma and sepsis may cause lifelong, static motor impairment (cerebral palsy) and mental retardation, as well as deafness.

As a result of research data and the increasing pressure for early diagnosis, the National Institutes of Health Consensus Development Conference in 1993 endorsed a universal newborn hearing screening program. The American Academy of Pediatrics (AAP) now recommends universal screening of infants with the goal of screening of all infants by 3 months of age. Every state has established Early Hearing Detection and Intervention (EHDI) programs to provide audiologic screening (23,24). Today, nearly 93% of all newborn infants in the United States complete hearing screening before discharge. As result, the average age that hearing loss is confirmed has dropped to 2 to 3 months (25).

In the past, newborn hearing screening received criticism because of the high rate of false positives, which resulted in unwarranted parental anxiety. Recently, the testing performance has improved, and now the average failure rate is less than 0.5%. About half of these infants whose results are false positives actually have normal hearing. To minimize anxiety, the euphemism "refer" was adopted to characterize failed screening tests (26). Counseling the parent about abnormal screening results should avoid creating anxiety. At the same time, the approach should not belittle the screening results to ensure that the parents bring their child for repeated testing in a few weeks.

The AAP recommends using one of two screenings: the auditory brainstem response (ABR) or the otoacoustic emissions (OAE) test. The ABR test measures average neural response to repetition of a large number of sound signals of the same pitch and intensity. The OAE test detects movements of outer hair cells of the cochlea with evoked sounds. Most hospital nurseries use both methods as part of a two-stage screening protocol. The OAE is most commonly used first for screening, as it is simpler to use in the nursery, but this test more frequently produces false-positive results. If the baby fails, then testing is repeated with the more-sensitive ABR test.

If newborn hearing screening is not done or if the child has a progressive hearing loss after initially passing the newborn screen, parents may be unaware that their infant has a hearing loss until the infant fails to reach language milestones, shows communication challenges, or fails school hearing tests. Therefore the AAP additionally recommends formal hearing screening for all children at 3, 4, and 5 years of age and then every 2 to 3 years until adolescence to identify children in whom a hearing loss may develop. In addition, children who have persistent middle ear effusions for more than two months should undergo screening. Usually the more severe or rapid onset of the hearing loss, the earlier its identification is possible.

Diagnosis of Hearing Loss

Audiologists perform a series of tests and construct an audiogram that shows the severity, sensitivity, thresholds, and frequencies of the hearing loss. These data will also allow the audiologist to recommend appropriate auxiliary aids, such as hearing aids and cochlear implants, and make the referral to early-intervention and support groups. The spectrum of hearing loss ranges through mild (25- to 45-dB loss); moderate (45- to 65-dB loss); severe (65- to 85-dB loss); profound (85- to 130-dB loss); and total (no residual hearing).

With increasing severity of hearing loss, distinguishing between the elements of spoken language becomes more difficult. Even a hearing loss of 15 dB during early childhood can impair speech perception, delay speech acquisition, and impair school performance. Children with borderline hearing loss (16 to 25 dB) may miss 10% of speech in a noisy environment, such as in a classroom, and have impaired interaction with peers. Children with a mild hearing loss may miss up to 50% of speech in a noisy classroom and, because of school and social difficulties, may lose self-esteem. Moderate hearing loss can cause significant problems with communication.

Although deaf children must undergo special testing for learning disabilities, proper assessment and methods for correction are thought to be lacking (27,28). Certain combinations of tests would be useful for education and vocational, as well as psychiatric counseling (29). Neuropsychiatric testing should be done by a trained professional who has experience and understands the deaf culture and language to avoid misunderstandings and misdiagnosis.

All options should be considered for the hearing-impaired child: hearing aids, cochlear implants, speech therapy, sign language, special education, mainstream education, and one-on-one instruction. Once diagnosed, children with hearing loss require close monitoring by an audiologist, yearly audiologic evaluations to monitor the level of hearing loss, and evaluations of auxiliary aids. Many schools require yearly evaluations for the Individual Education Program (IEP) for special education support. Although hearing will not improve with growth, deaf and hard-of-hearing children often learn to adapt. For optimal auditory–verbal development, comprehensive collaboration among the medical specialists, educators, and the family is vital.

Initial Parental Reaction

More than 95% of deaf children are born to hearing parents who have little or no knowledge of or experience with deafness (30). Most of these parents may be initially shocked and need to grieve the loss of their "normal" child. They may feel overwhelmed by the voluminous and sometimes conflicting information about deafness, early intervention, education, communication methods, and cochlear implants. Some parents never overcome these emotional hurdles or do so later in their child's life. Their feeling of loss may recur during their deaf child's life, especially if they wonder about schooling, graduation, higher education, work, and marriage. To lessen the impact, parents reach out to understand, accept, and advocate for their deaf child. The needs of siblings should not be overlooked. The deaf child must receive significant attention, including speech therapy, audiology appointments, and language tutoring. This extensive and time-consuming support often has an effect on the siblings and wider family. Families with access to adequate resources and support during early intervention experience decreased stress and, therefore, lower risk for socioeconomic problems. Nevertheless, challenging situations—family, home, school, work, community, and social— will persist throughout life. These stresses do not become easier with age; however, they become more manageable as the deaf child develops strategies and learns to advocate for himself.

Cultural Aspects of Deafness

Critchley (31) wrote, in 1967, that deafness impairs not only the learning of speech, but also the acquisition of vocabulary, comprehension of concepts, and learning of literary skills. These deficits can adversely affect the deaf child's social development and self-esteem. Despite advances, he saw deaf children segregated and social and educational differences splitting the community. The amount and quality of communication with family and society is positively correlated with self-esteem development (32,33).

Currently, some deaf individuals, informally affiliated as the "Deaf Culture" (34,35) contend that medical and other professional people tend to view deafness as "pathological," "abnormal," and a disability. They celebrate the birth of a deaf child who may share in the culture (35,36). Some members consider the terms "deafness" and "hearing impairment" to be offensive because of their emphasis on "impairment" or "disability." They consider themselves a society with its own preferred language, American Sign Language (ASL), which follows certain rules of interacting (37). They sometimes view attempts at integrating deaf children into mainstream society as forcing them into the hearing world where they are never equal and often seen as inferior.

Early Intervention

The key to success is early diagnosis and early intervention. As soon as the diagnosis is confirmed, infants with hearing loss should immediately partake in early-intervention services. However, it can take an average of 1 year before intervention begins (39). The selection of physicians, audiologists, and other appropriate therapists can be confusing and overwhelming to the family of the hearing-impaired child. Health insurance companies do not always cover the costs of hearing aids and cochlear implant surgery. Finances and appointments can hinder the child's prompt access to sound and communication. Late diagnosis and intervention hamper the acquisition of fundamental linguistic, social, and cognitive skills that provide the foundation for schooling and success in society. Early-intervention services include those addressed to the family. Some families choose to participate in support groups. Some may prefer to learn sign from a deaf adult who visits their home, whereas others prefer to attend a sign-language class.

Deaf children require early, individualized intervention to help establish communicative expression, receptive language, and a strong foundation of language. Profoundly deaf infants who received systematic family-centered intervention scored significantly better on measures of familial stress, developmental level, and communication ability than did those who received less-systematic intervention (40). Similarly, infants identified with hearing loss and early intervention initiated by 6 months of age, functioned within normal limits of expressive and receptive language when they were tested at about 26 to 36 months (21,41). Overall, the method matters less than early access to language for socioemotional development and academic achievement.

Access to Language and Communication

Language deprivation is the most profound consequence of deafness (10). However, no single communication approach works for all hearing-impaired children. Some deaf children with considerable residual hearing may depend on heavily auditory input if they have optimal amplification. However, most deaf children are "visual learners" to compensate for the limited hearing.

Models of development suggest that language arises through successive organizational adaptations and that early stages require extraction of acoustic representations from speech streams (42). A deaf child does not readily learn grammatical rules of spoken language. Social cognition and emotional needs drive the progression of language development (42). Hence a child who does not hear does not understand or learn age-appropriate language fluency. Self-expression is difficult for all children and even more difficult for children with hearing loss. Moreover, when difficulty interacting in a spontaneous way is encountered, secondary problems arise, such as learning difficulties, attention problems, social isolation, and depression (43). Many deaf adults never master language and read, on average, at a fourth-grade level (44). The average reading level has most likely improved in recent years because of the success of early-intervention programs. Interestingly, deaf college students from deaf families tend to do better academically, averaging an 11th-grade reading level, because of earlier access to language and good parent–child communication (3).

Poor language skills result in the deaf child experiencing loneliness, academic failure, and diminished self-worth (45). Conversely, several factors contribute to healthier self-esteem among deaf children and adolescents: parents who have a positive attitude toward deafness; availability of clear and accessible communication within the home; and whether the deaf child or adolescent identifies with others within the deaf community and has a rich sense of language and heritage as part of a vital cultural group (45). Interestingly, one study found that deaf and hard-of-hearing children had a more than twofold higher rate of injury regardless of age, race, and sex (46). Further studies are needed to determine if the sensory disability and its comorbidities make the children more prone to injury; children and parents of this population tend to seek more treatment; or the language barrier impedes full comprehension of warning signs. Effective communication and education is needed to reach out to children with hearing loss, and their specific language must help them be more aware and understanding of their surroundings (Table 17.4).

Speech Therapy and Mainstreamed Education

Deaf children must go through years of arduous speech training to produce phonemes and combine them into spoken words. They learn English essentially as a second language. Their outcomes are extremely varied. Sometimes time in speech training might have been better spent learning ASL as the primary language. In addition, many hearing family

TABLE 17.4 APPROACHES IN DEAF EDUCATION

Oral–aural: teaching the child to speak and use residual hearing

Bilingual–bicultural: ASL as language of access and instruction, with emphasis on teaching written and spoken English as a second language

Cued speech: combined speech and hand cues make English phonemes visible to the deaf child and develop receptive skills that enhance the understanding of spoken English. Cued speech incorporates eight hand shapes and four hand locations near the face to supplement the movements of lips, teeth, and tongue, thereby eliminating the ambiguities of speech reading.

Simultaneous communication (Sim-Com) (a.k.a. Signed Supported Speech–SSS): Both a spoken language and a manual language are used simultaneously. However, the concept of using two languages at the same time is rarely relayed perfectly, and the non-native language degrades in clarity

Total communication (TC): The use of different methods of communication (signed, oral, auditory, written, and visual aids) in the classroom, depending on the student's needs, abilities, and preferred mode of communication

---

members fail to become proficient in sign language or communicate in an effective way with the deaf child to engage the child in abstract semantic context. These problems can lead to a profound communication mismatch between the deaf child and hearing family that can affect the parent–child relationship and have detrimental psychosocial consequences (42).

Even if a deaf child is mainstreamed and appears to be doing well with speech, language, and academic performance, parents and teachers should examine the child's social and emotional well-being. Children and teenagers rarely see difference as a virtue, and deafness is no exception (43). Parents and teachers should address the following questions: Does the deaf child have friends, the ability to make new friends, and interact comfortably with the surrounding environment? Is the deaf child picking up language incidentally? How does the child explain the deafness and, if present, auxiliary aids to others? Is the child truly participating in the classroom, whether in the mainstream or in specialized schools? Is the child ostracized or accepted as someone who happens to use an auxiliary aid?

Adolescence poses another challenge because information about the world begins to surface through peers rather than through parents and family. Does the child have both deaf and hearing friends? Does the child continue to use the cochlear implant or hearing aids or both regularly (47)? Does the child acquire age-appropriate language fluency (48)? What kind of jobs does the child obtain? Does the hearing-impaired child have future goals? As the child grows and experiences different stages of Erickson's psychosocial development—latency, adolescence, and young adulthood—the understanding of the hearing loss becomes deeper and more abstract. If the child already has low self-esteem and low language, this becomes more challenging. The child may be teased and feel ashamed. Psychotherapy can play an important role in the child's well-being and help prevent manifestations of childhood difficulties from carrying on to adulthood.

Whether the child is raised in an oral or signing environment (or a combination of the two), deafness has a reverberating effect on emotional well-being. Deafness does not cause emotional disorders but can exaggerate them. In addition, the degree of deafness alone does not appear to be a risk factor in predicting psychiatric disorders in deaf children (49). The invisible nature of deafness often creates miscommunication and misunderstanding between individuals that can burden the deaf or hard-of-hearing child.

Emotional problems can be revealed in different ways. The child can become innerfocused as a result of reduced stimulation from the outside world and "feel different" from peers. Consequently, a negative self-dialogue can arise and lead to feelings of isolation, low self-esteem, sadness, and eventually depression (43). At the same time, if a signing deaf child is asked if he is "depressed," he may not comprehend the actual meaning of the word "depressed." A better strategy is to ask multiple questions about feelings, by using visual metaphors or drawing a timeline. Children can also react to hearing loss with "externalizing, impulsive, or acting-out behaviors that can be mistaken for attention-deficit disorder (ADD) or attention-deficit hyperactivity disorder (ADHD) (50,51). Language deprivation correlates with disruptive behavior (50).

Psychiatric Comorbidity

Of 37,407 American deaf school children surveyed by the Gallaudet Research Institute (GRI) in 2004 through 2005 (the last year of data available), 58% had no additional impairments; but 1.8% had comorbid developmental delay; 1%, autism; 9.2%, learning disability; 6.3%, ADHD; 9.5%, speech or language impairment; 8.2%, mental retardation; and 1.9%, "emotional disturbance" (52). Other studies showed a prevalence rate of 22% to 31% deaf children with mild to severe psychiatric disturbances along with a higher prevalence of neurological disorders, whereas the hearing control group had a 9.7% incidence rate (32,53).

Surveying individuals who acquired deafness in adolescence or later, Mahapatra (54) found psychiatric illnesses significantly more frequently among them than among controls. Moreover, he found that depressive illness was the predominant condition among those with psychiatric illness, but that psychosomatic illness was not more frequent among those with or without deafness (55). Watt and Davis (56) not only found that depression was more prevalent among deaf residential school adolescents, but also that they were prone to boredom when unable to engage in and follow conversations with other people. However, once the language needs of deaf children were addressed, mild but not severe depression was found to be more prevalent (57).

Psychosis seems no more prevalent among deaf children than among hearing children. However, Brown et al. (58) reported an association of deafness due to prenatal rubella exposure, usually in the first trimester, with the development of nonaffective psychosis in adulthood. Similarly, Thewissen (59) found an association between psychosis and hearing loss.

Shapira et al. (60) reported a possible association of prelingual deafness and the subsequent development of bipolar disorder. When schizophrenia develops in deaf individuals who rely on sign language, their communication disorder is reflected in their sign language (61). Schizophrenia within the deaf community appears to be roughly equivalent to the general population prevalence, although no reliable data confirm this (62). Interestingly, deaf schizophrenic patients report experiencing "voices." Researchers believe the "voice" hallucinations depend on the individual's sensory experience (residual hearing or before hearing loss) and language modality, which imprint the neural connections of the subvocal feedback loops.

Children with autistic-spectrum disorders, unlike otherwise normal deaf children, do not attempt to circumvent their inability to communicate with hand and facial gestures. Nevertheless, children with autistic-spectrum disorders should undergo hearing tests. Comparing deaf autistic individuals with hearing autistic individuals, Roper et al. (63) found no difference in their symptoms; however, autism was diagnosed later in deaf than in hearing autistic children. They concluded that the deafness did not cause autism. When testing autistic children, Rosenhall et al. (64) found mild to moderate hearing loss in 7.9% and pronounced or profound bilateral hearing loss in 3.5%. These rates of hearing losses are comparable to those found in mentally retarded populations, but much higher than those in the general population.

Many factors may precipitate, exaggerate, or even mimic ADHD, which affects 6.3% of American deaf school children. Kelly et al. (65) reported that the prevalence of ADHD in children in a state residential school for the deaf is similar to that in hearing children, but children with acquired hearing loss—as compared with those with congenital onset hearing loss—carry an increased risk for ADHD. Moreover, those authors thought that deaf children were particularly vulnerable to the detrimental effects of ADHD (51). They also pointed out that in these children, language/communication disorders, auditory processing disorder, and temporal-sequential processing disorder may mimic ADHD. In addition, the cause of the deafness (congenital rubella, for example) may be the cause of neurological impairment. The treatment of ADHD in deaf and hard-of-hearing children requires nonpharmaceutical management, stimulants, or both (51).

Although the GRI found a 9.2% comorbidity of learning disabilities in deaf and hard-of-hearing children, Kelly et al. (65), reviewing the literature, reported an incidence of 4% to 7%. In any case, certain behaviors in deaf children as the shared manifestations of ADHD and learning disabilities are likely to lead to diagnostic confusion.

The assessment and treatment of deaf children requires a multidimensional approach that includes cultural sensitivity, unrestricted communication access, understanding of child development, and a thorough medical and psychiatric evaluation. Awareness of the historical, social, and political forces contributing to deafness would help psychiatrists. Psychiatrists' appreciation of how deafness has influenced family life, peer-group, and academic adjustment may prompt them to use a "biopsychosocial" approach in dealing with "narcissistic vulnerabilities," defenses, and language-processing difficulties (66). With all these issues, deaf children and their families may benefit from meeting other deaf children, adults, and families with similar experiences. Proper psychological evaluation of a deaf child has been controversial as to whether to test both verbal and visual modalities and how to best test all aspects of intelligence in the presence of a language delay (10,11). The professional performing the test may not be fluent in the child's language of signing, or an interpreter is relaying the answers, which may skew the true results. Most important, the testing should be done in the preferred, most accessible communication mode of the patient, whether it is signing, lipreading, cued speech, or written. The professional should have a good understanding of deaf language, culture, and its communication challenges to avoid misdiagnosing the child as mentally retarded or learning disabled. Professionals experienced in working with the deaf should be able to separate the hearing loss from the core of the problems and not automatically assume it is the main problem. If a sign-language interpreter is used for the testing or any psychotherapy appointments, the interpreter should be a qualified, nationally certified interpreter and not a parent or friend.

Perspectives of community psychiatry, which emphasizes prevention, reduction, and relief of psychiatric illness, may help in organizing mental-health and rehabilitation services for deaf individuals to avoid psychopathological changes (32). Because emotional and behavioral characteristics of deaf children can be misconstrued as "pathology," appropriate diagnosis and treatment can be hindered (67). For example, the unique nature of ASL can make a deaf person appear psychotic if not properly understood (68).

Hearing Aids and Cochlear Implants

Hearing aids are prostheses that fit on the outside of the ear(s) and amplify sound but do not always improve speech discrimination. For example, using a hearing aid is like listening to a radio station filled with static: turning up the volume on the dial does not improve the voice clarity. Unlike eyeglasses that can completely correct vision, neither hearing aids nor cochlear implants completely correct hearing.

Individuals using a cochlear implant wear an external processor that, via a magnet, transmits signals to an internal processor under the scalp. The internal processor receives signals and transmits them through wires to microelectrodes that have been surgically implanted in the cochlea to stimulate the auditory nerve. Cochlear implants surpass hearing aids in sound input and quality. Increasing numbers of deaf children and adults are undergoing cochlear-implant surgery and are showing improved function and integration into the hearing society.

Children who were implanted before the age of 2 years demonstrated a nearly threefold greater rate of developing age-normal speech and language skills than do children who received an implant at 4 years of age (69–72). Most recently, Shin (73) reported that at 6 months after cochlear implant, deaf children had a marked increase in nonverbal cognitive functions and working memory. In addition, implants were associated with improvements in mood, social ability, self-esteem, and other psychological parameters.

Infants as young as 6 months have undergone cochlear implantation, but this entailed risks from the surgery, anesthesia, and immaturity of the skull. The FDA currently approves cochlear implants for children 12 months of age and older. Recent studies, which have shown a high degree of plasticity of the central auditory pathways after early bilateral implantation (74), support an earlier implantation (6–12 months) for optimal development of the central auditory pathways. Current research evidence shows that bilateral cochlear implants further enable sound localization and understanding of speech in a noisy environment, which is less achievable with unilateral implants (75).

A cochlear implant is not a simple surgery. It involves a comprehensive multidisciplinary assessment. The evaluation looks at the individual's medical and psychosocial background and the family's commitment to structured therapy to assure optimal results. The deaf individual undergoes an audiologic examination with and without amplification and radiological imaging of the temporal bones to evaluate the anatomy of the cochlear and auditory nerves. The outcomes are largely determined by the duration of deafness, age at cochlear implantation, educational setting, form of communication, family structure and support, access to therapy, speech-language development, and cognitive/motor/social development (76).

Future generations may be able to repair and regenerate hair cells and apply gene therapy to correct mutations. Researchers have identified stem cells that express the genes essential for hair cell development, but have not yet figured out how to position and "turn on" the regeneration of the sensory neurons in the human ear.

Summary

Improved genetic testing helps explain the physiology and predict capabilities with hearing aids and cochlear implants. Modern education and technology have enabled the deaf to achieve better speech, auditory, and academic skills than ever before. The technology permits the diagnosis of deafness in neonates. Infants with hearing loss are being equipped with digital hearing aids or cochlear implants or both that maximize auditory stimulation and auditory brain development during the critical period. Hearing aid and implant technology continue to improve volume and sound quality, which enable the deaf to hear with greater clarity and better speech discrimination. Still, the technology cannot replicate natural hearing.

Deafness is not just a medical diagnosis, but a multidimensional experience and cultural phenomenon. Early intervention is imperative in reducing the long-term detrimental effects of hearing loss, the worst of which is language deprivation. Hearing loss also threatens children's cognitive, emotional, and social development. It carries psychiatric comorbidity. Parents must consider how their own issues affect their child. Clinicians must be culturally sensitive, empathetic, and open-minded to the experience of each deaf or hard-of-hearing person.

Questions

1. What part of development is most affected by deafness?
   A. social development
   B. cognitive development
   C. perceptual visual development
   D. language development

2. What disorder is often overdiagnosed in deaf children?
   A. bipolar disorder
   B. schizophrenia
   C. ADHD
   D. delusional disorder

3. What percentage of deaf children are born to hearing parents?
   A. 50%
   B. 95%
   C. 15%
   D. none

4. According to the latest research, by what age should a child receive a cochlear implant for best outcome?
   A. 7 years
   B. 15 years
   C. 6–12 months
   D. 10 years

5. What infectious agent is the most common cause of prelingual deafness in the United States today?
   A. rubella
   B. scarlet fever
   C. cytomegalovirus
   D. tuberculosis

6. Children with hearing loss have increased risk of which of the following?
   A. depression
   B. language delay
   C. low self-esteem
   D. poor speech abilities
   E. all the above

7. What is the most common cause of congenital hearing loss?
   A. environment
   B. idiopathic
   C. syndrome
   D. nonsyndromic genetic

8. What is the most common syndrome with a comorbid hearing loss?
   A. Waardenburg
   B. Pendred
   C. Usher
   D. Treacher–Collins
   E. Mondini malformation

9. If a newborn fails the hearing screen, what should be done?
   A. refer to an ENT
   B. repeat the testing within 4–6 weeks
   C. referral to early intervention
   D. Nothing; reassure the parents it is probably fluid in ear canal.
   E. genetic testing

10. What percentage of newborns who fail the hearing screen have a true, confirmed hearing loss?
    A. 0.5%
    B. 5%
    C. 0.25%
    D. 1%

11. Which screening tests do most newborn nurseries use?
    A. OAE ABR
    B. ABR
    C. CT
    D. MRI

12. The American Academy of Pediatrics recommends that infants and children be screened if they have had exposure to the following:
    A. history of bacterial meningitis
    B. parental concerns regarding hearing and language development
    C. history of significant head trauma
    D. exposure to ototoxic medications
    E. all the above

Answers

1. D
2. C
3. B
4. C
5. C
6. E
7. D
8. B
9. B
10. A
11. A
12. E

REFERENCES

1. Infants test for hearing loss–United States, 1999-2001 *MMWR Morb Mortal Wkly Rep.* 2003;52:981–984.
2. King BH, Hauser PC, Isquith PK. Neuropsychiatric aspects of blindness and severe visual impairment, and deafness and severe hearing loss in children. In: Coffey CE, Brumback RA, eds. *Textbook of pediatric neuropsychiatry*. Washington, DC: American Psychiatric Association, 2005:397–423.
3. Hauser PC. Deaf readers' phonological encoding: an electromyogram study of convert reading behavior. *Dissert Abstr Int.* 2001;62:4B (UMI No. AAI3012772).
4. Teele DW, Klein JO, Chase C. Otitis media in infancy and intellectual ability: school achievement, speech, and language at age 7. *J Infect Dis.* 1990;162:685.
5. Sharma A, Martin K, Roland P, et al. P1 latency as a biomarker for central auditory development in children with hearing impairment. *J Am Acad Audiol.* 2005;654–673.
6. Kral A, Tillein J. Brain plasticity under cochlear implant stimulation. *Adv Otorhinolaryngol.* 2006;64:89–108.
7. Proksch J, Bavelier D. Changes in the spatial distribution of visual attention after early deafness. *J Cogn Neurosci.* 2002;14:687–701.
8. Fine I, Finney EM, Boynton GM, Dobkins KR. Comparing the effects of auditory deprivation and sign language within the auditory and visual cortex. *J Cogn Neurosci.* 2005;17:1621–1637.
9. Bavelier D, Brozinsky C, Tomann A, et al. Impact of early deafness and early exposure to sign language on the cerebral organization for motion processing. *J Neurosci.* 2002;21:8931–8942.
10. Braden JP, Jordan IK. *Deafness, deprivation and IQ*. New York: Springer, 1994.
11. Maller SI. Intellectual assessment of deaf people: a critical review of core concepts and issues. In: Marshark M, Spencer PE, eds. *Oxford handbook of deaf studies, language, and education*. New York: Oxford University Press, 2003:.
12. Toriello HV, Reardon W, Gorlin RJ. *Hereditary hearing loss and its syndromes*. Oxford: Oxford University Press, 2004.
13. Forge A, Becker D, Casalotti S, Edwards J. Gap in the inner ear: comparison of distribution patterns in different vertebrates and assessment of connexin composition in mammals. *J Comp Neurol.* 2003;467:207–231.
14. Schimmenti LA, Martinez A, Fox M, Crandall B. Genetic testing as part of the early hearing detection and intervention (EHDI) process. *Genet Med.* 2004;6:521–525.
15. Castillo FJ, Rodriguez-Ballesteros M, Martin Y, Arellano B. Heteroplasmy for the 1555A>G mutation in the mitochondrial 12S rRNA gene in six Spanish families with non-syndromic hearing loss. *J Med Genet.* 2003;40:632–636.
16. Hori A, Kataoka S, Saki K, et al. Valproic acid-induced hearing loss and tinnitus. *Intern Med.* 2003;42:1153–1154.
17. Barbi M, Binda S, Caroppo S, Ambrosetti U. A wider role for congenital cytomegalovirus infection in sensorineural hearing loss. *Pediatr Infect Dis J.* 2003;22:39–42.
18. Cunningham M, Cox EO, the Committee on Practice and Ambulatory Medicine and the Section on Otolaryngology and Bronchoesophagology. Hearing assessment in infants and children: recommendations beyond neonatal screening. *Pediatrics.* 2003;111:2:436–440.
19. Polat F. Factors affecting psychosocial adjustments of deaf students. *J Deaf Stud Deaf Educ.* 2003;8:325–339.
20. Yoshinaga-Itano C, Sedey AL, Coulter DK. Language of early, and later-identified children with hearing loss. *Pediatrics.* 1998;102:1161–1171.
21. Yoshinaga-Itano C. Early intervention after universal neonatal hearing screening: impact on outcomes. *Ment Retard Dev Dis Rev.* 2003;9:252–266.
22. Caselli MC, Volterra V. From communication to language in hearing and deaf children. In: Volterra V, Erting CI, eds. *From gesture to language in hearing and deaf children*. 2nd ed. Washington, DC: Gallaudet University Press, 1994:263–277.
23. White K. The current status of EHDI programs in the United States. *Ment Retard Dev Dis Res Rev.* 2003;9:79–88.

24. National Center for Hearing Assessment and Management (NCHAM). State UNHS summary statistics accessed, April 18, 2006 at http://www.infanthearing.org/status/unhsstate.html.
25. Harrison M, Roush J, Wallace J. Trends in age of identification and intervention. *Ear Hear.* 2003;24:89–95.
26. Morton CC, Nance WE. Newborn hearing screening: a silent revolution. *N Engl J Med.* 2006;354:2151–2164.
27. Roth V. Students with learning disabilities and hearing impairment: Issues for the secondary and postsecondary teacher. *J Learn Disabil.* 1991;24:391–397.
28. Soupkup M, Feinstein S. Identification, assessment, and intervention strategies for deaf and hard of hearing students with learning disabilities. *Am Ann Deaf.* 2007;152:56–62.
29. Morgan A, Vernon M. A guide to the diagnosis of learning disabilities in deaf and hard-of-hearing children. *Am Ann Deaf.* 1994;139:358–370.
30. Mitchell RE, Karchmer MA. Chasing the mythical ten percent: parental hearing status of deaf and hard of hearing students in the United States. *Sign Lang Stud.* 2002;4:138–163.
31. Critchley E. The social development of deaf children. *J Laryngol Otol.* 1967;81:291–307.
32. Schlesinger HS, Meadow KP. *Deafness and mental health: a developmental approach.* Department of Health, 1971.
33. Bat-Chava Y. Sibling relationships for deaf children: the impact of child and family characteristics. *Rehabil Psychol.* 2003;47:73–91.
34. King JF. When a child is born deaf. *Contemp Pediatr.* 2006;73–80.
35. Schlesinger H. The acquisition of bimodal language. In: Schlesinger IM, Namir L, eds. *Sign language for the deaf.* New York: Academic Press, 1978:.
36. Austen S, Crocker S. *Deafness in mind: working psychology with deaf people across the lifespan.* London: Whurr, 2004:3–20.
37. DeGutis DL. Evaluating and treating deaf children and adolescents. *Am Acad Child Adolesc Psychiatry News.* 2007;80–81.
38. Hintermair M. Parental resources, parental stress, and socioemotional development of deaf and hard of hearing children. *J Deaf Stud Deaf Educ.* 2006;11:493–510.
39. Strong CJ, Clark TC, Johnson D, et al. SKI*HI home-based programming for children who are deaf or hard of hearing: recent research findings. *Infant-Toddler Interv.* 1994;4:25–36.
40. Greenberg MT. Family stress and child competence: the effects of early intervention for families with deaf infants. *Am Ann Deaf.* 1983;128:407–417.
41. Apuzzo ML, Yoshinaga-Itano C. Identification of hearing loss after age 18 months is not early enough. *Am Ann Deaf.* 1998;143:380–387.
42. Geers AE. Speech, language and reading skills after early cochlear implantation. *JAMA.* 2004;291:2378–2380.
43. Kaland M, Salvatore K. The psychology of hearing loss. http://www.asha.org/about/publications/leader-online/archives/2002/ql/020319d.htm. 2004, Nov. 30.
44. Holt JA, Traxler CB, Allen TE. *Interpreting the scores: a user's guide to the 9th edition* Stanford Achievement Test for educators of deaf and hard-of-hearing students *(Gallaudet Research Institute technical report 97-1).* Washington, DC: Gallaudet University Press, 1997.
45. Bat-Chava Y. Antecedents of self-esteem in deaf people: a meta-analytic review. *Rehabil Psychol.* 1993;38:221–234.
46. Mann JR, Zhou L, McKee M, McDermott S. Children with hearing loss and increased risk of injury. *Ann Family Med.* 2007;5:528–533.
47. Christiansen JB, Leigh IW. *Cochlear implants in children: ethics and choices.* Washington, DC: Gallaudet University Press, 2002.
48. Hauser PC, Wills KE, Isquith PK. *Hard-of-hearing, deafness, and being deaf: treating neurodevelopmental disabilities.* New York: The Guilford Press, 2006:119–131.
49. Hindley P, Kitson N. *Mental health and deafness.* London: Whurr, 2000.
50. Glickman NS, Gulati S. *Mental health care of deaf people: a culturally affirmative approach.* Mahwah, NJ: Lawrence Erlbaum, 2003:74–76.
51. Kelly D, Forney J, Parker-Fisher S, Jones M. Evaluating and managing attention deficit disorder in children who are deaf or hard of hearing. *Am Ann Deaf.* 1993;138:349–357.
52. Gallaudet Research Institute. *Regional & national summary report of data from 2004–2005 annual survey of deaf/HOH and youth.* Washington, DC: GRI, Gallaudet University, 2005.
53. Freeman R, Maulkin S, Hastings J. Psychosocial problems of deaf children and their families: a comparative study. *Am Ann Deaf.* 1975;121:391–403.
54. Mahapatra SB. Psychiatric and psychosomatic illness in the deaf. *Br J Psychiatry.* 1974;125:450–451.
55. Mahapatra SB. Deafness and mental health: psychiatric and psychosomatic illness in the deaf. *Acta Psychiatry Scand.* 1974;50:596–611.
56. Watt JD, Davis FE. The prevalence of boredom proneness and depression among profoundly deaf residential school adolescents. *Am Ann Deaf.* 1991;136:409–413.
57. Leigh IW, Robins CJ, Welkowitz J, Bond RN. Toward greater understanding of depression in deaf individuals. *Am Ann Deaf.* 1989;134:249–254.
58. Brown AS, Cohen P, Greenwald S, Susser E. Nonaffective psychosis after prenatal exposure to rubella. *Am J Psychiatry.* 2000;157:438–443.
59. Thewissen V, Mylin-Germeys I, Bentall R, et al. Hearing impairment and psychosis revisited. *Schizophr Res.* 2005;76:99–103.
60. Shapira NA, DelBello MP, Goldsmith TD, et al. Evaluation of bipolar disorder in inpatients with prelingual deafness. *Am J Psychiatry.* 1999;156:1267–1269.

61. Thacker AJ. Formal communication disorder: sign language in deaf people with schizophrenia. *Br J Psychiatry.* 1994;165:818–823.
62. Atkinson JR. The perceptual characteristics of voice-hallucinations in deaf people: insights into the nature of subvocal thought and sensory feedback loops. *Schizophr Bull.* 2006;32:701–708.
63. Roper L, Arnold P, Monteiro B. Co-occurrence of autism and deafness: diagnostic considerations. *Autism.* 2003;7:245–253.
64. Rosenhall U, Nordin V, Sandstrom M, et al. Autism and hearing loss. *J Autism Dev Disord.* 1999;29:349–357.
65. Kelly D, Forney J, Parker-Fisher S, Jones M. The challenge of attention deficit disorder in children who are deaf or hard of hearing. *Am Ann Deaf.* 1993;138:343–348.
66. Feinstein CB. Early adolescent deaf boys: a biopsychosocial approach. *Adolesc Psychiatry.* 1983;11:147–162.
67. Pollard R. Psychopathology. In: Marschark M, Clark D, eds. *Psychological perspectives on deafness.* Vol 2. Mahwah, NJ: Lawrence Erlbaum, 1998:171–197.
68. Ecans J, Elliot H. The mental status examination. In: Elliot H, ed. *Mental status assessment of deaf clients: a practical guide.* Boston: Little Brown, 1987.
69. Geers AE. Speech, language and reading skills after early cochlear implantation. *Arch Otolaryngol Head Neck Surg.* 2004;130:634–638.
70. Waltzman S, Cohen N. Cochlear implantation in children younger than two years old. *Am J Otol.* 1998;19:158–162.
71. Geers AE, Nicholas J, Sedey A. Language skills of children with early cochlear implantation. *Ear Hear.* 2003;24:46S–58S.
72. Svirsky M, Teoh S, Neuburger H. Development of language and speech perception in congenitally, profoundly deaf children as a function of age at cochlear implantation. *Audio Neurotol.* 2004;9:224–233.
73. Shin MS, Kim SK, Kim SS, et al. Comparison of cognitive function in deaf children between before and after cochlear implant. *Ear Hear.* 2007;28(2 suppl):22s–28s.
74. Bauer PW, Sharma A, Martin K, Dorman M. Central auditory development in children with bilateral cochlear implants. *Arch Otolaryngol Head Neck Surg.* 2006:132:1133–1136.
75. Murphy J, O'Donoghue G. Bilateral cochlear implantation: an evidence-based medicine evaluation. *Laryngoscope.* 2007;117:1412–1218.
76. Papsin BC, Gordon KA. Cochlear implants for children with severe-to-profound hearing loss. *N Engl J Med.* 2007;357:2380–2387.

CHAPTER 18

Neuromuscular Disorders

HOWARD L. GEYER AND NAALLA D. SCHREIBER

Unlike most chapters in this book, which focus on conditions that affect the central nervous system (CNS), this one focuses on conditions that affect the peripheral nervous system (PNS). While the CNS consists of the brain and spinal cord, the PNS consists of the nerves, muscles, and neuromuscular junctions (NMJ). Neurologists refer to conditions that affect the PNS as neuromuscular disorders. Some disorders affect both the CNS and PNS and may lead to changes in cognition, behavior, or emotion in addition to signs and symptoms of PNS disease—as highlighted in this chapter.

Children and adolescents with neuromuscular disorders typically come to the attention of psychiatrists for one or more of three reasons. First, psychiatrists can play a crucial role in the management of emotional or behavioral manifestations or sequelae of the disorder. In particular, children with neuromuscular disorders can suffer from anxiety disorders, depression, or significant behavioral problems that may or may not be related to cognitive disability.

Second, a psychiatrist can help family members cope with the psychosocial consequences of disorders that potentially impact children's behavior, coping mechanisms, and functional status. Hereditary diseases can be particularly disruptive to normal family dynamics. The parents of an affected child may have unresolved guilt related to passing on a genetic illness to their child and may also feel conflicted about having additional children. Siblings may have concerns about their own risk of developing the disease or may feel neglected because the affected child seems to receive a disproportionate amount of parental attention. Psychiatrists can help parents or siblings by providing psychotherapy and, when needed, pharmacotherapy.

Finally, psychiatrists acquainted with neuromuscular conditions may aid in proper diagnosis. For example, patients with neuromuscular disease are sometimes misdiagnosed as "psychogenic" and referred for psychiatric care. Such a misdiagnosis is especially likely when patients' symptoms fluctuate or appear episodically, as in myasthenia gravis (MG) or periodic paralysis. A knowledgeable, astute psychiatrist may be able to identify dysfunction of the nervous system as an organic condition and ensure that the patient receives the appropriate treatment.

The majority of neuromuscular conditions exclusively affect the PNS and spare the CNS. Consequently, cognition is normal in most of these disorders, and the prevalence of major psychiatric illness is not significantly elevated. For example, children with polio, spinal muscular atrophy, and MG do not have cognitive impairment or psychiatric disturbance directly attributable to their condition—despite potentially devastating impairment in motor function. In contrast, weakness due to cerebral dysfunction (as in cerebral palsy) is often accompanied by cognitive abnormalities.

Anatomy and Physiology of the Peripheral Nervous System

The PNS transmits efferent information from the CNS to effectors, such as muscles and glands. It also carries afferent information to the CNS from the body and its environment. Disruption of efferent pathways often results in motor impairment, typically weakness. At the same time, damage to afferent pathways may produce sensory symptoms, particularly numbness and unpleasant sensations like spontaneously occurring pain.

The motor system controlling voluntary movement of skeletal muscle[1] consists of two populations of neurons: the lower motor neurons (LMNs), which innervate muscles, and the upper motor neurons (UMNs), which terminate by forming synapses with the cell bodies of LMNs. The cell bodies of the UMNs are located in the motor strip of the cerebral cortex. Their axons form the corticospinal tracts, which descend through the white matter of the cerebral hemispheres and brainstem. In the medulla, the corticospinal tracts decussate (cross to the opposite side) and descend in the spinal cord.

On terminating in the spinal cord, each UMN axon synapses with the cell body of an LMN located in the anterior horn of the spinal gray matter. Axons of LMNs leave the spinal cord via the ventral nerve roots and then travel peripherally, joining fibers carrying afferent information to form a mixed spinal nerve. The motor axons continue peripherally in these nerves and ultimately end in a nerve terminal in close proximity to the skeletal muscle.

The nerve terminal contains synaptic vesicles, packets that hold the neurotransmitter acetylcholine. When an action potential propagated along a motor nerve reaches the nerve terminal, electrochemical changes (mediated by calcium ions) cause the vesicles to fuse with the presynaptic membrane and release acetylcholine into the NMJ. The acetylcholine diffuses across the synaptic cleft and binds to receptors in the postsynaptic membrane located on the muscle. This binding results in electrochemical changes (mediated by sodium and potassium ions) that trigger a muscle contraction.

In contrast to motor pathways, which enable us to move, the somatosensory system permits us to detect various physical stimuli that can be perceived as touch, pain, cold, vibration, and other sensations. Specialized organs that detect the stimuli, called receptors, are located in the skin and elsewhere. They convert the physical stimuli into electrical signals that travel toward the CNS along sensory fibers.[2] These fibers join motor axons to form mixed nerves. The sensory axons carry afferent signals into the spinal cord via the dorsal roots. Sensory information travels to the brain chiefly through two tracts that ascend in the white matter of the spinal cord: the dorsal columns (which carry information about vibration, joint position, and light touch sensations) and the spinothalamic tracts (which mediate pain and temperature as well as light touch sensations).

In the lower cervical region, the mixed spinal nerves continue peripherally as the brachial plexus, a complex network of axons whose numerous branches provide motor and sensory innervation to the upper extremities (as well as frustration to students of anatomy). A similar structure, the lumbosacral plexus, innervates the lower extremities.

---

[1] Glands and smooth and cardiac muscle are not under voluntary control but are governed by the autonomic nervous system, which is not discussed in this chapter.

[2] The somatosensory system, which conveys information from receptors in skin, muscles, joints, and viscera, can be distinguished from the *special senses*, such as vision, hearing, taste, and smell. Not all aspects of the text's description of the somatosensory system are applicable to the special senses.

Principles of Diagnosis: Anatomic Localization

Disease processes can attack the PNS anywhere along its course. As they do when diagnosing CNS disease, neurologists try to localize a PNS lesion on the basis of the patient's symptoms and signs. This section describes the relationships between various sites of pathology and the clinical patterns they produce.

Because lesions of either the CNS or PNS may produce sensory or motor signs and symptoms, neurologists usually begin their evaluation of a patient by trying to determine whether the pathology is in the CNS or PNS (or both). Pathology in the brain or spinal cord causes motor symptoms and signs characteristic of UMN dysfunction. Causes of such pathology are diverse; examples include stroke, trauma, tumor, and multiple sclerosis. In addition to weakness, UMN damage can also produce spasticity, increased deep tendon reflexes (DTRs), and Babinski signs. Moreover, lesions of the brain may also produce cognitive changes.

With lesions of the LMN, hypotonia (decreased muscle tone) and decreased or absent DTRs typically accompany weakness. The specific findings, of course, depend on the site of the lesion in the PNS (Table 18.1). Diseases that exclusively affect anterior horn cells, such as poliomyelitis or spinal muscular atrophy, result in atrophy, weakness, and loss of DTRs. Although these illnesses may cause devastating weakness, they do not produce cognitive impairment. Involuntary twitching movements of muscles, fasciculations, are most characteristic of these disorders of the anterior horn cell but can occur with any lesion of the LMN.

Injury of motor axons, which can result from a plethora of conditions, can occur anywhere along their course through nerve root, plexus, or peripheral nerve. Injuries may occur in single nerves or combinations of nerves. Moreover, because motor fibers travel with sensory fibers along much of their course, sensory abnormalities, such as pain, numbness, or tingling often accompany weakness.

TABLE 18.1 CLINICAL-ANATOMICAL LOCALIZATION OF NEUROMUSCULAR DISORDERS

Site of Pathology	Name of Syndrome	Examples	Sensory vs. Motor	Tendon Reflexes	Other
Anterior horn cell	Motor neuronopathy	SMA, poliomyelitis	Pure motor	Decreased	Fasciculations
Nerve root	Radiculopathy	Herniated disc, meningitis	Sensorimotor	Decreased	Often painful
Plexus	Plexopathy	Tumor, radiation injury	Sensorimotor	Decreased	
Nerve	Neuropathy	Guillain-Barré syndrome, hereditary neuropathies	Sensorimotor	Decreased	Distal > proximal
Neuromuscular junction	None in common use	Myasthenia gravis, botulism	Pure motor	Variable	May be prominent in ocular or facial muscles
Muscle	Myopathy	Muscular dystrophies, inflammatory myopathies	Pure motor	Usually normal	Proximal > distal

SMA, spinal muscular atrophy.

Neurologists often differentiate abnormalities of peripheral nerve, neuropathies, from conditions affecting other segments of the axon. For example, nerve root involvement, or radiculopathy, may result from a herniated disc or an infection in the spinal subarachnoid space. Plexopathy involves the brachial or lumbosacral plexus, either completely or in a patchy distribution. Pathology in the root, plexus, or nerve typically causes muscle atrophy and weakness along with pain, numbness, or tingling. In addition, DTRs mediated by an affected nerve or nerve root will be depressed or absent.

Some processes such as focal entrapment affect an individual peripheral nerve (mononeuropathy). Generalized conditions such as diabetes can diffusely affect the PNS (polyneuropathy). Some conditions tend to affect several individual nerves (mononeuropathy multiplex).

Disruption of the NMJ, which occurs in botulism and MG, results in a pure motor syndrome without sensory features. It can cause generalized weakness or weakness restricted to one anatomical region. For example, MG often causes ptosis and weakness of extraocular muscles, but DTRs usually remain normal.

A wide variety of pathological processes may produce muscle disorders, myopathies. Neurologists recognize many causes of myopathy; etiologic categories include genetic, inflammatory, infectious, endocrine, metabolic, and toxic causes. The sections pertaining to specific diseases present details on each of these categories.

Approach to the Patient with Suspected Neuromuscular Disease

HISTORY

In neurology, as in psychiatry, the patient's history remains the most important element of the evaluation. Although the examiner should endeavor to obtain as much information as possible directly from the patient, the child's parents will often provide the majority of the information. The following components of the history deserve special mention.

Chief complaint

Children with neuromuscular disorders commonly present with weakness, numbness, tingling, gait difficulty, or ataxia. Neurologists seek to elicit a detailed description of the symptoms and should not accept at face value all terminology used by patients or their parents. For example, patients may state that they feel "weak" when in fact their problem is stiffness, rigidity, or incoordination. Similarly, because some terms, such as "numbness" and "dizziness," have a variety of meanings, neurologists will ask a patient reporting such symptoms to describe them in greater detail. One technique is to ask patients and their parents to describe tasks that might be impeded by the symptoms.

Chronology of present illness

The time course of an illness often differentiates among etiologies. For example, trauma, infections, intoxications, and conversion reactions emerge acutely, over minutes to days. A subacute onset evolving over days to weeks typifies many systemic conditions, such as autoimmune, endocrine, and nutritional disorders. A chronic time course may suggest a genetic or metabolic abnormality. Because some conditions tend to progressively worsen while others are static, neurologists always try to determine if a patient's symptoms are progressing or remaining stable. In addition, the patient's age at the time the symptoms began should be ascertained, as many disorders have a typical age at onset.

As an example, consideration of the time course helps narrow the differential diagnosis of acute childhood paralysis. Hyperacute paralysis—developing over hours—is most often associated with hyperkalemia or hypokalemia or intoxication (such as with insecticides). It can also be psychogenic, perhaps triggered by an intolerable or disturbing thought or situation. In paralysis developing over days to weeks, Guillain-Barré syndrome (GBS) is the most common culprit. Other diagnoses to consider include transverse myelitis, botulism, MG, acute inflammatory diseases of muscle, infection of anterior horn cells by viruses (such as enteroviruses or, in endemic areas, polio), tick paralysis, and exposure to various neurotoxins. Rare causes include acute intermittent porphyria and diphtheria (1,2).

Medical history (including medications)

When approaching a patient with a possible neuromuscular disorder, neurologists attempt to identify comorbid medical conditions. Neuromuscular disorders may result from underlying medical illness, such as neuropathy due to leprosy, or from the treatment of medical illnesses, such as chemotherapy-induced neuropathy. Also, because some neuromuscular disorders involve other organs, evidence of such nonneurological involvement may serve as a clue to the diagnosis. Likewise, a single systemic illness may injure the PNS along with other systems. For example, MG may occur in conjunction with other autoimmune disorders.

Social history

Many substances of abuse, including alcohol, cocaine, and heroin, can damage the PNS. Glue sniffing, which is prevalent among adolescents, can cause neuropathy because users inhale toxic hexacarbons. Industrial exposures, to heavy metals for example, can also produce neuropathy.

Perinatal history

Physicians should note birth complications, including prematurity and large birth weight (macrosomia). Particularly when evaluating a hypotonic (floppy) infant, they should attempt to determine if fetal movements were decreased during the third trimester, suggesting that weakness was present *in utero.*

Development

Children with neuromuscular disorders may be delayed in attaining gross or fine motor milestones. On the other hand, coexisting impairment of language or other cognitive domains raises the likelihood of cerebral palsy or other brain pathology. Clinicians use instruments such as the Denver Developmental Screening Test (Denver Developmental Materials, Inc, Denver, CO) and its derivatives to assess whether children have achieved developmental milestones at the appropriate time and in the usual sequence.

Family history

Identifying an inherited disorder is critical for making an accurate diagnosis and providing genetic counseling. Physicians should ascertain whether family members are affected and, if so, attempt to determine the pattern of inheritance. Autosomal dominant conditions affecting the PNS include many types of hereditary neuropathy and certain myopathies, including myotonic dystrophy, facioscapulohumeral dystrophy, and one type of myotonia congenita. X-linked disorders include Duchenne and Becker muscular dystrophies and several varieties of hereditary neuropathy. Exclusively maternal transmission suggests a mitochondrial disorder, such as **m**itochondrial encephalomyopathy, **l**actic **a**cidosis, and **s**troke (MELAS) or **m**yoclonic **e**pilepsy and **r**agged-red **f**ibers (MERFF). Even if a child has no obviously affected family member, parental consanguinity may suggest that the child has a genetic disorder with autosomal recessive inheritance.

PHYSICAL AND NEUROLOGICAL EXAMINATION

Because some neuromuscular disorders are associated with systemic manifestations, physicians should perform a thorough general as well as neurological examination. They should always measure head circumference: an abnormally large head (macrocephaly) or a small head (microcephaly) suggests a cerebral cause for a patient's symptoms. Dysmorphic facies may be diagnostic of a particular syndrome, especially in genetic disorders. For example, the face of patients with myotonic dystrophy type 1 has been described as shaped like a hatchet. Other neuromuscular conditions can be associated with organomegaly, endocrinopathy, scoliosis, or abnormalities of cardiac conduction, joints, or skin. Nerves may become enlarged (and may be palpable) in leprosy or in hereditary neuropathies (due to repeated demyelination and remyelination).

The neurological examination of the child with suspected neuromuscular disease naturally focuses on the PNS. Nevertheless, physicians should always include tests of the child's mental status because in some neuromuscular disorders, changes in cognition accompany the PNS abnormalities. These cognitive changes are variable and can manifest as learning disorders or frank mental retardation.

Cranial nerves

Examination of the cranial nerves is described in detail in Chapter 1. Cranial nerves can be disrupted singly, in combination, or as part of a generalized polyneuropathy. Because most of the cranial nerves belong to the PNS, it is important to examine their function carefully in patients with suspected neuromuscular disease. In particular, the complaint of diplopia (double vision) often reflects weakness of eye movement (external ophthalmoparesis), which can result from damage to the oculomotor (CN III), trochlear (CN IV), and/or abducens (CN VI) nerves. Ptosis (drooping of the eyelid) uncommonly results from myopathy affecting muscles that elevate the eyelid; more often it is due to dysfunction of CN III or the sympathetic fibers that innervate those muscles or the NMJ that joins CN III to the muscles. Disturbance of facial sensation may reflect trigeminal nerve (CN V) dysfunction. Palsy of the facial nerve (CN VII) causes drooping of the face, such as in Bell's palsy. Impaired auditory or vestibular function may suggest a lesion of the vestibulocochlear nerve (CN VIII). Difficulty speaking (dysarthria) and/or swallowing (dysphagia) can result from lesions affecting the glossopharyngeal (CN IX) or vagus (CN X) nerves. Neck flexion and turning and shoulder shrugging may be weak if the spinal accessory nerve (CN XI) is affected. With damage to the hypoglossal nerve (CN XII), the tongue may be weak or atrophic and fasciculations may be present.

When examining a patient, it is important for neurologists to remember that cranial nerve function depends not only on the cranial nerves themselves but also on related structures, such as the brainstem, NMJ, and cranial muscles. For example, external ophthalmoparesis can result not only from dysfunction of the oculomotor, trochlear, and/or abducens nerves but also from problems in the brainstem, NMJ, or extraocular muscles. Unilateral facial weakness usually signifies palsy of the facial nerve, but facial diparesis may result from neuropathy or myopathy.

Motor and gait

The motor examination includes assessment of muscle bulk, tone, and power. Atrophy—loss of muscle bulk—characterizes disorders of the LMN. For example, the sequelae of a severe Erb's palsy may include atrophy of the deltoid and biceps muscles due to injury to C5 and C6 nerve roots. Likewise, hammer toes, flat feet (pes planus), or high-arched feet (pes cavus) from atrophy of the foot muscles may bespeak hereditary or other long-standing motor neuropathy, especially in older children and adolescents. Atrophy may also result from prolonged disuse. On the other hand, hypertrophy of muscles may result from overuse, which may be intentional (as in bodybuilding) or a consequence of repetitive involuntary movements such as dystonia (see Chapter 3). Some conditions cause pseudohypertrophy, in which muscle fibers are unchanged in size but fatty infiltration or increased connective tissue enlarge the muscle bulk. A classic example is the calves of boys with Duchenne muscular dystrophy (DMD), which become enlarged by fibrosis of the muscle. Other examples include glycogen storage diseases and endocrine disorders such as hypothyroidism and acromegaly.

Neurologists assess muscle tone, another element of the motor examination, by moving the patient's body parts through their range of motion and feeling for resistance. Decreased tone (hypotonia) is most closely associated with lesions of the LMN, but it also can occur with cerebral or cerebellar pathology. Increased muscle tone in children usually occurs in one of two forms. Spasticity is increased resistance to passive movement that is more pronounced when the movement is made quickly. In contrast, the resistance of rigidity does not change with varying speeds of movement. Spasticity is typical of damage to the UMN in the brain or spinal cord, while rigidity is most characteristic of disorders of the extrapyramidal system, most commonly the basal ganglia.

An important component of the motor examination is the assessment of power. In older children and adolescents, neurologists usually use manual muscle testing, in which the examiner asks the patient to contract a muscle group and grades the strength of the contraction along a 0 to 5 scale (Table 18.2). Children younger than 6 years often are unable to cooperate with formal testing, but even preschoolers may cooperate with requests to walk (including walking on heels and on toes), rise from a sitting position, or perform a deep knee bend. An astute examiner will glean a great deal of information simply by observing the patient.

Watching a child walk gives valuable information about muscle power as well other neurological functions (including vision, balance, and coordination). By the age of 13 to 18 months, most toddlers can walk steadily with only occasional falls. At 18 months, most children can stand unassisted from a sitting position. By 24 months, most children have mastered the skills of running and jumping (often to their parents' dismay). Table 18.3 lists some patterns of gait abnormalities commonly observed in children.

Recognizing the pattern of motor involvement as more prominent either proximally or distally is crucial in identifying its underlying cause. Children with proximal muscle

TABLE 18.2 MEDICAL RESEARCH COUNCIL SCALE FOR GRADING POWER DURING MANUAL MUSCLE TESTING

Grade 0	No contraction
Grade 1	Flicker or trace of contraction
Grade 2	Active movement, with gravity eliminated
Grade 3	Active movement against gravity
Grade 4	Active movement against gravity and resistance
Grade 5	Normal power

TABLE 18.3 SOME GAIT ABNORMALITIES SEEN IN CHILDREN

Type of Gait	Description	Possible Clinical Significance
Scissoring gait	Adduction of legs	Spasticity (often cerebral palsy or other spastic paralysis)
Toe-walking gait	Heels raised from floor	Spasticity; muscular dystrophy; heel pain; unequal leg length (if unilateral); behavioral mannerism
Steppage gait	Knee is lifted high and foot slaps on floor	Foot drop due to weakness of dorsiflexion
Waddling gait	Wide stance, trunk swings from side to side	Weakness of hip muscles (especially thigh abductors); hip disease (e.g., Legg-Calve-Perthes disease, slipped capital femoral epiphysis)
Ataxic gait	Clumsy, poor coordination	Cerebellar disease or sensory abnormalities
Antalgic gait	Decreased weight-bearing on affected leg	Pain elicited by bearing weight

weakness may have difficulty standing from a sitting position, and may need to use their hands to push on the floor and their knees, a maneuver known as Gowers sign (Fig. 18.1A–E). A child with foot drop is likely to have trouble walking on his or her heels.

In general, muscle disease produces weakness and atrophy that is most pronounced proximally, while polyneuropathy results in predominantly distal abnormalities because it affects the longest nerves most severely. Exceptions include myotonic dystrophy, which is associated with distal weakness.

Sensation

Examination of sensation is highly subjective and requires the cooperation of the patient. Young children may be unable to provide useful information on formal sensory testing, although dramatically different reactions to similar stimulation in discrete body parts may reflect differential sensation.

Lesions of the anterior horn cell, NMJ, and muscle do not result in sensory changes. In contrast, nerve and nerve root damage, as well as CNS pathology, can cause abnormalities in sensation. A major goal of the sensory examination is to identify an anatomic pattern of abnormalities because, in analogy with motor abnormalities, sensory changes can be very helpful in localizing the site of the lesion.

Testing sensation of stimuli in a variety of sensory modalities may demonstrate dissociation of sensory changes, such that some modalities are affected more than (or to the exclusion of) others. Testing multiple modalities can be helpful in localization, for, as mentioned previously, separate tracts in the spinal cord carry information about pain and temperature (spinothalamic tracts) and about vibration and joint position (dorsal columns). Although neurologists sometimes test sensation of light touch, pin prick, cold, hot, vibration, and joint position, performing such an exhaustive examination is rarely practical in young patients. Rather, the examiner must selectively test those modalities most likely to elicit information relevant to the individual patient.

Deep tendon reflexes

Although disorders of the UMN typically produce hyperreflexia (overly brisk reflexes), diseases of the LMN tend to result in hyporeflexia or absent reflexes (areflexia). In length-dependent neuropathies, in which the longest nerves are preferentially damaged, a characteristic early sign is a bilaterally decreased Achilles tendon reflex. More focal reflex abnormalities occur in association with mononeuropathy, mononeuropathy multiplex, and radiculopathy. Reflexes are largely spared in myopathies and NMJ disorders unless very severe weakness is present.

Chapter 18 / NEUROMUSCULAR DISORDERS 375

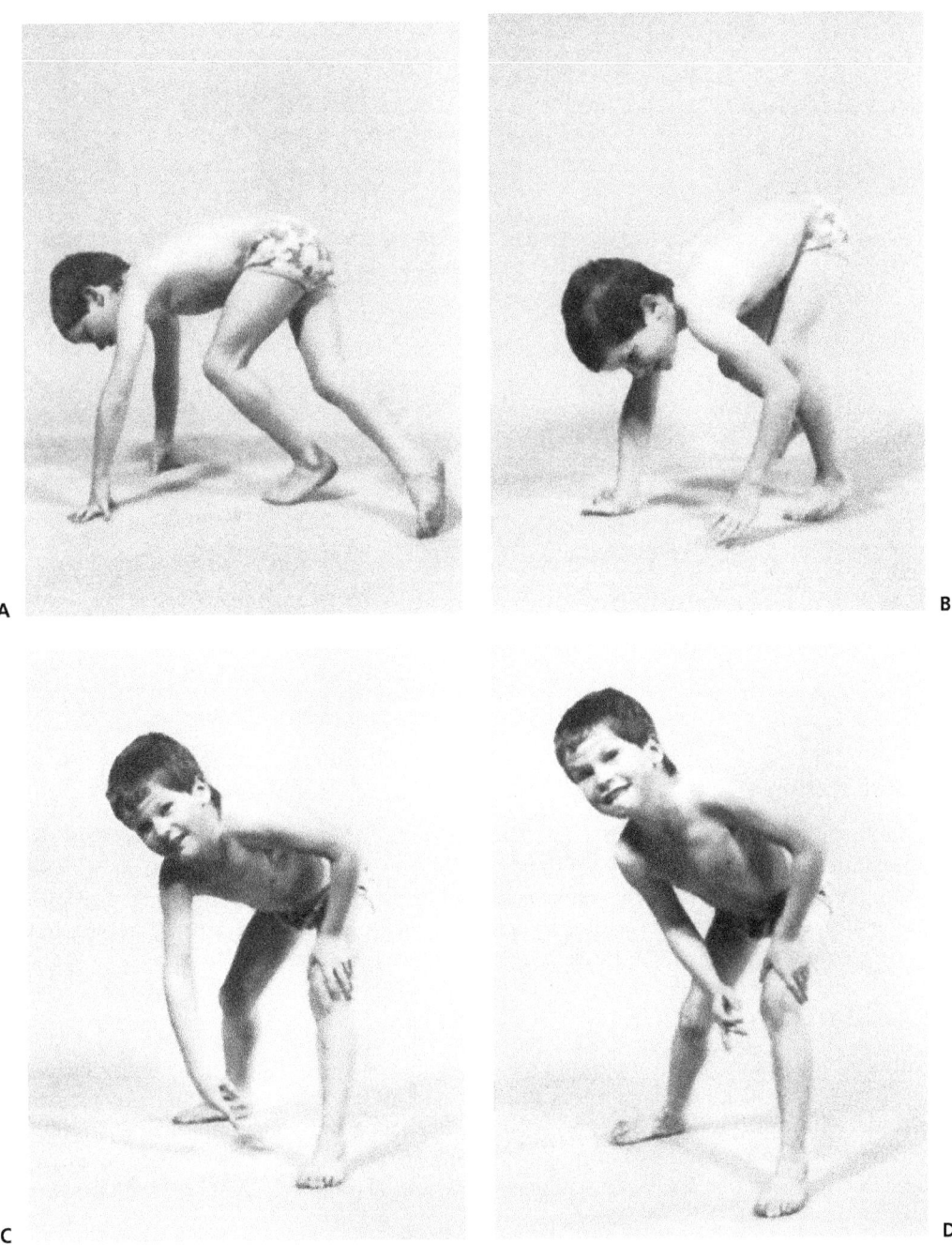

■ **FIGURE 18.1** Gowers sign is a classic finding in boys with Duchenne muscular dystrophy but may be present in children with proximal muscle weakness of any cause. In order to rise from a seated position on the floor, a child turns the body prone, then extends the arms and legs to raise the body **(A)**. The hands are brought closer to the feet, in order to bring the center of gravity above the feet **(B)**, and then one or both hands are used to push against the knees or thighs, enabling the child to straighten the back **(C–E)**. (From Bickley LS, Szilagyi P. *Bates' Guide to Physical Examination and History Taking*. 8th ed. Philadelphia: Lippincott Williams & Wilkins; 2003 with permission.)

E

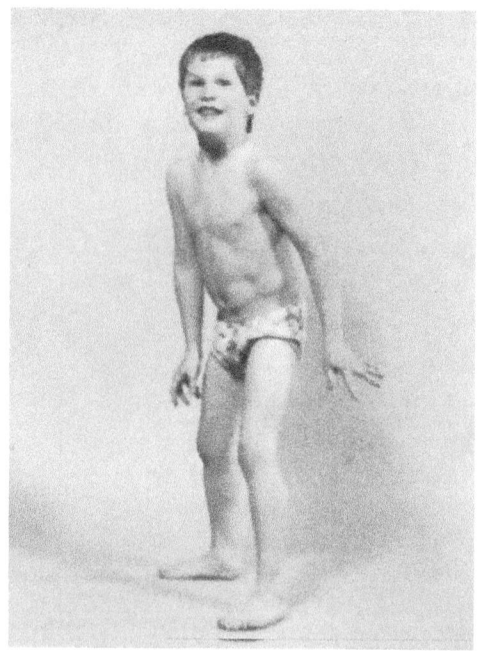

■ FIGURE 18.1 *(continued)*

Coordination

In most cases of ataxia in children, a CNS process is responsible. Nevertheless, PNS abnormalities that impair sensation of joint position can also result in ataxia. Most of these conditions are neuropathies that affect sensory fibers, either exclusively or together with motor fibers. A few conditions directly afflict the cell bodies of the sensory nerves, but these are rare, especially in children.

LABORATORY TESTING

Although the history and examination remain the mainstay of diagnosis, neurologists use ancillary testing to aid in diagnosis. Serum levels of muscle enzymes rise in many muscle disorders, including inflammatory myopathies, Duchenne and Becker muscular dystrophy, and muscle injury. Creatine phosphokinase (CPK) is the enzyme most commonly measured, but levels of aldolase, lactic acid dehydrogenase, alanine transaminase, and aspartate transaminase may also be elevated.

An indispensable tool in the diagnosis of many neuromuscular disorders is electrophysiologic testing, which helps not only with localizing the affected area of the PNS but also with determining its severity and the underlying pathophysiology. Nerve conduction studies (NCS), one of two components of this testing, involve electrical stimulation of sensory and motor nerves and measurement of various parameters of the resulting action potentials. Because pathological processes disrupt these parameters in different ways, analysis of the pattern of abnormalities can aid in identifying the underlying disorder. Neuropathy is an example of a condition in which NCS results are often abnormal. Specialized techniques, such as repetitive nerve stimulation, are useful in diagnosis of NMJ disorders like MG.

The second component of electrodiagnostic testing is electromyography (EMG), in which a clinician inserts a needle into the patient's muscle in order to record the electrical activity present in the muscle. Many abnormalities of the PNS can be detected with EMG, including motor neuron disease, neuropathies, NMJ disorders, and myopathies.

Neurologists may consider performing a Tensilon test if they suspect a patient has a NMJ disorder, such as MG. In this test, the neurologist gives the patient an intravenous injection of edrophonium (Tensilon), a short-acting acetylcholinesterase inhibitor, while observing its effect on weak muscles. Edrophonium inhibits the degradation of acetylcholine, producing an increase in acetylcholine at the NMJ, which transiently reverses weakness in MG patients. Because its effect is brief, lasting no more than a few minutes, edrophonium is useful for diagnosis but not for treatment. (Longer-acting cholinesterase inhibitors are used therapeutically.) Although neurologists usually perform this test when they suspect MG, it is important to keep in mind that other disorders may show "false positives." For example, injection of edrophonium ameliorates weakness in disorders of anterior horn cells.

In cases when noninvasive techniques are insufficient to permit a definitive diagnosis, a muscle biopsy for histologic examination may be helpful. Using a variety of techniques to examine such specimens, experienced neuropathologists often can give very specific information about the underlying disorder. On occasion, nerve biopsy may aid diagnosis of certain types of neuropathy.

In recent years, advances in molecular genetics and immunology have revolutionized the diagnosis of many hereditary neuromuscular disorders. Genetic testing now permits a specific diagnosis of many illnesses, whereas traditional methods yield only nonspecific findings. As a result, the need for invasive testing has significantly diminished. As researchers continue to elucidate the molecular basis of these disorders, genetic testing undoubtedly will play an increasingly larger role in diagnosis.

General Principles of Management of Patients with Neuromuscular Disorders

For a minority of neuromuscular conditions, specific treatment interventions are available. For example, infections of the PNS may be responsive to appropriate antibiotic regimens. Corticosteroids are effective both as anti-inflammatory drugs and as immunosuppressant agents. Other therapeutic options effective in dysimmune conditions include plasma exchange and infusion of human intravenous immunoglobulin (IVIG). Long-acting cholinesterase inhibitors like pyridostigmine (Mestinon) are useful in managing MG. Although not currently available, gene therapy may come to play a large role in treating neuromuscular disorders.

Although the future holds promise, at this time the management of most neuromuscular disorders remains purely supportive. For example, when treating patients who have pain, neurologists employ conventional analgesics as well as agents that suppress neuropathic pain. A neurologist may refer patients to a physiatrist to assess their need for assistive devices, such as orthotics, or to prescribe physical therapy and related treatments.

Many patients with neuromuscular disorders may benefit from a psychiatric consultation. In particular, psychiatrists can help by treating comorbid mood and anxiety disorders, attention deficit hyperactivity disorder, or behavioral manifestations of mental retardation. Furthermore, neuropsychological testing may identify cognitive deficits that can aid in the allocation of appropriate educational resources. In addition, as mentioned previously, psychiatrists or other mental health professionals can help parents and siblings cope with the impact of serious physical illness on the family structure.

Specific Diseases, by Anatomic Classification

ANTERIOR HORN CELL

Formerly, poliomyelitis was a common cause of acute anterior horn cell disease, but because of the Global Polio Eradication Initiative, this disease is now rare; fewer than 2000 cases were reported worldwide in the year 2006, mostly in the four countries in which polio remains endemic. Most exposed individuals are asymptomatic, but a minority develops fever and signs of meningeal irritation, such as headache and stiff neck, followed in 2 to 5 days by asymmetrical weakness. Patients often have severe muscle pain, and fasciculations. Their legs are affected more than their arms. When cranial muscles become weak, patients develop difficulty with speech, swallowing, and respiration. Despite the severe and extensive weakness, patients' cognition remains normal. The white blood cell (WBC) count in the cerebrospinal fluid (CSF) is elevated, and antibodies to poliovirus can be detected in serum and CSF. Stool cultures may be positive for poliovirus. There is no specific therapy for polio.

Other viruses, including enteroviruses, echoviruses, and coxsackie viruses, can infect anterior horn cells and cause a clinical presentation similar to polio. In New York City in 1999, there was an outbreak of West Nile virus (WNV), which never before had been reported in the Western hemisphere. Although less susceptible to severe neurological disease than adults, children infected by WNV may develop encephalitis or flaccid paralysis that clinically resembles polio (3). A WNV-induced neuropathy resembling GBS has also been reported in adults. The diagnosis of WNV depends on serologic studies in serum and CSF. There is no specific treatment; prevention depends on limiting transmission through control of the mosquito population.

Some conditions affecting anterior horn cells have a more chronic time course. The most common chronic disorder of anterior horn cells in children is spinal muscular atrophy (SMA). It is the second most common genetic disease of childhood, affecting 1 in 6,000 to 10,000 live births (4). The most common form is inherited in an autosomal recessive pattern and is associated with mutations in the *SMN1* gene on chromosome 5q, although rare forms of SMA arise from mutations in other genes.

Neurologists distinguish subtypes of SMA based on severity and age at onset. In general, earlier onset is correlated with clinically more severe disease. Newborns with congenital SMA are born with joint contractures, are unable to move, and have respiratory failure and hypotonia; they usually die by one month of age. Infants with SMA type I (Werdnig-Hoffman disease) develop severe weakness and hypotonia within the first few months of life, and most die in the first two years of age due to weakness of respiratory muscles. SMA type II begins somewhat later than type I but often by 18 months; children with type II never stand and tend to survive into childhood. SMA type III (Kugelberg-Welander disease) begins in childhood and is milder; patients typically survive into adulthood, and often can stand independently (but may not be able to walk). SMA type IV, the mildest type, can have juvenile or adult onset.

Features common to all forms of SMA include weakness that is more prominent proximally than distally, decreased reflexes, and fasciculations that may be especially prominent in the tongue. Importantly, intelligence is normal in all of these conditions. Even babies with SMA type I demonstrate normal intellect in their alert, interactive faces. Relative to the general population, SMA carries no increase in psychiatric comorbidity. However, SMA has a profound impact on family structure, and nonaffected siblings demonstrate remarkably high rates of psychopathology (5).

In the past, neurologists had to rely on investigations such as electrodiagnostic testing and muscle biopsy to diagnose SMA, but genetic testing has revolutionized the diagnosis of these conditions and has almost entirely supplanted the use of invasive tests.

Amyotrophic lateral sclerosis (ALS), or Lou Gehrig disease, the most common disease of anterior horn cells in adults, is very rare in children but childhood- and juvenile-onset variants do exist. Although most cases of adult-onset ALS are sporadic, the majority of children with ALS have a hereditary condition.

PERIPHERAL NERVE

Disorders that injure nerves can do so anywhere along their course: at the level of the nerve root, the plexus, or the terminal peripheral nerve. Diseases that occupy the spinal subarachnoid space, such as infectious or neoplastic meningitis, can affect the nerve roots as they exit the spinal cord. Other conditions preferentially affect the distal ends of the longest nerves, producing a length-dependent neuropathy.

Nerves can be damaged in two possible ways: axons can be disrupted, or the myelin sheath that coats the axons can be damaged. Categorizing neuropathies on the basis of this distinction, neurologists differentiate between axonal neuropathies and demyelinating neuropathies. (A few disease processes cause a combination of the two.) They also classify neuropathies as acute, subacute, or chronic on the basis of their time course. Most hereditary neuropathies have a chronic, slowly progressive course, while acquired neuropathies tend to present in an acute or subacute fashion.

Acute neuropathies

Among the most dramatic neuropathies is a group of conditions collectively known as GBS, the most common of which is acute inflammatory demyelinating polyneuropathy (AIDP). AIDP is rapidly progressive and can be life threatening, but prognosis is good if it is promptly diagnosed and treated. It affects patients of all ages and is thought to result from antibody-mediated attack against the myelin that insulates peripheral nerves. In many cases, a prodromal respiratory or gastrointestinal illness (most typically gastroenteritis due to *Campylobacter jejuni*) precedes onset of neurological symptoms by 1 or 2 weeks. Classically, numbness and weakness begin in the feet and rapidly spread proximally. Muscles of respiration may become weak, as may muscles innervated by cranial nerves. The disease may progress for up to 4 weeks, after which it stabilizes.

The diagnosis of GBS should be considered in any patient with rapidly progressive weakness and numbness. On examination, deep tendon reflexes are depressed or absent. Except in rare cases, mental status is unaffected, although severely debilitated adult GBS patients in the intensive care setting can manifest mood, anxiety, and psychotic symptoms (6). Helpful laboratory tests include analysis of CSF, in which the protein rises to high levels but the cell count remains normal (albuminocytologic dissociation). NCS demonstrate slowing of conduction velocity, especially in motor nerves, along with other abnormalities.

Treatment of GBS includes supportive care, which may require intubation and assisted ventilation. In recent years, plasmapheresis and administration of IVIG have both been demonstrated to hasten recovery in adults with GBS. Despite limited data on their use in children, pediatric neurologists have adopted these therapies to treat affected children. About 80% of children recover to the point of being able to walk independently.

Although GBS is the most common acute neuropathy, clinicians must consider other etiologies in its differential diagnosis. A number of infectious agents can cause acute neuropathy. Lyme disease in the United States is caused by infection with the spirochete *Borrelia burgdorferi*, transmitted by the bite of the *Ixodes* tick. It occurs most commonly in the northeastern states in late summer and early fall. The characteristic erythema migrans rash is a classic early finding but may not be present. Neurological manifestations, which occur in up to 40% of infected patients, may include involvement of both the CNS and PNS. Facial palsy and aseptic meningitis are the most common neurological findings in children

(7). Polyradiculopathy (involvement of multiple nerve roots) and polyneuropathy also occur, beginning in the acute stage or after a delay of months to years. Fever, headache, and joint pains are common, as is fatigue (especially in adults). Diagnosis depends on enzyme-linked immunosorbent assay (ELISA) with confirmation by Western blot. Neurological Lyme disease usually requires treatment with intravenous antibiotics.

Another tick-borne cause of neuropathy is tick paralysis, caused by the bite of the *Dermacentor* tick. Children are affected more often than adults. Weakness begins within hours to days of attachment of the tick to the skin, followed by rapid progression. Cranial nerves are often involved, and quadriplegia and respiratory failure may occur. Removal of the tick results in rapid recovery.

Diphtheria is a rare cause of neuropathy in the United States, thanks to widespread immunization. Viruses, such as Epstein-Barr virus (EBV) and human immunodeficiency virus (HIV), can produce neuropathy. In addition, many of the antiretroviral drugs used to treat HIV infection are also toxic to nerves.

Many toxins can cause chronic neuropathy, but acute toxic neuropathy is uncommon unless the exposure is very substantial. Heavy metals (such as mercury or arsenic), organophosphates used as insecticides, and toxins in the buckthorn fruit are some causes of acute-to-subacute neuropathy. Glue sniffing exposes abusers to *n*-hexane, a toxic hexacarbon that produces subacute sensorimotor neuropathy. In many cases of acute intoxication, involvement of other systems such as skin or gastrointestinal tract is more prominent than the neuropathy.

Acute intermittent porphyria, a hereditary (autosomal dominant) metabolic disorder, can cause attacks of acute neuropathy, usually in postpubertal patients. These attacks usually begin with abdominal pain, followed by weakness that may be severe enough to compromise breathing. In addition, CNS findings often occur, including seizures and psychiatric disturbances such as psychosis, depression, anxiety, or mental status changes. Elevated levels of porphobilinogen and delta-aminolevulinic acid in the urine confirm the diagnosis. Treatment of attacks with intravenous carbohydrates and/or hemin preparations has been advocated, but the best management involves prevention of attacks by avoidance of medications and situations known to trigger them. Barbiturates, phenytoin, alcohol, and many oral contraceptives are particularly likely to precipitate attacks; other agents that have been implicated include amitriptyline, imipramine, carbamazepine, and valproate.

Chronic neuropathies

The majority of chronic neuropathies in children are inherited. Hereditary neurophathies usually present in childhood but sometimes do not manifest until adulthood. Neurologists classify the hereditary neuropathies on the basis of three characteristics: the type(s) of nerve fiber involved (motor, sensory, and/or autonomic), the primary pathophysiology (axonal or demyelinating), and the inheritance pattern (dominant, recessive, X-linked, or mitochondrial). The overall prevalence of these disorders is approximately 30 per 100,000 individuals. Some hereditary conditions cause neuropathy along with other manifestations, which may include CNS involvement.

Traditionally, neurologists use the eponym Charcot-Marie-Tooth disease (CMT) to refer to hereditary motor-sensory neuropathies that occur without identifiable metabolic disturbances. Numerous subcategories of CMT are now recognized, including axonal and demyelinating neuropathies, with dominant, recessive, and X-linked patterns of inheritance. CMT1 comprises several dominantly inherited conditions with abnormal myelin; this is the most common group, accounting for approximately 50% of CMT patients. Dominantly inherited axonal neuropathies, categorized as CMT2, are next most common.

Axonal and demyelinating types of CMT with X-linked inheritance have been described, as have many rarer forms of the disease.

Patients with CMT typically have symmetrical weakness and atrophy in the distal legs and (less prominently) arms that worsen progressively but slowly. In most cases, onset is in the first through third decades but may be delayed until adulthood. Often the first symptoms are difficulty walking or frequent falling, and ankle sprains are common. As the neuropathy progresses, decreased power in the tibialis anterior muscle causes weakness of ankle dorsiflexion, leading to foot drop; this may result in steppage gait, in which the patient lifts the leg high to ensure that the toes clear the ground. Hand weakness may result in impairment of hand writing or of using buttons and zippers.

Both neurological and orthopedic abnormalities may be present on physical examination. The legs have been described as resembling stork legs or inverted champagne bottles due to atrophy of the distal leg muscles. Hammer toes (curling of the toes) and pes cavus (high-arched feet) may develop. DTRs are decreased or absent, and sensation (especially of vibration and joint position) is impaired. In some cases, nerves (such as the peroneal nerve) become enlarged—sometimes to the extent that neurologists can palpate them.

Specific diagnosis traditionally depended on careful characterization of a patient's family history to determine the pattern of inheritance, along with NCS to characterize the pathology as axonal or demyelinating. On occasion, nerve biopsy was performed. In recent years, the specific gene defect underlying many varieties of CMT has been identified, and molecular techniques have greatly improved the diagnosis of these conditions.

Many genetic conditions in addition to CMT result in neuropathy. Examples include metabolic disorders such as Krabbe disease and metachromatic leukodystrophy (MLD); these recessively inherited disorders tend to affect the myelin of the CNS, leading to mental retardation, visual impairment, and spasticity. Patients with juvenile-onset MLD can present with behavioral symptoms including problems with attention or hyperactivity, affective lability, or a schizophreniform-like psychosis. These children frequently also have learning disorders and cognitive dysfunction. Refsum disease is a metabolic disorder that classically begins in childhood with demyelinating neuropathy, deafness, ataxia, retinitis pigmentosa, and skin ichthyosis. Some hereditary ataxias, most notably Friedreich ataxia, are accompanied by neuropathy. The category of hereditary motor neuropathy (HMN) comprises various conditions now often considered forms of distal SMA. A variety of types of hereditary sensory neuropathy (HSN) have been described, many associated with abnormalities of the autonomic nervous system (called hereditary sensory and autonomic neuropathies, HSANs). Mitochondrial disorders associated with neuropathy include mitochondrial neurogastrointestinal encephalomyopathy (MNGIE) and neuropathy, ataxia, and retinitis pigmentosa (NARP).

No treatment is known to reverse or arrest the progression of hereditary neuropathies. Physiatrists and physical therapists can help by recommending appropriate exercise and by providing appropriate devices, such as a cane, crutches, or ankle-foot orthoses. Orthopedic surgery may be necessary to correct foot deformities. As with all inherited conditions, genetic counseling should be offered to families of patients with hereditary neuropathies. Children should have comprehensive psychiatric evaluations to determine the need for psychotherapy, medication, and educational accommodations. Parents of affected children may benefit from supportive psychotherapy and, when necessary, grief counseling.

Chronic neuropathies can also be acquired. Exposure to toxic substances either as an accident or as part of a medical regimen can lead to neuropathy. Many medications are toxic to nerves and can cause iatrogenic neuropathy. Whereas most psychotropic medications are generally not associated with neuropathy, exposure to lithium either in acute intoxication or with chronic treatment can produce neuropathy involving both sensory and motor fibers. Other medications that can cause neuropathy include disulfiram, phenytoin, nitrous oxide, vitamin B_6, some antibiotics (isoniazid, chloramphenicol, nitrofurantoin, metronidazole), and many antiretroviral and antineoplastic agents. Chronic exposure to heavy metals often leads to neuropathy. Notably, while lead intoxication is associated with neuropathy in adults, in children it is more likely to cause mental retardation, learning disabilities, and other symptoms of CNS toxicity.

A rare cause of neuropathy in childhood is chronic inflammatory demyelinating polyneuropathy (CIDP), in which symmetrical proximal and distal weakness progresses over 8 weeks or longer. Like in AIDP, reflexes are absent or diminished, and sensory symptoms are common. Electrophysiologic studies indicate nerve demyelination, and examination of the CSF reveals albuminocytologic dissociation. CIDP can be successfully treated with oral corticosteroids, IVIG, or plasma exchange, and many neurologists choose IVIG as first-line therapy in children with CIDP. Although most children respond to therapy, relapses may occur.

NEUROMUSCULAR JUNCTION

MG is a group of disorders in which transmission at the neuromuscular junction is disrupted. The most common form is an autoimmune disorder in which antibodies are formed against the acetylcholine receptor (AChR) on the postsynaptic muscle membrane. These antibodies interfere with neuromuscular transmission, resulting in weakness. The thymus gland is thought to play an important role in formation of these antibodies, and many patients with MG have associated thymic abnormalities (including hyperplasia and thymoma).

The peak incidence of autoimmune MG is in the second and third decades, when it affects females more than males. (Another peak in the sixth to eighth decade affects mostly men.) Extraocular muscles tend to be involved early, and the first symptoms often include ptosis or diplopia. Although weakness may remain restricted to the extraocular muscles, most patients develop weakness of other muscles, often producing dysarthria, dysphagia, facial weakness, or symmetrical proximal limb weakness. Involvement of respiratory muscles constitutes a life-threatening emergency. A characteristic feature of MG is weakness that fluctuates: power that is normal at one moment may worsen with muscle use due to depletion of acetylcholine stores from the presynaptic nerve terminal. Sensation and mental function are normal in MG.

Several methods are available for confirming the diagnosis of MG. Serum antibodies to the AChR can be measured, although a subset of patients with MG are "seronegative" (meaning they do not have antibodies to the acetylcholine receptor). It is now known that some "seronegative" MG patients have antibodies to other proteins (such as MuSK) found at the NMJ, and these can be assayed if AChR antibodies are absent.

A Tensilon (edrophonium) test can help confirm the diagnosis of MG. As mentioned previously, edrophonium is a short-acting inhibitor of the enzyme acetylcholinesterase. An intravenous injection of edrophonium reduces the enzymatic degradation of acetylcholine, prolonging its presence at the NMJ and consequently improving muscle strength for a few minutes. Although useful in conjunction with clinical judgment and other investigations, the Tensilon test is not entirely sensitive or specific for the diagnosis of MG.

Two of the tests used to diagnose MG are performed in a neurophysiology laboratory. In repetitive nerve stimulation, a motor nerve is repeatedly stimulated and the electrical response in the muscle it innervates is measured. Stimulation at a rate of two to three stimulations per second normally results in a comparable response to each stimulus. In MG, a "decremental" pattern may be elicited, in which, due to depletion of acetylcholine, successive responses are smaller than earlier ones. Another test, single-fiber EMG, examines action potentials from muscle fibers innervated by the same motor neuron. In MG, the latencies of these action potentials are more variable than in normal individuals. Single-fiber EMG is the most sensitive test for diagnosing MG but is less widely available.

Management of autoimmune MG involves symptomatic treatment as well as therapies aimed at the underlying immune mechanism. Pyridostigmine (Mestinon), a long-acting oral acetylcholinesterase inhibitor, is usually effective at improving weakness when taken several times daily. Neurologists may also prescribe medications that suppress the patient's immune system in order to modulate the underlying disease process. Corticosteroids are the most widely used, but chronic use is associated with numerous systemic adverse effects in addition to significant psychiatric dysfunction, including depression, mania, or even psychosis. Other potentially useful immunosuppressant agents include azathioprine and mycophenolate. Thymectomy, a surgical procedure, is often performed in patients with MG. Its exact role is not clearly defined but is most likely to be useful in seropositive patients with generalized MG and in patients with thymoma. Other treatment options include plasma exchange and IVIG, both of which produce beneficial but short-lived effects.

Pregnant women with MG may transmit AChR antibodies across the placenta. Consequently, their babies may be born with transient neonatal MG. Findings include generalized weakness, poor feeding, and a weak cry. Most babies spontaneously improve within weeks, but brief treatment with pyridostigmine is sometimes required. This condition should be distinguished from congenital MG, a group of disorders resulting from various rare molecular defects of the NMJ.

Another cause of dysfunction of the NMJ is botulism, which results from the toxin of the gram-positive bacillus *Clostridium botulinum*. Ingestion of food contaminated with either the bacterial spores themselves or the toxin they produce causes acute onset of diffuse weakness. A common scenario occurs when infants ingest foods such as raw honey that contains the spores; due to the immaturity of the flora in the infant gastrointestinal tract, the bacteria multiply and produce toxin. The toxin is taken up by motor nerve terminals and interferes with the release of acetylcholine.

Botulism causes weakness of extraocular, bulbar, and limb muscles, as well as autonomic abnormalities. Common presenting signs and symptoms include hypotonia, poor feeding, weak cry, pupillary dilatation, ptosis, and constipation. DTRs are depressed but sensation and cognition are not affected. Repetitive nerve stimulation at a rapid stimulation rate demonstrates an "incremental" pattern, in which successive motor action potentials increase in amplitude. *Clostridia* may grow in stool culture, and the toxin can be identified in stool or serum, although constipation may limit the availability of stool specimens.

Treatment of botulism involves supportive care, which includes appropriate hydration and nutrition; mechanical ventilation may be necessary. Patients often improve spontaneously over weeks to months. Antibiotics are not effective, and while an equine antitoxin is available, its risks outweigh its benefits in infants with botulism. Recent data suggest that botulism immune globulin is safe and effective in treatment of infant botulism (8,9). To help prevent infant botulism, the American Academy of Pediatrics recommends that infants younger than 1 year not be fed honey.

MUSCLE

Many pathological processes can result in myopathy. Inherited myopathies include muscular dystrophies, congenital myopathies, channelopathies, and metabolic myopathies (including mitochondrial myopathies). Acquired causes include infectious, inflammatory, endocrine, and toxic (including iatrogenic) processes.

In general, myopathies result in weakness that is more prominent proximally than distally. Proximal leg weakness may interfere with functions such as rising from a sitting position or climbing stairs; proximal arm weakness may cause difficulty combing hair or brushing teeth. Sensation is preserved, unless concurrent neuropathy or CNS pathology is present. In many cases, serum levels of muscle enzymes such as CPK are elevated. With EMG testing, characteristic features of myopathy, including short-duration, low-amplitude motor unit action potentials, are often present.

Muscular dystrophies

The muscular dystrophies are a group of genetic myopathies in which defects in structural muscle proteins lead to muscle degeneration with progressive wasting and weakness. They vary significantly in severity, anatomical distribution, age at onset, and inheritance pattern.

Duchenne and Becker muscular dystrophies

These are X-linked disorders with progressive symmetrical proximal weakness beginning in childhood. In DMD, the structural protein dystrophin is absent or nearly absent in muscle. DMD begins by the age of 5 years with gait dysfunction, including toe walking, frequent falls, and difficulty running or climbing stairs. The presence of Gowers sign reflects the presence of proximal muscle weakness (Fig. 18.1A–E). The calf muscles become enlarged and the Achilles tendons shorten, leading to toe-walking. Power in the arms and legs declines throughout childhood. Most boys require a wheelchair by the age of 12 years. Cardiomyopathy and hypoventilation are common and often lead to death in the third decade, especially if complicated by an intercurrent pulmonary illness.

Cognitive dysfunction is relatively common in patients with DMD. The mean full-scale intelligence quotient (IQ) is 80, and almost 35% of children fall in the mentally retarded range [defined as full-scale IQ less than 70 (10)]. Many children with normal IQ manifest reading disorders and may have additional problems with learning and memory. The cognitive deficits are static and do not correlate with neuromuscular disease severity.

Because of the chronic and progressive nature of DMD, leading ultimately to an early death, children with DMD and their families are under high levels of both physical and psychological stress. This significant burden leads to higher levels of depression in children and their parents (11). Social isolation, issues around dying, and physical dependency complicate the emotional health of DMD patients. At the same time, parental depression is related to caregiver burden, family dysfunction, feelings of guilt, and unresolved grief (12,13).

The serum CPK is markedly elevated in DMD, and muscle biopsy shows absent (or severely reduced) dystrophin content. Current diagnosis rests on molecular genetic testing, which is highly sensitive for identifying mutations in the gene coding for dystrophin and has essentially obviated the need for muscle biopsy.

Treatment with oral corticosteroids has a favorable but short-lived effect on both muscle strength and function (14). The side effects of steroids include weight gain, cushingoid appearance, and excessive hair growth. Behavioral effects may also occur. Management also consists of ventilatory support in patients with hypoventilation, early screening for cardiomyopathy (with echocardiography and electrocardiography) and appropriate treatment, and use of physical therapy, exercise, and assistive devices.

In Becker muscular dystrophy, muscle dystrophin is reduced to a lesser extent than in DMD. It is clinically similar to DMD but is less severe, with later age at onset and longer survival. Some patients have cognitive dysfunction, emotional difficulties, and behavioral problems that can predate neuromuscular involvement (15).

Myotonic dystrophy

Neurologists recognize two types of myotonic dystrophy; type 2 is also known as proximal myotonic myopathy (PROMM). Type 1 (DM1) is the most common hereditary neuromuscular disease in adults. It is inherited in autosomal dominant fashion, and demonstrates anticipation, such that onset is earlier and severity is greater in successive generations. Many neurologists have seen families in which a patient with mild myotonic dystrophy has a child with more severe involvement and a grandchild with devastating congenital myotonic dystrophy.

The classic presentation of DM1 is weakness and wasting of muscles in the face, neck, and distal limbs beginning in the second or third decade. Myotonia, delayed muscle relaxation after voluntary contraction, can be demonstrated on physical examination, but it is usually not bothersome to the patient. Over years, the weakness progresses and becomes more diffuse. Many systemic features commonly accompany DM1, including frontal balding, a hatchet-shaped face, cataracts, disordered sleep, and endocrine, cardiac, and pulmonary abnormalities.

In congenital DM1, infants (usually of mothers with DM1) show decreased movement in utero and are born with hypotonia and respiratory insufficiency requiring mechanical ventilation. Mean verbal IQ in patients who survive into childhood is 56, and these children manifest problems with emotion regulation and social interactions (16).

Patients with juvenile-onset DM1 (age at onset younger than 10 years) suffer from markedly delayed motor development, although the cognitive deficits are less pronounced (mean global IQ of 61 and mean verbal IQ of 75). Even children with normal-range IQ can demonstrate evidence of significant learning difficulties, especially in reading and spelling (17). Many children and adolescents with juvenile DM1 have associated psychopathology, most commonly ADHD and anxiety disorders (18). In fact, children with juvenile DM1 may initially present with school or behavioral problems and minimal neuromuscular disease.

Neurologists suspect the diagnosis of DM1 on the basis of family history and characteristic clinical features. In the past, EMG and muscle biopsy served as the basis for diagnosing DM1, but genetic testing has replaced these procedures as the definitive diagnostic test. Classically, EMG shows myopathic features as well as electrical myotonia (runs of motor unit action potentials that wax and wane in amplitude and frequency). When it is performed, muscle biopsy shows atrophy and internally located nuclei.

Management of DM1 is mostly directed at identifying and treating the associated systemic features. Physiatrists and physical therapists can help promote function and provide appropriate assistive devices. Physicians can prescribe mexiletine to minimize myotonia although this is usually not very bothersome to patients. Psychiatrists can help manage mood symptoms and behavioral problems with medication and psychotherapy.

Congenital muscular dystrophies

These disorders present in the neonatal period with hypotonia, joint contractures, and diffuse weakness and atrophy. Examples include merosin deficiency, muscle-eye-brain syndrome, Walker-Warburg syndrome, and Fukayama congenital muscular dystrophy. Mental retardation occurs in many but not all of these disorders. Magnetic resonance imaging (MRI) of the brain may be abnormal even in individuals with normal intelligence. Although treatment is mostly supportive, physical therapy is useful in management of the contractures.

Other muscular dystrophies

Several other categories of muscular dystrophy can begin in childhood. Limb-girdle muscular dystrophies are a group of conditions with autosomal dominant or autosomal recessive inheritance that cause progressive proximal muscle weakness and wasting. Severity and age at onset are highly variable. Some forms involve cardiac muscle, and a few can be associated with mental retardation, but this is not a prominent feature of this group of disorders. Facioscapulohumeral muscular dystrophy is an autosomal dominant condition causing progressive weakness that begins in the shoulders and face, followed by the foot dorsiflexors and other leg muscles. Hearing loss and retinal disease are common but cognition is normal. The rate of progression and the extent of disability vary among patients. Emery-Dreifuss muscular dystrophy consists of contractures, slowly progressive weakness, and cardiomyopathy inherited in X-linked, autosomal dominant, or (rarely) autosomal recessive fashion. No specific treatment is available for any of the muscular dystrophies mentioned in this paragraph, but physical therapy may be helpful.

Congenital myopathies

Several myopathies occurring in infancy, usually presenting with neonatal hypotonia, are not classified as dystrophies because the clinical course tends to be nonprogressive and muscle degeneration is not present on biopsy. These include central core disease, myotubular (centronuclear) myopathy, nemaline rod myopathy, and congenital fiber-type disproportion myopathy. Some are associated with severe weakness and lead to early death due to respiratory insufficiency, while others may cause minimal disability. Pattern of inheritance and clinical features may suggest possible disorders but rarely permit a specific diagnosis; in the past, muscle biopsy was needed for diagnosis but recently genetic tests for some of these myopathies have become available. Cognition is normal in most of these conditions, although some (such as myotubular myopathy) may be associated with mental retardation.

Channelopathies

Normal function of the CNS and PNS depends on precisely controlled movement of ions across cell membranes. Physiologically important ions such as sodium, chloride, calcium, and potassium are transported through specialized channels which open or close in response to electrochemical signals. Disorders of these ion channels—known as channelopathies—can be inherited (due to mutations in the genes that code for them) or acquired (mostly due to toxic or autoimmune processes that interfere with their function).

Clinically, channelopathies are highly diverse. In the CNS they can produce migraine, epilepsy, or ataxia, while in the PNS they can disrupt nerve, NMJ, or muscle. One feature common to these disorders is the paroxysmal nature of the symptoms: episodes or attacks tend to be separated by asymptomatic intervals. As mentioned previously, the intermittent nature of these disorders may lead clinicians to the erroneous conclusion that a patient's symptoms are not organic.

Muscle channelopathies usually result in myotonia (delayed muscle relaxation after contraction) or periodic paralysis. Inherited channelopathies associated with myotonia include myotonia congenita and paramyotonia congenita (caused by mutations in genes encoding chloride and sodium channels, respectively).[3] Myotonia congenita occurs in autosomal dominant and autosomal recessive forms, begins in childhood, and is often associated with muscle hypertrophy. The myotonia is exacerbated by cold or rest and improves with repeated contraction (the warm-up phenomenon). Paramyotonia congenita has autosomal dominant inheritance, begins in infancy, and worsens with cold or

---

[3] Chloride channel abnormalities are also thought to be responsible for the myotonia in myotonic dystrophy.

(unlike myotonia congenita) with exercise. Mexiletine can be used to treat the myotonia associated with these conditions.

Several genetic forms of periodic paralysis result from mutations in genes that code for sodium, calcium, or potassium channels. All demonstrate an autosomal dominant pattern of inheritance, and most are associated with abnormally high or low serum potassium levels during attacks. Hypokalemic periodic paralysis, the most common type, begins in the second decade of life. Attacks of moderate to severe limb weakness lasting hours to days can be triggered by a meal rich in carbohydrates and are treated by oral potassium. In hyperkalemic periodic paralysis, which begins in the first decade, attacks of weakness are more frequent and shorter in duration than those of hypokalemic periodic paralysis. The episodes vary in severity and may tend to follow exercise. Inhaled albuterol can be used to lower serum potassium and terminate an acute attack.

Metabolic myopathies (including mitochondrial myopathies)

Adenosine triphosphate (ATP) is the primary source of energy for muscle contraction. Much of the ATP used by muscle comes from metabolism of glycogen and fatty acids. Glycogen is converted to pyruvate, which is transported into mitochondria and converted to acetyl-CoA. Similarly, fatty acids are transported into mitochondria where they undergo beta-oxidation to acetyl-CoA. In the mitochondria, acetyl-CoA undergoes oxidative metabolism via the Krebs cycle, producing ATP. Deficiency of an enzyme in pathways responsible for the metabolism of these substrates can lead to myopathy.

Some metabolic myopathies may present in infancy with hypotonia. Metabolic myopathies that begin in childhood, adolescence, or adulthood sometimes cause weakness but also may result in exercise intolerance or cramps. Strenuous exercise may cause muscle breakdown, leading to myoglobinuria, in which muscle proteins are released into the urine, turning it the color of tea or cola.

Several metabolic myopathies are associated with deficiency of enzymes involved in glycogen metabolism. Acid maltase deficiency (Pompe disease), inherited in autosomal recessive fashion, may present in infancy with hypotonia and cardiomegaly or may begin in childhood or adulthood with slowly progressive proximal limb weakness. Enzyme replacement therapy is now available. Myophosphorylase deficiency (McArdle disease) also demonstrates autosomal recessive inheritance, but exercise-induced muscle aches and cramps may predominate over weakness. Myoglobinuria is common. No specific treatment is available. Other metabolic myopathies result from deficiency of other enzymes involved in glycogen metabolism.

Disorders of fatty acid metabolism can result from deficiency of carnitine, a protein necessary for transport of fatty acids into mitochondria. Carnitine deficiency can be genetic or may result from a variety of conditions (including treatment with valproic acid) that cause carnitine to be lost. Typically, proximal weakness begins in childhood and progresses slowly. Oral carnitine supplementation may be effective. Deficiency of very long chain acyl-CoA dehydrogenase, an enzyme involved in beta-oxidation of lipids in mitochondria, causes episodes of exercise-induced muscle pain and myoglobinuria.

Many mitochondrial disorders have been identified, with highly diverse clinical presentations. Because mitochondria play a crucial role in energy generation, disorders of mitochondria affect organ systems that require large amounts of energy, including brain and muscle. The term *mitochondrial encephalomyopathy* reflects the concurrent involvement of brain and muscle in these conditions. CNS manifestations may include seizures, mental retardation, deafness, and ataxia. Muscle manifestations may include weakness, exercise intolerance, and cardiomyopathy. Neuropathy may also be present. Short stature and hearing loss are other features that may be associated.

Some mitochondrial disorders begin in infancy, while others have onset in adulthood. Mitochondria contain their own DNA, which an individual inherits entirely from his or her mother. Consequently, disorders resulting from mutations in mitochondrial genes are transmitted from a woman to her offspring. However, because some components of mitochondria are encoded by genes in the nucleus, some mitochondrial disorders demonstrate autosomal (dominant or recessive) inheritance.

The typical mitochondrial myopathy begins in childhood and produces symmetrical proximal weakness and exercise-induced muscle pain. Many patients also have progressive external ophthalmoplegia and/or ptosis. Pigmentary retinopathy or neuropathy may be associated, and mental retardation may be present. Seizures may also occur, as in MERRF.

Mitochondrial myopathies may also be associated with psychiatric symptoms including mood and psychotic symptoms in addition to delirium or dementia. Psychiatric symptoms may be the initial manifestation of the disorder. A recent case report describes an adolescent male who presented with mania that progressed into a neurological syndrome suggestive of MELAS (19).

The serum CPK level in patients with mitochondrial myopathies is not always elevated, although a level that is normal at rest may rise with muscular exertion. Lactate levels are usually elevated; if normal in blood, physicians should measure lactate levels in CSF. Muscle biopsy shows a variety of changes, which may include the characteristic ragged-red fibers, reflecting clumping of abnormal mitochondria in muscle fibers. Molecular genetic testing is available for some mitochondrial disorders. No specific treatment is available for mitochondrial myopathies.

Inflammatory (including infectious) myopathies

Many acquired processes can cause inflammation of muscle, or myositis. Dermatomyositis and polymyositis are immune-mediated disorders with prominent muscle involvement. Dermatomyositis is the most common inflammatory myopathy in children, affecting boys more often than girls. It is thought to result from an autoimmune attack against small blood vessels in skin, muscle, nerve, and visceral organs. Some patients experience a prodromal illness with fever and upper respiratory symptoms. More often, the first symptom is rash. Other dermatologic manifestations are variable but may include edema, purple discoloration of the eyelids, and scaly erythema on the extensor surfaces of joints. Many children also develop subcutaneous calcified nodules. Symmetrical muscle pain and weakness begin proximally but usually become generalized; this progression can be rapid or insidious. Joint contractures, especially at the ankles, may occur. The CNS remains unaffected.

Children with dermatomyositis usually have elevated CPK levels, and the EMG shows myopathic changes and spontaneous activity. Muscle biopsy classically demonstrates perifascicular atrophy.

If not treated adequately, dermatomyositis is associated with significant morbidity and mortality, usually due to infarction in the gastrointestinal tract. High-dose corticosteroids should be administered as early as possible. Although the dose should be tapered to minimize side effects, treatment generally should be continued for at least 2 years. Unlike adults with dermatomyositis, who often require long-term steroid treatment, children who undergo gradual withdrawal tend not to relapse. If steroids are ineffective or produce intolerable side effects, neurologists consider adjunctive therapies such as IVIG, plasmapheresis, methotrexate, and other immunosuppressant medications.

Polymyositis is an inflammatory myopathy that mostly affects adults, although adolescents also can be affected. Typically, symmetrical proximal muscle weakness and pain develop over months. It may be idiopathic or accompany systemic inflammatory disorders such as sarcoidosis or collagen-vascular diseases like systemic lupus erythematosus, scleroderma, or mixed connective tissue disease. There is no rash associated with polymyositis. As in dermatomyositis, CPK is usually elevated and EMG demonstrates myopathy with spontaneous activity. Muscle biopsy classically shows inflammatory changes. Corticosteroids are the mainstay of therapy.

A number of infectious agents can cause myositis. Benign acute childhood myositis causes sudden onset of calf pain and gait dysfunction, mostly in school-age boys (20). In many cases it seems to be related to influenza or other viral infections, and is often self-limited. Lyme disease frequently causes myalgias, but rarely it can also cause myositis. Focal muscle abscesses can result from bacterial infections, such as *Staphylococcus aureus*, and tuberculosis. Children who eat undercooked meat may ingest parasites, most often trichinosis, which form cysts in muscle and lead to local muscle pain and swelling. Immunosuppression due to HIV infection may lead to bacterial, fungal, viral, or parasitic myositis. HIV infection also causes a variety of other myopathies, including a syndrome closely resembling polymyositis.

Endocrine myopathies

Hypothyroidism can cause progressive proximal muscle weakness and hypertrophy, along with lethargy, decreased energy, delayed growth, and cold intolerance. In addition, hyperthyroidism can result in painless proximal weakness. Hypoactivity or hyperactivity of parathyroid or adrenal glands can also lead to myopathy. In general, endocrine myopathies respond favorably to treatment of the underlying endocrinopathy.

Toxic (including iatrogenic) myopathies

A variety of toxins may result in myopathy, including many substances prescribed by physicians. Virtually all antipsychotic drugs have been associated with elevated serum CPK levels, reflecting breakdown of muscle; severe cases result in neuroleptic malignant syndrome, while mild cases may be entirely asymptomatic. Amphetamines and lithium are other causes of muscle breakdown. Use of phenytoin has been reported to cause inflammatory myopathy in adolescents, presumably as part of a hypersensitivity reaction. Proximal muscle weakness and atrophy are frequent side effects of chronic corticosteroid use, and intravenous administration of high-dose steroids also can produce acute myopathy. The antiemetic ipecac can cause a myopathy that also involves cardiac muscle. Other myotoxic drugs include the antiretroviral agent zidovudine (AZT), the immunosuppressant cyclosporine, and the antimalarial drugs chloroquine and hydroxychloroquine. Intramuscular injections can cause focal myopathy.

Not all myotoxins are prescribed by physicians. Alcohol is toxic to muscle, and alcohol abusers often develop a chronic myopathy that includes cardiomyopathy. Also, binge drinking can result in acute myopathy. The venom injected by the bite of some pit vipers and other snakes, or by massive stinging events by hundreds of bees or wasps, can also be myotoxic.

HYSTERICAL PARALYSIS

Motor deficits are an uncommon presentation of conversion disorder in children. When they develop, their manifestations may be as extreme as flaccid quadriplegia. Adolescents with conversion disorder tend to have high levels of environmental stress (21). Treatment is mostly supportive and involves physical and occupational therapy in addition to psychotherapy. Psychotropic medication may also be indicated for comorbid mood or anxiety disorders. In one study, almost 85% of children had recovered function after 4 years although many of them continued to have mood or anxiety disorders (22).

The neurologist, in consultation with the psychiatrist, must distinguish between conversion disorder, factitious disorder, and malingering, as this determination will guide the clinician in the proper approach to the patient.

Summary

Many pathological processes affect the PNS. Neurologists rely on a careful history and physical examination to localize the dysfunction in the nervous system and narrow the possible causes. Judicious use of laboratory testing helps to confirm a diagnosis; increasingly, techniques of molecular genetics are proving useful in the diagnosis of hereditary neuromuscular conditions, and as our understanding of the genetics of neuromuscular disorders continues to advance, more tests undoubtedly will become available.

Psychiatrists can contribute to the care of children with neuromuscular disorders by helping to manage the cognitive, emotional, and behavioral abnormalities that accompany some of these conditions, in addition to providing much-needed support for chronically ill patients and their families.

Questions

1. A 15 year old tells her pediatrician that she has noted intermittent double vision and difficulty swallowing for the past 2 months. Detailed neurological examination is normal. Any of the following would be a reasonable next step EXCEPT
   A. measure acetylcholine receptor antibodies in the serum.
   B. perform repetitive nerve stimulation.
   C. perform a Tensilon test.
   D. prescribe an antidepressant with anxiolytic properties.

2. Which of the following findings is most likely to be present in a patient with mental retardation and weakness?
   A. muscle atrophy
   B. fasciculations
   C. hyperreflexia
   D. neuropathy

3. Which of the following commonly affect(s) patients with Duchenne muscular dystrophy?
   A. learning disabilities
   B. mental retardation
   C. depression
   D. steroid-induced behavioral changes
   E. All of the above are common in patients with Duchenne muscular dystrophy.

4. Which of the following psychoactive medications is recognized as a cause of neuropathy?
   A. disulfiram
   B. amitriptyline
   C. chlorpromazine
   D. haloperidol
   E. tranylcypromine

5. A 5-year-old boy is noted to have a tendency to walk on his toes. Which of the following is the LEAST likely to be the cause of his toe-walking?
   A. Duchenne muscular dystrophy
   B. spasticity due to dysfunction of upper motor neurons
   C. a behavioral mannerism not related to neurological disease
   D. chronic inflammatory demyelinating polyneuropathy (CIDP)

6. Which of the following processes is most likely to cause sensory loss?
   A. neuropathy due to acute lithium intoxication

B. myopathy due to chronic use of haloperidol
C. exacerbation of myasthenia gravis due to use of a beta-blocker
D. wound botulism due to use of contaminated needles to inject drugs of abuse

Answers

1. D. The history is highly suggestive of myasthenia gravis (MG). It is characteristic of MG for the severity of symptoms to fluctuate, so it is not surprising that the examination in the doctor's office is normal. Measurement of acetylcholine receptor antibodies, repetitive nerve stimulation, Tensilon test, and single-fiber electromyography are all useful methods of making the diagnosis of MG.

2. C. Mental retardation indicates pathology of the central nervous system and suggests that associated weakness is due to dysfunction of upper motor neurons. Hyperreflexia is typical of such dysfunction, whereas atrophy and fasciculations are associated with lower motor neuron lesions.

3. E. All of these are commonly seen in boys with Duchenne muscular dystrophy.

4. A. Disulfiram, used in the treatment of alcoholism, causes a distal sensorimotor axonal neuropathy. Of historical interest is the antidepressant zimeldine, which was withdrawn from the market in 1983 because it was associated with increased risk of Guillain-Barré syndrome.

5. D. CIDP causes symmetrical proximal and distal weakness. All the others are potential causes of toe-walking.

6. A. Acute lithium intoxication can cause sensorimotor axonal neuropathy. Other neuromuscular disorders caused by lithium include myopathy and drug-induced myasthenia gravis. Disorders of muscle or the neuromuscular junction do not affect sensation.

REFERENCES

1. Jones HR Jr. Guillain-Barré syndrome: perspectives with infants and children. *Semin Pediatr Neurol.* 2000;7:91–102.
2. Schaumburg HH, Herskovitz S. The weak child—a cautionary tale. *N Engl J Med.* 2000;342:127–129.
3. Heresi GP, et al. Poliomyelitis-like syndrome in a child with West Nile virus infection. *Pediatr Infect Dis J.* 2004;23:788–789.
4. Ogino S, et al. Genetic risk assessment in carrier testing for spinal muscular atrophy. *Am J Med Genet.* 2002;110:301–307.
5. Laufersweiler-Plass C, et al. Behavioural problems in children and adolescents with spinal muscular atrophy and their siblings. *Dev Med Child Neurol.* 2003;45:44–49.
6. Weiss H, et al. Psychotic symptoms and emotional distress in patients with Guillain-Barré syndrome. *Eur Neurol.* 2002;47:74–78.
7. Bingham PM, et al. Neurologic manifestations in children with Lyme disease. *Pediatrics.* 1995;96:1053–1056.
8. Arnon SS, et al. Human botulism immune globulin for the treatment of infant botulism. *N Engl J Med.* 2006;354:462–471.
9. Thompson JA, et al. Infant botulism in the age of botulism immune globulin. *Neurology.* 2005;64:2029–2032.
10. Cotton S, Voudouris NJ, Greenwood KM. Intelligence and Duchenne muscular dystrophy: full-scale, verbal, and performance intelligence quotients. *Dev Med Child Neurol.* 2001;43:497–501.
11. Polakoff RJ, et al. The psychosocial and cognitive impact of Duchenne's muscular dystrophy. *Semin Pediatr Neurol.* 1998;5:116–123.
12. Abi Daoud MS, Dooley JM, Gordon KE. Depression in parents of children with Duchenne muscular dystrophy. *Pediatr Neurol.* 2004;31:16–19.
13. Morrow M. Duchenne muscular dystrophy—a biopsychosocial approach. *Physiotherapy.* 2004;90:145–150.
14. Manzur AY, et al. Glucocorticoid corticosteroids for Duchenne muscular dystrophy. *Cochrane Database Systematic Rev.* 2004, Issue 2. Art. No.: CD003725. DOI: 10.1002/14651858.CD003725.pub2.
15. North KN, et al. Cognitive dysfunction as the major presenting feature of Becker's muscular dystrophy. *Neurology.* 1996;46:461–465.
16. Roig M, et al. Presentation, clinical course, and outcome of the congenital form of myotonic dystrophy. *Pediatr Neurol.* 1994;11:208–213.
17. Cohen D, et al. Reading and spelling impairments in children and adolescents with

infantile myotonic dystrophy. *J Neurolinguistics.* 2006;19:455–465.
18. Goossens E, et al. Emotional and behavioral profile and child psychiatric diagnosis in the childhood type of myotonic dystrophy. *Genet Couns.* 2000;11:317–327.
19. Grover S, et al. Mania as a first presentation in mitochondrial myopathy. *Psychiatry Clin Neurosci.* 2006;60:774–745.
20. Mackay MT, et al. Benign acute childhood myositis: laboratory and clinical features. *Neurology.* 1999;53:2127–2131.
21. Ercan ES, Varan A, VeznedaroGlu B. Associated features of conversion disorder in Turkish adolescents. *Pediatr Int.* 2003;45:150–155.
22. Pehlivanturk B, Unal F. Conversion disorder in children and adolescents: a 4-year follow-up study. *J Psychosom Res.* 2002;52:187–191.

CHAPTER 19

The Diagnostic Approach to Neuropsychiatric Presentations

AUDREY M. WALKER, KAREN BALLABAN-GIL, NGOC NGUYEN, AND RANA JEHLE

The collaboration between pediatric neurology and child and adolescent psychiatry is crucial when patients present with symptoms at the interface of the two disciplines. Real-time team collaboration allows for effective assessment of difficult, diagnostically puzzling cases while also providing an excellent setting for the training of fellows in pediatric neurology, child and adolescent psychiatry, pediatric residents and medical students. At the Children's Hospital at Montefiore/Albert Einstein College of Medicine, pediatric neurologists and child and adolescent psychiatrists work in the outpatient and inpatient setting in such a team. This section presents two children who were seen by our interdisciplinary team and describes our approach to the assessment.

Case 1: A 14-Year-Old Girl with Sudden Onset of Auditory and Visual Hallucinations

PRESENTATION OF CASE

Rana Jehle, P.A. (physician's assistant, pediatrics, Children's Hospital at Montefiore)

A 14-year-old girl was seen in the pediatric neurology clinic because of the acute onset of visual and auditory hallucinations.

One month prior to presentation, the patient began to experience brief episodes of visual hallucinations, in which the "devil" appeared to her. At times, "Jesus with horns" would also appear. She also described auditory hallucinations, which were accompanied by the visual ones, in which she heard a "deep male voice" that she believed to be that of the devil; however, she did not report any words or phrases in that experience. The patient sometimes heard her own voice outside of her body. She feared during these episodes that she was "selling her soul to the devil." Initially, the episodes occurred exclusively at night; they subsequently occurred during wakefulness and became more frequent during the course of the month, eventually occurring multiple times during daytime as well. The episodes were not related to menses. The patient attempted to dispel the hallucinations with prayer, but eventually disclosed them to her parents. Fervent Roman Catholics, they first brought her to their parish priest, who advised the use of prayer and medals to ward off the phenomena. The hallucinations persisted and became more frequent, leading to worsening insomnia and anxiety. The patient became increasingly withdrawn, and insisted that she be permitted to sleep with her parents. Despite these disturbances, she continued to go to school.

Before this illness she had been an honors student in her eighth grade parochial school class and had many friends. Over the course of the month, her schoolwork deteriorated and she had difficulty concentrating. She became increasingly fearful with depressed mood and believed she was "going insane."

She had focal seizures, first diagnosed when she was 9 years old, which were frequently heralded by an aura of blurry vision and a "thumping" sensation on the left side of the head. One to 2 minutes after the aura, the seizures progressed to right-sided facial twitching, grunting, and retroversion of the eyes. The movements were followed by 1 to 2 minutes of whole body stiffening and shaking. The seizures occurred predominantly at night and were followed by postictal confusion, headache, and aphasia. They occurred two to three times per month with increased frequency during menses. Infrequently, a flurry of seizures would occur several times in a day, requiring treatment with lorazepam. The seizures had been refractory to carbamazepine therapy. Two prior magnetic resonance imagings (MRIs) showed hyperintense signal abnormality on the FLAIR sequences in the posterior and medial aspect of the left temporal lobe. The differential diagnosis of this finding includes cortical dysplasia versus a low-grade neoplasm.

The patient also had a history of asthma in the past but was on no medications for the asthma at the time of presentation.

There is no family history of psychiatric disorders. There is a history of seizure disorder (type unknown) in a paternal cousin.

The patient was being treated with oxcarbazepine 600 mg every morning and 900 mg every evening and lorazepam 2 mg as needed at the time of the current presentation.

On examination, the patient was a well-appearing, well-related adolescent girl. She was cooperative and pleasant. Her vital signs were blood pressure (BP) 113/57 mm Hg, temperature (T) 98.7°F, pulse (P) 68 beats per minute, and respiratory rate (RR) 20 breaths per minute. Mental status showed completely normal orientation, memory, reality testing, and concentration.

The general physical examination showed no abnormalities.

A complete laboratory workup, including electrolytes, complete blood count (CBC), thyroid function tests, and liver function tests, was normal. Urine pregnancy and serum toxicology tests were negative, but her urine drug screen was positive for benzodiazepines.

The patient was admitted to the epilepsy monitoring unit and a psychiatric consultation was requested.

DIFFERENTIAL DIAGNOSIS

What is the differential diagnosis of the acute onset of psychosis in an adolescent girl with epilepsy?

Karen Ballaban-Gil (Professor of Clinical Neurology and Pediatrics, Albert Einstein College of Medicine; Director of Training, Child Neurology, Albert Einstein College of Medicine)

1. New seizure manifestation. Because this adolescent has a history of complex partial seizures, we must consider that her new complaints may be related to her seizures.

Her current symptoms could represent either a new seizure manifestation or a psychosis occurring in the postictal or interictal period Alternatively, these symptoms may have resulted from "forced normalization." That is, in some patients with complex partial seizures, attaining seizure control leads paradoxically to deterioration of their neuropsychiatric status, including a schizophrenia-like psychosis (1, 2).

Seizures arising from the occipital lobe may produce visual symptoms including hallucinations. Elementary visual symptoms, the most common, consist of colored or multicolored circular patterns, such as spots, circles, and balls. Patients typically describe seeing multiple figures, and other shapes less frequently. Often they see an increased number of figures as the seizure progresses. The figures are usually unilateral, mainly in the temporal visual hemifield. Episodes of epileptic-induced visual hallucinations are brief, lasting anywhere from a few seconds through several minutes (3). Rarely, patients may have status epilepticus with prolonged visual symptoms. In this variant, visual hallucinations are stereotyped. Seizures that produce visual hallucinations may remain as simple partial seizures with only visual symptoms or they may progress to express other ictal symptoms, such as tonic and/or clonic motor activity.

Less commonly, patients may experience more complex visual hallucinations that can take the form of people, animals, objects figures, or scenes. The hallucinations may be familiar or unfamiliar, friendly or frightening. These hallucinations probably originate in the occipital parietal or occipital temporal junction areas (3). There are also rare reports of auditory and complex visual hallucinations associated with seizures of frontal or orbitofrontal origin (4,5).

Seizures arising from the temporal lobe, particularly the uncus, may cause olfactory or gustatory hallucinations. Seizures arising from neocortical temporal cortex may result in auditory hallucinations consisting of a buzzing sound, a voice or voices, or a muffling of ambient sounds.

Some patients with epilepsy exhibit delusions and/or hallucinations as a postictal phenomenon, although this has rarely been reported in children (6). In these cases, the hallucinations and delusions occur following one or a cluster of seizures. These patients are often confused and subsequently amnestic for events that occur during the seizure episode and postictal period (7,8). Seizures arising from the temporal lobe are most often associated with the development of postictal psychosis, but postictal psychosis has also been reported in association with frontal lobe seizures (9).

In this case, postictal psychosis is unlikely because there was no known change in the patient's seizure frequency prior to the onset of the symptoms, and she had very good recollection of the hallucinations. In addition, her cognition and consciousness were not impaired even during her hallucinations.

Likewise, as there was no reduction in her seizure frequency prior to the onset of these symptoms, forced normalization is not a likely explanation.

2. Psychiatric side effects of anticonvulsants. Some antiepileptic drugs (AEDs) cause psychiatric side effects, including psychosis (Table 19.1). In most cases of medication-induced neurocognitive and psychiatric reactions, the problems occur within a short time after the initiation of the AED. These adverse reactions occur with the newer AEDs as well as those that have been in long-term use. In this patient, as there was no recent change in the AED regimen, AED side effects are not a likely explanation of her symptoms.

TABLE 19.1 ANTIEPILEPTIC DRUGS AND THEIR PSYCHIATRIC SIDE EFFECTS

AED	PSYCHIATRIC SIDE EFFECTS
Levetiracetam	Behavioral symptoms including agitation, anxiety, apathy, depersonalization, depression, emotional lability, hostility, hyperkinesias, nervousness, neurosis, personality disorder, psychosis
Lamotrigine	Infrequent reports of depersonalization, hallucinations, hostility, hyperkinesias, mind racing, panic attacks, paranoia, personality disorder, psychosis, suicidal ideation
Zonisamide	Depression and psychosis, psychomotor slowing, difficulty with concentration, speech and language problems/word finding difficulties
Topiramate	Depression, mood problems, suicidal ideation, psychomotor slowing, difficulty with concentration/attention, speech and language problems/word finding difficulties
Carbamazepine	Visual hallucinations, confusion, depression with agitation
Oxcarbazepine	Psychomotor slowing, difficulty with concentration, speech or language difficulties
Phenytoin	Nervousness
Phenobarbital	Sedation, excitement, depression
Valproate	Depression, psychosis, aggression, hyperactivity, hostility, behavioral deterioration
Pregabalin	Anxiety, depersonalization, infrequent hallucinations, hostility, rare delusions, mania, paranoia, psychosis
Gabapentin	Infrequent hallucination, agitation, paranoia, suicidal ideation, psychosis
Felbamate	Agitation, aggression, infrequent hallucinations, suicidality
Tiagabine	Impaired concentration, confusion, speech and language problems

Data from *Physicians Desk Reference*. Montvale, NJ: Thompson; 2008.

Audrey Walker M.D. (Associate Clinical Professor of Psychiatry and Pediatrics, Albert Einstein College of Medicine; Director of Training, Child and Adolescent Psychiatry, Albert Einstein College of Medicine; Director of Child and Adolescent Psychiatry, Montefiore Medical Center)

This case presents a problem familiar to neurologists and psychiatrists who treat children and adolescents with epilepsy: the onset of mental status changes and altered behavior that involves perceptual disturbances, emotional activation, and functional and vegetative deterioration. These symptoms are seen in a number of psychiatric disorders that have their onset in childhood and adolescence as well as in complex partial seizures (CPS) and AED side effects (see previous). The ability to differentiate (a) the onset of a new psychiatric disorder in an epileptic adolescent from (b) the onset of PCS in an adolescent with epilepsy is further complicated by the fact that, like seizures, some psychiatric disorders have an episodic course.

Does epilepsy predispose to psychiatric problems? If so, does the chronicity of epilepsy and its psychosocial impact cause psychiatric comorbidity, much as would complicate other life-altering chronic illnesses? One of the problems in analyzing this case is the paucity of data on children and adolescents with epilepsy. If one considers only studies with children and adolescents, the data is scant. Yet, to extrapolate from the adult literature to children and adolescents has many pitfalls. The psychiatric diagnostic possibilities are different in children and adolescents compared with adults. The child's developing brain leads to variation in the expression of psychiatric symptoms compared to adults. In addition, adults with epilepsy who present for psychiatric assessment usually have had a longer duration of illness than children with epilepsy and thus have had more time to accumulate the psychosocial distress and psychiatric comorbidity associated with the disease. Given all these considerations, in this discussion, reference to the adult literature will be made only when there is a paucity of data pertaining to the child and adolescent population.

Several studies have demonstrated that children and adolescents with epilepsy have greater psychopathology compared to children with other chronic diseases (11,12). The prevalence of psychiatric comorbidity in children and adolescents with epilepsy was recently examined in a large population-based retrospective study (13). In this study of newly diagnosed cases of epilepsy, the prevalence of psychiatric comorbidities in patients 16 years of age or younger was 51%. When patients with mental retardation and pervasive developmental disorder (PDD) were eliminated from the group, the prevalence of psychiatric disorders was 40.4%. The most common psychiatric disorders in these children were attention deficit hyperactivity disorder (ADHD) (17%), and mood and adjustment disorders (10%). No cases of psychotic disorder were identified in this study. It is important to note, however, that as these children were newly diagnosed, the burden of coping with a chronic illness during development would not yet have delivered its full impact. A recent meta-analysis of 46 studies including 2,434 children with epilepsy (14) found that children with epilepsy were at increased risk for psychopathology, including internalizing and externalizing behavior problems compared with healthy controls and children with chronic diseases that did not involve the central nervous system. In these children with epilepsy, somatic complaints and attention problems were the most common symptoms. Although valuable, a weakness of this study is that the length of time from epilepsy diagnosis to assessment inevitably varies among the 46 studies culled, thereby conferring a nonuniform effect of the duration of chronic illness and its contribution to the development of secondary psychopathology. Overall, these more recent findings are in line with Rutter's Isle of Wight Study (15) that examined the entire child population of the Isle of Wight and found that the rate of psychiatric comorbidity for children with epilepsy to be 34.3%. Of note, in the Isle of Wight study, there were no cases of psychosis identified in children with epilepsy.

The differential diagnosis of the acute onset of psychotic symptoms in a teenager with epilepsy also includes schizophreniform disorder, anxiety and affective disorders, conversion disorder, and substance abuse disorder. In this case, the presence of severe anxiety, depressed mood, and alteration in vegetative functioning helps to narrow the diagnostic focus.

1. Schizophreniform disorder. A population-based cohort study (16) examined the risk of schizophrenia or schizophrenia-like psychosis in individuals ages 15 and older with epilepsy and concluded that a history of epilepsy was associated with an increased risk of schizophrenia or schizophrenia-like psychosis. People with epilepsy had almost 2.5 times the risk of schizophrenia and 3 times the risk of schizophrenia-like psychosis compared to the general population. All types of epilepsy significantly increased the risk of developing schizophrenia or schizophrenia-like psychosis. In this study, an association was found between the development of schizophrenia-like psychosis in patients with epilepsy and a family history of schizophrenia.

   In a retrospective study, the prevalence of interictal psychosis in patients with epilepsy was 4.7% (17) with a correlation between epilepsy originating in the temporal lobes and interictal psychosis. Caplan et al. (18) reported that 10% of children with complex partial seizures had interictal schizophrenia-like psychosis.

Several features of the history and diagnostic workup are helpful in determining whether this patient is presenting with a new seizure manifestation or a schizophreniform disorder:

1. Preexisting epilepsy diagnosis. When a patient with a history of epilepsy presents with new onset of psychotic symptoms, the clinician must consider that the new symptoms are related to the past history of seizures
2. Premorbid psychological signs and symptoms. Patients who later are diagnosed with schizophreniform disorder are more likely to present with a history of abnormal premorbid suspiciousness and poor peer relationships than patients with new onset seizures.
3. A family history of schizophrenia-spectrum disorders. This is more common in those patients who are later diagnosed with schizophreniform disorder than in patients later determined to have ictal psychosis (19).
4. Onset. The psychosis seen in seizures is typically more abrupt in onset than that seen in schizophreniform disorder.
5. Age of onset. Schizophreniform disorder is rare prior to mid-adolescence. The incidence of schizophreniform disorder peaks for men in the late twenties and even later for women.
6. Mental status examination. Patients with ictal or postictal psychotic symptoms are more likely to have appropriate affect and intact reality testing than patients with schizophreniform disorder. Visual hallucinations are more common in ictal psychosis compared with schizophreniform disorder in which auditory hallucinations and delusions are more commonly encountered (20,21). The patient also described an "out-of-body" experience (heard her own voice outside of herself), which has been associated with CPS of temporal origin (22).
7. Recovery and remission. Patients with ictal psychosis have good recovery and return to premorbid level of function compared with patients with schizophreniform disorder.

In this 14-year-old adolescent girl with a history of epilepsy, an acute onset of psychotic symptoms followed a high level of academic, social, and psychological functioning. There was no family history of schizophrenia-spectrum disorders. Her mental status examination was characterized by appropriate affect, preserved reality testing (e.g., she said that she thought she was "going crazy"), and visual hallucinations that were well formed and frequently accompanied by less frequent auditory hallucinations that were much less well formed, as well as an out-of body experience These features of the presentation indicate that physicians should consider an organic etiology of new-onset seizures as a more likely diagnosis than a schizophreniform presentation.

2. Anxiety, depression, and bipolar disorders. Anxiety and mood disorders are amongst the most common psychiatric comorbidity in children with epilepsy (14,23–25). Using a structured psychiatric interview format, Caplan et al. (23) studied 100 children aged 5 to 16 years with complex partial seizures and found that 33% had affective and anxiety diagnoses, with most children having anxiety disorder (63%) or comorbid affective/anxiety and disruptive disorders. (26.1%) Only 5.2% had depression alone as a diagnosis. These values are significantly greater than in normal subjects.

The relationship between bipolar disorder and epilepsy, particularly in children and adolescents, has been insufficiently studied. Plioplys et al. (26) noted that those studies that used structured psychiatric interviews in children with epilepsy did not find any cases of bipolar disorder. In the adult literature, although anxiety, mood, and affective disturbances are common, manic episodes are rarely reported. However, in a recent study, Ettinger et al. (27) found that bipolar symptoms were 1.6 to 2.2 times more common in adults with epilepsy than in adults with other chronic diseases and 6.6 times more common than in the healthy comparison group.

In this patient's presentation, several features guide the clinician in identifying whether the patient suffers from a comorbid anxiety or affective disorder rather than or in addition to an ictal or postictal phenomenon.

1. Family history. Children with epilepsy who later develop depressive or bipolar disorders have been found to have a significantly higher rate of positive family history for affective disorders than children with epilepsy who do not develop affective disorders (28,29).
2. Premorbid psychological signs and symptoms. Dunn et al. (24) found that in children with epilepsy, premorbid adjustment predicted the later development of depressive disorders. Specifically, a youth's negative attitude toward having epilepsy was found to be associated with the subsequent development of depressive disorders in adolescence.
3. Age of onset. Children with epilepsy who develop depressive disorders tend to develop them in adolescence or later compared with the development of other common psychiatric comorbidities seen in children with epilepsy, such as ADHD (28).
4. Course. The onset of seizures is acute. In contrast, affective and anxiety disorders tend to evolve over the course of weeks or more.
5. Response to treatment. Ictal symptoms of anxiety and depression would not be responsive to antidepressant medications. In contrast, interictal depressive disorders are responsive to selective serotonin reuptake inhibitors (SSRIs) (30).
6. Neurological examination. The neurological examination will not usually aid in clarifying the differential diagnosis because many patients with epilepsy, as well as those with an affective or anxiety disorder, have a normal interictal neurological examination.

This pubertal girl's presentation includes depressed mood, insomnia, social withdrawal, school refusal, and severe anxiety. It was heralded by the onset of auditory and visual hallucinations. However, this patient had no family history of affective disorders and her adjustment to her epilepsy diagnosis had been excellent. She had a history of compliance with AEDs and her seizure disorder had been stable prior to the onset of her hallucinations. There had been no recent change in the AED regimen. Her symptoms had an abrupt onset and visual hallucinations dominated the clinical picture. Based on these considerations, the index of suspicion for a new affective or anxiety disorder falls and suspicion for a new seizure presentation rises.

3. Conversion disorder. Conversion nonepileptic seizures (NES) are episodes of altered movements, sensations, or experiences that are similar to epileptic seizures but without associated abnormal brain discharges on electroencephalogram (EEG). Underlying psychological processes are considered to be causative factors in the production of conversion NES.

Conversion NES and epilepsy frequently occur concomitantly. The prevalence of conversion NES in adults with epilepsy is high, with estimates ranging between 9% to 50% of patients referred to epilepsy centers (31). Although there were few studies in this population, it had been thought in the past that the risk of conversion NES in children and adolescents with epilepsy was lower than in adults, Recently, Kotagal et al. (32) found that 15.2% of children and adolescents with epilepsy had co-occurring conversion NES. Vincentiis et al. (33) prospectively studied children ages 4 to 18 in an ambulatory epilepsy clinic and found a prevalence of 30.4% of these patients had conversion NES co-occurring with their epilepsy. This unusually high number is not representative of the general epilepsy population, as these children were attending a clinic specialized for epileptic children with psychiatric issues. Nevertheless, these studies strongly suggest that the prevalence of conversion NES in children and adolescents with epilepsy is higher than previously believed.

In this patient's presentation, aspects of the history and clinical examination are helpful in differentiating new epileptic presentation from the onset of conversion NES.

1. The patient and family denied any history of recent stressful events that may have caused anxiety and emotional distress that conversion symptoms are presumed to alleviate
2. Past history of physical or sexual abuse has been found to be much more common in patients with conversion NES compared with patients with epilepsy (34). An extensive history was taken and no evidence for physical or sexual abuse was identified in this presentation.
3. The presence of a model in the child's immediate environment can be important in the onset of new episodic events; however, when a child already has epilepsy, the semiology of the pre-existing seizure can serve as a model for a conversion NES. Notably, these recent episodes reported by the patient are quite different clinically from her original presentation of seizures several years ago.
4. Dissociative symptoms. Recent work suggests that dissociative symptoms are more common in patients with conversion NES than epilepsy (34,35). However, dissociative symptoms have been found to be more common in complex partial seizures than in other forms of seizure disorder (36,37). The Dissociative Experiences Scale (DES) (38) is a valid and reliable instrument for the screening of dissociative symptoms that is included as a standard part of the clinical assessment of all pediatric patients at the Children's Hospital at Montefiore in whom Conversion NES are being considered.
5. Clinical features of the episodes. Several symptoms common in conversion NES are uncommon in epilepsy: crying, screaming, cursing, combativeness, slow evolution of the episode, long duration of the episode, as well as extinction of the episode when the patient believes he is unobserved.

    Symptoms that are common in epilepsy but uncommon in conversion NES include: confusion after the episode, incontinence, tongue biting, and other types of self-injury. The clinician must regard these guidelines with caution as conversion NES can imitate many aspects of true epileptic seizures. In addition, certain seizure types, such as frontal lobe complex partial seizures, include atypical clinical features, such as agitation, vocalizations including screaming, motor behaviors including kicking, and forced running. These seizure manifestations can be confused with behavioral episodes.

6. Serum prolactin (PRL) measurement. Measurement of serum PRL can be used to aid in the differentiation of epileptic seizures from NES. Serum PRL levels concentration is elevated 10 to 20 minutes after a generalized tonic clonic seizure or partial complex seizures but not in Conversion NES. Chen et al. (39) concluded that a serum PRL assay is probably a useful adjunct for differentiating generalized tonic clonic seizures or CPS from NES, particularly when video EEG monitoring is not immediately available.
7. EEG results. A normal interictal EEG does not rule out the possibility that an event is a seizure. Nor would it confirm the diagnosis of NES. In roughly 50% of patients with CPS, the interictal EEG is normal (40).
8. Video EEG monitoring. Video EEG monitoring is currently considered to be the "gold standard" for the definitive differentiation of NES from epileptic events (41).
9. Failure to respond to AEDs. In the adult population, NES is the reason for 20% to 30% of cases of AED failure. It is suspected that similar statistics apply to the pediatric population (42). NES should be suspected in patients who present with episodic events that are considered to be seizures but are refractory to AEDs.

4. Substance abuse disorder. Studies on the prevalence of substance abuse in children and adolescents with epilepsy are lacking. In this case, the index of suspicion for a substance abuse disorder is low. The patient had an excellent level of functioning in the home and school setting. She had maintained excellent academic level, was well connected to her peers, and had a stable, attached relationship with her parents. There was no report of a change in her emotional or behavioral status. Urine and serum toxicology screens were both negative, except for benzodiazepines, which she was taking for seizure control. However, many substances of abuse can present with psychotic symptoms.

Substances of Abuse Associated with Psychosis (43)

1. Associated with abuse
   Substances Associated with Psychosis

   - Alcohol
   - Amphetamines
   - Anabolic steroids
   - Cannabis
   - Hallucinogens, including lysergic acid (LSD), mescaline (peyote) 3,4-methylenedioxymethamphetamine (MDMA, ecstasy), phencyclidine (PCP)
   - Inhalants
   - Ketamine
   - Meperidine

2. Substances, when withdrawn, associated with psychosis

   - Alcohol
   - Barbiturates
   - Benzodiazepines

Urine drug tests are typically ordered to detect recent use of illegal substances. At the Children's Hospital at Montefiore, the urine toxicology assay screens for the following substances: amphetamines, barbiturates, benzodiazepines, cannabinoids, cocaine, opiates, methadone, phencyclidine, and oxycodone. Although these assays are useful, the clinician must recognize their limitations. For example, ecstasy may not be detected in a routine urine toxicology screen even though amphetamines are part of the routine set of substances assayed. When a serum toxicology screen is ordered, the substance of concern must be specified. Thresholds that must be exceeded to produce a positive assay differ amongst different institutions. In addition, the creatinine value must be consulted to determine whether the possibility of diluted urine, excessive water ingestion prior to sample collection, or otherwise adulterated specimen should be considered. The clinician must be familiar with the length of time that a specific drug of abuse remains in the body after ingestion. For example, cocaine and its metabolites may be detected for up to 3 days after use, whereas marijuana, when use is chronic, can be detected for as long as one month.

HOSPITAL COURSE

The patient was admitted to the epilepsy monitoring unit.

Dr. Ballaban-Gil

Video-EEG monitoring was performed. The baseline EEG was abnormal with nearly continuous rhythmic and polymorphic theta activity in the left temporal region, as well as focal spikes in the left temporal region. During the monitoring, she experienced many of her typical hallucinations, including both visual and auditory ones. All her hallucinations were associated with rhythmic theta (4 to 4.5 Hz) activity in the left temporal region. Similar rhythmic theta activity was also present interictally. In addition, over a 6-day period she had 18 convulsions (complex partial seizures with secondary generalization), whose onset was electrically nonlocalizable.

A positron emission tomography (PET) scan, performed during the hospitalization, showed moderately decreased metabolism involving the left temporal lobe, most marked in the mesial aspect.

Dr. Walker

During the course of her admission to the epilepsy monitoring unit, the patient had a full psychiatric evaluation. Her mother confirmed the history that the patient had been academically successful until the onset of her symptoms and that she had excellent relationships with her family and peers. She denied any changes in the family constellation during the premorbid period. The patient had adapted well to her epilepsy diagnosis and had been compliant with AED regimen in the past. The patient was a cooperative, friendly young adolescent girl who had a broad range of affect appropriate to content. She was not experiencing auditory or visual hallucinations during the psychiatric interview but was able to describe them. She denied any symptoms of dissociation, and this history was confirmed with the DES scale, which showed minimal dissociative symptoms.

Dr. Ballaban-Gil

Because of the flurry of seizures, the patient was treated with intravenous (IV) fosphenytoin and then started on levetiracetam, which was rapidly titrated up to a dose of 1,500 mg per day. After attaining that dosage, all symptoms resolved, including the hallucinations and the convulsive seizures. The presence of the rhythmic activity associated with the hallucinations suggests an ictal etiology; however, because this same EEG discharge was present without associated clinical symptoms, this relationship is not definitive. Alternatively, given the frequency of her seizures (18 over 6 days), these symptoms could be a postictal phenomenon. The resolution of the episodes following the addition of a new AED confirms the ictal or postictal etiology of the events.

CLINICAL DIAGNOSIS

The final diagnosis in this patient is either simple partial seizures of left temporal origin or postictal phenomenon.

Case 2: A 13-Year-Old Girl with Amnesia after a Fall

PRESENTATION OF CASE

Ngoc Nguyen, M.D. (Pediatric psychosomatic fellow, Montefiore Medical Center/Albert Einstein College of Medicine)

A 13-year-old girl was brought to the emergency department at the Children's Hospital at Montefiore because of amnesia after a fall.

The patient had been in her usual state of good health until the day of admission when, according to her family, she went to the bathroom and slipped on water. Her sister noted after several minutes that the patient had not returned, went to look for her, and discovered her unresponsive on the floor of the bathroom. Her sister began to shake the patient in order to arouse her. She estimated that approximately 15 minutes elapsed between the time the patient left the room and the time she began to regain consciousness. As the patient regained consciousness, she was disoriented to person, place, and time. Although sleepy, she was able to speak and complained of lightheadedness, left temporal headache, and pain in her left arm. There was no evidence of incontinence or abnormal movements according to the family.

The patient's parents bought her to the emergency room (ER) by car. On arrival in the ER, the patient's VS were BP 139/80 mm Hg; P 82 beats per minute, regular; RR 22 breaths per minute; T +97.3°F, orally. She was noted to have a bruise over the left temporal region. Cardiac and pulmonary examinations were without abnormalities.

On mental status examination she was cooperative and alert but disoriented to person, place, and time. Attention was noted to be poor. Speech was monotonous and high-pitched. She seemed to have lost comprehension and expression in Spanish, and her use of English was unsophisticated for her age and her reported premorbid ability. (Her family reported that the patient had learned both Spanish and English since infancy.) Affect was constricted.

As previously noted, the patient had significant retrograde amnesia including loss of autobiographical information. She had no anterograde amnesia. The patient was hypersomnolent.

Neurological examination was otherwise normal. There were no focal neurological deficits. Gait and station, deep tendon reflexes, and cerebellar, motor, and sensory examinations were normal.

Further history was obtained. The patient was born in the United States. She was described as an "A" student with many friends.

Medical history is significant for Raynaud disease.

Psychiatric history is significant for self-cutting behavior and mood lability 1 year prior to the present admission. She also has a history of physical abuse in the past as well as a history of sexual abuse by an older male cousin in the year prior to the presenting complaints. She had no prior history of psychiatric assessment or treatment for these problems.

The family reported no evidence for ingestions of medicines or alcohol that day. There is no known history of substance abuse. On the day of admission, the patient had gone to a horror film with her sister and friends, after which she vomited in the movie theatre bathroom and said to her companions "Don't ever take me to anything like that again!"

On admission to the ER, laboratory tests were performed: urine/serum toxicology were negative, a serum pregnancy test was negative, and CBC and blood chemistries were also normal. Noncontrast head computed tomography (CT) and noncontrast MRI of the brain were normal.

The patient was observed in the ER for 24 hours. During this time, she remained amnestic to person, place, and time and did not recognize relatives and friends. She also seemed to have lost certain skills, such as the ability to brush her hair or bathe. She retained the ability to toilet herself. Personality changes were also noted: She was withdrawn and childlike, in stark contrast to her previous demeanor, which was described by her family as "outspoken" and "rebellious."

After 24 hours of observation, the patient was discharged for outpatient follow-up.

DIFFERENTIAL DIAGNOSIS

Acute onset of amnesia after head trauma

Karen Ballaban-Gil

1. Traumatic brain injury (TBI). Retrograde amnesia is the inability to remember prior events despite a normal level of consciousness. The most common cause of transient amnesia is acute head trauma with concussion. Usually, head trauma results in transient retrograde and anterograde amnesia. Typically, the extent of the amnesia roughly correlates with the duration of the loss of consciousness and patients who experience concussion with sustained loss of consciousness remain more neurocognitively impaired in the short term (<48 hours) but nearly all patients have full recovery of memory within a few days of the injury (44). Patients with posttraumatic amnesia have preserved autobiographical memories, such as remembering their name or date of birth (45).

    In this case, the history of apparent head trauma with loss of consciousness, substantiated by physical signs of trauma (bruising, etc.) makes this the most likely diagnosis. However, the loss of autobiographical information is atypical.

2. Seizure. Seizures can also result in retrograde amnesia, primarily during the postictal period. Seizures occur as a sequela in 6% of mild and 35 % of severe TBI in children (46). The postictal amnesia that results is typically brief.

    Pure amnestic seizures have been reported in patients with temporal lobe seizures. The only clinical manifestation of these seizures is the patient's inability to remember what occurs during the seizure, without loss of other cognitive functions. During these seizures, the individual is able to interact normally with their physical and social environment (47). These patients always have seizures with other semiologies, as well. As this patient has no history of seizures, this is an unlikely etiology of her current amnestic state.

3. Transient global amnesia (TGA). TGA can be seen in patients with migraine or vascular disease. In TGA, there is profound disturbance of short-term memory with preservation of immediate recall and long-term memory. Memory recovers spontaneously, usually within a few hours (48). The etiology of TGA is not certain, but may be caused by transient ischemia to the medial temporal lobes, which are supplied by branches of the vertebrobasilar system. Pediatric cases of TGA are extremely rare. It most often occurs in patients older than 50 years, as a result of vascular disease, but can occur with migraine headaches, particularly basilar migraine. The age of our patient and the loss of long-term memory in this case are inconsistent with this diagnosis.
4. Delirium. Delirium is an acute disturbance in level of consciousness, attention and focus, and cognition. The cognitive changes may include memory deficits, disorientation and language disturbance. Delirium develops over a period of hours to days and tends to fluctuate. Delirium may be caused by ingestion of medications and illicit drugs, including benzodiazepines, narcotics, amphetamines, antipsychotics, antidepressants, and alcohol. Anticholinergic medications such as antihistamines may also cause delirium. Sudden withdrawal from alcohol, benzodiazepines and barbiturates in long-term users can also result in delirium. Electrolyte abnormalities and infectious etiologies, including encephalitis or meningitis can result in delirium, as well. This patient did have changes in language function and drowsiness (i.e., depressed level of consciousness), so delirium must be considered. Appropriate laboratory investigations ruled out exposure to many substances, making this less likely, but still a possible diagnosis. Infectious etiology is unlikely in the absence of fever and other signs of systemic illness.

Audrey Walker M.D. and Ngoc Nguyen M.D.

N.N.

The most prominent feature of this case is the sudden onset of severe retrograde amnesia and disturbance of language function after head trauma. This history is significant also for the presence of sexual abuse by a male cousin in the year prior to the current presenting complaints and a past history of physical abuse. The patient had a history significant for mood lability and self-cutting behaviors in the year prior to presentation.

A.W.

Amnesia or memory loss is common following physical, chemical or emotional insults to the brain. Given the neurological and psychiatric signs and symptoms in the presentation, a number of possible etiologies must be considered.

1. Dissociate amnesia/conversion disorder. Dissociation is a disruption of the usually integrated functions of consciousness, memory, identity, or perception of the environment (49). Conversion disorder is an illness consisting of symptoms or deficits that effect voluntary motor or sensory functions, which suggest another medical condition, but that is judged to be due to psychological factors because the illness is preceded by conflicts or other stressors (50). The concepts of conversion and dissociation are based on the same psychological mechanism and can be traced back to the 19th century conceptualizations by Janet and Freud of hysterical neurosis. Both are understood

to be psychological defenses that allow painful affects and memories to be banished from conscious awareness. In *Diagnostic and Statistical Manual of Mental Disorders, 4th edition* (DSM IV), dissociative disorders and conversion disorders are classified separately. Both patients with dissociative disorders as well as patients with conversion disorders have high incidences of physical and sexual abuse histories compared with patients with other psychiatric disorders such as affective disorders, as well as compared with normal controls (51,52). Recent studies have demonstrated high degrees of conversion symptoms in patients with dissociative disorders (53) and that dissociation is very common in patients with conversion disorders (37,54). Based on this recent data as well as the historical and theoretical linkages between the two diagnoses, dissociative disorders and conversion disorder are considered together in the discussion of this patient's presentation.

Dissociative amnesia is characterized in *Diagnostic and Statistical Manual of Mental Disorders, 4th edition, text revision* (DSM IV TR) as an "inability to recall important personal information, usually of a traumatic nature, that is too extensive to be explained by ordinary forgetfulness" (49). This reversible memory impairment most commonly presents as a retrograde amnesia, particularly effecting aspects of personal history. General medical and neurological causes of amnesia, such as the effects of substance abuse, medications, or head trauma, must be ruled out for the diagnosis of dissociative amnesia to be made.

Dissociative amnesia is typically a transient amnesia that is more common in females. Yudofsky and Hales (55) has proposed guidelines for distinguishing dissociative amnesia from the memory loss accompanying neurological disease:

1. Type of amnesia. In dissociative amnesia, anterograde amnesia rarely occurs. In the amnesia that accompanies neurological disorders, both retrograde and anterograde amnesia is present.
2. Content of memory lost. In dissociative amnesia, details of personal identity and history are lost. By contrast, the amnesia that accompanies neurological disorders typically spares details of the personal history, identity, and early life events.
3. Indifference. In dissociative amnesia, the patient may show indifference to the deficit in contrast to the amnesia following neurological insult, where the patient is typically concerned.
4. Course of recovery. In dissociative amnesia, return of lost memory may be sudden, in contrast to the course of recovery after neurological insult, which follows a more stereotypical course in which more distant memories are recovered first, with memory for recent events returning later.

2. Substance or alcohol-induced amnesia

Ngoc Nguyen M.D.

A number of substances of abuse as well as alcohol can hamper memory function. Alcohol and benzodiazepines are sedative/hypnotics known to affect the brain's ability to lay down new memories (56). Most sedative-hypnotics, when used in high doses, encumber concentration and attention, the precursors of memory formation. The anterograde amnesia that results from excessive use of sedative/hypnotics is transient and resolves once the substance is eliminated.

In long-term alcohol abuse, Korsakoff syndrome may develop due to chronic thiamine deficiency. This amnestic syndrome is seen after many years of chronic alcohol use and is characterized by intact immediate recall but poor performance with time elapsed. The retrograde amnesia seen in Korsakoff's includes gaps in both recent and remote memory, which the patient may attempt to disguise with confabulation.

A.W.

There are a number of drugs of abuse that can cause amnesia including methylene dioxymethamphetamine (MDMA, Ecstasy), gamma hydroxybutyrate (GHB, G, Liquid Ecstasy), ketamine, and phencyclidine (PCP, Angel Dust). They are not routinely included in the urine and serum drugs screens and infrequent use may result in false negative screens due to nondetectable levels. Immunoassay assessment followed by gas chromatography or high-performance liquid chromatography is usually required to accurately establish the presence of these substances (57).

The index for suspicion for substance or alcohol abuse in this patient is low. There was no history of past use of drugs or alcohol. The patient's function at school and with her peers had not changed in the period prior to the current presentation. The possibility of an inadvertent ingestion exists. However, as the vital signs were stable throughout the described course and urine and serum toxicology screens were negative, this is an unlikely explanation for her profound retrograde amnesia.

CLINICAL COURSE

NN

The patient was observed in the ER for 24 hours. Her physical examination including vital signs remained unremarkable. The neurological examination was normal with the exception of persistent profound retrograde amnesia that included loss of autobiographical information. An EEG was performed, which was normal. The patient was discharged to outpatient follow-up with a presumed psychiatric etiology to her persistent retrograde amnesia.

Additional history was obtained during the outpatient psychiatric evaluation. The patient had engaged in superficial self-cutting of her arms during the year prior to the onset of the current presentation. During the same time period, she had become, at the age of 12 years, involved in a sexual relationship with an 18-year-old male cousin. This relationship had recently been terminated when the cousin decided to marry his pregnant girlfriend. The patient was described by her mother, who had only recently learned of this relationship, as "distraught" over the breakup.

Earlier on the day on which the patient presented to the ER, she had accompanied her sister and some friends to a movie. This movie was a violent one. The plot consisted of a group of friends who were lured into sexual exploitation and then serially murdered. Many of the scenes were sadistic and graphic. The patient became distraught and vomited in the bathroom of the theatre. Several hours later, the patient was found by her sister unconscious on the bathroom floor in her home.

Although the patient had only mild scalp contusions and the unremarkable emergency room course described previously, she had persistent retrograde amnesia for the first 3 months of psychiatric treatment. Most remarkable was the loss of memory for her own identity. In addition, her affect appeared depressed, she was frequently tearful and hypersomnolent. She continued to speak in a high-pitched, monotonous tone of voice.

The initial treatment aimed to engage the patient in a supportive psychotherapy. Eventually, the therapeutic approach included connecting affect to feelings. After 3½ months of weekly treatment, the patient began to rapidly regain her memory, beginning with the retrieval of autobiographical memory and memory of family members. The amnesia persisted only for the 3-hour time span spent at the movies on the day of admission.

CLINICAL DIAGNOSIS

Mild Traumatic Brain Injury followed by Dissociative Amnesia

Conclusion

The two cases presented in this section utilize an interdisciplinary approach to neuropsychiatric presentations in childhood and adolescence. This approach involves real-time collaboration between the pediatric neurologist and the child and adolescent psychiatrist. We emphasize the importance of obtaining a thorough, detailed description of neurological and psychiatric symptoms, a complete family history, and a comprehensive neurological and psychiatric examination that includes a detailed mental status examination. As these cases illustrate, the same neuropsychiatric symptoms can be observed in a number of neurological and psychiatric disorders and only the well-informed collaboration between the neurologist and psychiatrist will result in the timely identification and successful treatment of these complicated patients.

REFERENCES

1. Clemens B. Forced normalization precipitated by lamotrigine. *Seizure.* 2005;14:485–489.
2. Krishnamoorthy ES, Trimble MR, Kanner AM. Forced normalization at the interface between epilepsy and psychiatry. *Epilepsy Behav.* 2002;3:303–308.
3. Panayiotopoulos CP. Occipital lobe epilepsies. In: *A Clinical guide to Epileptic Syndromes and Their Treatment.* 2nd ed. London: Springer-Verlag; 2007:413–434.
4. La Vega-Talbot M, Duchowny M, Jayakar P. Orbitofrontal seizures presenting with ictal visual hallucinations and interictal psychosis. *Pediatr Neurol.* 2006;35:78–81.
5. Fornazzari L, et al. Violent visual hallucinations and aggression in frontal lobe dysfunction: clinical manifestations of deep orbitofrontal foci. *J Neuropsychiatry.* 1992;4:42–44.
6. Nissenkorn A, et al. Postictal psychosis in a child. *J Child Neurol.* 1999;14:818–819.
7. Logsdail S, Toone BK. Post-ictal psychosis: a clinical and phenomenological description. *Br J Psychiatry.* 1988;152:246–252.
8. Savard G, et al. Postictal psychosis after partial complex seizures: a multiple case study. *Epilepsia.* 1991;32:225–231.
9. Adachi N, et al. Inter-ictal and post-ictal psychosis in frontal lobe epilepsy: a retrospective comparison with psychosis in temporal lobe epilepsy. *Seizure.* 2000;9:328–335.
10. *Physicians Desk Reference.* Montvale, NJ: Thompson; 2008.
11. Austin J, et al. Childhood epilepsy and asthma: comparison of quality of life. *Epilepsia.* 1994;35:608–615.
12. Hoare P. The development of psychiatric disorders among schoolchildren with epilepsy. *Dev Med Child Neurol.* 1984;26:3–13.
13. Hedderick F, Buchhalter JR. Comorbidity of childhood-onset epilepsy and psychiatric and behavioral disorders: a population-based study. *Ann Neurol.* 2005;54(suppl): S115.
14. Rodenberg R, et al. Psychopathology in children with epilepsy: a meta-analysis. *J Pediatr Psychol.* 2005;30:453–468.
15. Rutter MG, Yule W. *A Neuropsychiatric Study in Childhood.* Philadelphia: Lippincott, Williams & Wilkins; 1970.
16. Qin P, et al. Risk for schizophrenia and schizophrenia-like psychosis among patients with epilepsy: population-based cohort study. *BMJ.* 2005;331:23–25.

17. Kanemoto K, Tsuji T, Kawasaki J. Reexamination of interictal psychoses based on DSM IV psychosis classification and international epilepsy classification. *Epilepsia.* 2001;42:98–103.
18. Caplan R, et al. Psychopathology in pediatric complex partial and primary generalized epilepsy. *Dev Med Child Neurol.* 1998;40:805–811.
19. Matsuura M, et al. A polydiagnostic and dimensional comparison of epileptic psychoses and schizophrenia spectrum disorders. *Schizophrenia Res.* 2004;69:189–201.
20. Ulloa RE, et al. Psychosis in pediatric mood and anxiety disorders clinic: phenomenology and correlates. *J Am Acad Child Adolesc Psychiatry.* 2000;39:337–345.
21. Caplan R. Thought disorder in childhood. *J Am Acad Child Adolesc Psychiatry.* 1994;33:605–615.
22. Blanke O, et al. Out-of-body experience and autoscopy of neurological origin. *Brain.* 2004;127:243–258.
23. Caplan R, et al. Depression and anxiety disorders in pediatric epilepsy. *Epilepsia.* 2005;46:720–730.
24. Dunn DW, Austin JK, Huster GA. Symptoms of depression in adolescents with epilepsy. *J Am Acad Child Adolesc Psychiatry.* 1999;38:1132–1145.
25. Hedderick R, Buchhalter JR. Comorbidity of childhood-onset epilepsy and psychiatric and behavioral disorders. *Ann Neurol.* 2003;54(S):S115.
26. Plioplys S, Dunn D, Caplan R. 10-year research update review: psychiatric problems in children with epilepsy. *J Am Acad Child and Adolesc Psychiatry.* 2007;46:1389–1402.
27. Ettinger A, et al. Prevalence of bipolar symptoms in epilepsy vs other chronic health disorders. *Neurology.* 2005;65:535–540.
28. Thome-Souza S, et. al. Which factors may play a pivotal role in determining the type of psychiatric disorder in children and adolescents with epilepsy? *Epilepsy Behav.* 2004;5:988–994.
29. Kudo T, et al. Manic episode in epilepsy and bipolar I disorder: a comparative analysis of 13 patients. *Epilepsia.* 2001;42:1036–1042.
30. Thome-Souza MS, Kuczynski E, Valente KD. Sertraline and fluoxetine: safe treatments for children and adolescents with epilepsy and depression. *Epilepsy Behav.* 2007;10:417–425.
31. Benbadis SR, Allen Hauser W. An estimate of the prevalence of psychogenic non-epileptic seizures. *Seizure.* 2000;9:280–281.
32. Kotagal P, et al. Paroxysmal non epileptic events in children and adolescents. *Pediatrics.* 2002;110:E46.
33. Vincentiis S, et al. Risk factors for psychogenic non epileptic seizures in children and adolescents with epilepsy. *Epilepsy Behav.* 2006;8:294–298.
34. Akyuz G, et al. Dissociation and childhood abuse history in epileptic and pseudoseizure patients. *Epileptic Disord.* 2004;6(3):187–192.
35. Prueter C, Schultz-Venrath V, Rimpau W. Dissociative and associated pathological symptoms in patients with epilepsy, pseudoseizures, and both seizure forms. *Epilepsia.* 2002;43:188–192.
36. Devinsky O, et al. Dissociative states and epilepsy. *Neurology.* 1989;39:835–840.
37. Alper K, et al. Dissociation in epilepsy and conversion nonepileptic seizures. *Epilepsia.* 1997;38:991–997.
38. Armstrong JG, et al. Development and validation of a measure of adolescent dissociation: the adolescent dissociative experiences scale. *J Nerv Mental Disorders.* 1997;185:491–497.
39. Chen DK, Yuen T, Fisher RS. Use of serum prolactin in diagnosing epileptic seizures. *Am Acad Neurol.* 2005;65:668–675.
40. Narayanan JT, Labar DR, Schaul N. Latency to first spike in the EEG of epilepsy patients. *Science.* 2008;17:34–41.
41. Reuber M, et al. Diagnostic delay in psychogenic non epileptic seizures. *Neurology.* 2002;58:493–495.
42. Andriola MR, Ettinger AB. Pseudoseizures and other non epileptic paroxysmal disorders in children and adolescents. *Neurology.* 1999;53:589–595.
43. Stern TA, et al. *Massachusetts General Hospital Handbook of General Hospital Psychiatry.* 5th ed. Philadelphia: Elsevier; 2004.
44. McCrea M, et al. Immediate neurocognitive effects of concussion. *Neurosurgery.* 2002;50:1032–1042.
45. Levin HS, et al. Impairment of remote memory after closed head injury. *J Neurol Neurosurg Psychiatry.* 1985;48:556–563.
46. Frey LC. Epidemiology of posttraumatic epilepsy: a critical review. *Epilepsia.* 2003;44(suppl 10):11–17.
47. Palmini AL, Gloor P, Jones-Gotman M. Pure amnestic seizures in temporal lobe epilepsy. Definition, clinical symptomatology and functional anatomical considerations. *Brain.* 1992;115:749–769.
48. Yamane K, et al. Basilar artery migraine associated with transient global amnesia. *J Neurol Neurosurg Psychiatry.* 1987;50:816–817.
49. American Psychiatric Association. *Diagnostic and Statistical Manual of Mental Disorders, 4th edition, text revision.* Washington DC: APA; 2000.
50. Sadock BJ, Sadock VA, eds. *Comprehensive Textbook of Psychiatry.* 8th ed. Philadelphia: Lippincott, Williams & Wilkins; 2005.
51. Atlas JA, Wolfson MA, Lipschitz DS. Dissociation and somatization in adolescent inpatients with and without history of abuse. *Psychol Rep.* 1995;76:1101–1102.
52. Sar V, et al. Childhood trauma, dissociation, and psychiatric comorbidity in patients with conversion disorder. *Am J Psychiatry.* 2004;161:2271–2276.
53. Maaranen P, et al. Factors associated with pathological dissociation in the general population. *Aust N Z J Psychiatry.* 2005;39:387–394.

54. Spitzer C, et al. Dissociative experiences and psychopathology in conversion disorders. *J Psychosomatic Res.* 1999;46:291–294.
55. Yudofsky SC, Hales RE, eds. *Essentials of Neuropsychiatry and Clinical Neurosciences.* Washington DC: American Psychiatric Publishing; 2004.
56. Curren HV. Tranquilising memories: a review of the effects of benzodiazepines on human memory. *Biol Psychiatry.* 1986;23(2):179–213.
57. Lowinson JH, Ruiz P, Millman RB, eds. *Substance Abuse: A Comprehensive Textbook.* 4th ed. Philadelphia: Lippincott Williams & Wilkins; 2005.

Glossary

accommodative esotropia eye convergence or "crossing," that occurs when individuals with hyperopia or "far-sightedness" attempt to fixate on near targets

acetylcholine a neurotransmitter; found at the neuromuscular junction [as well as certain central nervous system (CNS) synapses]

actigraphy method that uses an acceleration-sensitive device to measure activity levels that reflect sleep–awake states

acute disseminated encephalomyelitis (ADEM) a self-limited, monophasic, inflammatory immune-mediated disorder of the brain and spinal cord that often follows exanthematous or other infectious illnesses of childhood. Symptoms of that one event often mimic those of MS.

afferent directed from the periphery toward the central nervous system. Cf. efferent.

akathisia a sense of inner restlessness and the urge to move, manifest as uncontrollable motor restlessness, usually involving the legs primarily or exclusively

albuminocytologic dissociation the cerebrospinal fluid (CSF) profile in which the protein level is elevated but the cell count is low; characteristic of Guillain-Barré syndrome

amblyopia impaired or dim vision

American Sign Language (ASL) in the United States, the primary manual language recognized, with its own grammar and syntax. Countries may have their own distinct sign-language dialects.

anterior horn the area of the grey matter of the spinal cord that contains the cell bodies of lower motor neurons

anticipation a genetic characteristic in which the age at onset of a disease becomes progressively earlier in successive generations

antiretroviral drugs medications for the treatment of infection by retroviruses such as HIV; different classes act at different stages of the HIV life cycle.

applied behavior analysis (ABA) the design, implementation, and evaluation of environmental modifications to produce socially significant improvement in human behavior. ABA includes the use of direct observation, measurement, and functional analysis of the relations between environment and behavior. ABA uses antecedent stimuli and consequences, based on the findings of descriptive and functional analysis, to produce practical change (shapingbehavior.com). It is heavily dependent on the theories of operant conditioning. It does not refer to any specific application or implementation technique.

aprosodia a loss of the normal melodic intonation and cadence of speech, often caused by a nondominant-hemisphere lesion

Arnold–Chiari malformation anomalous development of the cervical spine and hindbrain such that the cerebellum herniates downward to varying degrees through the foramen magnum

ataxia lack of coordination; or a disorder with incoordination as a prominent feature

ataxic cerebral palsy nonprogressive motor dysfunction present from birth or beginning in early childhood, characterized by abnormalities in balance and position, precipitated by voluntary movement

attention-deficit hyperactivity disorder (ADHD) a common neuropsychiatric disorder with developmentally inappropriate levels of hyperactivity, impulsivity, and inattention

atonic (hypotonic) cerebral palsy nonprogressive motor dysfunction present from birth or beginning in early childhood, characterized by generalized muscular hypotonia that persists beyond age 2 to 3 years and is not secondary to disorder of muscle or peripheral nerve

auditory–verbal therapy in therapy of hard-of-hearing or deaf individuals, emphasis on using amplification of residual hearing and integrating sounds to learn to speak and lip-read

aura sensory or psychological symptom that is initial manifestation of some migraines or seizures

automatism during a seizure, the stereotyped, repetitive, purposeless behavior carried out in a state of impaired consciousness. Most often automatisms consist of chewing, lip smacking, or walking in a circle.

axonal neuropathy any disorder of nerves in which nerve fibers (axons) are disrupted

Babinski sign an abnormal response to stimulation of the plantar surface of the foot, characterized by extension of the great toes and fanning of the other toes. Although normal in an infant, it indicates CNS disease in an adult.

basal ganglia paired subcortical nuclei in the brain that are part of the extrapyramidal system and act to regulate movement; include the globus pallidi, caudate nuclei, and putamen

benign epilepsy syndromes varieties of epilepsy with childhood onset, associated with normal development, neurological examination, and brain MRI. These disorders carry a good prognosis for complete remission of seizures by late adolescence. The most common example is benign rolandic epilepsy.

bilingual–bicultural educational method of having two teachers, one hearing and one deaf, using the whole-language approach to build a solid foundation of ASL and written English skills

block designs a paradigm in which experimental conditions are separated into distinct sets, each of which is presented for an extended period

blood-oxygenation–level dependent (BOLD) imaging a functional magnetic resonance imaging technique that allows the imaging of active brain function based on the different magnetic properties of oxygenated and deoxygenated hemoglobin

bradykinesia slowness and loss of amplitude of spontaneous movement, classically associated with parkinsonism

bradyphrenia slowness of thought processes associated with parkinsonism

brainstem myoclonus myoclonus originating in the brainstem

bruxism unconsciously grinding one's teeth, often during sleep or periods of anxiety, but sometimes a stereotypie

cataracts a loss of transparency in the lens of the eye, resulting in impaired vision

CCTV-EEG continuous video-EEG monitoring system that records patients' clinical events and simultaneous EEG to document and classify seizures, correlate events with sleep–wake stages, localize epileptogenic foci, and document pseudoseizures

cerebral autosomal dominant arteriopathy (CADASIL) a genetically determined cerebrovascular disorder that causes migraine and stroke-like episodes. It is often included in the differential diagnosis of multiple sclerosis (MS) and hereditary stroke.

cerebral palsy abnormalities of muscle tone, movement, or posture resulting from a nonprogressive insult to the brain, occurring prenatally or in early childhood

cGy unit of radiation, previously called "rad"

channelopathies disorders, usually paroxysmal or episodic in nature, that have as their underlying pathological abnormality a defective ion channel

chemokines a small family of cytokines or proteins secreted by cells as chemical signals

chorea involuntary, continuous, abrupt, rapid, unsustained, irregular movements that flow randomly from one body part to another

clonus alternating contractions and relaxations of muscles produced by quick, forceful stretch of a muscle tendon about a joint. It is indicative of pyramidal tract, or upper motor neuron, dysfunction.

cochlear implant a surgically implanted electronic device within the cochlea that directly stimulates the auditory nerve and provides sound input to deaf or severely hard-of-hearing persons

comorbidity coexisting conditions, found on epidemiologic studies, without necessarily a causal relationship. For example, anxiety and depression are found commonly in migraine patients, but may or may not be the cause of migraines

complex motor tic an orchestrated sequence of simple motor tics or compulsive semipurposeful movements (touching, tapping, "evening up")

complex phonic tic compulsively uttered out-of-context syllables, words, phrases, or paroxysmal changes of prosody

conductive hearing loss type of hearing loss caused by failure of efficient conduction of sound waves through the outer ear, tympanic membrane, or middle ear ossicles

cones photoreceptor-type cells in the retina responsible for color vision

coprolalia a complex vocal tic consisting of out-of-context compulsive obscene, blasphemous, or otherwise socially inappropriate utterances

copropraxia complex motor tic consisting of compulsive, out-of-context, socially inappropriate or obscene gestures

cortical myoclonus myoclonus originating in the cortex; may evolve into a seizure

corticospinal tract the pathway containing the axons of upper motor neurons

cued speech a visual communication method that uses eight phonetic hand shapes in four different positions near the mouth to identify and distinguish the different speech sounds as a person speaks

cytokines a group of peptides or proteins that are used in organisms as signaling compounds. Similar to hormones and neurotransmitters, cytokines to allow cells to communicate with one another

Dandy Walker malformation cystic dilatation of the fourth ventricle, which shifts caudally and displaces cerebellar hemispheres, resulting in intermittent obstruction

Deaf capital "D" Deaf refers to the sociocultural group of people who grew up in the deaf world and consider themselves members of the "deaf community"

deaf lower case "d" deaf refers to the technical and medical diagnosis of hearing loss

delayed sleep-phase syndrome difficulty with both falling asleep and awakening at conventional times. Generally manifests as individuals routinely falling asleep in the early morning and awakening in the early afternoon

demyelinating neuropathy any disorder of nerves in which the myelin sheath is disrupted

diagnostic overshadowing erroneously attributing the symptoms of mental disorders to intellectual disability

diplopia double vision

disease-modifying therapies (DMTs) the principal approach to altering the course of MS, but not curing it. By blunting the immunological response, they decrease the frequency and severity of MS relapses and, to a lesser degree, lessen the accumulation of neurological impairments or disability

dorsal column a spinal-cord pathway carrying afferent information about sensory modalities, particularly vibration and joint position

dorsal stream projection from primary visual cortex toward parietal lobe structures that specializes in spatial perception and action planning

dysarthria disruption of the articulation of speech due to a pathological process within the CNS

dyskinesia any abnormal, hyperkinetic movement resulting from impairment of normal voluntary movement, usually due to extrapyramidal-system dysfunction

dyskinetic cerebral palsy nonprogressive motor dysfunction present from birth or early childhood, characterized by abnormal, involuntary fluctuations in muscle tone, resulting in rapid and writhing movements

dysphagia difficulty with swallowing

dystonia involuntary, sustained, or intermittent co-contractions of opposing muscle (agonists and antagonists) groups, resulting in twisting, writhing movements, coarse tremor, or abnormal postures

early intervention (EI) special services and resources provided for children (and families) identified as having or being at risk for developing a disability that will affect their development. The goal of EI is to remediate existing developmental problems and/or prevent further problems or delays

echolalia pathological repetition of another person's words or phrases, usually seen in association with frontal lobe dysfunction and Tourette syndrome

echophenomena compulsive repetition of others' words (echolalia) or gestures (echopraxia)

echopraxia a complex motor tic consisting of the compulsive echoing or mirroring of others' gestures or actions

echo-planar imaging (EPI) a pulse sequence commonly used in ƒMRI, in which the brain is rapidly imaged in slices

edrophonium (Tensilon) a short-acting cholinesterase inhibitor used as a diagnostic test for myasthenia gravis (i.e., the Tensilon test)

efferent directed from the central nervous system toward the periphery. Cf. afferent.

electroencephalography (EEG) technology that measures the electric potentials of the brain, usually via scalp electrodes

electromyography a neurophysiological test used to examine the electrical activity of muscle

encephalocele protrusion of brain tissue through the cranium due to a malformation of the brain and skull

encephalopathy disease of the brain

epigenetic nonmutational factors that modify the expression of a gene

epilepsy chronic clinical disorder characterized by recurrence of seizures

erythema migrans a rash typical of early Lyme disease

"evening-up" a "just right" phenomenon that involves symmetrical touching or arranging or repetition of actions an even number of times

event-related design a paradigm in which experimental conditions are presented as discrete events that may vary in their timing and order

executive function the application of cognitive control, such as planning and strategizing, to facilitate goal-directed behavior

extrapyramidal circuits or pathways within the brain, involving the basal ganglia, that modulate movement; lesions in the extrapyramidal circuits cause involuntary movement disorders, such as chorea, dystonia, ballism, rigidity, tremor, and bradykinesia

flair fluid attenuated inversion recovery (FLAIR) imaging. An MRI sequence that highlights lesions that abut cerebrospinal fluid (CSF) spaces. Used to identify small white matter lesions, gliosis, low-grade neoplasms, and those near CSF

fluorescent in situ hybridization process by which fluorescently labeled DNA probes are hybridized to chromosome preparations, allowing determination of microdeletion and/or analysis of subtelomeric region

foot drop weakness of dorsiflexors of the foot at the ankle

fovea central portion of retina where acuity is highest and receptor density greatest

functional behavioral assessment (FBA) assessment of behavior mandated in school settings to identify causes and consequences of a child's behavior problems before developing a formal intervention plan

functional connectivity analysis that measures correlations of activity between remote brain regions

functional magnetic resonance imaging (ƒMRI) the use of magnetic resonance imaging technology to measure active brain function

functional neuroimaging the use of neuroimaging technology to measure active brain function

genomics study of functions and interactions of all genetic material; the human genome is composed of 20,000 to 25,000 genes as well as noncoding genetic material

geste antagoniste term used to describe sensory tricks used by patients with primary forms of dystonia in which a slight sensory input temporarily relieves the dystonia (i.e., placing finger lightly on chin to straighten head in cervical dystonia)

glaucoma a condition of increased pressure within the eyeball, causing gradual loss of sight

go/no-go a task in which a series of cued simple motor responses (button push) are accompanied by occasional "no-go" cues requiring suppression of this motor response

Gower maneuver use of the hands to push on the floor and thighs to rise to a standing position, used by patients with proximal leg weakness. A classic finding in Duchenne muscular dystrophy

hard-of-hearing (HOH) mild hearing loss; HOH people tend to function well in the hearing world and usually can hear satisfactorily, except in certain environments, such as in noisy backgrounds.

highly active antiretroviral therapy (HAART) combination of several (usually three or four) antiretroviral drugs used to treat HIV/AIDS

hydrocephalus condition in which cerebrospinal fluid production exceeds absorption, or obstruction of the cerebrospinal fluid pathway, resulting in dilation of the cerebral ventricles, often associated with increased intracranial pressure

hyperactivity a state in which an individual is easily excitable and abnormally active

hyperexplexia an abnormally sensitive startle response in which startle results in a generalized myoclonic jerk; some forms are inherited defects in the glycine receptor.

hyperfractionated radiation a technique in which radiation is delivered twice daily or more frequently in smaller doses

hyperlexia a precocious ability to read words or an intense fascination with letters or numbers; sometimes seen with below-average ability to understand spoken language

hypertonia increased muscle tone

hypnic myoclonus myoclonus occurring at sleep onset that is often physiological

hypomimia diminished facial expression or "masked facies" seen in parkinsonism as a manifestation of bradykinesia

hypophonia diminished volume of speech, as seen in parkinsonism

hypotonia decreased muscle tone

ichthyosis a condition in which the skin is scaly, like that of a fish

immunosuppression reduction of the activation or efficacy of the immune system by a disease process or induced by treatments, such as steroids or radiation

impulsivity decreased ability to control or suppress actions

inattention a state in which an individual is easily distractible and has difficulty maintaining focus

induction the influence of one embryonic tissue on another, so that one tissue induces differentiation in the other

infantile exotropia/esotropia congenital misalignment of the eye outwardly (exotropia) or inwardly (esotropia)

jittering the randomization of the time intervals between events

"just right" phenomena a form of complex tic or compulsion wherein the individual feels the need to repeat an action or vocalization until it feels "just right" in terms of tactile or proprioceptive feel, sound, appearance (e.g., symmetry), or number

la belle indifference abnormal indifferent affect or inappropriate lack of concern in one's physical symptoms, observed in some patients with psychogenic movement disorders

lateral geniculate nucleus (LGN) visually responsive portion of the thalamus

leukodystrophy term for a group of white-matter genetic disorders that cause abnormal development or degeneration of CNS myelin. Their manifestations may mimic the clinical symptoms and MRI appearance of MS, but usually emerge in infancy or early childhood and have a relentlessly progressive course. Examples include adrenoleukodystrophy and metachromatic leukodystrophy.

leukoencephalopathy toxic damage to oligodendroglioma and myelin due to chemotherapy, especially methotrexate, with and without cranial radiation. CTs show calcifications in the basal ganglia, hypodense areas, and increased sulci. MRIs show increased T_2 signals that extend from the ventricles to the gray-matter/white-matter border. Clinical symptoms include dementia, seizures, ataxia, tremor, and long-tract signs.

limit-setting sleep disorder a type of behavioral insomnia characterized by bedtime delay tactics that occur predominantly when parents do not set and enforce consistent limits

longitudinal relaxation the process by which the net magnetization recovers along the longitudinal (parallel) axis as the nuclei realign with the static magnetic field after a radiofrequency (RF) pulse

lower motor neuron (LMN) a neuron in the peripheral nervous system whose cell body is located in the spinal cord (or brainstem) and whose axon terminates by forming a neuromuscular junction with a muscle

lumbosacral plexus a network of axons connecting lumbar and sacral nerve roots to terminal nerve branches

magnetic resonance imaging (MRI) technology that uses a series of radiofrequency (RF) pulses in combination with time-varying magnetic fields to image biological tissue

magnetoencephalography (MEG) technology that measures small magnetic-field changes caused by neuronal electrical activity

meningocele aperture in vertebral spine with protrusion of meninges

microarray glass, silicon wafers, or microsphere-sized beads on which hundreds or thousands of nucleic acid probes are deposited, allowing analysis of an entire genome

micrographia smallness of handwriting, usually seen in association with parkinsonism

mock scan a simulation designed to mimic the environment of an MRI scanner to acclimate patients for actual scanning

mononeuropathy any disorder affecting a single nerve

mononeuropathy multiplex any disorder affecting two or more individual nerves

motion artifacts blurring and ghosting of the images due to movement of the object being imaged

motor impersistence the inability to maintain persistent muscle tone, often seen in association with chorea [e.g., darting tongue (inability to maintain tongue protrusion)]

multiple sleep latency test (MSLT) a type of sleep study involving a series of standardized nap opportunities to measure daytime sleepiness; it is typically performed after overnight polysomnography. MSLT is frequently used to help diagnose narcolepsy.

myelomeningocele malformation in vertebral spine with protrusion of meninges and spinal cord, resulting in distal sensory and motor function

myoclonus brief, involuntary shock-like contractions of a group of muscles that can be caused by pathology at any level in the nervous system

myoglobinuria the presence of the muscle protein myoglobin in the urine, usually in association with muscle breakdown

myopathy any disorder affecting muscle

myositis inflammation of muscle

myotonia delayed relaxation of muscle after voluntary contraction or percussion

narcolepsy a chronic disorder characterized by excessive sleepiness, often seen as repeated naps or lapses into sleep throughout the day. Cataplexy, a hallmark of narcolepsy, is a sudden decrease or loss of motor tone, often precipitated by an emotional response, such as a surprise or hearing a joke, is a hallmark of narcolepsy.

neural circuits a group of interconnected neurons that are involved in specific brain functions

neuraxis radiation radiation to brain and spinal cord (craniospinal)

neurofibromatosis a neurocutaneous disorder manifested by skin lesions including café-au-lait spots, axillary and groin freckling, Lisch nodules, optic gliomas, CNS tumors

neuroimaging the use of various technologies to image the structure and/or active function of the brain

neuropathy any disorder affecting one or more nerve(s) or all nerves

neurulation refers to the bending of the neural placode to form the neural tube

non-nucleoside reverse transcriptase inhibitors (NNRTIs) another class of antiretroviral drugs used to treat HIV infection

nucleoside analogue reverse transcriptase inhibitors (NRTIs) the first class of antiretroviral drugs developed to treat HIV infection

null point the position in which a dystonic limb or neck can be placed that quiets the movements

nystagmus repetitive, slow drift of the eye(s) in one direction followed by a fast movement in the opposite direction

ocular dominance columns spatial organization of cells in primary visual cortex according to the eye that causes the strongest activation

oculogyric crisis an acute movement disorder in which the eyeballs forcefully deviate upward and the neck may forcefully extend; seen in postencephalitic parkinsonism and dystonic reactions to dopamine-blocking medications

oligoclonal bands (OCBs) immunoglobulins, which do not have a specific target, that are detectable in the cerebrospinal fluid (CSF) of many, but not all, MS patients. They also are detectable in the CSF in some infectious and inflammatory diseases.

oligodendrocytes the cells within the central nervous system that produce myelin. Schwann cells produce myelin in the peripheral nervous system

ophthalmoparesis weakness of eye movements

opportunistic infection infection caused by organisms that usually do not cause disease in a person with a healthy immune system but can affect persons with immunosuppression

optic chiasm the X-shaped structure formed on the inferior surface of the brain where the two optic nerves split and form the optic tracts

orientation columns spatial organization of cells in primary visual cortex according to the stimulus orientation or angle that causes the strongest response

palilalia compulsive repetition of one's own just-uttered words or phrases

PANDAS [Pediatric Autoimmune Neuropsychiatric Disorder Associated with Streptococcus] is a hypothesized condition characterized by prepubertal onset of the development or exacerbation of tics or obsessive–compulsive disorder (OCD), occurring in close temporal association with group A β-hemolytic streptococcal infection (GABHS); often accompanied by minor neurological abnormalities, such as choreiform movements (motor impersistence; irregular, small jerky, asymmetrical movements) or clumsiness

parakinesia camouflaging an abnormal involuntary movement by making it appear semipurposeful; normally seen in chorea

parasomnias undesirable experiences or physical events that occur during entry into sleep, within sleep, or during arousals from sleep. Sleepwalking, confusional arousals, and sleep terrors are examples.

parkinsonism a combination of rigidity, rest tremor, bradykinesia, and postural instability that results from extrapyramidal dysfunction

periodic limb movements in sleep episodes of highly stereotyped, repetitive limb movements that occur during sleep; if numerous, associated arousals may result in sleep disruption. The diagnosis is established with overnight polysomnography.

periventricular leukomalacia the most common pathological correlate of cerebral palsy; it represents injury of deep cerebral white matter.

phase coherence after radiofrequency (RF) pulse excitation, the nuclei all have identical dipole moments in the transverse plane, which decays rapidly as different nuclei rotate in the transverse plane at different speeds

plasmapheresis a procedure in which a patient's blood is removed, the plasma treated or replaced, and the remaining blood returned to the body; used in the treatment of autoimmune disorders

plexopathy any disorder affecting a plexus (such as the brachial or lumbosacral plexus)

polyneuropathy any disorder affecting multiple nerves or all of the nerves

polysomnography (PSG) a sleep study that uses multiple leads to record physiological parameters simultaneously (including EEG, eye movements, muscle activity, ECG, pulse oximetry, end-tidal carbon dioxide levels, airflow, and respiratory effort)

positive behavioral support (PBS) formal mandated intervention plan developed in a school setting to address behavior problems identified through functional behavioral assessment (FBA)

positron emission tomography (PET) an imaging technology in which a radioactive tracer isotope is attached to a metabolically active molecule and injected as a contrast to image active brain function

postlingual deafness the onset of deafness after language has been acquired

pragmatics set of rules governing the use of language in context, including intention; sensorimotor actions before, accompanying, and after the utterance; knowledge shared in the communicative pair of speakers; and the elements in the environment surrounding the message

prelingual deafness the onset of deafness before language has been acquired

premonitory urges or sensations somatic sensations or urges that precede and are often transiently relieved by the performance of a tic

primary dystonia disorders in which dystonia is the sole neurological abnormality (with exception of tremor) and for which no developmental, degenerative, or exogenous cause for the dystonia can be identified (e.g., generalized torsion dystonia, or DYT-1 dystonia)

primary visual cortex (V1) occipital lobe region that receives the largest projection from the lateral geniculate nucleus (LGN) and that is at the start of the cortical processing path for vision

propriospinal myoclonus myoclonus originating in the spinal cord; usually involves trunk flexion

prosody melody of speech determined primarily by modifications of pitch, quality, strength, and duration; perceived primarily as stress and intonational patterns

protease inhibitors (PIs) a class of medications used to treat retroviral infections, particularly HIV, that prevent viral replication by inhibiting the activity of protease, an enzyme required for assembly of new viral particles

pseudohypertrophy an apparent increase in muscle bulk that is actually due to increased bulk of another tissue or infiltration of muscle by fat cells

pseudoseizure (psychogenic seizure) (nonepileptic seizure) seizure-like event without underlying EEG abnormality that is a manifestation of a psychiatric disturbance, such as a conversion disorder, or of malingering

pseudotumor cerebri (benign intracranial hypertension or idiopathic intracranial hypertension) syndrome of headache, blurred vision, and increased intracranial pressure with papilledema without intracranial mass or hydrocephalus. If untreated, this disorder can lead to visual loss. Although termed "idiopathic," many cases are attributable to venous sinus occlusion, obesity, retinoic acid, and vitamin A or tetracycline toxicity.

ptosis drooping of an eyelid (or any other body part)

pyramidal tracts a term used interchangeably with corticospinal tract to describe the tracts in the brain that directly control movement and originate in the primary motor cortex and descend through the internal capsule and from the corticospinal tracts. They decussate (cross) in the ventral medulla. Pyramidal tract lesions cause weakness, hyperreflexia, and velocity-dependent hyperreflexia (spasticity).

radiculomyelitis disease of the spinal nerves that is characterized by pain that radiates from the spine outward (radially)

radiculopathy any disorder affecting one or more nerve root(s)

radiofrequency (RF) pulses electromagnetic pulses in a specific frequency range capable of exciting hydrogen electrons to a higher energy state

reaction-time variability a within-subject measure of the inconsistency in the latency of responding to stimuli

"rebound" exacerbation refers to flare-up of tics caused by too-rapid discontinuation or reduction in dose of an anti-tic medication

relapsing–remitting MS (RRMS) the most common course of MS in which signs and symptoms undergo exacerbations and remissions. Most children and adults initially experiencing RRMS eventually transition into a steady deterioration of a secondary progressive course.

response inhibition the suppression of contextually inappropriate actions that may interfere with goal-directed behavior

resting-state part of experiment when an individual is not engaged in a specific task

restless-legs syndrome a disorder associated with distressing paresthesias in the lower extremities, prompting an urge to move the legs. The diagnosis is based on subjective criteria.

retinal ganglion cells cells in the retina that send visual information to the brain via the optic nerve

retinitis pigmentosa any of several genetic disorders that affect the retina, causing progressive visual loss

retinopathy of prematurity (ROP) a disease of the eye that affects premature infants

retrocollis forced extension at the neck, resulting in an abnormal posturing of the head, sometimes seen as a form of tardive dystonia

rhizotomy surgical severing of the dorsal nerve root innervating a spastic muscle group

rigidity resistance to passive muscle stretch that is neither directional nor velocity dependent, and usually results from dysfunction of the extrapyramidal system

rods photoreceptor-type cells in the retina responsible for nighttime and achromatic (grayscale) vision

secondary dystonia disorders in which dystonia is symptomatic of an underlying disease process, insult, or exposure (e.g., dystonia secondary to dopamine-blocking medications)

secondary generalization of a seizure the evolution of a partial (focal) seizure into a generalized seizure

seizure clinical event caused by a self-limited hypersynchronous electrical discharge of cortical neurons

semantics study of meaning in language, including the relations between language, thought, and behavior

Semiology term used to describe the clinical manifestations of a seizure

sensorineural hearing loss type of hearing loss caused by damage, malfunction, or abnormality in the vestibulocochlear nerve, inner ear, or central auditory processing centers of the brain

signal-to-noise ratio the magnitude of the effect of interest (signal) divided by its variation (noise)

simple motor tics sudden, fleeting, or fragmentary movements, such as blinking, grimacing, or head jerking

simple phonic or vocal tics unarticulated sounds, such as throat clearing, sniffing, or grunting

single-nucleotide polymorphism (SNP) DNA sequence variation that occurs within a genome. The human genome contains about 10 million SNPs.

single-photon emission computed tomography (SPECT) technology in which a radioactive gamma-emitting tracer is attached to a metabolically active molecule and injected as a contrast to image active brain function

sleep-onset association disorder a type of behavioral insomnia in which inappropriate reliance occurs on specific conditions that facilitate a child's falling asleep; the absence of these conditions may result in prolonged sleep latency or nightly awakenings

spastic diplegia bilateral spasticity with lower extremities more severely affected

spastic hemiplegia spasticity of ipsilateral upper and lower extremities

spasticity (hypertonia) resistance to passive muscle stretch that increases with increased velocity, has directionality, and is normally due to dysfunction of the pyramidal system; typically associated with hyperactive deep tendon reflexes, clonus, and Babinski signs

spatial normalization a step in the neuroimaging processing stream in which an individual's brain image is deformed onto a template brain to facilitate interindividual comparisons

spatial resolution how well changes in an image can be distinguished across remote locations in space

spina bifida failure of vertebral fusion, which usually involves lumbar spine

spinothalamic tract an afferent pathway in the central nervous system carrying information about sensory modalities, such as pain and temperature

spreading depression decreased electrophysiological activity provoked by dysfunction cortex that spreads across the cerebral cortex. This process is purported to explain the progress of visual aura in migraines.

state regulation the ability to manage one's internal motivation

static encephalopathy nonprogressive brain dysfunction

steppage gait an abnormal pattern of walking in which a patient lifts his or her knee high in the air; characteristic of patients with foot drop and seen in those with peroneal nerve injury or tabes dorsalis

stereotypy repetitive, stereotyped, nonpurposeful gestures or movements of the hands that may be partially suppressible

stop signal a task in which a series of cued simple motor responses (button push) are accompanied by occasional "stop" cues requiring suppression of this motor response

strabismus abnormal eye alignment or squint

Sturge–Weber syndrome a neurocutaneous disorder involving hemifacial hemangioma in a trigeminal distribution, ipsilateral leptomeningeal vascular malformation, and contralateral neurological signs

subtelomeric rearrangement rearrangements leading to deletions of the functional end of the chromosome, thought to be responsible for a significant number of structural chromosomal abnormalities not previously detected with routine karyotype analysis

suppressibility the ability to suppress or delay the performance of a tic, albeit transient and often associated with increased tension or urge to tic and subsequent rebound of tics

susceptibility artifacts signal losses in BOLD ƒMRI images due to magnetic-field inhomogeneities near air–tissue interfaces

syntax the way in which words are assembled in a sentence to convey meaning

T$_1$ recovery (see longitudinal relaxation)

T$_1$-weighted images anatomical MR images that are sensitive to T$_1$ recovery

T$_2$ decay (see transverse relaxation)

T$_2$ relaxometry an ƒMRI technique that uses changes in resting cerebral blood flow to measure active brain function

T$_2$-weighted images anatomical MR images that are sensitive to T$_2$ decay

T$_2$* decay Similar to T$_2$ decay, but specifically sensitive to the BOLD contrast, commonly used in ƒMRI

T$_2$*-weighted images functional MR images that are sensitive to T$_2$* decay

tardive used to describe movement disorders that arise as a complication of prolonged (usually longer than 6 months) treatment with dopamine receptor–blocking drugs (e.g., tardive dyskinesias)

temporal resolution how well changes in an image can be distinguished over time

Tensilon see edrophonium

tics a heterogeneous group of spontaneous, brief, simple or complex movements or vocalizations that abruptly interrupt normal actions or speech and are usually associated with a preceding urge, partial suppressibility, and relief after performing the tic

transformed migraine combination of migraine and tension-type headaches causing chronic nonprogressive daily headache

transverse relaxation the process by which the net magnetization in the transverse (perpendicular) plane decreases as the nuclei lose their phase coherence after a radiofrequency (RF) pulse

tremor a rhythmic oscillatory movement produced by alternating or synchronous contractions of antagonist muscle groups

triptans orally, sublingually, or parenterally administered category of antimigraine medicines that activate a subpopulation of serotonin receptors. These medicines have not been FDA approved for young children.

tuberous sclerosis a neurocutaneous disorder that consists primarily of facial angiomas, multisystem hamartomas, cortical tubers, and subependymal astrocytomas, often associated with mental retardation and epilepsy

upper motor neuron (UMN) a neuron in the central nervous system whose cell body is located in the brain and whose axon terminates by forming a synapse with the cell body of a lower motor neuron. UMNs form the corticospinal (pyramidal) tract.

vasculopathy disease of the blood vessels

ventral stream projection from primary visual cortex toward temporal lobe structures that specialize in object, form, and color perception

verbal auditory agnosia inability to understand spoken words; pure-word deafness

verbal dyspraxia also referred to as childhood apraxia of speech; a nonlinguistic sensorimotor disorder of articulation characterized by the impaired capacity to program the speech musculature and the sequencing of muscle movements for the volitional production of phonemes (sounds)

visually evoked potentials (VEPs) electrical-activity patterns evoked by visual stimulation

volume of radiation extent of radiotherapy port (i.e., whole brain, focal, or craniospinal axis)

working memory the temporary storage and manipulation of information necessary for goal-directed behavior

Index

Page numbers in *italics* denote figures; those followed by "t" denote tables.

A

Acetaminophen
  in migraine, 162
Acetazolamide
  in movement disorders, 64
Acetylcholine, 368
Acid maltase deficiency, 387
Acoustic schwannoma, 30
Acquired immune deficiency syndrome. *See* HIV infection
Actigraphy
  in sleep disorders, 125
Acute disseminated encephalomyelitis, 315
Acute intermittent porphyria, 380
Adolescents
  delayed sleep phase syndrome in, 127
  excessive sleepiness in, 125
  headache in, 155
  juvenile myoclonic epilepsy in, 110
  pseudoseizures in, 104
  sleep patterns of, 141
  Tourette syndrome in, 79
Affective disorders, 40
  in multiple sclerosis, 313
Akathisia
  neuroleptic-induced, 67
Akinetopsia, 340
Albinism
  ocular, 336
Alcohol
  abuse of, 407
Alexander disease, 35
Alice in Wonderland syndrome, 161
Alpha-adrenergic agents
  in Tourette syndrome, 89–90
Amantadine
  in multiple sclerosis, 318
Amblyopia, 329, 332
  treatment of, 332–333
American Academy of Neurology (ANN), 18
Amitriptyline
  for migraine prophylaxis, 155, 163, 167
Amnesia
  after fall, 403–408
    clinical course of, 407–408
    clinical diagnosis of, 408
    differential diagnosis of, 404–407
    presentation of case, 403–404
  dissociative, 406
  transient global, 405
Amphetamines
  for attention deficit hyperactivity disorder, 93, 139
  as cause of myopathy, 389
  in epilepsy, 117
Amyotrophic lateral sclerosis, 379
Anencephaly, 232
Angiofibroma
  in tuberous sclerosis, 212–213, *213*, *214*
Anterior horn cell disease, 378–379
Anticholinergic drugs
  for dystonia, 54
  in movement disorders, 67

Anticonvulsants. *See* Antiepileptic drugs.
Antidepressants
  in epilepsy, 117, 118t
  in HIV infection, 296
  visual impairment and, 340
Antiemetics
  in migraine, 162
Antiepileptic drugs, 64, 112–113, *113*
  in dystonia, 54
  interactions with psychotropic drugs, 117, 118t
  psychiatric side effects of, 395, 396t
  psychotropic effects of, 117, 118t
  in sleep disorders, 134
Antihistamines
  in HIV infection, 297
Antioxidants
  in HIV infection, 292
Antipsychotics
  in intellectual disability, 257
Antiretroviral therapy
  in HIV encephalopathy, 289–291
Anxiety
  in epilepsy, 398
  in HIV infection, 296–297
  sleep disturbances in, 140–141
  in Tourette syndrome, 86
Artane. *See* Trihexyphenidyl
Arterial infarction, 33
Arteriovenous malformation, 32
Astrocytoma, 172, 175
  anaplastic, 174
  brainstem, 25–26, *26*
  cerebellar, 24–25, *25*, 182
  pilocytic, 174
  subpendymal giant cell, 216
  supratentorial, 26
Ataxias, 376
  episodic, 64
Atomoxetine
  in attention deficit hyperactivity disorder, 94
Attention deficit hyperactivity disorder, 39
  functional magnetic resonance imaging in, 193–199
  hearing disorder and, 360
  intellectual disability and, 251, 256
  in neurofibromatosis, 211
  periodic limb movement disorder and, 137–139
  response inhibition in, 193–198, *195*, 196t, *197*
  and resting state, 198–199
  and restless legs syndrome, 137–139
  sleep-disordered breathing and, 136–137
  sleep disorders and, 136–139
  structural changes in, 39
  Tourette syndrome and, 57, 80, 93–94
  traumatic brain injury and, 273
  treatment of
    examination of effects of, 199
    medications in, 139
    psychostimulants in, 117
    stimulants in, 93
Autism, 39
  deafness and, 359
  intellectual disability and, 251
  neuroimaging in, 39
  in tuberous sclerosis, 217
Avonex, 317
AZT, 290, 389

423

B

Baclofen
  in cerebral palsy, 230, 231
  in dystonia, 54
  in multiple sclerosis, 318
  in spasticity, 51–52
  in tic disorders, 91
Bardet-Biedl syndrome, 335
Basal ganglia, 47
Becker muscular dystrophy, 8, 371–372, 384
Benzodiazepines
  in cerebral palsy, 230
  in dystonia, 54
  in epilepsy, 112
  in HIV infection, 296
  in sleep disorders, 134
  visual impairment and, 340
Benztropine
  in movement disorders, 67
Betaseron, 317
Bipolar disorder, 40, 140
  and epilepsy, 398–399
  in HIV infection, 296
Blood-oxygenation-level-dependent response, 190, *190*
Bone lesions
  in neurofibromatosis, 210
Botulinum toxin
  in cerebral palsy, 230
  in dystonia, 54
  in Tourette syndrome, 58, 91
Botulism, 383
  signs and symptoms of, 383
  treatment of, 383
Bradykinesia, 48
Brain
  development of
    hearing loss and, 354
    immaturity of, 270
Brain injury
  in child abuse, 22
  primary
    mechanisms/physics of, *266*, 266–267, *267*
  traumatic, 265–280, 404
    academic achievement following, 274
    attention deficit hyperactivity disorder and, 273
    behavioral profile of, 272
    classification of, 269–271, 270t
    clinical course of, 268–269, *269*
    executive functions following, 273
    imaging of, 267–268
    intelligence quotient scores after, 272
    language pathology and, 273–274
    memory following, 273
    neurobehavioral outcome of, 271–273
    pathophysiology of, 265–266
    psychiatric disorders in, 272
    recovery from
      prognostic factors in, 271t
    treatment of
      postacute, 274–275
Brain tumors, 171–188
  age distribution of, 171
  case histories of, 182–184
    cerebellar astrocytoma, 182
    craniopharyngioma, 183–184
    oligodendroglioma, 182–183, 184
  classification of, 171
  headache and, 172–173, 174
  imaging of, 22–23, 175
    posterior fossa, 23–26
      atypical teratoid/rhabdoid tumors, 24
      brainstem astrocytoma, 25–26, *26*
      cerebellar astrocytoma, 24–25, *25*
      ependymoma, 25
      medulloblastoma, 23–24, *24*
    supratentorial, 26–28
      astrocytoma, 26
      craniopharyngioma, 27, *27*
      ependymoma, 26–27
      pineal region tumors, 27–28, *28*, *29*
  incidence of, 22, 171
  long-term treatment effects, 177–180
    endocrinopathy, 177
    neurocognitive deficits, 178–179
    neurological status, 177
    oncogenesis, 177–178
    psychiatric status, 179–180
    psychosocial functioning, 179
    radiation-induced dementia, 178
  midline, 174
  neuorological evaluation in, 175
  in neurofibromatosis, 210, *211*
  posterior fossa, 175
  prognosis for, 171, 172, 177–178
  seizures and, 174
  signs and symptoms of
    localizing, 174–175
    nonlocalizing, 172–173
  treatment of, 176
    chemotherapy, 176
    neurocognitive approaches to, 181
    psychosocial and neuropsychiatric, 180–184
    radiation therapy, 176
    surgical resection, 176
  visual pathways and, 335
Brainstem
  gliomas of, 26, *26*, 209
Bupropion
  in HIV infection, 296

C

Café-au-lait spots, 205–206, *206*
Canavan disease, 35
Carbamazepine
  in chorea, 61
  in epilepsy, 394
  in intellectual disability, 257
  in movement disorders, 64
  in seizures, 113
  in sleep disorders, 134
  visual impairment and, 340
Carbatrol. *See* Carbamazepine
Carbidopa-levodopa
  in cerebral palsy, 230
  in dystonia, 55
Carnitine deficiency, 387
Case histories
  of amnesia after fall, 403–410
  of attention deficit hyperactivity disorder, 138–140
  of auditory and visual hallucinations, 393–403
  of brain tumors, 182–184
  of chorea, 61–62
  of Duchenne muscular dystrophy, 8
  of dystonia, 55
  of narcolepsy, 135–136
  of obstructive sleep disorder, 132
  of psychogenic movement disorder, 66
  of sleep disorder, 127, 129
  of tremor, 49–50
  of tuberous sclerosis, 217–219
  of Wilson disease, 7–8
Cataracts
  congenital and developmental, 327–328
Cavernous malformations, 31
Central nervous system infection, 34
  HIV-related, 281
  opportunistic, 288–289
Central nervous system tumors
  in neurofibromatosis type 1, 208–209, *209*

Cerebral anomalies
  congenital. *See* Congenital cerebral anomalies
Cerebral autosomal dominant arteriopathy with subcortical infarcts and leukoencephalopathy (CACDASIL) 316
Cerebral palsy, 7, 225–231
  atonic, 228–229
  birthweight and, 226, 226t
  classification of, 227, 227–229
  diagnosis of, 226, 229
  dyskinetic, 227, 228
  etiology of, 226
  functional outcome in, 229
  gestational age and, 226, 226t
  language problems in, 229–230
  psychiatric disorders in, 229
  spastic, 227, 227
  spastic diplegic, 227, 227–228, 228
  spastic hemiplegic, 227, 228
  treatment of, 230–231
Cerebral visual impairment, 334
Cerebrospinal flow studies, 15
Channelopathies
  myotonia in, 386
  symptoms of, 386
Charcot-Marie-Tooth disease, 380–381
Charles Bonnet syndrome, 339
Chemotherapy
  in brain tumors, 176
  oncogenesis due to, 177–178
Chiari malformations, 18, 19, 37
Child abuse, 21–22, 23
Chorea, 59–62
  causes of, 59
  clinical features of, 59
  differential diagnosis, 60, 61t, 81
    from dystonia, 52
  drug-induced, 60, 81
  evaluation of patient with, 62
  genetic forms of, 82
  neurobehavioral symptoms of, 60
  postinfectious, 81
  Sydenham, 59
  treatment of, 60
Chronotherapy, 127
Citalopram
  in HIV infection, 296
Clonazepam
  in dystonia, 54
  in HIV infection, 296
  in myoclonus, 64
  in seizures, 114–115
  in Tourette syndrome, 58
Clonidine
  in attention deficit hyperactivity disorder, 139
  in drug-induced movement disorders, 67
  in intellectual disability, 257
  in spasticity, 51
  in Tourette syndrome, 58, 89–90
Clozapine
  in tardive dyskinesia, 68
  in Tourette syndrome, 57
Cochlear implants, 361
Cognitive subtraction, 190
Compulsions
  instruments for assessing, 87–88
  in Tourette syndrome, 80
Computed tomography
  angiography, 13–14, 14
  brain tumors on, 175
  of head, 13
Concussion, 20
Congenital cerebral anomalies, 36–37
  Chiari malformations, 37
  Dandy-Walker syndrome, 37
  heterotopia, 37
  holoprosencephaly, 37, 38
  imaging of, 36
  lissencephaly, 37, 37
  polymicrogyria, 37
  schizencephaly, 37
Congenital heart disease, 32
Conversion
  nonepileptic seizures
    and epilepsy, 400–401
Conversion disorders, 65, 94, 337, 389–390
  epileptic seizures in, 399
Coordination examination, 376
Copaxone, 317
Coprolalia, 56
Corpus callosum agenesis, 231–232
Cortical auditory evoked potentials, 349, 350–351
Cortical tubers
  in tuberous sclerosis, 216, 216
Corticosteroids
  in inflammatory myopathies, 388–389
  in muscular dystrophies, 384
Cranial nerves
  examination of, 2, 3t, 372
Craniopharyngioma, 27, 27, 175, 183–184
Creatinine phosphokinase, 376
Cyclophosphamide (Cytoxan), 317
Cyclosporine, 389
Cyproheptadine
  for migraine prophylaxis, 155, 163
Cysticercosis, 34
Cytomegalovirus, 288

D

Dandy-Walker malformation, 235
Dandy-Walker syndrome, 37
Dantrolene
  in cerebral palsy, 230
Deafness. *See* Hearing loss
Deep-brain stimulation
  in dystonia, 54
  in tic disorders, 92
Deep tendon reflexes, 374
  commonly tested, 4t
Delirium, 297, 405
Dementia
  in HIV infection, 297
  radiation-induced, 178
Demyelinating disease, 36
Depakene, Depakote. *See* Valproic acid
L-Deprenyl, 292
Depression
  in brain tumor, 173
  in epilepsy, 398
  in hearing impairment, 359
  in HIV infection, 295–296
  in multiple sclerosis, 313, 318
  in muscular dystrophies, 384
  in Tourette syndrome, 86
  visual complaints and, 338
Dermatomyositis, 388
Desipramine
  for attention deficit hyperactivity disorder, 94
Desmoplastic neuroepithelial tumors, 174
Developmental delay
  use of term, 243
Diazepam
  in epilepsy, 112
Diffusion tensor imaging, 15–16
Diffusion weighted imaging, 15
Dihydroxy-ergotamine
  in migraine prophylaxis, 155
Dilantin. *See* Phenytoin
Diphenhydramine
  in migraine, 162–163
  in movement disorders, 67
Diphtheria, 380

Dopamine-depleting agents
  in Tourette syndrome, 90–91
Dopamine-receptor blockers
  tardive dyskinesia and, 83
  in Tourette syndrome, 57, 90–91
Duchenne muscular dystrophy, 8, 371–372, 384
  clinical course of, 384
  cognitive dysfunction in, 384
  diagnosis of, 384
  treatment of, 384
Dysembryoplastic neuroectodermal tumor, 19, 20
Dyskinesias, 64
  tradive dyskinesias, 67, 83
Dysmyelinating diseases, 35
Dystonia, 48, 52–55
  case history of, 55
  clinical features of, 52
  definition of, 52, 82
  differential diagnosis of, 52, 53t
    from chorea, 52
  early-onset, 83
  etiologic classification of, 52
  genetic form of, 52–53
  in movement disorders, 48
  primary vs. secondary, 53
  treatment of, 54–55
  voluntary movements and, 83

E

Edrophonium, 377, 382
Electroencephalogram
  in epilepsy, 106, 106–107
Electromyograms
  in sleep studies, 124
Emery-Dreifuss muscular dystrophy, 386
Emotional factors
  in hearing impairment, 358–359
  in visual impairment, 342
Encephalocele, 232
Encephalomyelitis
  acute disseminated, 315, 315t
  disseminated, 35
Encephalopathy(ies)
  clinical manifestations of, 283t, 283–284
  epileptic, 111
  following radiation therapy, 177
  HIV-related, 282–283
  posterior reversible, 35
  static, 51–52, 225–242
Endocrine dysfunction
  brain tumors and, 174
Endocrine myopathies, 389
Ependymoma, 172, 175
  posterior fossa, 25
  supratentorial, 26–27
Epilepsy, 6, 103–121
  acute onset of psychosis in
    differential diagnosis of, 394, 397
  age-related syndromes of, 107t, 107–108
  alternative therapy in, 116
  anxiety, depression, and bipolar disorders in, 398
  antidepressants in, 117, 118t
  attention deficit hyperactivity disorder and, 397
  auditory and visual hallucinations in
    clinical diagnosis in, 403
    differential diagnosis of, 394–402
    hospital course in, 402–403
    presentation of case, 393–394
  autosomal dominant nocturnal frontal lobe, 133
  behavioral manifestations of, 117–119
  benign occipital, 111
  benign partial syndromes, 110–111
    with centrotemporal spikes, 110–111
    rolandic, 110–111
  benign syndromes of, 108–109
  bipolar disorder and, 398–399
  childhood absence, 109–110
  complex partial, 108, 109t
  with complex partial seizures, 82
  depression in, 398
  etiology and diagnosis of, 105–107, 106
  generalized benign, 109–110
  juvenile myoclonic, 63, 110
  learining disorders in, 111, 117, 119
  mental status changes in, 396
  and migraine, 161
  neuropsychiatric comorbidities of, 116–119
  occipital, 339
  psychosis in, 394, 397
  seizure classification in, 103–105
  and sleep disorders, 133–134
  substance abuse disorder in, 401
  syndromes of, 107–108
  treatment of, 112–113
  with typical absence seizures, 82
Epileptic encephalopathies, 111
Epstein-Barr virus, 380
Ergotamine
  for migraine, 162
Esotropia, 322
  accommodative, 330, 330–332
  infantile, 330
Ethosuximide
  for seizures, 114
Eye
  anatomy of, 323–325, 325
  and cerebral visual pathways
    disorders of, 335–336
  disorders of, 327–334

F

Facioscapulohumeral dystrophy, 386
Flaccid quadriplegia, 389
Fluoxetine
  for obsessive-compulsive behaviors, 92
Fluphenazine
  in Tourette syndrome, 57
Fluvoxamine
  in obsessive-compulsive disorder, 92
  in sleep disorders, 140
Focal cortical resection
  in seizures, 250
Fosphenytoin
  in epilepsy, 402
Fragile X syndrome
  intellectual disability and, 246, 252
Freckling, 206, 207
Frontal sinus infection, 34
Functional magnetic resonance imaging. *See* Magnetic resonance imaging, functional

G

Gabapentin
  in migraine prophylaxis, 155
  in seizures, 115
Gait
  abnormalities of, 4, 4t
  defects of, 7, 8
  examination of, 3–4, 4t
Gait defects, 373, 374t
Galactosemia, 335
Gamma hydroxybutyrate, 407
Germ cell tumors, 27
Germinomas, 27

Glasgow Coma Scale, 20, 270t
Glatiramer acetate, 317
Glaucoma
    angle-closure, 340
    congenital/juvenile, 328–329
Glioblastoma multiforme, 172
Glioma(s), 171–172, 175
    brainstem, 26, *26*, 209
    following radiation therapy, 177
    of optic pathways, 29, 208, *209*
Glue-sniffing, 380
Gowers sign, *375–376*, 384
Guanfacine
    in intellectual disability, 257
    in Tourette syndrome, 58, 89–90
Guillain-Barré syndrome, 371, 379

H

HAART, 291–292
Habit reversal therapy
    in tic disorders, 91
Hallucinations
    auditory and visual, 393–403
    in epilepsy. *See* Epilepsy, auditory and visual hallucinations in
    seizures and, 395
    visual, 338–340
Hallucinogen perception disorder, 339–340
Haloperidol
    in Tourette syndrome, 57, 90
Hamartomas
    in tuberous sclerosis, 30
Head circumference
    in brain tumor, 173
    in Rett syndrome, 59
Head trauma, 19–21, *21*
    child abuse and, 21–22
Headaches, 151–170
    acute generalized, 158
    acute recurrent, 154t
    alternative medicine in, 164
    brain tumors and, 172–173, 174
    chronic progressive, 154, 155t, 164–165, 165–167
    classification of, 152–154, *153*
    depression and, 152
    differential diagnosis of, 153, 153t
    epilepsy and, 161
    evaluation in, 156t, 156–157
    history of, 151
    imaging in, 17–18, *19*, 157
    laboratory studies in, 157
    management of, 161–164
    migraine. *See* Migraine
    pathophysiology of, 154–155
    physical examination in, 156–157
    prevalence of, 151–152
    prognosis in, 164
    psychological interview in, 157–158
    retinal, 161
    tension-type, 154
    treatment of
        long-term management in, 166–167
        prophylactic, 163, 164t
        psychological evaluation in, 166
Hearing
    anatomy of, 349–350
    development of, 350–351
    lack of
        impairments due to, 351
    of newborn
        sceening and diagnosis of, 353–355
    sceening of
        situations requiring, 353, 353t
Hearing aids, 351, 360

Hearing loss
    assessment and treatment in, 360–361
    brain development and, 354
    central, 350
    communication in, 357
    conductive, 350
    congenital, 349–365
    cultural aspects of, 356
    diagnosis of, 355
    early intervention in, 356–357
    education in, 357–359, 358t
    etiologies of, 351–353
    hearing aids in, 351
    language deprivation in, 357
    learning disorders in, 350–351, 354, 355, 357, 359, 360
    neonatal
        risk factors for, 352t, 352–353
    nonsyndromic, 351
    parental reaction to, 355–356
    peripheral, 350
    sensorineural, 350
    speech therapy in, 357–359
    syndromic, 351, 352t
Heavy metal–induced neuropathy, 380
Hematoma
    subdural, 22, *23*
Hemodynamic response, 190, *190*
Hemorrhage
    subarachnoid, 18
Hepatolenticular degeneration, 7
Hereditary sensory neuropathy, 381
Heterotopia, 37
Hip displacement
    in cerebral palsy, 230–231
HIV infection, 19
    attention-deficit hyperactivity disorder in, 295
    behavioral disorders in, 295
    cerebrospinal fluid studies in, 286
    clinical manifestations of, 282–285
    CNS involvement in, 34
        antiretroviral therapy in, 289–291
        cerebrovascular disease in, 289
        diagnosis of, 286
        neuropathology of, 286–287
        symptomatic treatment of, 292–293
        treatment of, 289–293
    confidentiality and, 298
    developmental and psychosocial issues in, 298
    disclosure in, 298–299
    drug therapy in
        neuropsychiatric side effects of, 294t
    encephalopathy related to
        clinical manifestations of, 283t, 283–284
    end of life in, 299
    epidemiology of, 282
    medication adherence in, 299
    mood disorders in, 295–297
    myelopathies in, 300
    myopathies in, 300
    neuropathogenesis of, 287–288
    neuroprophylaxis in, 291–292
    neuroprotection in, 292
    neuropsychiatric aspects of, 281–308
    neuroradiologic findings in, 285–286
    psychiatric assessment in, 293
    psychiatric disorders in, 293–295
    secondary CNS disorders in, 288–289
HIV virus, 380
Holoprosencephaly, 37, *38*
Human immunodeficiency virus infection. *See* HIV infection
Huntington disease, 47
Hydrocephalus, 235–237
    anomalies associated with, 237
    "arrested," 236

Hydrocephalus (continued)
  causes of, 236, 236t
  CFS shunting for, 236
  complications of, 237
  noncommunicating vs. communicating, 235
  normal-pressure, 237
  progressive
    shunt placement in, 236
  psychiatric consultation for, 237–238
  signs and symptoms of, 237
Hydroxychloroquine, 389
Hyperopia
  correction of, *331*, 331–332
  optics of, *330*, 330–331
Hypertension
  in neurofibromatosis 1, 210
Hysteria, 337
Hysterical paralysis, 389–390

I

Imaging. *See* Neuroimaging
Immunoglobulin therapy
  in multiple sclerosis, 317
Infections. *See also* Central nervous system infections
  hearing impairment due to, 353
  multiple sclerosis vs., 315
Inflammatory demyelinating polyneuropathy, 379, 382
Insomnia, 125–126
Intellectual disability, 243–259
  adaptive behavior in, 254–255
  attention deficit hyperactivity disorder and, 251, 256
  and autism, 251
  behavior problems in, 252
  cerebral palsy and, 254
  clinical assessment in, 245
  definition of, 243
  diagnostic challenges in, 252–253
  diagnostic guidelines in, 244
  dual diagnosis in, 250–251
  education in, 255
  etiology of, 244–245
  functional behavioral assessment in, 256
  genetic syndromes in
    psychopathology of, 252
  genetic testing in, 245–246
  intellectual limitations in, 247–249
  intelligence testing in, 253–254
  intervention in, 253
  learning and interaction styles in, 249
  metabolic testing in, 247, *248*
  in muscular dystrophies, 384, 386
  neuroimaging in, 246–247
  positive behavioral support in, 256
  presentation of, 247
  prevalence of, 244
  prognosis in, 255
  psychiatric disorders in, 250–251
  psychopharmacology in, 256–257
  psychotherapy in, 257–258
  resources for information on, 259t
  seizures and, 249–250
  terminology in, 243–244
  vulnerability to maltreatment in, 253
  working with families in, 258
Interferons
  in multiple sclerosis, 317, 317t

J

Janz syndrome, 110

K

Keppra. *See* Levetiracetam
Ketamine, 407
Klonopin. *See* Clonazepam
Korsakoff syndrome, 407
Krabbe disease, 381
Kugelberg-Welander syndrome, 378

L

Lamictal. *See* Lamotrigine
Lamotrigine
  in HIV infection, 296
  in movement disorders, 64
  in seizures, 115, 250
Landau-Kleffner syndrome, 111–112
Language disorders
  in deafness, 357
Learning disorders
  in epilepsy, 111, 117, 119
  in hearing impairment, 350–351, 354, 355, 357, 359, 360
  in neurofibromatosis 1, 211–212
  in static encephalopathy, 238
Leigh disease, 35
Lennox-Gastaut syndrome, 111
Leukoencephalopathy(ies)
  neurogenetic, 316
  progressive multifocal, 34
Leukomalacia
  periventricular, 226–227
Levetiracetam
  in dystonia, 54
  in epilepsy, 402
  in myoclonus, 64
  in seizures, 115, 250
  in tic disorders, 91
Levine-Critchley syndrome, 83
Levodopa
  in dystonia, 54, 55
Limb-girdle dystrophy, 385–386
Lisch nodules, 209
Lissencephaly, 37, *37*
Lithium
  as cause of myopathy, 389
  in HIV infection, 296
  in intellectual disability, 257
  neuropathy and, 381–382
  visual impairment and, 340, 341
Liver transplant
  in Wilson disease, 51
Lorazepam, 394
  in epilepsy, 112
  in HIV infection, 296
Lou Gehrig disease, 379
Lower motor neurons, 368
Lyme disease, 379–380
Lymphangioleiomyomatosis
  in tuberous sclerosis, 215

M

Magnetic resonance imaging, 14–15
  brain tumors on, 175
  functional, 16, 189–193
    advantages of, 191
    in attention deficit hyperactivity disorder, 193–199
    caveats of, 192–193
    limitations of, 191–192
    task design in, 190
  in multiple sclerosis, 310–311, *311*
Magnetic resonance spectroscopy, 16
Malingering, 337–338
McArdle disease, 387

Medulloblastoma, 23–24, 24, 172, 175
MELAS syndrome, 388
Melatonin
  in attention deficit hyperactivity disorder, 139
  in sleep disorders, 134
  in tardive dyskinesia, 69
Memantine, 292
Memory loss. See Amnesia
Meningitis
  complications of, 34
  imaging in, 34, 34
  tuberculous, 34
Meningocele, 233, 233
Mental retardation. See Intellectual disability
MERRF syndrome, 388
Mestinon, 383
Metabolic disorders, 35
  involving eyes, 335
  myopathies, 387–388
Metachromatic leukodystrophy, 381
Methotrexate, 388
Methylene dioxymethamphetamine, 407
Methylphenidate
  in attention deficit hyperactivity disorder, 93,139–140
  in epilepsy, 117
  in HIV infection, 296
  in intellectual disability, 256
Methylprednisolone
  in chorea, 61
Methysergide
  in migraine prophylaxis, 155
Metoclopramide
  acute dystonic reactions to, 67–68
Mexiletine, 385, 387
Midazolam
  in epilepsy, 112
Migraine, 6–7, 152
  acute recurrent, 158–159
  with aura, 159
  basilar artery, 160
  clinical features of, 155
  complex, 159
  confusional, 160
  epidemiology of, 151–152, 154t
  as familial disorder, 155–156
  hemiplegic, 159
  ophthalmoplegic, 160
  pathogenesis of, 155
  prophylaxis of, 155
  treatment of
    nonpharmacological, 163–164
    pharmacological, 162–163
    prophylactic medications in, 163, 164t
    symptomatic, 162, 162t
    symptomatic abortive, 163, 163t
  visual aura in, 338
  without aura, 159
Minocycline, 292
Mitochondrial disorders
  multiple sclerosis vs., 316
  myopathies, 387–388
  neurogastrointestinal encephalopathy, 381
Mitoxantrone, 317
Modafil
  in multiple sclerosis, 318
Molecular imaging, 16
Motor examination, 373, 373t, 375–376
Movement disorders, 47–76
  classification of, 47
  drug-induced, 67–69
  dyskinesias, 67
  parkinsonism, 48
  paroxysmal, 64–65
  psychogenic, 65–66
  tics, 55–58
  tone abnormalities in, 51–55
  Wilson disease, 47, 50–51
Moya moya disease, 14
Mucopolysaccharidoses, 335
Multiple sclerosis, 309–321
  affective disorders in, 313
  behavioral problems in, 312–313
  classification of, 311–312
  cognitive and academic concerns in, 313
  definition of, 309
  demographic features of, 310
  depression in, 313, 318
  diagnosis of, 310
  differential diagnosis of, 315t, 315–316
  disease course in, 311–312
  genetics and, 314
  MRI findings in, 310–311, 311
  pathology and pathogenesis of, 314–315
  prognostic factors in, 312
  psychosocial concerns in, 313
  relapses in
    treatment of, 317
  signs and symptoms of, 310
  symptomatic therapy in, 318
  treatment of, 316–317
    disease-modifying, 317, 318t
Multiple sleep latency test, 124
Munchausen-by-proxy syndrome, 338
Munchausen syndrome, 338
Muscle biopsy, 377
Muscle relaxants
  in dystonia, 54
Muscular dystrophies, 384–386
  Becker, 8, 384
  congenital, 385
  Duchenne, 8, 384
  Emery-Dreifuss, 386
  facioscapulohumeral, 386
  limb-girdle, 385–386
  myotonic, 385
Musculoskeletal examination, 2–3
Myasthenia gravis, 370, 382
  age at onset, 382
  diagnosis of, 382
    repetitive EMG stimulation for, 382–383
    Tensilon test in, 382
  etiology of, 382
  neurologic examination for, 382
  treatment of, 383
Myelomeningocele, 233, 234
Myoclonic seizures, 63
Myoclonus, 62–64
  categories of, 62
  clinical features of, 62
  definition of, 62
  differential diagnosis of, 63t
  hypnic, 62
  myoclonic jerks in, 82
  opsoclonus-myoclonus, 63
  treatment of, 63
Myoclonus-dystonia, 54
Myoglobinuria, 387
Myopathies
  congenital, 386
  endocrine, 389
  inflammatory acquired, 388
  metabolic, 387–388
  muscular dystrophies, 384–386
  toxic, 389
Myophosphorylase deficiency, 387
Myositis, 388
Myotonia congenita, 386
Myotonic dystrophy, 385
  clinical presentation of, 385
  cognitive deficits in, 385
Myotoxins, 389

N

Narcolepsy, 135
Natalizumab, 317
Nefazodone
  visual impairment and, 340
Neoplasms
  intracranial, 22–28
  multiple sclerosis vs., 315–316
Nerve conduction studies, 376
Neural tube defects, 232–234, 233
Neuritis of third nerve, 160
Neuroacanthocytosis, 83
Neurocysticerosis, 105
Neuroectodermal tumor
  dysembryoplastic, 19, 20
Neurofibromatosis, 29–30
  clinical presentation of, 29
  neurological manifestations of, 30
  type 1, 29–30
    and attention deficit hyperactivity disorder, 211
    café-au-lait macules and freckling in, 205–206, 206,207
    cardiovascular abnormalities in, 210
    central nervous system tumors in, 208–209, 209
    clinical features of, 205–206, 206, 207
    cognitive and behavioral manifestations of, 210
    learning disabilities in, 210–211
    neurofibromas in, 207, 207–208, 208
    ocular manifestations of, 209
    peripheral nerve sheath tumors and, 209
    skeletal manifestations of, 210
  type 2, 29–30
Neuroimaging
  computed tomography, 13–14, 21
  functional, 189–203
  of head trauma, 19–21, 21
  for headaches, 17–18, 19
  magnetic resonance imaging, 14–15, 21
  techniques of, 13–17
Neuroleptic malignant syndrome, 389
Neuroleptics
  in Tourette syndrome, 57
Neurological disorders
  psychiatric comorbidities of, 6–7
Neurological examination, 1–2
  in brain tumors, 175
  clues on, 5–6
  in neuromuscular disorders, 372–376
  for psychiatrist, 1–12
Neuromuscular disorders, 367–392
  anterior horn disease, 378–379
  chronic neuropathies, 380–382
  chronology of illness in, 370–371
  family history in, 371–372
  history taking in, 370–372
  juvenile myasthenia gravis, 370, 382
  laboratory testing in, 376–377
  localization of, 369t, 369–370
  management in, 377
  medical history in, 371
  motor examination in, 373, 373t, 375–376
  neurological examination for, 372–376
  peripheral nerve disease in, 369t, 369–370, 379–382
  physical examination for, 372–376
  psychiatric consultation in, 377
  sensation examination in, 374
Neuromuscular junction
  disruption of, 370, 372, 382–373
Neurontin. See Gabapentin
Neuropathies
  acute, 379–380
  chronic, 380–382
  medications causing, 381–382
Night terrors, 128

Nightmares, 129
Nimodipine, 292
Nonsteroidal anti-inflammatory drugs
  in migraine, 162
Novantrone, 317

O

Obsessions
  instruments for assessing, 87–88
Obsessive-compulsive disorder, 40
  cognitive-behavioral therapy in, 93
  Tourette syndrome and, 57, 80, 92–93
  treatment of, 92–93
Obstructive sleep apnea syndrome, 130–132
  causes of, 130
  conditions associated with, 130–131
  prevalence of, 130
  treatment of, 131
Occipital epilepsy, 339
Ocular albinism, 336
Olanzapine
  in Tourette syndrome, 57, 90–91
Oligodendrogliomas, 172, 174, 182–183, 184
Oncogenesis
  radiation and chemotherapy-induced, 177–178
Opsoclonus-myoclonus syndrome, 63
Optic nerve hypoplasia, 336
Optic pathway
  gliomas of, 29, 208, 209
Oxcarbazepine, 394
  in intellectual disability, 257
  in movement disorders, 64
  in seizures, 115

P

Pain disorders
  in HIV infection, 297
PANDAS, 56, 60, 85, 86, 95
Papilledema, 173, 341
Papillorenal syndrome, 335
Parakinesia, 59
Paralysis
  hysterical, 389–390
Paramyotonia congenita, 386–387
Parasomnias
  arousal, 127–129
    cause of, 128
    management of, 128–129
    patterns of, 127–128
    nightmares, 129
Parkinsonism
  clinical features of, 48
  differential diagnosis of, 48
Paroxetine
  in obsessive-compulsive disorder, 92
Paroxysmal movement disorders, 64–65
Paroxysmal nonepileptiform disorders, 104, 105t
Paroxysmal torticollis, 160
Paroxysmal vertigo, 160
Pediatric autoimmune neuropsychiatric disorder.
  See PANDAS
δ-Penicillamine
  in Wilson disease, 51
Penicillin
  in Sydenham chorea, 60
Perfusion imaging, 15
Periodic limb movement disorder, 134
  attention deficit hyperactivity disorder and, 137–139
Peripheral nerve sheath tumors
  malignant, 209, 218

Peripheral nervous system, 367
  anatomic localization of, 369t, 369–370
  anatomy and physiology of, 368
  diseases of, 379–382
Petit mal seizures
  in epilepsies, 82
Phakomatoses, 28–31
Phencyclidine, 407
Phenobarbital
  in epilepsy, 112–113, 114
Phenothiazines
  visual impairment and, 341
Phenytoin
  as cause of myopathy, 389
  in epilepsy, 112, 114
  in movement disorders, 64
  in sleep disorders, 134
Pimozide
  in Tourette syndrome, 57, 90, 91
Pineal region tumors, 27–28, *28, 29*
Plexopathy, 370
Poliomyelitis, 369, 378
Polymicrogyria, 15, 37
Polymyositis, 388–389
Polysomnography, 124, 130, *130, 131*
Pompe disease, 387
Porphyria-induced polyneuropathy, 380
Positron emission tomography, 16, 191
Post-traumatic stress disorder, 141
  following brain tumor, 180–181
  in HIV infection, 296–297
Prader-Willi syndrome
  behaviors in, 252
Precocious puberty, 174–175
Prematurity
  ophthalmic complications of, 333–334
Primidone
  in tremor, 50
Propranolol
  in tremor, 50
Pseudoarthrosis, 210
Pseudoseizures, 104
Pseudotumor cerebri, 165, 341
Psychogenic movement disorders, 65–66
Psychosis
  in epilepsy, 394, 397
  substances of abuse associated with, 401–402
Psychosocial interventions
  in Tourette syndrome, 94–95
Psychostimulants
  in attention deficit hyperactvity disorder, 117
Pyridostigmine
  for myasthenia gravis, 383

Q

Quetiapine
  in tardive dyskinesia, 68
  in Tourette syndrome, 57, 90–91

R

Radiation exposure, 17
Radiation therapy
  in brain tumors, 176
  oncogenesis due to, 177–178
Rebif, 317
Reflexes
  examination of, 3, 4t
Renal artery stenosis
  in neurofibromatosis, 210
Repetitive transcranial magnetic stimulation
  in tic disorders, 92
Reserpine
  in tardive dyskinesia, 68

Restless legs syndrome, 134
  attention deficit hyperactivity disorder and, 137–139
Retina
  development of, 324
Retinitis pigmentosa, 381
Retinopathy of prematurity, 333–334
Rett syndrome, 40
  clinical features of, 59
Rhabdomyoma
  in tuberous sclerosis, 214
Rhizotomy
  in cerebral palsy, 231
Rigidity
  in parkinsonism, 52
Risperidone
  in chorea, 60–61
  in Tourette syndrome, 90–91

S

Schizencephaly, 37
Schizophrenia
  childhood-onset, 39
  in hearing impairment, 359
Schizophreniform disorder, 397–398
School performance
  in hearing impairment, 355
  tics and, 86, 95
Seizures, 18–19, *20*
  absence (petit mal), 82
  amnestic, 404
  brain tumors and, 174
  classification of, 103–104, 104t
  differential diagnosis of, 82
  febrile, 18
  and hallucinations, 395
  in intellectual disability, 249–250
  in neurofibromatosis, 210
  nonepileptic, 104–105
  nonfebrile, 18–19
  during sleep, 133–134
  temporal lobe, 82
  in tuberous sclerosis, 216
Selective serotonin reuptake inhibitors
  in epilepsy, 117
  in HIV infection, 296
  in intellectual disability, 257
  in obsessive-compulsive disorder, 92
Selegeline, 292
Sensory examination, 274
Separation anxiety
  in HIV infection, 296
Septo-optic dysplasia syndrome, 336
Sertraline
  in obsessive-compulsive disorder, 92
  visual impairment and, 340
Shagreen patches, 213–214, *214*
Sinemet. *See* Carbidopa-levodopa
Sinus infection
  frontal, 34, *34*
Skin
  abnormalities of, 5, 5t
  in neurofibromatosis, 205–208
  in phakomatoses, 28–31
  in tuberous sclerosis complex, 212–214, *213, 214, 215*
Skull fracture, 20, *21*
Sleep
  age-related changes in, 125
  assessment of, 124
  seizures and, 133–134
  stages of, 123, *124*
Sleep-disordered breathing, 130–132
  attention deficit hyperactivity disorder and, 136–137
Sleep disorders, 123–149
  assessment of, 124–125
  attention deficit hyperactivity disorder and, 136–139

Sleep disorders (continued)
  circadian rhythm, 126–127
  confusional arousals, 128
  delayed sleep phase syndrome, 126–127
  electrical status epilepticus of sleep, 133
  excessive sleepiness, 124
    narcolepsy, 135
  insomnia, 125–126
  limit-setting, 126
  neuropsychiatric disorders associated with, 140–141
  parasomnias
    arousal, 127–129
    nightmares, 129
  periodic limb movements, 134
  sleep-onset association, 126
  sleep terrors, 128
Sleepwalking, 128
Sodium valproate
  in epilepsy, 112, 113–114
  in migraine prophylaxis, 155
Somatosensory system, 368
Somnambulism, 128
Spasticity, 51–52
Spectroscopy
  magnetic resonance, 16
Speech therapy
  in deafness, 357–359
Spina bifida, 232–233, 233
Spinal muscular atrophy, 369, 378
Staring spells
  differential diagnosis of, 109t
Static encephalopathy, 51
Stereotypies, 59, 81
Steroids
  as cause of myopathy, 389
  in HIV infection, 292
  in multiple sclerosis, 317
Strabismus, 329–333
Stroke, 32
Sturge-Weber syndrome, 30
Subacute sclerosing panencephalitis, 63
Subarachnoid hemorrhage, 18
Subdural hematoma, 22, 23
Subependymal nodules
  in tuberous sclerosis, 216
Substance abuse
  in HIV infection, 297
Substance abuse disorder
  in epilepsy, 401
Substances of abuse
  associated with psychosis, 401–402
Sulpride
  in tic disorders, 31
Sydenham chorea, 59

T

Tardive dyskinesia, 67, 83
Tegretol. *See* Carbamazepine
Tensilon test, 377, 382
Teratoid/rhabtoid tumors
  atypical, 24
Tetrabenazine
  in tardive dyskinesia, 68
  in tic disorders, 91
  in Tourette syndrome, 57–58
Tetrathiomolybdate
  in Wilson disease, 51
Thymectomy, 383
Tiagabine
  in sleep disorders, 134
Tiapride
  in tic disorders, 91
Tic disorders, 77–101. *See also* Tourette syndrome
  clinical features of, 85–87
  conditions associated with, 77
  differential diagnosis of, 80–84
  evaluation of, 87
  Tourette syndrome, 58, 77–101
  transient
    diagnostic criteria in, 78
  treatment of, 88–92, 93–94
Tics
  causes of, 56
  clinical phenomenology of, 79–80
  definition of, 55, 78
  motor, 56, 78
  natural history of, 79–80
  phonic, 56, 78
  prevalence of, 77
  stress and, 55–56
  suppression of, 55
  transient vs. chronic, 77
  vocal, 78
Tick paralysis, 380
Tizanidine
  in multiple sclerosis, 318
  in spasticity, 51
Topiramate (Topomax)
  in dystonia, 54
  in migraine prophylaxis, 155
  in seizures, 115–116, 250
  visual impairment due to, 340
Torticollis
  paroxysmal, 160
Tourette syndrome, 40–41, 77–101
  during adolescence, 79
  age of onset of, 77
  assessment in, 85–87
  attention deficit hyperactivity disorder and, 57, 80, 93–94
  behavioral manifestations of, 78
  comorbid disorders in, 80, 86, 92–94
  compulsion in, 80
  diagnosis of, 56, 56t, 79
  differential diagnosis of, 80–84
  etiology of, 84–85
  family factors and, 87
  genetic factors in, 56, 84
  history taking in, 85–86
  instruments for assessing, 87–88
  long-term course and prognosis for, 57
  obsessive-compulsive behaviors in, 57, 80, 92–93
  perinatal factors in, 84
  physical and neurological findings in, 57
  prevalence of, 77–78
  psychosocial interventions in, 94–95
  race and sex distribution of, 77–78
  school and social adjustment in, 86, 95
  severity of, 79
  stereotypical movements in, 81
  and tic disorders, 77–101
  tics of, 79, 89
  treatment of, 88–92
    behavior-modifying drugs in, 58
    education, coping, and adapting, 57, 88
    emerging methods of, 91–92
    medication principles in, 89–91
    targets of, 88
    tic-suppressing drugs in, 57–58
Tremor, 49–50
  cerebellar, 49
  classification of, 49
  clinical features of, 49
  definition of, 49
  diagnosis of, 50
  dystonic, 50
  essential, 49
Trihexyphenidyl
  in cerebral palsy, 230
  in dystonia, 54
Trileptal. *See* Oxcarbazepine

Triptans
  in migraine, 162, 163
Tuberous sclerosis complex, 30–31, 212–219
  cardiac manifestations of, 214
  case histories of, 217–219
  chromosome abnormalities in, 30
  clinical diagnostic criteria for, 213t
  cognitive and behavioral manifestations of, 216–217
  cutaneous lesions in, 212–214, *213, 214, 215*
  diagnostic studies in, 30
  intracranial manifestations of, 216
  neuroradiological imaging in, 30–31
  ophthalmological lesions in, 215
  pulmonary manifestations of, 215
  renal manifestations of, 215

U

Upper motor neurons, 368

V

Valproate
  in epilepsy, 112, 113–114
  in tic disorders, 91
Valproic acid
  in intellectual disability, 257
  in movement disorders, 64
  in myoclonus, 64
  in sleep disorders, 134
  in Sydenham chorea, 60–61
Vascular malformations, 31, 32
  arteriovenous, 31, 32
  cavernous, 31
  venous, 31
Vascular occlusive disease, 32–33
  sickle cell disease and, 32
  stroke, 32
Vasculitis
  multiple sclerosis vs., 316
Venous malformations, 31
Verapamil
  for migraine prophylaxis, 155
Vertigo
  paroxysmal, 160
Vidovudine, 290, 389
Vigabatrin
  visual impairment due to, 340–341
Vision
  abnormal development of, 327
  normal development of, 323–327
Vision disorders
  brain tumors and, 174
  nonorganic, 336–338
Visual functions
  cortical structures and, 326
  subcortical structures and, *325*, 325–326
Visual hallucinations, 338–340

Visual impairment
  cerebral, 334
  development and neuropsychology of, 323–343
  education in, 341, 342
  motor development in, 341
  psychosocial impact of, 341–342
Visual maturation
  delayed, 334–335
Visual pathways
  brain tumors involving, 335–336
  and eye
    disorders involving, 335–336
Visual system
  binocular vision and, 326
  developing
    anatomy and physiology of, 323–327
  motion perception and, 326–327
  perception of color, shape, and form, 327
  visual acuity and, 326
  visual field size and, 326
Vitamin deficiency diseases, 316
Vomiting
  brain tumors and, 173
  cyclical, 160–161
Von Hippel-Lindau disease, 31
von Recklinghausen disease. *See* Neurofibromatosis, type 1

W

Wernig-Hoffman disease, 378
West Nile virus, 378
Whiplash/shaking injury syndrome, 22
White matter diseases, 35
Williams syndrome, 252
Wilson disease, 7–8, 35, 47, 48, 50–51, 68
  diagnostic tests for, 51
  differential diagnosis of, 50–51
  inheritance pattern for, 7
  neurologic findings in, 8
  psychiatric features of, 7
  symptoms of, 8
  treatment of, 51
Withdrawal emergent dyskinesia, 68

Y

Yale Brown Obsessive Compulsive Scale, 87
Yale Global Tic Severity Scale, 87

Z

Zarontin. *See* Ethosuximide
Ziprasidone
  in Tourette syndrome, 57, 90, 91
Zonisamide (Zonegran)
  in seizures, 116, 250